Psychiatric Issues in Epilepsy

A Practical Guide to Diagnosis and Treatment

Psychiatric Issues in Epilepsy

A Practical Guide to Diagnosis and Treatment

Alan B. Ettinger, M.D.

Associate Professor, Department of Neurology
Albert Einstein College of Medicine
Bronx, New York
and
Chief, EEG Division and Comprehensive Epilepsy Center
Director, Huntington Hospital Epilepsy Monitoring Program
Long Island Jewish Medical Center
New Hyde Park, New York

Andres M. Kanner, M.D.

Associate Professor, Departments of Neurological Sciences and Psychiatry
Rush Medical College
and
Associate Director, Section of Epilepsy and Clinical Neurophysiology
Director, Laboratory of Electroencephalography and Video-EEG Telemetry
Department of Neurological Sciences
Rush Presbyterian-Saint Luke's Medical Center
Chicago, Illinois

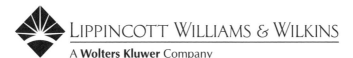

LIPPINCOTT WILLIAMS & WILKINS
A **Wolters Kluwer** Company
Philadelphia • Baltimore • New York • London
Buenos Aires • Hong Kong • Sydney • Tokyo

Acquisitions Editor: Charles W. Mitchell
Developmental Editor: Raymond E. Reter
Production Editor: John C. Vassiliou
Manufacturing Manager: Colin J. Warnock
Cover Designer: Mark Lerner
Compositor: Lippincott Williams & Wilkins Desktop Division
Printer: Edwards Brothers

© 2001 by **LIPPINCOTT WILLIAMS & WILKINS**
530 Walnut Street
Philadelphia, PA 19106 USA
LWW.com

Printed in the USA

Library of Congress Cataloging-in-Publication Data

Psychiatric issues in epilepsy : a practical guide to diagnosis and treatment / editors,
Alan B. Ettinger, Andres M. Kanner.
   p. ; cm.
  Includes bibliographical references and index.
  ISBN 0-7817-2176-8
   1. Epilepsy—Psychological aspects. 2. Epileptics—Mental health. I. Ettinger, Alan B.
II. Kanner, Andres M.
  [DNLM: 1. Epilepsy—cimplications. 2. Epilepsy—psychology. 3. Mental
Disorders—diagnosis. 4. Mental Disorders—etiology. 5. Mental Disorders—therapy. WL
385 P974157 2001]
  RC372 .P757 2001
  616.8′53′0019—dc21

                                     00-067143

10 9 8 7 6 5 4 3 2 1

I dedicate this book to the memory of my beloved mother, Lillian Ettinger, whose kindness and love for others, and whose valiant struggle against illness was an inspiration for devoting my efforts to studying and improving the quality of life of my patients.

Alan B. Ettinger, M.D.

An unending and selfless support of my beloved wife Hilary and my daughters Lesley-Ann and Lauren Amanda was paramount in the achievement of this work. I therefore dedicate this book to them!

Andres M. Kanner, M.D.

Contents

Contributing Authors

Joan K. Austin, D.N.S., R.N., F.A.A.N.   *Distinguished Professor, Indiana University School of Nursing, 1111 Middle Drive, Indianapolis, Indiana 46202*

John J. Barry, M.D.   *Assistant Professor, Department of Psychiatry, Stanford University Medical Center, 401 Quarry Road, MC5723, Stanford, California 94305*

Donna C. Bergen, M.D.   *Associate Professor, Department of Neurological Sciences, Rush Medical College, 1725 West Harrison Street, Chicago, Illinois 60612*

Ahmad Beydoun, M.D.   *Associate Professor and Director, Clinical Neurophysiology Laboratories and Epilepsy Program, Department of Neurology, University of Michigan Health System, 1500 East Medical Center Drive, UH 1B300/0036, Ann Arbor, Michigan 48109*

Dietrich P. Blumer, M.D.   *Professor, Department of Psychiatry, University of Tennessee, Memphis–Health Science Center, 135 North Pauline, Suite 633, Memphis, Tennessee 38105; Active Staff, Departments of Psychiatry and Neurology, Baptist Medical Center, 899 Madison Avenue, Memphis, Tennessee 38146*

Elizabeth S. Bowman, M.D.   *Professor, Department of Psychiatry, Indiana University School of Medicine; Consulting Psychiatrist, Epilepsy Clinic, Indiana University Hospital, 550 North University Boulevard, 541 Clinical Drive, Indianapolis, Indiana 46202*

Janice M. Buelow, Ph.D., R.N.   *Director, Rush Epilepsy Education and Outreach Program, Department of Neurology, Rush Presbyterian-Saint Luke's Medical Center, 1653 West Congress Parkway, Chicago, Illinois 60612*

Keith Davies, M.D., F.R.C.S.   *Associate Professor, Department of Neurosurgery, University of Tennessee, Memphis, 847 Monroe, Suite 427, Memphis, Tennessee 38163; Neurosurgeon, Semmes-Murphey Clinic, 930 Madison Avenue, Suite 600, Memphis, Tennessee 38103*

Orrin Devinsky, M.D.   *Professor, Department of Neurology, Neurosurgery, and Psychiatry, New York University; Director, New York University-Mount Sinai Epilepsy Center, 403 East 34th Street, New York, New York 10016*

Oscar Doval, M.D.   *Visiting Scholar, Department of Neuropsychiatry, University of Illinois, Chicago, 912 South Wood Street, Chicago, Illinois 60612; Chief, Division of Neuropsychiatry, Grupo Medico Humana, Caracas, Venezuela*

David W. Dunn, M.D.   *Associate Professor, Department of Psychiatry and Neurology, Indiana University; Director, Child and Adolescent Psychiatry Clinics, Riley Hospital for Children, 702 Barnhill Drive, Indianapolis, Indiana 46202*

Alan B. Ettinger, M.D.   *Associate Professor, Department of Neurology, Albert Einstein College of Medicine, 1410 Pelham Parkway South, Bronx, New York 10473; Chief, EEG Division and Comprehensive Epilepsy Center; and Director, Huntington Hospital Epilepsy Monitoring Program, Long Island Jewish Medical Center, 270-05 76th Avenue, New Hyde Park, New York 11040*

Shirley M. Ferguson, M.D. *Professor Emerita of Psychiatry, Department of Psychiatry, Medical College of Ohio, 3120 Glendale Avenue, Toledo, Ohio 43614*

Carol Estwing Ferrans, Ph.D., R.N., F.A.A.N. *Associate Professor, College of Nursing, University of Illinois at Chicago, 845 South Damen Avenue, Chicago, Illinois 60612*

Marlis Frey, R.N., M.S.N., C.G.N.P. *Nurse Practitioner, Department of Neurology, Rush Presbyterian-Saint Luke's Medical Center, 1725 West Harrison Street, Chicago, Illinois 60612*

Pilar Garcia-Damberre, M.D. *Attending Physician, Department of Psychiatry, Hospital de la Princesa, Diego de Leon 62, Madrid, Spain 28006*

Moises Gaviria, M.D. *Professor, Departments of Psychiatry and Neurosurgery, University of Illinois, Chicago, 912 South Wood Street, Chicago, Illinois 60612*

Patricia A. Gibson, M.S.S.W. *Assistant Professor, Department of Neurology, Wake Forest University, Medical Center Boulevard, Winston Salem, North Carolina 27157*

Antonio Gil-Nagel, M.D. *Director of Epilepsy Program, Department of Neurology, Hospital Ruber Internacional, La Maso 38, Mirasierra, Madrid, Spain 28034*

Christopher L. Grote, Ph.D. *Assistant Professor, Department of Psychology, Rush Medical College; Psychologist, Department of Psychology, Rush Presbyterian-Saint Luke's Medical Center, 1653 West Congress Parkway, Chicago, Illinois 60612*

Sandra D. Hamberger, R.C.S.W. *Social Work Consultant, Comprehensive Epilepsy Center, Long Island Jewish Health Systems, 270-05 76th Avenue, New Hyde Park, New York 11040*

W. A. Hauser, M.D. *Professor, Department of Neurology and Public Health, G.H. Sergievsky Center College of Physicians and Surgeons, Columbia University; Attending Physician, New York Presbyterian Hospital, 630 West 168th Street, New York, New York 10032*

Dale C. Hesdorffer, Ph.D., M.P.H. *Assistant Professor, Department of Public Health (Epidemiology), G.H. Sergievsky Center, Columbia University, 630 West 168th Street, New York, New York 10032*

Thomas J. Hoeppner, Ph.D. *Associate Professor, Department of Neurological Sciences, Rush Medical College, 1653 West Harrison Street, Chicago, Illinois 60612*

Nga Huynh, Pharm.D. *Department of Pharmacy, Stanford University Medical Center, 401 Quarry Road, Stanford, California 94305*

Andres M. Kanner, M.D. *Associate Professor, Departments of Neurological Sciences and Psychiatry, Rush Medical College; Associate Director, Section of Epilepsy and Clinical Neurophysiology; Director, Laboratory of Electroencephalography and Video-EEG Telemetry, Department of Neurological Sciences, Rush Presbyterian-Saint Luke's Medical Center, 1653 West Congress Parkway, Chicago, Illinois 60612*

Ruben Kuzniecky, M.D. *Professor, Department of Neurology, University of Alabama at Birmingham; Director, Epilepsy Center, University of Alabama at Birmingham Hospital, 1719 6th Avenue South, Birmingham, Alabama 35294*

Christos C. Lambrakis, M.D. *Assistant Professor, Department of Neurology, New York Medical College, Grasslands Road, Valhalla, New York 10595; Epileptologist, Northeast Regional Epilepsy Group, Hackensack University Medical Center, 20 Prospect Avenue, Hackensack, New Jersey 07601*

Marcelo E. Lancman, M.D. *Associate Professor, Department of Neurology, New York Medical College, Grasslands Road, Valhalla, New York 10595; Director, Epilepsy Program, Saint Agnes Hospital, 305 North Street, White Plains, New York 10605*

Anna Lembke, M.D. *Research Fellow, Department of Psychiatry and Behavioral Sciences, Stanford University, 401 Quarry Road, Stanford, California 94305*

Susan M. Palac, M.D. *Assistant Professor, Department of Neurological Sciences, Rush Medical College, 600 South Paulina Street; Epileptologist, Department of Neurological Sciences, Rush Presbyterian-Saint Luke's Medical Center, 1653 West Congress Parkway, Chicago, Illinois 60612*

Erasmo A. Passaro, M.D. *Assistant Professor, Director, Adult Epilepsy Laboratory, Department of Neurology, University of Michigan; Attending Neurologist, Department of Neurology, University of Michigan Health System, 1500 East Medical Center Drive, Ann Arbor, Michigan 48109*

Mark Rayport, M.D.C.M., Ph.D. *Professor Emeritus, Departments of Neurological Surgery and Radiology, Medical College of Ohio, Mulford Library 331; Honorary Medical Staff, Departments of Neurosurgery and Radiology, Medical College of Ohio Hospital, Toledo, Ohio 43614*

Anthony L. Ritaccio, M.D. *Associate Professor, Department of Neurology, New York University Medical Center; Epileptologist, New York University-Mount Sinai Epilepsy Center, 403 East 34th Street, New York, New York 10016*

Amity Ruth, Ph.D. *Neuropsychology Fellow, Department of Psychiatry, Cognitive Neurology and Alzheimer's Disease Clinic, Northwestern University Medical School, 320 East Superior Street, Chicago, Illinois 60611*

Steven C. Schachter, M.D. *Associate Professor, Department of Neurology, Harvard Medical School; Medical Director, Office of Clinical Trials and Research, Beth Israel Deaconess Medical Center, 330 Brookline Avenue, Boston, Massachusetts 02215*

Angela Scicutella, M.D., Ph.D. *Assistant Professor, Department of Psychiatry, Albert Einstein College of Medicine, 1300 Morris Park Avenue, Bronx, New York 10461; Attending Neuropsychiatrist, Department of Geriatric Psychiatry, Long Island Jewish Medical Center, 270-05 76th Avenue, New Hyde Park, New York 11040*

Clifford A. Smith, Ph.D. *Postdoctoral Fellow, Department of Psychiatry, Weill Medical College of Cornell University, 525 East 68th Street, Box 147, New York, New York 10021*

Michael C. Smith, M.D. *Associate Professor, Department of Neurological Sciences, Rush Medical College; Director, Rush Epilepsy Center, Department of Neurological Sciences, Rush Presbyterian-Saint Luke's Medical Center, 1653 West Congress Parkway, Chicago, Illinois 60612*

Alan L. Steinberg, M.D. *Assistant Professor, Department of Geriatrics and Psychiatry, State University of New York at Stony Brook, Stony Brook, New York 11790*

Michael I. Steinhardt, Psy.D. *Neuropsychologist, Pediatric Neuroscience Institute, Hackensack University Medical Center, 20 Prospect Avenue, Hackensack, New Jersey 07601*

Deborah Weisbrot, M.D. *Assistant Professor and Director, Child and Adolescent Outpatient Clinic, Department of Psychiatry and Behavioral Sciences, State University of New York at Stony Brook, Stony Brook, New York 11794*

Preface

The close relationship between epilepsy and psychiatric processes has been recognized since antiquity; yet, systematic research of psychiatric aspects of epilepsy has a short history that has lagged behind many other domains of epilepsy research. A striking example is the existence of only one double-blind placebo-controlled study (in 1979) assessing efficacy of antidepressant agents for depression in epilepsy (1), in spite of the atypical presentations of depression in this disorder and the unexplored potential risks of these agents in the presence of seizures. Similarly, minimal systematic studies have evaluated treatment of psychosis and epilepsy. The paucity of such studies has contributed to the clinician's timidity toward using psychotropic drugs in epilepsy, leaving many psychiatric complications of epilepsy untreated. The lack of rigorous studies and reliance upon anecdotal experience has also translated into minimal availability of specific comprehensive guides for making practical diagnostic and management decisions. *Psychiatric Issues in Epilepsy: A Practical Guide to Diagnosis and Treatment*, therefore, attempts to organize our current knowledge of psychiatric aspects of epilepsy, to critically analyze salient investigations in medical literature, to highlight what is not known, and to provide practical recommendations wherever possible for diagnosis and management.

In *Psychiatric Issues in Epilepsy*, we emphasize many fascinating elements of the complex relationship between epilepsy and psychiatric disorders. For example, although it is intuitive that depression is a direct consequence of the experience of having seizures, published evidence suggests that depression may in fact be a risk factor for epilepsy (an observation of Hippocrates in the fourth century BC) perhaps due to the existence of common pathogenic mechanisms for both disorders (2).

Other examples of this complicated relationship are emphasized throughout this book. The action of neurotransmitters like serotonin and norepinephrine on the kindling model of partial epilepsy parallels that of affective disorder models. Thus, a decrease of these neurotransmitters can facilitate the kindling process, just as neurotransmitter synaptic depletion can result in symptoms of depression and vice versa. Psychiatrists and neurologists nowadays find themselves swapping pharmacologic therapies, using antiepileptic drugs (AEDs) to replace lithium in the prophylactic treatment of bipolar disorders, and taking advantage of antimanic and antidepressant properties of drugs like valproic acid and lamotrigine. In fact, when AEDs are now introduced, they are almost immediately assessed for their potential psychotropic properties.

Another interesting issue noted throughout this book concerns the relation between seizure frequency with psychiatric symptoms. For example, some authors suggest the need to achieve a seizure-free state to avert the recurrence of episodic psychotic symptoms. In other patients, seizure freedom is associated with a reactivation of a psychotic process, or *de novo* development of psychosis. Up to 25% of epilepsy patients may experience a transient depressive episode after undergoing a temporal lobectomy, unrelated to the extent of seizure control. Recent epidemiologic data reveals that rapidly-achieved seizure control and AED discontinuation is not necessarily associated with a future devoid of psychosocial problems. Conversely, new surgical treatments of specific epileptic syndromes have been followed by the remission of previously developed psychopathology, suggesting the possible existence of "paraictal psychiatric disorders." All of these examples illustrate the vast complexity and close association between psychiatric phenomena and epilepsy in dire need of investigation.

This book also emphasizes previously neglected psychological needs of epilepsy patients. Thankfully, in the last decade, neurologists and epileptologists have recognized the need to address quality-of-life issues in the assessment of their patients. Chapters 19–22 address assessment and management of these psychosocial concerns.

We hope *Psychiatric Issues in Epilepsy: A Practical Guide to Diagnosis and Treatment* will further the curiosity of health professionals involved in the management of patients with epilepsy, and enhance an interdisciplinary dialogue and collaboration that is (alas!) often (and without reason) absent (i.e., between psychiatrists and neurologists). Since psychiatric issues in epilepsy pose frequent challenges in the routine evaluation and management of patients with seizures, we also hope that this book will be an invaluable reference for a wide variety of healthcare providers including epileptologists, general neurologists, psychiatrists, neuropsychologists, general practicioners, and social workers, among many other disciplines.

REFERENCES

1. Robertson MM. Depression in patients with epilepsy: an overview and clinical study. In: Trimble MR, ed. *The psychopharmacology of epilepsy.* New York: John Wiley & Sons, 1985:65–82.
2. Lewis AJ. Melancholia: a historical review. *J Ment Sci* 1934;80:1–42.

Psychiatric Issues in Epilepsy

A Practical Guide to Diagnosis and Treatment

1

Introduction

Alan B. Ettinger and *Andres M. Kanner

*Huntington Hospital Epilepsy Monitoring Program, Long Island Jewish Medical Center,
New Hyde Park, New York 11040; and *Department of Neurological Sciences, Rush Presbyterian-
Saint Luke's Medical Center, Chicago, Illinois 60612*

Despite the fact that a close relationship between epilepsy and psychiatric disorders has been recognized since antiquity, it remains one of the least explored areas in the epilepsy literature. The reasons for the relative lack of systematic research in this area of epilepsy are not clear. The problem is real and is reflected by the following observations: (a) Only a few of the epilepsy programs have on their team a psychiatrist with expertise in the field of epilepsy. Thus, psychiatric evaluations are carried out during the course of a neuropsychological battery of tests. (b) The relative absence of psychiatrists' input into the evaluation and management of patients with epilepsy is reflected in the almost complete absence of experience with the use of psychotropic drugs in these patients. To give one example of this peculiar phenomenon, to date there has been only one controlled study evaluating the effect of antidepressant drugs for treatment of major depression in patients with epilepsy.

Psychopathology, cognitive deficits, and psychosocial problems are frequent among patients with epilepsy. As we comment in Chapter 3, even patients who reach a seizure-free state and can discontinue taking antiepileptic drugs (AEDs) are at risk of comorbidity in these domains. In a population-based study, Sillanpaa et al. (1) suggested that patients with uncomplicated epilepsy may not fare as well as controls in vocational training, marriage or living with a partner, employment, and socioeco-

nomic status. In addition, these authors found that patients who have remained seizure-free *off AEDs since childhood* had a worse outcome than controls in levels of achievement in primary education, marriage (or living with a partner), and having children. Camfield et al. (2) assessed the social outcome after the age of 18 years in a population-based prospective study of 337 children with partial epilepsy and *normal intelligence.* Social isolation was recorded in 16%, financial dependency in 30%, and unemployment in 30%. Clearly, these two population-based studies demonstrate a greater vulnerability of patients with epilepsy, even in the absence of any cognitive impairment or when an optimal seizure control (i.e., seizure freedom off AEDs) is achieved.

In their review of epidemiologic considerations of depression, psychosis, and epilepsy (Chapter 2), Hauser and Hesdorffer illustrate the relatively high prevalence of psychopathology in the general population and the even higher morbidity among patients with epilepsy. They provide thought-provoking data suggesting that the relationship between epilepsy and depression is not unidirectional, as previously believed, but bidirectional. That is, not only is epilepsy a risk factor for depression, but depression appears to be a potential risk factor for epilepsy as well. Interestingly enough, a similar observation was made by Hippocrates in the fourth century BC when he wrote: "epileptics become melancholic and melancholic epileptics. . ."

In Chapter 3, Kanner and Weisbrot remind us that psychopathology in epilepsy frequently is unrecognized. Clinicians on the frontlines of the initial evaluation of epileptic patients have a crucial opportunity to identify symptoms of concern, and Chapter 3 provides a practical set of questions that can be integrated routinely into the initial assessment. These authors also highlight a differential diagnostic approach to psychiatric symptoms, including a consideration of intrinsic effects of the underlying central nervous system disorder, AED effects, and psychosocial factors.

Clinicians frequently encounter epileptic patient complaints about dysfunction in memory, attention, concentration, and language. Neuropsychological testing (Chapter 4) is invaluable in providing objective quantification of deficits, sorting out potential etiologies, and assessing the psychiatric contributions to these impairments. Neuropsychological testing is an integral part of the epilepsy surgery evaluation and can assist in the distinction of epileptic from psychogenically determined nonepileptic seizures (pseudoseizures). Neuropsychological testing also includes personality assessments such as the Minnesota Multiphasic Personality Inventory (MMPI), which complements the psychiatric interview.

Although psychopathology and epilepsy are fraught with numerous controversies, most experts agree that depressive symptomatology is a particularly frequent problem among epileptic patients. Clinicians may be most familiar with the diagnosis of major depressive disorder, but Barry et al. (Chapter 5) highlight a more subtle form of depression common to epileptic patients, termed "interictal dysphoric disorder." Clinician awareness of depression risk factors, such as family history of depression or antiepileptic barbiturate therapy, can lead to important interventions on behalf of these patients. Practical clinical issues also arise regarding the fear of eliciting seizures by using antidepressant agents that have the potential to lower seizure thresholds; therefore, discussions of the comparative risks among many currently available choices are especially valuable for the health care provider. The clinician needs to be familiar with potential drug interactions, including the risk of inducing drug toxicity or reducing drug efficacy; these issues are highlighted in Chapter 5. Electroconvulsive therapy (ECT) sometimes is required to treat refractory depression, and the clinician will find the discussion emphasizing the safety of ECT, even in epileptic patients, to be reassuring.

In Chapter 6, Rayport and Ferguson provide a thought-provoking approach to the very complex topic of the psychosis of epilepsy. They propose the existence of "episodic" and "nonepisodic" psychoses of epilepsy as an alternative classification of this psychiatric comorbidity. They provide case examples rich in detail that demonstrate the close relationship between the status of seizure control and the risk of psychopathology. They also review the controversial notion of an inverse relationship between seizure frequency and exacerbation of psychosis, termed "forced normalization".

Commonly associated with depression, anxiety symptoms are very frequent in epileptic patients. In Chapter 7, Sciutella provides a pragmatic approach to the assessment of anxiety, citing a number of physical symptoms that should be surveyed. A classification of anxiety symptoms is described in relation to the phases of epilepsy, and the reader is told that fear may be either a manifestation of a seizure or an interictal phenomenon. Differential diagnosis must be considered, because other diseases, such as panic disorder, may mimic the symptoms of ictal fear. Anxiety also may be induced iatrogenically by withdrawal of antiepileptic agents. Health care providers frequently are asked whether stress and anxiety can induce seizures; Chapter 7 lends clarity to this controversial relationship. Pharmacologic and nonpharmacologic treatments are noted, and the clinician is cautioned to remind patients to avoid abrupt withdrawal of benzodiazepines, which can produce severe withdrawal symptoms.

Disruptive behavioral disorders, including attention-deficit/hyperactivity disorder (ADHD), oppositional defiant disorder

(ODD), and conduct disorder, are common behavioral disorders in children. The clinician is likely to wonder whether these disruptive disorders are encountered more commonly in epileptic patients, and, if so, how their presentations and treatments differ in epileptic versus nonepileptic children. Dunn addresses these issues in Chapter 8. He suggests that children with epilepsy are at increased risk of ADHD or at least many of its symptoms, but evidence is lacking to definitively associate epilepsy with the latter two behavioral syndromes. Pediatricians should be prepared to address the increased risk of behavioral and academic problems encountered in epileptic children. An assortment of specific standardized questionnaires, including the Child Behavior Checklist or the Child and Adolescent Symptom Inventories, can be invaluable for screening for these symptoms. Dunn notes an important distinction between ictal or postictal aggressive behavior and ODD/conduct disorder. He also notes the relative safety of stimulant medications without significantly reducing seizure threshold.

In Chapter 9, Weisbrot and Ettinger provide an overview of psychiatric symptoms and disorders (depression, anxiety, and psychosis) in pediatric epileptic patients, addressing the primary care physician who is likely to encounter patients with these symptoms. They emphasize that, left unrecognized, these problems may lead to persistent emotional distress and have a profound adverse effect on academic, social, and emotional functioning. This chapter also reviews treatment issues, including psychopharmacologic management, psychotropic effects of AEDs, drug interactions, and the risks of AED reduction of seizure threshold, which all are relevant for the primary care physician.

In Chapter 10, Ritaccio and Devinsky clarify the debate surrounding the controversial "temporal lobe epilepsy personality syndrome," citing methodologic limitations in the medical literature. This chapter gives the clinician a thoughtful perspective on many negative traits and stigmas that unfortunately have been attributed to epileptic patients, while re-

minding the clinician that other psychiatric disturbances, including depression and psychosis, should be addressed carefully.

In Chapter 11, Kanner and Kuzniecky look at the family of postictal psychiatric symptoms and disorders, as well as psychopathology, as an expression of paraictal disorders. The latter include disorders whose principal psychiatric pathology appears and remits with the onset and eradication of epileptic activity.

Psychiatric issues are an integral part of the care of patients with mental retardation, especially in the face of a comorbid epileptic disorder. In Chapter 12, Ettinger and Steinberg highlight the common diagnostic challenge of distinguishing aberrant behaviors from seizures. They also address concerns about reducing seizure threshold when administering psychotropic agents, minimizing medication-related side effects, and attempting to treat both behavioral difficulties and seizures. Although there are relatively few studies focused on this area, the authors attempt to present a clinically relevant synthesis of the related medical literature.

In Chapter 13, Schachter tackles the disputed association of epilepsy and aggressive or violent behavior by raising questions about whether aggression is due to occurrence of the epileptic seizure, the associated brain damage that may be the cause of seizures, socioeconomic factors, or medications. A complicated literature debates this issue, and the clinician must become well acquainted with this topic because aggression may be encountered in patients who are restrained during ictal or postictal confusional states, in postictal psychosis, and occasionally during interictal periods.

Epilepsy typically is considered a disorder that develops early in life, yet the incidence of epilepsy increases sharply in the elderly, even exceeding incidence rates of childhood. This lends particular importance to dedicating a discussion of psychiatric issues in epilepsy as they pertain specifically to older age groups. Despite a paucity of studies in this regard, Frey (Chapter 14) presents a practical summary of psychiatric disturbances in this increasingly important segment of the epilepsy population, focusing on depression, anxiety, and psychosis. Frey's discussion undoubtedly will inspire researchers to develop future research to enhance our understanding of this poorly studied area.

For the estimated 20% to 30% of epileptic patients with seizures unsatisfactorily controlled by AED therapy, serious consideration should be given to a surgical evaluation. Although it is intuitive that depressive symptoms would resolve among epileptic patients successfully treated with focal resections, such as temporal lobectomy, Blumer and Davies (Chapter 15) note the diversity of outcomes as well as the *de novo* development of depression.

The recent introduction of new AED therapies raises new challenges for clinicians selecting therapies for specific epileptic patients. Individual drug efficacy is of paramount importance, but knowledge of potential positive and negative drug properties, especially psychotropic effect, also is essential in the choice of specific agents. Beydoun and Passaro (Chapter 16) review our current knowledge of these psychiatric AED properties, complementing the discussion of these effects in mentally retarded epileptic patients (Chapter 12).

Whereas Chapter 21 provides the clinician with tools for surveying quality of life in epilepsy, Gil-Nagel and Garcia-Damberre (Chapter 19) give real-life examples of quality-of-life difficulties in school, the workplace, social gatherings, and other public environments. They offers suggestions for social interventions that address a number of these concerns.

In Chapter 20, Gibson describes the utility of social services to address many of the concerns raised in quality-of-life assessments. Clinicians can greatly enhance patient care by taking advantage of social services for epileptic patients, including education, counseling, and patient and family advocacy. Many issues that are not necessarily addressed adequately in the typical physician office visit may be considered by the social worker who will discuss patient concerns, including financial duress, driving and occupation restrictions, employment discrimination, scholastic difficulties, self-esteem problems, patient fears, stigma, and the desire to optimize independent living.

It is intuitive that the primary goal of epilepsy treatment is to control seizures. Only recently has the medical community acknowledged the importance of targeting the other physical, psychological, and social effects of this disorder. The clinician will find the discussion by Buelow and Estwing Ferrans (Chapter 21) on quality of life in epilepsy of practical utility, particularly in the selection of invaluable assessments that can be integrated readily into the clinical evaluation of epileptic patients.

In Chapter 22, Austin focuses on the psychosocial aspects of pediatric epilepsy, including their relevance to the overall management of childhood epilepsy. Provocative issues, including the impact of epilepsy on psychological development, on family relations, and in the school setting, will be useful for discussions that clinicians will want to have with epileptic children and their parents.

In Chapter 23, Bergen and Hamberger review our limited knowledge of issues of sexuality in epilepsy. A striking element of this topic is the profound paucity of literature on this subject. Attempts to collect anecdotal reports from therapists or physicians caring for epileptic patients revealed how infrequently health care providers inquire about the impact of epilepsy on quality-of-life issues related to sexuality. This chapter hopefully will motivate care providers to devote time to investigating these potential problems in our epileptic patients.

Although the temporal lobe is the most common single site for partial seizures, frontal lobe dysfunction is a frequent contributor to neurobehavioral complications of epilepsy, including cognitive and mood disorders, and occurs even in the presence of extrafrontal seizure foci. In Chapter 17, Doval et al. highlight the diverse manifestations of frontal lobe dysfunction and provide the clinician with a summary of specific neurobehavioral syndromes to be aware of in clinical practice.

In Chapter 18, Hoeppner and Smith provide a basic science perspective to psychopathology in epilepsy, presenting animal models that help us understand the fundamentals of neuronal elements of emotional behavior relevant to epilepsy.

Pseudoseizures are psychogenically determined nonepileptic episodes that mimic the manifestations of epileptic seizures. The daunting clinical challenge of distinguishing epileptic phenomena from pseudoseizures is reviewed comprehensively by Lancman et al. in Chapter 24. These authors note that as many as 30% of patients referred to tertiary epilepsy centers have pseudoseizures as a cause for seizure intractability. Misdiagnosis of pseudoseizures can result in persistent and inappropriate exposure to AEDs and their associated toxicities and, on some occasions, other potentially harmful interventions such as intubation. This chapter argues for a comprehensive approach that, when appropriate, utilizes multiple diagnostic modalities to render a diagnosis.

Whereas a vast literature focuses on the diagnosis of pseudoseizures, relatively few studies address underlying psychiatric diagnoses, treatment, and outcome. Bowman (Chapter 25) and Kanner et. al. (Chapter 26) address these equally important topics. Bowman notes that nonpsychiatric clinicians still "need to know the comorbid psychiatric illness when explaining pseudoseizures to patients, screening of psychiatric emergencies in these patients, and making referrals for mental health care." For mental health professionals, an understanding of psychiatric morbidity is essential for sorting out numerous comorbid psychiatric disorders. Although the clinician may suspect many pseudoseizure patients produce the phenomena volitionally (e.g., malingering), nonvolitional disturbances, including conversion and dissociative disorder, are much more common.

In the context of recent research on outcome, Kanner et al. (Chapter 26) provide a practical algorithmic approach to revealing the diagnosis of pseudoseizures to patients. Although a clear understanding of underlying psychiatric diagnoses is prerequisite to the design of appropriate treatments, this chapter should inspire sorely needed rigorous research into the utility of different treatments for this disorder.

In this book, we attempt to present the most relevant data in the field of psychiatric aspects of epilepsy and to provide this information from a practical perspective. We hope this text will be of use to all health professionals involved in the management of patients with epilepsy.

REFERENCES

1. Sillanpaa M, Jalava M, Kaleva O, et al. Long-term prognosis of seizures with onset in childhood. *N Engl J Med* 1998;338:1715–1722.
2. Camfield C, Camfield P, Smith B, et al. Biologic factors as predictors of social outcome of epilepsy in intellectually normal children: a population-based study. *J Pediatr* 1993;122:869–873.

2

Psychosis, Depression, and Epilepsy

Epidemiologic Considerations

W. A. Hauser and Dale C. Hesdorffer

Department of Public Health, G.H. Sergievsky Center, Columbia University, New York, New York 10032

There has been a presumed association between mental illness and epilepsy since the earliest medical writings. This association also has been linked to socially inappropriate activities such as criminality. There may be misperceptions about the relationship between psychopathology (e.g., psychosis) and epilepsy, and efforts to dispel this notion—at least in the minds of the general population—have been a focus of lay epilepsy organizations. Although mechanisms are not well understood, clinical, anatomic, and neurochemical studies seem to confirm an association between epilepsy and major psychiatric illness.

From an epidemiologic standpoint, one must first consider the frequency of each of these conditions before one can consider whether an unusual association exists between two conditions. Both epilepsy and major psychosis are conditions affecting a substantial proportion of the population. Incidence and cumulative incidence provide the most useful information in evaluating the joint occurrence of disease.

Unfortunately, there are few incidence studies of both epilepsy and psychosis. Studies that allow evaluation of the joint probabilities of epilepsy and psychosis and that allow one to distinguish time order are virtually nonexistent.

FREQUENCY OF EPILEPSY

Prevalence

Prevalence is a measure of the number of cases of a disease existent in the population at a particular point in time. The prevalence of *epilepsy (recurrent unprovoked seizures)* shows wide variation across studies, but prevalence generally ranges from 4 to 10 per 1,000 population (1–4). This two- to three-fold variation is related in part to varying definitions, but it also is related to true differences in frequency across populations. The prevalence of epilepsy generally is higher in developing countries than in industrialized nations. In industrialized countries, prevalence tends to increase with advancing age, reaching a peak in the oldest age groups. In contrast, prevalence in developing countries is highest in young adults. These prevalence cases are characterized by chronicity and thus are highly selected. They also are characterized by survival from diagnosis. Population-based prevalence cases are akin to cases seen in general medical or neurologic clinics. They generally have much less severe disease than cases seen at tertiary referral centers. This difference in severity must be taken into account when considering reports of coexistence of psychosis and epilepsy, because most are generated from these tertiary referral centers.

Incidence

There are only a few total population incidence studies of epilepsy. The incidence of epilepsy in industrialized countries is about 50 per 100,000 population per year (5,6). The incidence in developing countries probably is double this rate (3,4,7). Regardless of geographic area, there is an excess incidence in males, and only about 35% of cases have a clearly identified antecedent. In industrialized countries, incidence is high in children up to 1 year and in the elderly. This contrasts with developing countries, where incidence generally peaks in childhood and few new-onset cases are identified in adults after the age of 50 years.

Cumulative Incidence

Because of remission, the lifetime prevalence of epilepsy is considerably higher than the prevalence of active epilepsy. The cumulative incidence is germane to the assessment of comorbidity for two conditions such as psychiatric disease and epilepsy, and it is an estimate of lifetime prevalence. As used here, cumulative incidence is an assessment of the risk to have developed epilepsy through a particular age. For a condition such as epilepsy, in which there is little excess mortality (at least for cases of unknown cause), the cumulative incidence should approximate the prevalence of a lifetime history of the condition. In developed countries, the cumulative incidence of epilepsy is about 1% through age 20 years and about 5% through age 80 years (1); the cumulative incidence for all seizure disorders ranges from 10% to 20% through age 80 years. The cumulative incidence in developing countries is higher through the adult years.

FREQUENCY OF MAJOR PSYCHIATRIC DIAGNOSES

In industrialized countries, diagnosis of a major psychiatric illness of some type can been expected in at least 50% to 60% of the population during their lifetime (lifetime prevalence) (8). Substance abuse or dependence (alcohol in 15% to 25% of the population or tobacco in about 30% of the population) accounts for a large proportion of cases, but a substantial proportion of the population at some time can be expected to be diagnosed with other major disorders, including psychosis (9).

Frequency of Schizophrenia

Prevalence

The point prevalence of schizophrenia ranges from 1 to 3 per 1,000, but overall there is a ten-fold variation in frequency, with higher prevalence reported in studies from developing countries (10). In studies from the United States, prevalence in those over age 18 years probably is 5 per 1,000, and "lifetime" prevalence is around 6 to 7 per 1,000 (11).

Incidence

Using strict diagnostic criteria, incidence ranges from 7 to 14 per 100,000 (12–14). There seems to be little geographic variation in developed countries. Males may have an earlier onset of schizophrenia, although gender-specific incidence is similar or demonstrates a slight male excess overall. Incidence is higher in migrants of color to Great Britain when compared to whites or to the population of their native countries (15–17). There is a question of decreasing incidence of schizophrenia in recent years, although the combination of coding changes in clinical practice and reduced hospitalization rates causes difficulty in interpreting the apparent reduced frequency.

Nonaffective remitting psychosis is of interest because of its similarity to ictal or postictal psychotic states (18). The incidence is about 6 per 100,000 in developed countries and is about twice as high in females as males. The incidence is increased ten-fold in developing countries over that in developed countries.

Frequency of Depression

Prevalence

Community-based studies suggest a point prevalence of depression of 2% to 4%, although estimates are higher in studies of selected populations (8,19–21). Prevalence is higher in females, and point prevalence is highest in the adult population. Prevalence increases as one goes from community to primary care settings to inpatients. (This may be a phenomenon of importance in studies of psychiatric disease and epilepsy.) The lifetime prevalence of major depression approaches 20% in some studies and is higher in females (22).

Incidence

Incidence based on first episode or first treatment for major depression varies markedly among studies (14,23–25). Incidence has been reported to be 1 to 2 per 1,000 per year in males and 3 to 5 per 1,000 in females. Incidence is consistently higher in females than in males. In the epidemiologic catchment area studies, an incidence of 2% per year was reported and varied by age and gender. There are time trends in incidence, with an increasing incidence in middle-aged males reported in more recent studies. In Sweden, cumulative incidence to age 70 years was 27% in males and 46% in females. In studies from the United States, cumulative incidence was reported to be about 17%

Bipolar Disorders

The prevalence and presumably the incidence of bipolar disorders are about 10% of the rates for major depression.

PSYCHIATRIC DISORDERS IN PEOPLE WITH EPILEPSY

A number of cross-sectional studies have evaluated the frequency of psychiatric disturbances in people with epilepsy. Most studied has been the association between depression

and epilepsy. There is a perception that depression is more common in people with epilepsy, but these reports generally are from referral centers, fail to take into account the time order of the two conditions, and do not have a comparison group. Studies from select populations of people with epilepsy suggest that suicide is more frequent in those with epilepsy than in the general population. This observation was confirmed in two recent population-based studies of mortality in people with epilepsy (26,27). The question of time order of depression and the occurrence of epilepsy has seldom been addressed. It appears that clinicians generally assume that the epilepsy caused the depression, but this is not a valid conclusion that can be drawn from cross-sectional studies.

Depression Prior to the Diagnosis of Epilepsy

Many cross-sectional studies have examined the association between depression and epilepsy, but these studies are not useful for establishing whether epilepsy leads to depression or depression leads to epilepsy. Only four studies examined the temporal relationship, and in only three was an appropriate comparison group identified. In a hospital case series of 51 patients with late-onset epilepsy and possible psychiatric diagnosis, Dominian et al. (28) noted that 16% had a history of depression before the initial seizure. This hospitalized group probably represents more severe forms of epilepsy, and there was no control group.

In a population-based, case-control study of patients with newly diagnosed adult-onset epilepsy, depression was found to be seven times more common among cases than among age- and sex-matched controls ($p = 0.03$) (29). When analyses were restricted to cases with a "localized onset" seizure, depression was 17 times more common among cases than among controls ($p = 0.002$). Because patients responded to the questionnaire 4 to 6 weeks after the diagnosis of their first seizure, it is possible that responses were not limited to depression preceding the first diagnosis of epilepsy.

In a population-based, case-control study of incidence of cases of epilepsy of unknown cause in older adults, Hesdorffer et al. (30) noted that *Diagnostic and Statistical Manual of Mental Disorders, Revised Third Edition* (DSM-III-R) depression before the date the patient's initial seizure came to medical attention was 3.7 times more common among cases than among controls after adjusting for medical therapies for depression. This increased risk was more prominent among cases with partial-onset seizures. Among cases, major depression occurred closer to the index date than for controls, suggesting that pathophysiology leading to depression may lower seizure threshold.

A recent study of new-onset epilepsy among children in Iceland demonstrated that depression meeting DSM-IV criteria occurred four times as often among cases with epilepsy than among age- and gender-matched controls (31). A complex interaction between antidepressive therapy and epilepsy was observed in adults in Iceland. In older adults, depression was a risk factor for epilepsy; in young adults, epilepsy seemed to be correlated with therapy rather than DSM-IV depression (32).

These studies all demonstrate a consistent increased risk of epilepsy subsequent to diagnosis of depression. Although consistent with causation, it seems likely that common antecedents are responsible for coexistence of the two conditions.

Depression and Other Neurologic Disorders

Epilepsy is not the only neurologic condition for which depressive illness imparts increased risk. At least two studies reported a higher than expected risk of depression before the onset of Parkinson's disease. In a study of consecutive patients with Parkinson's disease, Mayeux et al. (33) found that 20% were depressed before the onset of clinical symptoms. Similarly, in a study of the effect of lev-odopa treatment on idiopathic Parkinson's disease, 22% of 178 cases were severely depressed prior to disease onset (34). Depression that precedes the onset of Parkinson's disease may represent a symptom associated with striatal nigral degeneration, or the accompanying neurotransmitter changes may increase the risk of disease by making the brain vulnerable to other insults (35).

In multiple sclerosis patients, depression has been reported months or even years before the onset of clinical symptoms. Matthews (36) and Goodstein and Ferrell (37) each reported three cases with multiple sclerosis in whom depression heralded the onset of other more typical neurologic symptoms. These authors argued that depression is as much a neurologic symptom of multiple sclerosis as gait disturbance. Depression occurred in 26% of multiple sclerosis patients prior to symptom onset, but in no controls with other chronic neurologic conditions matched for age, sex, and degree of disability (38).

Depression also may be a risk factor for Alzheimer's disease. Recent studies clearly demonstrated an association between risk of epilepsy and dementia in general and Alzheimer's disease in particular. The EURO-DEM collaborative reanalysis of 11 case-control studies of NINCDS-ADRDA or DSM-III diagnosed Alzheimer's disease found that a history of depression at least 1 year before the onset of Alzheimer's disease was more common among late-onset cases than among controls (39). Alzheimer's cases diagnosed after 70 years of age were more than four times more likely to be diagnosed with depression within 10 years of disease and twice as likely to be diagnosed with depression more than 10 years before Alzheimer's disease.

The consistency and strength of the association between prior depression and subsequent neurologic diseases of the brain, including epilepsy, are compelling. It is difficult to attribute this association to a prodrome of the neurologic disorder, because the association between depression and these neurologic diseases remains, even when limited to depression occurring many years prior to neurologic diagnosis. The prevalence of depression prior to developing epilepsy is remarkably consistent across these diseases: 21% prior to their first unprovoked seizure; 20% to 22% of patients prior to the onset of idiopathic Parkinson's disease (33,34); and 26% of patients prior to onset of multiple sclerosis (38). These numbers suggest that alterations in neurotransmitter function associated with depression may increase susceptibility to other diseases of sclerosis.

Other Psychiatric Conditions Preceding Epilepsy

Schizophrenia

Clinical observations early in the last century suggested an inverse relationship between epilepsy and schizophrenia. It was these observations that led to the institution of convulsive therapy, initially with camphor and later with electroconvulsive therapy (ECT), as a treatment for major psychosis. There have been few epidemiologic studies confirming or refuting these contentions. In a case-control study of new onset epilepsy in older adults, a prior diagnosis of schizophrenia was protective of developing epilepsy.

In a case-control study of psychiatric illness in developing countries, epilepsy in children increased the risk of schizophrenia by a factor of 2 (40). Febrile seizures were not associated with an increased risk of epilepsy. This association may explain the apparent protective effect of schizophrenia for epilepsy in studies of adults.

Manic-Depressive Disorders

In studies of older adults in Rochester, Minnesota one case met DSM-III-R criteria for mania prior to the onset of epilepsy; no controls were affected (41). There do not appear to be any other studies addressing time order of these two conditions.

Substance Abuse

Alcohol abuse and heroin use have been identified as risk factors for epilepsy (42–44).

For alcohol abuse, the risk of developing epilepsy increases in a dose-related fashion. One would expect that people with a history of substance abuse disorders would be overrepresented in the group of people with newly diagnosed epilepsy, although DSM-IV definitions have not been applied to any studies.

EPILEPSY AND PSYCHIATRIC DISORDERS OF UNCERTAIN DIRECTIONALITY

Using data from a population-based survey of psychiatric disturbances, there was a twofold (nonsignificant) increased risk of "seizures" and major psychoses. There is no other information given about the nature of the disturbance in those with a diagnosis of seizures. In these same communities, panic disorder and "seizures" coexist five times more frequently than would be expected by chance (45). The observation could be spurious due to overlap of symptoms in the two disorders. In addition, the questions used to identify those with seizures clearly would not distinguish those with epilepsy from those with acute symptomatic seizures. This data, as with those from most other studies of epilepsy in people with psychiatric disorders, do not all consider the establishment of time order, and definitions of epilepsy would not conform to those used in most contemporary studies of epilepsy.

PSYCHOSIS FOLLOWING A DIAGNOSIS OF EPILEPSY

There are selective psychoses that present as an initial diagnosis more frequently in, or may be unique to, people with an established diagnosis of epilepsy. Most of the reports deal with the highly select population with intractable epilepsy seen at referral centers and/or potential candidates for epilepsy surgery. Although extrapolation to the general population with epilepsy may not be appropriate, study of such cases clearly can lead to improved understanding of basic mechanisms for both conditions and ultimately to appropriate interventions.

Schizophrenia-Like Psychosis of Epilepsy

A schizophrenia-like psychosis has been described in individuals with epilepsy (46–48). There are differences in the psychological and symptom profiles of these individuals and the more typical cases of schizophrenia, hence the term "schizophrenia-like." It has been suggested that the condition is unique to those with temporal lobe epilepsy, particularly those with left temporal foci (49). Psychosis may increase with increasing seizure frequency, and most cases had epilepsy of relatively long duration. It has been suggested that limbic pathology either produced by or associated with epilepsy is responsible for the aberrant psychiatric state, possibly related to modifications of dopaminergic pathways (50).

These findings may be related in part to selectivity of study populations. Most reports come from surgical centers where patients with chronic epilepsy are likely to be seen. In a clinicopathologic study comparing patients with chronic epilepsy, patients with schizophrenia, and patients with epilepsy and psychosis, pathologic changes were more severe in those with psychosis and epilepsy and not limited to the temporal lobe, and seizure type was not different when patients with epilepsy alone were compared to those with psychosis and epilepsy.

Psychotic States Precipitated or Prevented by Ictal Phenomena

There are situations, presumably rare, in which psychosis can be attributed directly to the seizures or their consequences.

Ictal Psychosis

Ictal or periictal psychosis generally is identified in the context of chronic and intractable epilepsy, although it certainly is possible that an ictal or postictal psychotic episode may occur in less refractory cases, or even in those with an undiagnosed seizure disorder (51). The acute psychotic episode may be an extension of the ictal perceptions or aura, but it may be prolonged and may be misdiagnosed. Given the very low incidence in industrialized countries and the close temporal sequence between seizure and psychotic state, there seems little question regarding the causal association. There is little information on the actual frequency of such events in the general epilepsy population.

Interictal Psychoses

Interictal psychoses in patients with chronic and intractable epilepsy have received considerable attention. They are generally termed "schizophreniform" because they do not meet usual DSM criteria for schizophrenia.

Alternating Psychosis

In some individuals, a theoretical and somewhat controversial reciprocal relationship may exist between seizures and psychosis (52). According to this concept, as a convulsive disorder becomes better controlled, aberrant thought processes start or intensify (53,54). Mechanisms to explain these alternating psychoses (and the electroencephalographic [EEG] correlate of forced normalization) remain uncertain but may be related to modification of neurochemical balance or seizure-related electrical brain activity. This phenomenon has been used to explain the association between vigabatrin use and psychosis (55).

Psychoses Following Epilepsy Surgery

On long-term follow-up, psychosis following temporal lobectomy seems particularly frequent, even after discounting cases with preoperative psychosis (56). There may be laterality issues in the development of psychosis, with risk being higher in those with right-sided surgical interventions. The role of surgical intervention is difficult to evaluate, given the presumed increased risk of psychosis in the absence of surgery and the long duration between the surgery and the development of psychosis in many cases.

TREATMENT OF PSYCHOSIS AND RISK OF EPILEPSY

An alternative explanation for an association between convulsive disorders and antecedent psychosis relates to treatments for the latter conditions. The association of many of the therapies with seizures is suggested but not necessarily established, and the association with recurrent unprovoked seizures has seldom been explored.

Antidepressant Use and Seizures

Depression and its neurochemical correlates may make the brain more vulnerable to seizures; alternatively, treatments for depression could explain the observed relationship. Antidepressants may increase the risk of seizures, perhaps due to inhibition of serotonin reuptake at the synaptic cleft. Tricyclic antidepressants, selective serotonin reuptake inhibitors, and neuroleptics can cause seizures. In animal studies, low doses of imipramine or amitriptyline raise the seizure threshold of mice; high doses of imipramine induce clonic seizures (57). Imipramine, amitriptyline, nortriptyline, maprotiline, and desipramine increase spike activity of perfused guinea pig hippocampal slices in a dose-dependent fashion that differs for each antidepressant (58).

Two percent of all patients seen for seizures by the Neurology Service at San Francisco General Hospital between June 1973 and November 1982 were believed to have suffered seizures due to drug toxicity. Thirty percent were attributed to antidepressant or neuroleptic medication. Jabbari et al. (59) reviewed the charts of 186 patients admitted to Walter Reed Army Medical Center during 1982 who satisfied DSM-III-R criteria for depression. Only one patient (2.2%), who had no computed tomographic evidence of brain pathology and no history of prior seizures in his medical record, developed a seizure while taking tricyclic antidepressants. Greenblatt et al. (60) reported no seizures during a randomized clinical trial comparing imipramine, phenelzine, isocarboxazid, ECT, and placebo for treatment of depression. Seizures have been reported as a potential complication of all of the selective serotonin reuptake inhibitors, but these effects have been studied less systematically. The Boston Collaborative Drug Surveillance Program reported no seizure associated with antidepressant use (61). (Given the incidence of epilepsy, at least one case would have been expected in the Boston study.)

These animal studies and clinical series are informative about the relationship between antidepressants and provoked or acute symptomatic seizures, but they provide no longitudinal data to test possible associations between these drugs and epilepsy. In the case-control studies conducted by Hesdorffer et al. (30), there was a two-fold increased risk of epilepsy among those taking tricyclic antidepressive medication. This risk was not significant after adjusting for depression.

Neuroleptics and Seizures

Neuroleptics are associated with an increased risk of seizures (57). In a study of 859 patients treated with phenothiazines, 1.2% developed seizures (62). The incidence of seizures was dose dependent: 9% among patients on high-dose therapy and 0.5% among patients on low-dose therapy. Most seizures occurred when therapy began or when the dose of phenothiazine was increased. A high proportion of patients who were prescribed clozapine were reported to have seizures (63). The Boston Collaborative Drug Surveillance Study found a low risk (0.12%) of seizures due to neuroleptic drugs (64). These data again provide no information regarding the association between these agents and the development of epilepsy. In the case-control study of Hesdorffer et al. (30), a history of having been prescribed a phenothiazine was 1.6 times more common among newly diagnosed cases of epilepsy than among controls in univariate analysis (95% confidence interval [CI] 1.0 to 2.5). In multivariate analysis, use of these compounds was no longer significant (odds ratio = 1.3, 95% CI = 0.8 to 2.2). Although 29.6% of depressed cases and 21.4% of depressed controls were prescribed a phenothiazine prior to the date of diagnosis of epilepsy, phenothiazine exposure was not completely concordant with psychiatric diagnoses; 44% of individuals prescribed phenothiazines had no psychiatric diagnosis.

Electroconvulsive Therapy and Epilepsy

Interest in the relationship between ECT and spontaneous seizures began after Goddard observed that repeated daily brief subconvulsive electrical stimulation applied to specific regions of the brain eventually provokes seizures in animals (65). This kindling persists through a stimulus-free year. Spontaneous seizures can result in the absence of gross pathologic brain changes after more than 300 stimulations in the rat and 50 stimulations in the cat and baboon. Thus, kindling results in permanent transsynaptic alterations in brain function in the absence of gross tissue damage (66).

In kindling, electrical current is applied through implanted depth electrodes, whereas ECT uses surface electrodes. Ramer and Pinel (67) experimentally mimicked ECT by giving electroconvulsive shocks to rats. Electroconvulsive shock therapy causes between-treatment alterations in the EEG; in some cases, these changes can persist for as long as 3 months after the last treatment. Weiner (68) reviewed 21 studies of the persistence of EEG changes following ECT and concluded that, in seven studies, a small percentage of patients had EEG changes that persisted longer than 3 months after the last ECT (range 3 months to 1 year); a large number of ECT treatments predicted the persistence of EEG changes.

During a cycle of ECT treatments, seizure threshold increases (69). Increasing seizure thresholds seem incompatible with the hypothesis that ECT can lead to development of spontaneous seizures. However, spontaneous seizures have occurred in cats during a course of ECT despite an elevated seizure threshold (70,71), indicating that the amount of current needed to evoke a seizure during ECT may not be the same as the threshold for "intrinsic" seizures. Sackeim et al. (69) observed an increase in seizure threshold during a course of ECT treatments but a decrease at the beginning of the next course of ECT. Therefore, animal and human studies support both the antiepileptic and the convulsant capabilities of ECT.

Whereas recent literature suggests that ECT can be utilized safely in patients with depression and epilepsy, two published studies report an increased risk of unprovoked seizure following ECT. Blackwood et al. (72) interviewed 166 patients under the age of 70 years who had undergone at least one ECT course in 1971 or 1976 to determine whether or not they experienced subsequent seizures. A mean of 18 months had elapsed between the last ECT and the interview. Three patients (1.8%) experienced a first unprovoked seizure after they began ECT. The authors, incorrectly comparing the incidence of unprovoked seizures to the seizure prevalence in the general population, concluded that ECT does not augment the risk of developing seizures. In fact, their incidence is more than 36 times the expected. Devinsky and Duchowny (73) reviewed all published cases of spontaneous seizures following ECT. The average annual incidence of seizures after ECT was 114 per 100,000, which is almost three times greater than the incidence of unprovoked seizures among adults in Rochester, Minnesota (6).

In univariate analysis of a case-control study of older adults with new-onset epilepsy, cases were 4.7 times more likely than controls to have received ECT (95% CI = 1.2 to 18) (30). This effect diminished and was not significant in multivariate analysis.

SUMMARY

There appears to be considerable evidence to support the hypothesis that the convulsive disorders, psychiatric illness in general and psychosis in particular, coexist more frequently than expected by chance. Most of the studies cannot establish time order. It is important to clarify the relationship, but proper studies of incidence cohorts of patients with psychiatric disease and with convulsive disorders is necessary. The few studies of incidence cohorts of epilepsy suggest that depression is a risk factor for epilepsy and that schizophrenia is protective in adults. Childhood epilepsy is a risk factor for schizophrenia. Cross-sectional studies, which are much more difficult to interpret, may confirm these findings and may suggest an association with panic. Psychosis—nonpersistent and schizophrenic-like—appears to occur with increased frequency in people with epilepsy. The relationship seems to increase with increasing severity of disease regardless of how it is measured, but is based on select patient groups. Studies that use improved definitions, limit results to the first event, and have appropriate controls are necessary for proper interpretation of the findings.

REFERENCES

1. Hauser WA, Annegers JF, Kurland LT. Prevalence of epilepsy in Rochester, Minnesota: 1940–1980. *Epilepsia* 1991;32:429–445.
2. Cowan LD, Leviton A, Bodensteiner JB, et al. Problems in estimating the prevalence of epilepsy in children: the yield from different sources of information. *Paediatr Perinat Epidemiol* 1989;3:386–401.
3. Rwiza HT, Kilonzo GP, Haule J, et al. Prevalence and incidence of epilepsy in Ulanga, a rural Tanzanian district: a community-based study. *Epilepsia* 1992;33:1051–1056.
4. Placencia M, Sander JW, Roman M, et al. The characteristics of epilepsy in a largely untreated population in rural Ecuador. *J Neurol Neurosurg Psychiatry* 1994;57:320–350.
5. Ólafsson E, Hauser WA, Luðvigsson P, et al. Incidence of epilepsy in rural Iceland: a population-based study. *Epilepsia* 1996;37:951–955.
6. Hauser WA, Annegers JF, Kurland LT. Incidence of epilepsy and unprovoked seizures in Rochester, Minnesota: 1935–1984. *Epilepsia* 1993;34:453–468.
7. Lavados J, Germain I, Morales A, et al. A descriptive study of epilepsy in the District of El Salvador, Chile 1984–1988. *Acta Neurol Scand* 1992;91:718–729.
8. Anthony JC, Eaton WW, Henderson AS. Psychiatric epidemiology. *Epidemiol Rev* 1995;17:240–242.
9. Anthony JC, Warner LA, Kessler RC. Comparative epidemiology of dependence on tobacco, alcohol, controlled substances, and inhalants: basic findings from the National Comorbidity Survey. *Exp Clin Psychopharmacol* 1994;2:244–268.
10. Stefánsson JG, Lindal E, Björnsson JL, et al. Period prevalence rates of specific mental disorders in an Iceland cohort. *Soc Psychiatry Psychiatr Epidemiol* 1994;29:119–125.
11. Kessler RC, Gonagle KA, Zhao S, et al. Lifetime and 12 month prevalence of DSM-III-R psychiatric disorder in the United States: results from the National Co-Morbidity Survey. *Arch Gen Psychiatry* 1994;51:8–19.
12. Bhugra D, Leff J, Mallett R, et al. Incidence and outcome of schizophrenia in whites, African-Caribbeans and Asians in London. *Psychol Med* 1997;27:791–798.
13. Suvisaari JM, Haukka JK, Tanskanen AJ, et al. Decline in the incidence of schizophrenia in Finnish cohorts born from 1954 to 1965. *Arch Gen Psychiatry* 1999;56:733–740.
14. Newman SC, Bland RC. Incidence of mental disorders in Edmonton: estimates of rates and methodological issues. *J Psychiatr Res* 1998;32:273–282.
15. McNaught AS, Jeffreys SE, Harvey CA, et al. The Hampstead Schizophrenia Survey 1991. II: Incidence and migration in inner London. *Br J Psychiatry* 1997;170:307–311.
16. Mahy GE, Mallett R, Leff J, et al. First-contact incidence rate of schizophrenia on Barbados. *Br J Psychiatry* 1999;175:28–33.
17. Hickling FW, Rodgers-Johnson P. The incidence of first contact schizophrenia in Jamaica. *Br J Psychiatry* 1995;167:193–196.
18. Susser E, Wanderling J. Epidemiology of nonaffective acute remitting psychosis vs. schizophrenia: sex and sociocultural setting. *Arch Gen Psychiatry* 1994;51:294–301.
19. Murphy JM, Laird NM, Monson RR, et al. A 40-year perspective on the prevalence of depression: the Stirling County Study. *Arch Gen Psychiatry* 2000;57:209–215.
20. Ohayon MM, Priest RG, Guilleminault C, et al. The prevalence of depressive disorders in the United Kingdom. *Biol Psychiatry* 1999;45:300–307.
21. Blazer DG, Kessler RC, McGonagle KA, et al. The prevalence and distribution of major depression in a national community sample: the National Comorbidity Survey. *Am J Psychiatry* 1994;151:979–986.
22. Wittchen HU, Knauper B, Kessler RC. Lifetime risk of depression. *Br J Psychiatry Suppl* 1994 Dec;16–22.
23. Murphy JM, Laird NM, Monson RR, et al. Incidence of depression in the Stirling County Study: historical and comparative perspectives. *Psychol Med* 2000;30:505–514.
24. Eaton WW, Anthony JC, Gallo J, et al. Natural history of Diagnostic Interview Schedule/DSM-IV major depression. The Baltimore Epidemiologic Catchment Area follow-up. *Arch Gen Psychiatry* 1997;54:993–999.
25. Rorsman B, Grasbeck A, Hagnell O, et al. A prospective study of first-incidence depression. The Lundby study, 1957–72. *Br J Psychiatry* 1990;156:336–342.
26. Nilsson L, Tomson T, Farahmand BY, et al. Cause-specific mortality in epilepsy: a cohort study of more than 9,000 patients once hospitalized for epilepsy. *Epilepsia* 1997;38:1062–1068.
27. Rafnsson V, Olafsson E, Hauser WA, et al. Mortality among people with unprovoked seizures. *Neuroepidemiology (in press)*.

28. Dominian MA, Serafetinides EA, Dewhurst M. A follow-up study of late-onset epilepsy: II. Psychiatric and social findings. *Br Med J* 1963;1:431–435.

29. Forsgren L, Nystrom L. An incident case-referent study of epileptic seizures in adults. *Epilepsy Res* 1990;6: 66–81.

30. Hesdorffer DC, Hauser WA, Annegers JF, et al. Major depression is a risk factor for seizures in older adults. *Ann Neurol* 2000;47:246–249.

31. Hesdorffer D, Ludvigsson P, Hauser WA, et al. Depression is a risk factor for epilepsy in children. *Epilepsia* 1998;39[Suppl 6]:222.

32. Hesdorffer DC, Olafsson E, Ludvigsson P, et al. Antidepressive use may explain the relationship between depression and epilepsy. *Epilepsia* 1999;40[Suppl 7]:86.

33. Mayeux R, Stem Y, Rosen J, et al. Depression, intellectual impairment and Parkinson's disease. *Neurology* 1983;31:645–650.

34. Shaw KM, Lees AJ, Stern GM. The impact of treatment with levodopa on Parkinson's disease. *Q J Med* 1980; 49:283–293.

35. McNamara ME. Psychological factors affecting neurological conditions: depression and stroke, multiple sclerosis, Parkinson's disease, and epilepsy. *Psychosomatics* 1991;32:255–267.

36. Matthews WB. Multiple sclerosis presenting with acute remitting psychiatric symptoms. *J Neurol Neurosurg Psychiatry* 1979;42:859–873.

37. Goodstein RK, Ferrell RB. Multiple sclerosis presenting as depressive illness. *Dis Nerv Sys* 1977;38: 127–131.

38. Whitlock FA, Siskind MM. Depression as a major symptom of multiple sclerosis. *J Neurol Neurosurg Psychiatry* 1980;43:861–865.

39. Jorm AF, Van Diujn CM, Chandra V, et al. Psychiatric history and related exposures as risk factors for Alzheimer's disease: a collaborative re-analysis of case-control studies. *Int J Epidemiol* 1991;20[Suppl 2]:S43.

40. Jablinsky A, Sartorius N, Ernberg G, et al. Schizophrenia: manifestations, incidence, and course in different cultures. A World Heath Organization ten-country study. *Psychol Med Monogr Suppl* 1992;20:1–97.

41. Hesdorffer DC, Hauser WA, Annegers JF, et al. Psychiatric diagnoses preceding unprovoked seizures in adults: a population-based case-control study. *Epilepsia* 1992;33[Suppl 3]:16.

42. Ng SKC, Hauser WA, Brust JC, et al. Alcohol consumption and the risk of new onset seizures. *N Engl J Med* 1988;319:666–673.

43. Leone M, Bottacchi E, Beghi E, et al. Alcohol use is a risk factor for a first generalized tonic-clonic seizure. The ALCE (Alcohol and Epilepsy) Study Group. *Neurology* 1997;48:614–620.

44. Ng SKC, Brust JCM, Hauser WA, et al. Illicit drug use and the risk of new-onset seizures. *Am J Epidemiol* 1990;132:47–57.

45. Neugebauer R, Weissman MM, Ouellette R, et al. Comorbidity of panic disorder and seizures: affinity or artifact? *J Anxiety Disord* 1993;7:21–35.

46. Trimble MR. The schizophrenia-like psychosis of epilepsy. *Neuropsychiatry Neuropsychol Behav Neurol* 1992;5:103–107.

47. Bruton CJ, Stevens JR, Frith CD. Epilepsy, psychosis, and schizophrenia: clinical and neuropathologic correlations. *Neurology* 1994;44:34–42.

48. Mendez MF, Grau R, Doss RC, et al. Schizophrenia in epilepsy: seizure and psychosis variables. *Neurology* 1993;43:1073–1077.

49. Gold JM, Hermann BP, Randolph C, et al. Schizophrenia and temporal lobe epilepsy: a neuropsychological analysis. *Arch Gen Psychiatry* 1994;51:265–272.

50. Ring HA, Trimble MR, Costa DC, et al. Striatal dopamine receptor binding in epileptic psychoses. *Biol Psychiatry* 1994;35:375–380.

51. Umbricht D, Degreef G, Barr WB, et al. Postictal and chronic psychoses in patients with temporal lobe epilepsy. *Am J Psychiatry* 1995;152:224–231.

52. Schiffer RB. Epilepsy, psychosis, and forced normalization. *Arch Neurol* 1987;44:253.

53. Wolf P. Acute behavioral symptomatology at disappearance of epileptiform EEG abnormality: paradoxical or "forced" normalization. In: Smith DB, Treiman DM, Trimble MR, eds. Neurobehavioral problems in epilepsy. *Adv Neurol* 1991;55:127–142.

54. Wolf P, Trimble MR. Biological antagonism and epileptic psychosis. *Br J Psychiatry* 1985;146:272–276.

55. Sander JW, Hart YM, Trimble MR, et al. Vigabatrin and psychosis. *J Neurol Neurosurg Psychiatry* 1991;54:435–439.

56. Leinonen E, Tuunainen A, Lepola U. Postoperative psychoses in epileptic patients after temporal lobectomy. *Acta Neurol Scand* 1994;90:394–399.

57. Zaccara O, Muscas C, Messori A. Clinical feature, pathogenesis and management of drug-induced seizures. *Drug Safety* 1990;5:109–151.

58. Luchins DI, Oliver AP, Wyatt RJ. Seizures with antidepressants: an in vitro technique to assess relative risk. *Epilepsia* 1994;25:25–32.

59. Jabbari B, Bryan GE, Marsh EE, et al. Incidence of seizures with tricyclic and tetracyclic antidepressants. *Arch Neurol* 1985;42:480–481.

60. Greenblatt M, Grosser GH, Wechsler H. Differential response of hospitalized patients to somatic therapy. *Am J Psychiatry* 1964;121:935–943.

61. Anonymous. Drug-induced convulsions: Report from Boston Collaborative Drug Surveillance Program. *Lancet* 1972;2:677–679.

62. Logothetis J. Spontaneous epileptic seizures and electroencephalographic changes in the course of phenothiazine therapy. *Neurology* 1967;17:869–877.

63. Haller E, Binder RL. Clozapine and seizures. *Am J Psychiatry* 1990;147:1069–1071.

64. Messing RO, Closson RG, Simon RP. Drug-induced convulsions: a 10-year experience. *Neurology* 1984;34: 582–586.

65. Adams RE. Does kindling model anything clinically relevant? *Biol Psychiatry* 1990;27:249–279.

66. Racine R. Kindling: the first decade. *Neurosurgery* 1978;3:234–252.

67. Ramer D, Pinel JP. Progressive intensification of motor seizures produced by periodic electroconvulsive shock. *Exp Neurol* 1977;51:421–433.

68. Weiner RD. The persistence of electroconvulsive therapy-induced changes in the electroencephalogram. *J Nerv Ment Dis* 1930;168:224–228.

69. Sackeim HA, Decina P, Prohovnik I, et al. Anticonvulsant and antidepressant properties of electroconvulsive therapy: a proposed mechanism of action. *Biol Psychiatry* 1983;18:1301–1310.

70. Essig CF, Groce ME, Williamson EL. Reversible elevation of electroconvulsive threshold and occurrence of

spontaneous convulsions upon repeated stimulation of the cat brain. *Exp Neurol* 1961;4:37–47.

71. Essig CF, Flanary HG. The importance of the convulsion in the occurrence and rate of development of electroconvulsive threshold elevation. *Exp Neurol* 1966; 14:448–452.

72. Blackwood DHR, Cull RE, Freeman CPL, et al. A study of the incidence of epilepsy following ECT. *J Neurol Neurosurg Psychiatry* 1980;43:1098–1102.

73. Devinsky O, Duchowny MS. Seizures after convulsive therapy: a retrospective case survey. *Neurology* 1983; 13:921–925.

3

Psychiatric Evaluation of the Patient with Epilepsy

A Practical Approach for the "Nonpsychiatrist"

Andres M. Kanner and *Deborah Weisbrot

*Department of Neurological Sciences, Rush Presbyterian-Saint Luke's Medical Center, Chicago, Illinois 60612; and *Department of Psychiatry and Behavioral Sciences, State University of New York at Stony Brook, Stony Brook, New York 11794*

Should every patient with epilepsy undergo a psychiatric evaluation? A brief review of any chapter of this book would be sufficient to convince the most nonpsychologically oriented clinician of the need to include a psychiatric assessment in the evaluation of any patient with epilepsy. Indeed, compared to controls, these patients are at higher risk of suffering from affective, anxiety, and psychotic disorders, as well as attention-deficit disorders. Despite this fact, psychopathology among epileptics goes unrecognized, even when the severity of the psychiatric disorder is having a significantly negative impact on the patient's quality of life (1).

Much of the psychiatric and neuropsychological data on epilepsy published to date are gathered in tertiary care centers, where patients with the more severe forms of epilepsy are evaluated and treated. Yet, in a population-based study, Sillanpaa et al. (2) suggested that patients with uncomplicated epilepsy may not fare as well as controls in vocational training, marriage or living with a partner, employment, and socioeconomic status. In addition, these authors found that patients who remained seizure-free off antiepileptic drugs (AEDs) since childhood had a worse outcome than controls in levels of achievement in primary education, marriage (or living with a partner), and having children. Camfield et al. (3) as-

sessed the social outcome after the age of 18 years in a population-based prospective study of 337 children with partial epilepsy and normal intelligence. Social isolation was recorded in 16%, financial dependency in 30%, and unemployment in 30%. Clearly, these two population-based studies demonstrate a greater vulnerability of patients with epilepsy, even in the absence of any cognitive impairment or when an optimal seizure control (i.e., seizure freedom off AEDs) is achieved.

The underrecognition of psychiatric and psychosocial problems in patients with epilepsy is a sad reality, with serious negative consequences to their quality of life. We do not believe that every patient with epilepsy should be referred to the psychiatrist for evaluation. However, a psychiatric and psychosocial assessment should be carried out by the physician responsible for the management of the seizure disorder (i.e., internist, pediatrician, adult or pediatric neurologist, or epileptologist) at the time of the initial diagnostic evaluation of the epileptic seizure disorder. Consultation with the psychiatrist or neuropsychologist should be considered at the discretion of the treating physician, after the initial assessment.

The aim of this chapter is to provide some guidelines on how to approach the evaluation of psychopathology in patients with epilepsy.

In addition, we intend to provide the nonpsychiatrist with a model that can be used to carry out such evaluations in the office. We also discuss the role of psychiatric rating scales in the overall assessments of these patients.

HOW TO APPROACH PSYCHOPATHOLOGY IN PATIENTS WITH EPILEPSY

From an Etiopathogenic Perspective

Psychiatric symptoms in epilepsy are the expression of at least three important processes: (i) an intrinsic epileptic process resulting from neurochemical and neurophysiologic changes in the limbic circuit; (ii) an expression of the iatrogenic potential of many of the AEDs used in these patients; and (iii) an expression of a reactive process to a chronic disorder that demands multiple adjustments. Psychiatric symptoms also can result from the interaction between two or all three processes. Accordingly, the occurrence of any psychiatric or psychosocial phenomena must be placed in the context of these possible scenarios.

We cite some examples of depressive disorders in epilepsy to illustrate these points. The expression of depressive disorder as an intrinsic process of the seizure disorder is exemplified by the higher incidence of interictal depression among patients with partial seizure disorders that involve the limbic circuitry (i.e., partial seizures of temporal lobe origin) (4–10). This incidence is higher than that of patients with generalized seizure disorders (11–17). In addition, patients with auras consisting of psychic symptoms have a higher rate of depression than patients with partial seizure without auras or whose auras consist of motor, sensory, or autonomic symptoms (18). Thus, it is clear that involvement of limbic neuroanatomic structures constitutes a risk factor for depression among patients with epilepsy.

With respect to the iatrogenic process responsible for psychiatric symptoms among patients with epilepsy, it is well known that all AEDs can cause psychiatric symptoms in these patients, some more than others (19,20).

Phenobarbital is known to cause depression (21–27) and to be associated with the occurrence of suicidal ideation (24), as well as of suicidal and parasuicidal behavior (28,29). Primidone, tiagabine, topiramate, vigabatrin (30–32), and felbamate (33) are among the other AEDs known to frequently cause symptoms of depression. We also observed severe symptoms of depression with lamotrigine in five of 90 patients taking this drug on a monotherapy regimen (unpublished data). AEDs with mood-stabilizing properties, such as carbamazepine and valproic acid, occasionally can cause similar problems (20).

There are two other iatrogenic processes that can result in psychiatric symptoms. The first process is through the discontinuation of AEDs with mood-stabilizing properties in patients with underlying psychiatric disorders that have been under control with these AEDs. Thus, episodes of depression, mania, or panic attacks have been reported from the discontinuation of AEDs such as carbamazepine or valproic acid (34). The second process can result from the pharmacokinetic interaction between an enzyme-inducing AED and a psychotropic drug. Specifically, AEDs such as carbamazepine, phenytoin, primidone, and phenobarbital induce the metabolism of most antidepressants and antipsychotic drugs. Hence, the addition of one of these AEDs in the presence of a psychotropic drug will result in a drop of the serum concentrations of the latter, which, in turn, may cause the recurrence of a psychiatric process that had been well controlled by the psychotropic drug at higher serum concentrations.

Included among the psychosocial factors known to mediate the occurrence of depression are the following: (i) the patient's lack of acceptance and poor adjustment of his or her epilepsy (35); (ii) the stigma associated with the diagnosis of epilepsy and the well-known discrimination to which these patients are subjected (36–38); (iii) the lack of control in one's life caused by the random occurrence of epileptic seizures (39,40); and (iv) the patient's lack of social support and the need to make significant adjustments in lifestyle, such as relinquishing driving privileges or changing jobs to ensure that seizure precautions are closely observed. These are just a few of the obstacles that the epileptic patient must face on a daily basis (36,41–45). The ability to cope with these obstacles often is hampered by the psychological and psychiatric problems that are not infrequent among the epileptic patient. For example, neuropsychological studies have shown that even epileptic patients with a normal intelligence have a lower degree of flexibility of mental processing than normal controls (46–48).

From the Perspective of Its Temporal Relation to Seizures

Psychopathology can be classified according to the temporal relationship between the presentation of psychiatric symptoms and the seizure occurrence into (i) ictal symptoms (the psychiatric symptoms are a clinical manifestation of the seizure), (ii) periictal symptoms (symptoms precede and/or follow the seizure occurrence), and (iii) interictal symptoms (symptoms occur independently of the seizure occurrence). For example, ictal depression is the expression of a simple partial seizure (or "aura") or of the beginning of a complex partial seizure in the form of one or more depressive symptoms. These depressive symptoms are experienced by the patient before the epileptic activity has spread to subcortical and/or contralateral structures, causing loss of consciousness. It has been estimated that 25% of patients with auras have a variety of psychiatric symptoms as their principal clinical manifestation; 15% of these involve affect or mood changes (49,50). In some series, ictal anxiety and fear are the most common types of ictal affect, followed by ictal depression (50). At times, mood changes represent the only expression of simple partial seizures, and consequently they may be difficult to recognize as epileptic phenomena. These mood changes typically are brief, stereotypic, occur out of context, and are associated with other ictal phenomena.

Periictal psychiatric symptoms typically precede and/or follow seizure occurrence (50–54). At times, prodromal symptoms of depression may extend for hours or even days prior to the onset of a seizure (55). Postictal psychiatric symptoms are the most frequent presentation of periictal symptoms. They may present as isolated symptoms or in clusters mimicking psychiatric disorders, i.e., postictal psychosis or depression. The postictal period comprises the time period from the moment of recovery of consciousness following a seizure up to 5 days. Clinicians must remember that psychiatric symptomatology often may appear following a 12- to 48-hour symptom-free period after regaining consciousness. The incidence of postictal psychiatric symptoms has not been determined; however, in a recently completed study, we found the presence of postictal symptoms of depression in 48 of 100 patients with poorly controlled partial seizure disorders, with a median duration of 24 hours (56). Interestingly, postictal symptoms of depression can outlast the ictus for up to 2 weeks (51) and, at times, have led patients to suicide (57–61). Postictal psychotic symptoms were identified in 8% of patients (56).

Interictal psychiatric symptomatology is the most common presentation of psychiatric disorders among patients with epilepsy (13). For example, although the real prevalence of interictal depression is unknown, some clinical investigations showed that 20% of temporal lobe epilepsy patients became interictally depressed and that up to 62% of patients with intractable complex partial seizures had a history of depression, which may be episodic in nature (62,63).

WHAT PSYCHIATRIC SYMPTOMS SHOULD BE ASSESSED IN EVERY EVALUATION?

Every initial evaluation must gather information pertaining to the following six domains:

1. The patient's understanding of what epilepsy is, and of his or her seizure disorder in particular

2. Presence of psychiatric symptoms or disorders, per se
3. The impact of epilepsy on the patient's professional life, interpersonal relationships, and in the family dynamics
4. The acceptance (or rejection) of the epilepsy by the patient and his or her family
5. Any past psychiatric history that preceded the onset of the seizure disorder
6. Any family psychiatric history.

Ideally, information should be gathered from the patient and a close relative who knows the patient well, as patients often may minimize or deny certain personality traits that may be the source of interpersonal problems and that may have a direct impact on his or her quality of life.

Given their relatively high prevalence in epileptic seizure disorders, clinicians should always inquire about the presence of symptoms of depression and anxiety disorders; including panic attacks and attention-deficit disorder, during both interictal and postictal periods.

In the following section, we include two sets of questions that can serve as a model to screen psychiatric and psychosocial problems associated with the seizure disorder in adults and children, respectively. These sets of questions are not intended to be a complete psychiatric questionnaire aimed at eliciting all types of psychiatric symptoms. They reflect a "quadre" of questions that are designed to identify, during an initial assessment, the presence of the more frequent types of psychopathology encountered in adults and children with epilepsy. In our experience, these sets of questions can be administered over a relatively short period of time, while conducting a diagnostic evaluation in the office, and provide rather broad psychosocial and psychiatric profiles of the patient.

Adult Questionnaire

Introductory Comments

It is not uncommon for patients with epilepsy to experience a variety of difficulties in their daily activities and/or in their relations with others. Sometimes patients with epilepsy may experience psychological symptoms, such as symptoms of depression or anxiety. Some of these symptoms may be caused by the medication they take to control their seizures. Other times, these symptoms may be related to the electrical and chemical changes caused in the brain by the seizure disorder, and other times these symptoms may result from the difficulties encountered by the patient in coping with this disease.

Understanding of Epilepsy

1. Can you first tell me what is your understanding of epilepsy and of your particular seizure disorder?
2. Do you have any fears or concerns with respect to your seizures and whether they could cause any harm to you?
3. Can you tell me how has having seizures changed your daily life?
4. How has it changed your life with your spouse/parents/friends?
5. How has it changed your life at work/school?
6. Do you think that you have fully accepted having epilepsy?
7. Do you think your parents/spouse/family/friends/ have accepted that you have epilepsy?

I am now going to ask you a series of questions regarding several psychological symptoms that patients with epilepsy may experience. Tell me if you have experienced any of these symptoms:

Symptoms of Depression

1. Are you having difficulty finding pleasure in activities you used to enjoy?
2. Do you have to push yourself now to do things that you used to enjoy in the past?
3. Do people get on your nerves for things that never used to bother you before?
4. Do you have little tolerance for people?
5. Do you notice that your mood changes without any apparent reason? For exam-

ple, one day you are happy, and without any reason you get moody, cranky, and cannot enjoy anything the next day?

6. Do you feel so bad that you feel completely hopeless?
7. Do you feel that there is nothing you can do to feel better about yourself?
8. Do you sometimes wish you were dead?
9. Do you think about ways of harming yourself?
10. Do you find yourself crying for things that never made you cry before?

Symptoms of Anxiety

1. Do you worry about things you never worried about before?
2. Do you fear that something bad will happen to your loved ones, even though you know there is nothing to worry about?
3. Does your heart start beating fast, out of the blue, and you feel like you cannot catch your breath and that something terrible is going to happen to you, like having a heart attack, a stroke, etc.?
4. Do you get frightened of being left alone or leaving the house by yourself?

Difficulties with Attention, Concentration, and Impulsivity

1. Are you having a hard time concentrating? Do you notice that you get easily distracted?
2. Do you have to read things several times before you feel that you have finally learned them?
3. Do you find that you are making decisions without thinking about the consequences? Have you been acting impulsively?
4. Do you have a hard time focusing on one thing at a time? As if you had to jump from one thing to the other without finishing anything?
5. Are you having a hard time getting organized in your activities?

Psychotic Symptoms

1. Do you find that your mind is playing tricks on you? For example, do you feel that people in the street are staring at you and talking about you?
2. Do you feel that someone is going to hurt you?
3. Are you hearing voices when no one is around?

Symptoms of Mania

1. Do you suddenly get a burst of energy, where you feel like you can do anything you want?
2. Do your thoughts race from one to the other, to the point where you have difficulty verbalizing everything that is going on in your head?

Vegetative Symptoms

1. Have you noticed a change in your sleeping pattern?
2. Have you noticed a change in your appetite?
3. Have you noticed a change in your sexual drive?

Child and Adolescent Questionnaire

Children and adolescents do not respond well to a checklist or highly structured list of questions. This often evokes "yes" or "no" answers or monosyllabic responses. The clinician will be much more successful if he or she can develop a friendly, flexible, and relaxed approach with the young person. A sense of humor is also an asset in a skillful interviewer to put the child at ease. As in the adult questionnaire presented earlier, this list *in no way* represents a complete mental status examination. These questions are offered as a guideline of critical issues that need to be addressed in a psychiatric assessment of children and adolescents. The level of questions should always be formulated according to level of maturity of the child or adolescent, i.e., some older adolescents can be given the adult questions, whereas some younger adolescents will require that questions be phrased as if for a younger child. Many of the questions listed are similar to those utilized in Rutter's classic Isle of Wight study.

Understanding of Epilepsy

1. What is epilepsy?
2. Do you know what kind of epilepsy you have?
3. How does it feel to have epilepsy? Is there anything about having epilepsy that worries you?
4. How are things at school? Has having epilepsy caused problems for you in your class?
5. Do other kids tease you because you have epilepsy?
6. What about at home or with your friends? Has epilepsy caused problems for you there?
7. Does having epilepsy stop you from doing things that you want to do? Give an example.

Aggression

1. What things make you mad? How mad do you get? What do you feel like doing when you are mad?
2. Do you ever want to hurt anyone? . . . Kill anyone?
3. Do you have trouble with your temper?
4. Do you get into fights? . . . Frequently?

Mood

1. How is your mood (make sure child knows this concept) most of the time?
2. Do you get into bad moods where, for no reason, you are mad at everyone?
3. Are there things you enjoy, or is it hard to have fun?
4. Have you ever felt really high or hyper for more than a few hours (not drug induced)?
5. How do you feel about yourself? Do you like yourself?

6. Have you ever felt so bad you wished you could disappear? . . . Die?
7. Have you ever tried to hurt or kill yourself? . . . What did you do? . . . What happened?

Anxiety

1. What kind of things do you worry about?
2. Do you ever find yourself getting nervous or panicky for no reason. If yes, when?
3. Does your head ever feel funny when you get nervous? Do you feel light-headed?
4. Do you ever worry that something will happen to you or to your parents?
5. Do you get very homesick or worried if your parent(s) leave?

Inattention, Distractibility, Hyperactivity, and Conduct

1. Do you have trouble sitting still at school?
2. Do you have to get up and down a lot?
3. Is it hard to pay attention?
4. What thing is the hardest in school? The easiest?
5. How do you get along with your teacher?
6. Do you talk back to the teacher or break the rules?

Psychotic Symptoms

1. Sometimes, when people are feeling low, they get the feeling that other people are looking at them or talking about them or laughing at them. Do you ever feel like that? . . . Or, do you ever feel people are generally against you?
2. Has it ever seemed to you that the world around you has changed in some strange way that you cannot quite figure out, as if things had become unreal?
3. Have you ever felt like you were in a different place than you really were?
4. Have you ever felt that you had special "gifts" or "powers," such as being able to talk directly to God, putting your hand in a fire and not being burned, or being able to predict the future?

Obsessions and Compulsions

1. Is there anything that comes to your mind and goes over and over, and you cannot get rid of it even though it bothers you or does not make sense?
2. Have you ever stayed home from school because you were worried or afraid that someone might get sick, become hurt, or die, or that you might get sick or hurt? . . . Other reasons?
3. Do you sometimes find yourself doing things that seem silly, like touching things or washing over and over again?
4. After you have done something, do you go back and check again to see if it is all right even though you know it is?

Physical and/or Sexual Abuse

This is a complex area that requires significant interviewing skills. It is important for the nonpsychiatrist to be willing to consider the possibility that molestation and abuse can occur. The clinician needs to be aware of his or her own feelings about sexuality. Questions about sexual abuse should be part of a routine review of symptoms. The clinician can ask questions framed in a general way and give the child permission to speak about very difficult topics, such as those in the questions that follow. Do not ask leading questions.

1. Do you have any concerns about your body?
2. Do you know anyone who has ever experienced sexual or physical abuse?
3. Has anyone ever touched you in a way that made you feel uncomfortable?

Questions Specifically for Adolescents

1. Are you sexually active?
2. Are you using any drugs that have not been prescribed? What about alcohol?

Far from being irrelevant or optional, clinicians must consider the fact that the information gathered in a psychiatric assessment has direct relevance to the actual management of a seizure disorder. For example, patients with a past psychiatric history of depression or attention-deficit disorder will be at risk of recurrence of such disorders with the use of certain AEDs, such as barbiturates, topiramate, or certain benzodiazepines. By the same token, clinicians who are alert to affective symptoms in their patients may decide to choose an AED with mood-stabilizing properties that could prevent seizures and act as a prophylactic agent against the recurrence of depressive disorders.

USE OF RATING SCALES IN PATIENTS WITH EPILEPSY

In the next section, we review some of the frequently used self-report rating scales. Many neurologists have tried to save time in their evaluation of psychopathology in the patient with epilepsy by side stepping the actual psychiatric interview with the completion of self-rating questionnaires and rating scales designed to identify a variety of psychiatric conditions. Although there is no doubt that such instruments can be of assistance in the evaluation of these patients, we believe that they should *never* be used instead of the direct interview with the patient and his or her family. Following are some of the reasons.

A. Open discussion between the clinician and the patient and his or her family members is the only way to demystify and clarify many erroneous ideas about psychopathology and epilepsy, which often are at the core of the rejection of the diagnosis of epilepsy by both patients and family members.

B. In an informal interview setting, the clinician can get a "feeling" for the patient's awareness of his or her own psychological and cognitive difficulties. It allows the clinician to predict the occurrence of potential problems that may result from having to take medication on a daily basis and cope with a diagnosis of epilepsy, above all, when the patient comes from cultural environments where such a disorder is fraught with taboos and misinformation.

C. Most rating scales and self-report questionnaires are developed to identify psychopathology in nonepileptic patient populations. Accordingly, the sensitivity and specificity of these instruments may not apply in the same manner to the epileptic patient. For example, the Hamilton Rating Scale for Depression does not inquire about irritability, which is a pivotal symptom in the depressive disorder of the epileptic patient. Furthermore, on self-report measures, some patients may be endorsing items that potentially reflect side effects to their AEDs rather than actual symptoms of psychiatric disorders.

D. Psychiatric rating scales are like thermometers: they can be used to tell if the patient has a "fever"; however, they do not tell much about the specific illness. In discussing a patient's responses to a checklist with him or her, it is not infrequent to discover that the person meant something quite different from what he or she endorsed on the self-report measure. This is particularly true for child or parent checklists. Although rating scales can be very helpful in guiding initial interviews or tracking the course of treatment response, they should never be used to make diagnosis in the absence of a clinical interview.

E. Ultimately, there is no substitute for a thoughtful interview with a patient, and the best rating scale is one based on a checklist of the individual patient's symptoms.

Nonetheless, rating scales can be valuable in supplying clinical data to help in making what are often difficult psychiatric diagnoses. The information obtained from a self-report questionnaire can be helpful in guiding a clinical interview toward particular problem areas. In a neurology practice, the self-report measures can help the clinician decide whether a referral to a psychiatrist is indicated.

Useful Self-Report Measures for Adults with Epilepsy

The following scales are representative samples of self-report measures. For practical clinical use, they do not require interpretation by a psychologist or a psychiatrist. A complete list of available self-report measures,

structured interviews, and other clinician-administered assessments is beyond the scope of this chapter. The reader is referred to reference 66 for further discussions of this topic. Included in the following is a list of a number of measures that are used frequently by the authors and have been found to be of clinical value on a regular basis.

Minnesota Multiphasic Personality Inventory: Self-report personality inventory with ten clinical scales (hypochondriasis, depression, hysteria, psychopathic deviance, malefemale, paranoia, psychasthenia, schizophrenia, mania, and social introversion) and three validity scales. The administration time is about 40 to 90 minutes (67).

Adult Self-Report Inventories-4: The Adult Self-Report Inventories are symptom inventories that can be used as a guide for conducting clinical interviews. They include the behavioral symptoms of more than two dozen psychiatric disorders described in the American Psychiatric Association's *Diagnostic and Statistical Manual of Mental Disorders, Fourth Edition* (DSM-IV). There are parallel versions of the Adult Self-Report Inventories that are designed to obtain information from both patients and significant others. These inventories take approximately 15 to 20 minutes to complete. Items are grouped according to diagnostic categories (68).

Hopkins Symptom Checklist (SCL-90 Revised): The SCL-90 is used to evaluate a broad range of psychopathology. It consists of 90 items and usually can be completed in less than 30 minutes. The scoring system includes nine symptom scales (somatization, obsessive-compulsive behavior, interpersonal sensitivity, depression, anxiety, hostility, phobic anxiety, paranoid ideation, and psychoticism) and three global indexes. This scale has documented validity and has been used in many treatment studies of mood disorders and schizophrenia (69).

Beck Depression Inventory (BDI): The BDI is the most commonly used self-rating scale for depression. There are 21 items scored on a scale from 0 to 3 according to how the patient feels at the current time. The BDI has been found to correlate well with other ratings of depression, such as the Hamilton Depression Scale (HAM-D) used by psychiatrists to rate depression. The scale is sensitive to change and has been used in clinical drug trials (70).

Yale-Brown Obsessive Compulsive Scale (Y-BOCS): This is the most widely used scale for rating obsessive-compulsive symptoms. It includes a symptom checklist as well as a ten-item scale that is rated by clinicians. It has been shown to be a highly reliable instrument that is sensitive for measuring changes in the severity of obsessive-compulsive symptoms (71).

Quality of Life in Epilepsy (QOLIE): The recent development of self-report quality-of-life inventories for adult epileptic patients are 15- or 31-item measures that assess the impact of epilepsy on a variety of psychosocial issues, including a patient's self-esteem and relationships with others. Many physicians may find the abbreviated ten-item QOLIE measure to be the most efficient for use in the clinical setting. The QOLIE-10 assesses worries related to seizures, emotional well-being, energy/fatigue, cognitive function, medication effects, social function, and overall quality of life. The QOLIE-10 can be obtained free of charge by contacting the publisher (72).

Useful Self-Report Measures for Children and Adolescents with Epilepsy

CSI-4 (Child Symptom Inventories): The Child Symptom Inventories are screening instruments for the behavioral, affective, and cognitive symptoms of more than a dozen DSM-IV childhood disorders. There are Child Symptom Inventories for three different age groups: Early Childhood Inventory-4 (ages 3 to 5 years), Child Symptom Inventory-4 (ages 5 to 12 years), and Adolescent Symptom Inventory-4 (ages 12 to 18 years). There is a self-report measure for adolescent patients: Youth's Inventory-4 (ages 12 to 18 years) (73).

Child Behavior Checklist (CBCL): Developed by Thomas M. Achenbach, this scale evaluates pathologic behaviors and social competence in children ages 4 to 16 years. Forms are available for teachers, parents, and children. It is one of the most widely used scales for both clinical use and research (74).

Children's Depression Inventory (CDI): This is a 27-item self-report questionnaire that can be given to 7- to 17-year-olds. It is currently one of the most widely used instruments for monitoring depression in children. Each question includes three statements of increasing severity (75).

Multidimensional Anxiety Scale for Children (MASC): This is a scale for children and adolescents designed to assess symptoms of anxiety. The 39 items are scored on a scale from 0 to 3 as follows: 0 = never true about me; 1 = rarely true about me; 2 = sometimes true about me; 3 = often true about me (76,77).

Connors' Parent/Teacher Rating Scales: This scale identifies behavior problems through parent and teacher report. It is available in three versions: a 93-item version, a 48-item version, and a ten-item screening version. It is used in children ranging in age from 3 to 17 years (78).

Leyton Obsessional Inventory-Child Version (LOI-CV; Short Form): This questionnaire is a 20-item inventory with "yes/no" responses adapted from the adult version to assess obsessive-compulsive symptoms (79).

Quality-of-Life Scales for Children and Adolescents: (see description of the Adult QOLIE). The Pediatric Quality-of-Life Enjoyment and Satisfaction Questionnaire (PQ-LES-Q) is a 15-item measure that assesses the quality of life in children and adolescents. This scale focuses on the child's or adolescent's views about general health, well-being, and feelings about the medical condition. Response categories range from "very poor" to "very good." In addition, an adolescent version of the Adult Quality of Life in Epilepsy Inventory has recently been developed (80,81).

CONCLUSIONS

Psychopathology often is unrecognized by clinicians in patients with epilepsy, yet this type of comorbidity accounts for much of the poor quality of life of these patients. It is the responsibility of the clinician treating the seizure disorder to identify the psychosocial impact of epilepsy on his or her patients, as well as the presence of any psychiatric disorders or risk factors that would facilitate their occurrence. This type of assessment can be followed by a referral for a complete psychiatric evaluation. Enhanced appreciation of the multifactorial contributors to psychiatric disturbances, including effects of the underlying central nervous system disorder, relation to seizures, medication effects, and psychosocial influences, should heighten the awareness of clinicians to these problems. Strategic utilization of key questions and selected self-report measures can help alert the clinician to psychiatric distress and the need for further evaluation and treatment but should never be used as the sole diagnostic screening tool.

REFERENCES

1. Wiegartz P, Seidenberg M, Woodard A, et al. Co-morbid psychiatric disorder in chronic epilepsy: recognition and etiology of depression. *Neurology* 1999;53[Suppl 2]:S3–S8.
2. Sillanpaa M, Jalava M, Kaleva O, et al. Long-term prognosis of seizures with onset in childhood. *N Engl J Med* 1998;338:1715–1722.
3. Camfield C, Camfield P, Smith B, et al. Biologic factors as predictors of social outcome of epilepsy in intellectually normal children: a population-based study. *J Pediatr* 1993;122:869–873.
4. Mendez M, Cummings J, Benson D, et al. Depression in epilepsy. Significance and phenomenology. *Arch Neurol* 1986;43:766–770.
5. Indaco A, Carrieri P, Nappi C. Interictal depression in epilepsy. *Epilepsy Res* 1992;12:45–50.
6. Dongier S. Statistical study of clinical and electroencephalographic manifestation of 536 psychotic episodes occurring in 516 epileptics between clinical seizures. *Epilepsia* 1959/1960;1:117–142.
7. Septien L, Giroud M, Didi-Roy R. Depression and partial epilepsy: relevance of laterality of the epileptic focus. *Neurol Res* 1993;15:136–138.
8. Roy A. Some determinants of affective symptoms in epileptics. *Can J Psychiatry* 1979;24:554–556.
9. Stevens J. Interictal clinical manifestation of complex partial seizures. In: Penry J, Daly D, eds. Complex partial seizures and their treatment. *Adv Neurol* 1975; 11:85–112.
10. Altshuler L. Depression and epilepsy. In: Devinsky O, Theodore W, eds. *Epilepsy and behavior.* New York: Wiley-Liss, 1991:47.
11. Robertson, M. Epilepsy and mood. In: Trimble M, ed. *Epilepsy, behavior and cognitive function.* New York: John Wiley and Sons, 1988:145.
12. Robertson M. Depression in patients with epilepsy reconsidered. In: Pedley T, ed. *Recent advances in epilepsy, Volume 4.* Edinburgh: Churchill Livingstone, 1988:205.
13. Robertson M. Depression in patients with epilepsy: an overview. *Semin Neurol* 1991;11:182–189.
14. Robertson M. Depression in patients with epilepsy: an overview and clinical study. In: Trimble M, ed. *The psychopharmacology of epilepsy.* New York: John Wiley and Sons, 1985:65.
15. Robertson M. Ictal and interictal depression in patients with epilepsy. In: Trimble M, ed. *Aspects of epilepsy and psychiatry.* New York: John Wiley and Sons, 1986:213.
16. Robertson M. The organic contribution to depressive illness in patients with epilepsy. *J Epilepsy* 1989;2: 189–230.
17. Robertson M. Depression in epilepsy. In: Trimble M, ed. *Women and epilepsy.* New York: John Wiley and Sons, 1991:223.
18. Mendez M, Engebrit D, Doss R. The relationship of epileptic auras and psychological attributes. *J Neuropsychiatry Clin Neurosci* 1996;8:287–292.
19. Collaborative Group for Epidemiology of Epilepsy. Reactions to antiepileptic drugs: a multicenter survey of clinical practice. *Epilepsia* 1986;27:323–330.
20. McConnell H, Duncan D. Treatment of psychiatric comorbidity in epilepsy. In: McConnell H, Snyder P, eds. *Psychiatric comorbidity in epilepsy.* Washington, DC: American Psychiatric Press, 1998:245.
21. Robertson M, Trimble M, Townsend H, et al. The phenomenology of depression in epilepsy. *Epilepsia* 1987;28:364–372.
22. Robertson M. Carbamazepine and depression. *Int Clin Psychopharmacol* 1987;2:23–35.
23. Wyler A, Richey E, Hermann B. Comparison of scalp to subdural recordings for localizing epileptogenic foci. *J Epilepsy* 1989;2:91–96.
24. Brent D, Crumrine P, Varma R. Phenobarbital treatment and major depressive disorder in children with epilepsy. *Pediatrics* 1987;80:909–917.
25. Ferrari N, Barabas G, Matthews W. Psychological and behavioral disturbance among epileptic children treated with barbiturate anticonvulsants. *Am J Psychiatry* 1983; 140:112–113.
26. Smith D, Collins J. Behavioral effects of carbamazepine, phenobarbital, phenytoin and primidone. *Epilepsia* 1987;28:598.
27. Barabas G, Matthews W. Barbiturate anticonvulsants as a cause of severe depression. *Pediatrics* 1988;82:284–285.
28. Mackay A. Self-poisoning: a complication of epilepsy. *Br J Psychiatry* 1979;134:277–282.
29. Hawton K, Fagg J, Marsack P. Association between epilepsy and attempted suicide. *J Neurol Neurosurg Psychiatry* 1980;43:168–170.
30. Ring H, Reynolds E. Vigabatrin and behavior disturbance. *Lancet* 1990;335:970.

31. Ring H, Heller A, Farr I. Vigabatrin: rational treatment for chronic epilepsy. *J Neurol Neurosurg Psychiatry* 1990;53:1051–1055.

32. Ring H, Reynolds E. Vigabatrin. In: Pedley T, ed. *Recent Advances in epilepsy,* Volume 5. Edinburgh: Churchill Livingstone, 1992:177.

33. McConnell H, Duffy J, Cress K. Behavioral effects of felbamate. *J Neuropsychiatry Clin Neurosci* 1994;6: 323.

34. Ketter TA, Post RM, Theodore WH. Positive and negative psychiatric effects of antiepileptic drugs in patients with seizure disorders. *Neurology* 1999;53[Suppl 2]:S53–S67.

34. Chaplin J, Yepez R, Shorvon S. A quantitative approach to measuring the social effects of epilepsy. *Neuroepidemiology* 1990;9:151–158.

35. Dell J. Social dimension of epilepsy: stigma and response. In: Whitman S, Hermann B, eds. *Psychopathology in epilepsy:* social dimensions. New York: Oxford University Press, 1986.

36. Jacoby A. Felt versus enacted stigma: a concept revisited. *Soc Sci Med* 1994;38:269–274.

37. Scambler G. Sociological aspects of epilepsy. In: Hopkins A, ed. *Epilepsy.* New York: Demos, 1987.

38. DeVellis R, DeVellis B, Wallston B. Epilepsy and learned helplessness. *Basic Appl Soc Psychol* 1980;1: 241–253.

39. Hermann B, Whitman S. Psychosocial predictors of interictal depression. *J Epilepsy* 1989;2:231–237.

40. Dodrill C. Neuropsychology. In: Laidlaw J, Richens A, Chadwick D, eds. *A textbook of epilepsy,* 4th ed. London: Churchill Livingstone, 1993.

41. Craig C, Oxley J. Social aspects of epilepsy. In: Laidlaw J, Richens A, Oxley J, eds: *A textbook of epilepsy,* 3rd ed. London: Churchill Livingstone, 1988.

42. Goldstein J, Seidenberg M, Peterson R. Fear of seizures and behavioral functioning in adults with epilepsy. *J Epilepsy* 1990;3:101–106.

43. Mittan R. Fear of seizures. In: Whitman S, Hermann B, eds. *Psychopathology in epilepsy:* social dimensions. New York: Oxford University Press, 1986.

44. Roth D, Goode K, Williams V. Physical exercise, stressful life experience, and depression in adults with epilepsy. *Epilepsia* 1994;35:1248–1255.

45. Brown S, Reynolds E. Cognitive impairment in epileptic patients. In: Reynolds E, Trimble M, eds. *Epilepsy and psychiatry.* Edinburgh: Churchill Livingstone, 1981:147.

46. Sorensen A, Hansen H, Hogenhaven H. Ego functions in epilepsy. *Acta Psychiatr Scand* 1988;78:211–221.

47. Matthews C. The neuropsychology of epilepsy: an overview. *J Clin Neuropsychol* 1992;14:133–143.

48. Brown S, Reynolds E. Cognitive impairments in epileptic patients. In: Reynolds E, Trimble M, eds. *Epilepsy and psychiatry.* Edinburgh: Churchill Livingstone, 1981:147.

49. Ardila A, Montanez P, Bernal B. Partial psychic seizures and brain organization. *Int J Neurosci* 1986;30: 23–32.

50. Williams D. The structure of emotions reflected in epileptic experiences. Brain 1956;79:29–67.

51. Weil A. Depressive reactions associated with temporal lobe uncinate seizures. *J Nerv Ment Dis* 1955;121: 505–510.

52. Mulder D, Daly D. Psychiatric symptoms associated with lesions of the temporal lobe. *JAMA* 1952;150: 173–176.

53. Reynolds J. *Epilepsy:* its symptoms, treatment and relation to the chronic convulsive diseases. London: Churchill, 1861.

54. Weil A. Ictal emotions occurring in temporal lobe dysfunction. *Arch Neurol* 1959;1:87–97.

55. Perrine K, Congett S. Neurobehavioral problems in epilepsy. *Neurol Clin North Am* 1994;12:129–152.

56. Soto A, Kanner A, Hershkowitz L. Postictal psychiatric symptoms in patients with poorly controlled seizures: a prevalence study. *Epilepsia* 1997;38[Suppl 8]:155.

57. Betts T. Depression, anxiety, and epilepsy. In: Reynolds E, Trimble M, eds. *Epilepsy and psychiatry.* New York: Churchill Livingstone, 1981:60.

58. Mendez M, Doss R. Ictal and psychiatric aspects of suicide among epileptics. *Int J Psychiatry Med* 1992;22: 231–238.

59. Mendez M, Lanska D, Manon-Espaillet R. Causative factors for suicide attempts by overdose in epileptics. *Arch Neurol* 1989;46:1065–1068.

60. Hancock J, Bevilacqua A. Temporal lobe dysrhythmia and impulsive or suicidal behavior. *South Med J* 1971;64:1189–1193.

61. Anatassopoulos G, Kokkini D. Suicidal attempts in psychomotor epilepsy. *Behav Neuropsychol* 1969;1: 11–16.

62. Currie S, Heathfield K, Henson R. Clinical course and prognosis of temporal lobe epilepsy. A survey of 666 patients. *Brain* 1971;92:173–190.

63. Blumer D, Zielinski J. Pharmacologic treatment of psychiatric disorders associated with epilepsy. *J Epilepsy* 1988;1:135–150.

64. Rutter M, Graham P. The reliability and validity of the psychiatric assessment of the child: I. interview with the child. *Br J Psychiatry* 1968;114:563–579.

65. Rutter M, Graham P, Yule WA. *A neuropsychiatric study in childhood.* Philadelphia: JB Lippincott, 1970.

66. Marder SR. Psychiatric rating scales. In: Kaplan HI, Sadock BJ, eds. *The comprehensive textbook of psychiatry,* 6th ed., Volume 1. Baltimore: Williams & Wilkins, 1995:619–635.

67. Hathaway SR, McKinley JC. *The Minnesota Multiphasic Personality Inventory manual,* revised ed. New York: Psychological Corporation, 1989.

68. Gadow KD, Sprafkin J. *The symptom inventories:* an annotated bibliography. Stony Brook, NY: Checkmate Plus, 1998.

69. Derogatis LR, Cleary PA. Confirmation of the dimensional structure of the SCL-90: a study in construct validation. *J Clin Psychol* 1977;33:981–989.

70. Beck AT, Ward CH, Mendelson M, et al. An inventory for measuring depression. *Arch Gen Psychiatry* 1961;4:561–571.

71. Goodman WK, Price LH, Rasmussen SA, et al. The Yale-Brown Obsessive Compulsive Scale, I: development, use, and reliability. *Arch Gen Psychiatry* 1989;46:1006–1011.

72. Cramer JA, Perrine K, Devinsky O, et al. A brief questionnaire to screen for quality of life in epilepsy: the QOLIE-10. *Epilepsia* 1996;37:577–582.

73. Nolan EE, Volpe RJ, Gadow KD, et al. Development, gender and comorbidity differences in clinically referred children with ADHD. *J Emotion Behav Disord* 1999;7:11–20.

74. Achenbach TM, Edelbrock CS. *Child behavior checklist.* Burlington, VT: TM Achenbach, 1986.

75. Kovacs M. Children's Depression Inventory (CDI). *Psychopharmacol Bull* 1985;21:995–998.

76. March J. *Manual for the Multidimensional Anxiety Scale for Children (MASC).* Toronto, Ontario: Multi-Health Systems, 1998.

77. March JS, Parker JDA, Sullivan K, et al. The Multidimensional Anxiety Scale for Children (MASC): factor structure, reliability, and validity. *J Am Acad Child Adolesc Psychiatry* 1997;36:554–565.

78. Conners CK. *The Conners' Ratings Scales.* Austin, TX: Pro-Ed, 1985.

79. Berg C, Rapoport J, Flament M. The Leyton Obsessional Inventory-Child Version. *J Am Acad Child Psychiatry* 1986;25:84–91.

80. Cramer JA, Westbrook LE, Devinsky O, et al. Development of the quality of life in epilepsy inventory for adolescents: the QOLIE-AD-48. *Epilepsia* 1999;40:1114–1121.

81. Sabaz M, Cairns DR, Lawson JA, et al. Validation of a new quality of life measure for children with epilepsy. *Epilepsia* 2000;41:765–774.

4

Neuropsychological Evaluation of the Patient with Seizures

Christopher L. Grote, *Clifford A. Smith, and †Amity Ruth

Department of Psychology, Rush Presbyterian-Saint Luke's Medical Center, Chicago, Illinois 60612;
Department of Psychiatry, Weill Medical College of Cornell University, New York, New York 10021;
and †Department of Psychiatry, Cognitive Neurology and Alzheimer's Disease Clinic, Northwestern University Medical School, Chicago, Illinois 60611

Neuropsychological investigations of patients with epilepsy have led to some of the most important discoveries of brain–behavior relationships, which include the critical role of the hippocampal formations in memory, plasticity of speech and language, and hemispheric specialization of cognitive functioning (1).

The usual purpose for referring a patient with epilepsy for neuropsychological evaluation is to assist in diagnosis and to plan appropriate treatments for the individual patient. The goal of this chapter is to acquaint the health professional with the most common issues confronting a neuropsychologist when consulted in epilepsy cases. We review the types of typical referral questions, the means of assessment, and the possible implications of findings for each of the following types of patient with epilepsy: (i) the adult with epilepsy, including candidates for surgical treatment; (ii) the patient with suspected nonepileptic psychogenic paroxysmal events; and (iii) the child with epilepsy. Neuropsychologists also participate in the intracarotid sodium amytal "Wada" procedures to evaluate lateralization of speech and memory functions (2) and in clinical trials of experimental anticonvulsants (3), but these topics are beyond the scope of this chapter.

NEUROPSYCHOLOGICAL EVALUATION OF THE ADULT WITH EPILEPSY

The brain is electrophysiologically dysfunctional during a seizure, which, in turn, interferes with cognitive and psychological functions (4). Addionally, at least one study has suggested that subclinical epileptiform activity occurring during interictal periods may cause further cognitive and psychological disturbance (5). Not surprisingly, complaints of memory, attention, concentration, and language dysfunction are common in epileptic patients. These problems are thought, in turn, to contribute to the increased prevalence of psychosocial and psychiatric problems noted in these patients. Because of these various cognitive and psychological disruptions, neuropsychologists often are called upon to aid in clinical care and treatment planning.

Approximately 10% of patients with epilepsy become sufficiently medically intractable to be considered for surgical therapy (6). Recent decades have seen a marked increase in the number of patients with epilepsy undergoing surgery, most typically temporal lobe surgery, in an attempt to alleviate their seizures. An estimated 80% of patients undergoing anterior temporal lobectomy experience total or partial seizure remission (7). However, the benefits of improved seizure control must be weighed against the possibility of postoperative declines in cognition or behavior (8). The most commonly reported postoperative cognitive complication is a decline in the ability to learn and recall new material, particularly verbal stimuli such as stories or word lists (9). Nearly half of patients undergoing dominant temporal lobe resections experience clinically significant losses in verbal memory functioning (10).

Accordingly, neuropsychologists have come to play an important role in the preoperative and postoperative evaluations of epilepsy surgery candidates. The next section of this chapter reviews commonly used neuropsychological tests and how they can be used to provide valuable information regarding the localization and lateralization of epileptogenic foci. We also review the importance of establishing a baseline assessment of the patient's cognitive and psychological function, and how a neuropsychological evaluation can be used to help predict postoperative seizure and cognitive outcome (8).

Commonly Used Neuropsychological Tests

Not every epilepsy center utilizes the exact same battery of tests, but certain psychometric instruments tend to be used with some uniformity. These include measures of intelligence, language, memory, visuospatial, motor, attention and concentration, and executive functioning (Table 4.1). In addition to psychometric evaluation, the neuropsychologist's interview can help document psychosocial functioning and concerns.

Although tests of general intelligence are poor predictors of postsurgical seizure outcome, they are able to provide a frame of reference in which to evaluate broad cognitive domains. The Wechsler Adult Intelligence Scales (WAIS), including the current version (WAIS-III), are the most commonly used measures of general intelligence. These mea-

TABLE 4.1. *Commonly used assessment measures*

Intelligence
  Wechsler Adult Intelligence Scales (WAIS-R, WAIS-III)
  Stanford-Binet Scale
  Raven's Progressive Matrices
Achievement
  Wide Range Achievement Tests (WRAT-R, WRAT-III)
  Woodcock-Johnson Psychoeducational Battery-Revised: Tests of Achievement
  Wechsler Individual Achievement Tests
Attention/concentration
  Digit span
  Spatial span
  Stroop test
  Digit symbol
  Symbol search
Executive functions
  Wisconsin Card Sorting Test
  Trails B
  Category test
  Similarities
Language
  Boston Naming Test
  Controlled oral word association
  Animal naming
Memory
  Wechsler Memory Tests (WMS-R, WMS-III)
  California Verbal Learning Test
  Rey Auditory Verbal Learning Test
Visuospatial
  Block design
  Picture completion
  Picture arrangement
  Object assembly
Motor/sensory
  Dichotic listening test
  Grooved pegboard
  Finger tapping

sures are composed of a number of subtests designed to assess general knowledge, expressive vocabulary, verbal attention, abstraction, comprehension, and visuospatial construction and perception. These subtests provide an overall assessment of the individual's cognitive functioning (full-scale IQ), as well as verbal and performance IQ scores, and "index" scores that measure verbal and nonverbal ability, working memory, and processing speed. Assessment of learning and memory are essential, because these abilities often are affected by epilepsy. Although a number of instruments have been developed to measure these skills, perhaps the Wechsler Memory Scale (WMS) has been used with the greatest frequency. The third version (WMS-III) incorporates prose and paired learning subtests to assess learning and recall of auditorily presented material. Face recognition and character recall subtests are used to test memory for visually presented material. These measures are administered with an immediate and delayed recall format, which permits the neuropsychologist to assess learning and retention of this material. In addition, the WMS-III incorporates a task of visual attention (spatial span), a task of working memory (letter-number sequencing), and optional list learning and figure learning tasks. The WMS-III and WAIS-III were costandardized. This allows the clinician to report the frequency that particular memory-IQ discrepancies occurred in the standardization study.

In addition to these tasks, measures designed to assess cognitive flexibility and abstraction (e.g., Wisconsin Card Sorting Test), fine motor control (e.g., grooved pegboard), sensory function (e.g., dichotic listening), and working memory (e.g., paced auditory serial addition test) may be incorporated. Finally, a crucial component of the neuropsychological evaluation is the assessment of personality and psychosocial functioning. Based on the perceived risk for postoperative psychological deterioration, many centers consider the presence of psychosis, severe depression, personality disorders, or frequent pseudoseizures as contraindicative to surgery (11). However, as noted, when taking prevalence rates into consideration, the risk of developing postsurgical psychopathology is not beyond what would be expected in the population at large (12). Yet, even with this, a thorough presurgical psychological evaluation is necessary as the psychosocial stressors associated with seizures and surgery are significant (13). Of the objective measures available to the neuropsychologist, the Minnesota Multiphasic Personality Inventory (MMPI; and the current revision, MMPI-2) is the most commonly used measure of psychopathology. Both measures have been shown to validly assess the level of psychopathology in epileptic patients (14,15). The measure is designed to broadly assess an individual's level of psychological and personality adjustment.

Interpretation of Neuropsychological Test Scores, Including Their Ability to Lateralize/Localize Cerebral Dysfunction

It is relatively easy to administer and score neuropsychological tests. The challenge lies in interpretation. Although certain neurocognitive deficits have been associated with specific anatomic correlates, one must be cautious when drawing conclusions about structural dysfunction from neuropsychological test data. Test performance frequently varies across different measures and domains. When performance is variable, assumptions about particular cognitive deficits can be more difficult. Conclusions about impairment typically should not be based on a patient's poor performance on a single measure. Instead, inferences about cognitive impairments or localized/lateralized cerebral dysfunction should be based on the convergence of all data, including imaging results, individual and family history, other chronic health issues, medication effects, psychosocial factors, and personality and neuropsychological test scores.

Interpretation of neuropsychological profiles of patients with epilepsy often will involve cases of temporal lobe dysfunction. This is not surprising, as the site of epileptiform activity in the majority of patients with partial complex seizures is the hippocampus (16). Memory and learning disorders are common in epileptic patients regardless of epileptic focus (17). However, patients whose epileptic activity originates in the temporal lobe are especially likely to display pronounced memory difficulties (18), although the extent of memory deficits in these patients may vary, depending on the integrity of the hippocampi and their adjacent temporal structures (19).

It has been suggested that lateralization of cerebral dysfunction in patients with temporal lobe epilepsy preferentially influences the type of memory deficit. That is, left-sided foci produce deficits in verbal memory (20) and right-sided foci produce visual memory deficits

(21,22). However, lateralization of memory deficits is equivocal, and conflicting results have been reported. Some studies showed that patients with right-sided epileptic activity do not demonstrate greater impairment on nonverbal memory tests when compared to patients with a left hemisphere focus (23,24). It also was demonstrated that some patients with left-sided temporal lobe epilepsy show impairment for both verbal and nonverbal material (18).

Patients with temporal lobe epilepsy often have cognitive deficits other than those related to learning and memory abilities. This is because of the numerous afferent and efferent pathways connecting brain areas. A myriad of neurocognitive functions associated with these pathways can be disrupted during epileptic activity. A recent review (25) reported that epilepsy surgery candidates, most of whom have seizures of temporal lobe origin, have a mean IQ of only 90, which places them at about the 25th percentile in comparison to the general population. This general diminution of ability may be due to the fact that the temporal lobes are connected to the frontal lobe system by a series of neural pathways that are responsible for memory, language, and attentional abilities (26,27). Deficits in attention, working memory, and other abilities typically associated with the frontal lobe system have been noted in patients with temporal lobe epilepsy, as well as in the general epileptic population (28).

Patients with seizures of frontal lobe origin may be at risk of a variety of cognitive deficits, because this region has involvement in motor, sensory, perception, attention, personality, language, and memory functions (29). One study found that patients with frontal lobe epilepsy performed more poorly than patients with temporal lobe epilepsy on tests of attention, psychomotor speed, memory span, and concept formation (30). Other investigators were unable to find a consistent pattern of neuropsychological test results in subjects with frontal lobe epilepsy (31). Conversely, poor performance on purported measures of executive function do not necessarily imply dysfunction of the frontal lobes. For example, a review of the Wisconsin Card Sorting Test found weak evidence that frontal lobe patients performed more poorly on this test in comparison to nonfrontal patients. It was concluded that there was insufficient justification to use only the Wisconsin Card Sorting Test as a clinical or research marker of frontal lobe dysfunction. This highlights the value of administering several measures in each cognitive domain to ensure reliable and accurate data.

Individuals with epileptic foci in the occipital or parietal regions are especially likely to show deficits in visuospatial, perceptual, and constructional abilities (32). One study investigating surgical outcome in occipitotemporal epileptic patients found general and diffuse neurocognitive deficits (33).

In summary, neuropsychological testing can be useful in confirming lateralized or localized cerebral dysfunction. These inferences are most likely to be accurate when there is concordant evidence from more than one neuropsychological test that an area of cognition is impaired. A test score alone is not a diagnosis, nor does it necessarily imply dysfunction of a particular area of the brain. Accurate inferences about the significance of a psychological test score will increase when it is interpreted in the context of other test scores, educational and occupational factors, the patient's history, and findings from medical and imaging studies.

Baseline Neuropsychological Assessment of the Adult Epilepsy Surgery Candidate

As the diagnosis of epilepsy typically is based on a patient's clinical history and electroencephalogram, neuropsychology plays a limited role in the actual diagnosis. However, the neuropsychological evaluation provides supplementary information by identifying cognitive patterns that are consistent with patterns of cognitive dysfunction associated with either focal or diffuse epileptic activity (34). Repeat neuropsychological evaluations in the preoperative phase can provide some indication of the effects of epilepsy or medications on the patient's cognition and behavior across time, as there is some evidence that ongoing seizures (35), increased seizure frequency (36), and extended use of antiepileptic medication (37) all may have deleterious effects on cognition. Preoperative evaluations also are necessary if the effect of surgery on cognition or behavior is to be examined.

Use of Preoperative Neuropsychological Data to Predict Postoperative Seizure and Cognitive Outcome

The ideal outcome of epilepsy surgery is the complete amelioration of all seizures. Because surgery does not eliminate all seizures in all cases, selection criteria have been developed to identify patients most likely to benefit from this intervention. Demographic variables, such as age of seizure onset, seizure history, electrographic characteristics, and radiologic variables, have been shown to be predictive of postoperative status (38). There is some evidence that preoperative neuropsychological data help predict seizure outcome (39).

Seizure control following epilepsy surgery must be weighed carefully against possible postoperative cognitive decrements, particularly verbal memory (9,40,41). The most useful predictor of postsurgical cognitive decline is the presurgical functional capacity of the tissue to be resected (42). Baseline neuropsychological testing by itself is a relatively weak predictor of postoperative outcome. However, when combined with magnetic resonance imaging data about the size and health of the hippocampal region, in addition to the side of surgery, this information is useful in predicting which patients are at risk of significant postoperative decline in verbal memory. Chelune (40) demonstrated that patients who did not have evidence of magnetic resonance imaging atrophy of the left hippocampus and who had average or better baseline verbal memory were at the highest risk of postoperative verbal memory decline. All eleven such patients in that study who later underwent left temporal lobectomy demonstrated a significant decline in verbal memory on follow-up testing.

Left temporal lobectomies also put a patient at risk of postoperative decrements in confrontation naming ability (43). Examination of 217 patients who underwent left (speech-dominant) anterior temporal lobectomy showed impairment on the Boston Naming Test before surgery, but postoperative naming test scores were then about 8% lower than those obtained preoperatively. This investigation did not examine if preoperative naming scores were predictive of changes in naming ability following surgery, but it did note that greater naming declines were seen among patients with later age of seizure onset.

The influence of test-retest practice effects must be considered when the postoperative scores of patients with epilepsy are examined. Increases of 3.3, 7.9, and 5.8 points on verbal, performance, and full-scale IQ scores, respectively, were reported for a nonsurgical group of 105 patients with epilepsy after a 5-year test-retest interval (44). Investigators have used measures of "reliable change" to address this issue (45). This allows the clinician to determine if postoperative changes in cognitive test scores exceed, or do not approach, what would be expected from the effect of having twice taken a battery of tests within 6 to 12 months' time.

Preoperative and postoperative patients with epilepsy also have psychological difficulties, including depression, phobic, panic, and psychosexual disorders (12,46). Although improved seizure control following surgery may improve psychological functioning, postoperative onset of psychosis and anxiety disorders have been reported, particularly for those with both chronic presurgical psychotic disturbances and ongoing postsurgical seizures (47). However, there is some evidence that the surgical treatment of epilepsy does not increase the overall risk of psychopathology among medically intractable patients (12).

NEUROPSYCHOLOGICAL EVALUATION OF THE PATIENT WITH NONEPILEPTIC SEIZURES

It has been estimated that 20% of patients at epilepsy referral centers have nonepileptic seizures (48). As recently reviewed by Krumholz (49), the term "nonepileptic seizures" (NES) can refer to a wide variety of disorders that are mistaken for epilepsy but which are due to causes other than abnormal electrical discharges in the brain. These disorders include both physiologic and psychological disorders. Examples of the former include cardiac, vascular, and movement disorders (50). If physiologic disturbances, including electroencephalographic abnormalities, can be ruled out in a patient presenting with nonepileptic events, then a psychological or psychiatric diagnosis may be in order. Reference to the *Diagnostic and Statistical Manual of Mental Disorders, Fourth Edition* (DSM-IV) (51) indicates that the most appropriate diagnosis typically will be conversion disorder with seizure or convulsion. However, Bowman (52) recently pointed out that some cases of apparent NES are classified more appropriately as panic disorder or posttraumatic stress disorder. The possibility of comorbid psychiatric diagnoses, including affective, anxiety, dissociative, somatoform, and personality disorders, also needs to be considered. The consulting neuropsychologist can assist in the evaluation of the patient with NES by contributing to the assessment of the psychiatric diagnosis. Of course, this type of consultation might instead be performed by a psychiatrist or by other physicians familiar with the DSM-IV. What other or possibly unique skills might a neuropsychologist bring to this evaluation? In the rest of this section, we will review the following aspects of patients with nonepileptic events: (i) neuropsychological characteristics; (ii) assessment and diagnosis of insufficient effort; (iii) personality assessment; and (iv) assessment of psychosocial stressors.

Neuropsychological Characteristics of the Patient with Nonepileptic Events

Patients with NES and no concomitant epilepsy often have impaired neuropsychological performance. Wilkus and Dodrill (53) administered a battery of neuropsychological

tests to 25 such patients. They reported that 51.6% of resulting scores fell outside of normal limits, but they found no important differences in neuropsychological functioning between matched subgroups of psychogenic seizure patients and their epileptic counterparts. A more recent study (54) compared intelligence and neuropsychological test scores of 44 patients with "pure pseudoseizures" against those of nine patients with "mixed pseudoseizures and epilepsy." The two groups did not differ significantly on measures of intellectual ability, as they achieved IQ scores of 95.4 and 92.7, respectively. Similarly, the two groups did not differ significantly on the Halstead Impairment Index (HII), a global measure of cognitive impairment (55). Overall, this study found that 63% of all subjects obtained an HII in the "impaired" range. A third neuropsychological study (56) similarly found patients with either epilepsy or NES to be impaired compared to normal controls. Again, no differences were noted between the epilepsy and NES groups, but further analysis of the data suggested that the impairment in the NES group was related to emotional factors, as indicated by analyses of the MMPI-2. Other investigators, however, found that 20% to 30% of patients with nonepileptic events have a significant history of head trauma (57,58). Although the etiology of nonepileptic events is beyond the scope of this review, it remains a fact that NES patients are at risk of poor performance on neuropsychological tests. Therefore, detailed assessment of neuropsychological and emotional functioning may be useful in describing the cognitive strengths and weaknesses of these patients and in estimating the etiology of any deficits.

Assessment and Diagnosis of Insufficient Effort

Patients with nonepileptic events typically are not thought to be deliberately or intentionally producing their seizures. Instead, NES often is thought to be a manifestation of a patient's inability to cope with stressful events or memories. Previous studies pointed out that NES can be secondary to conflicts with family members (59) or precipitated by traumatic life events (60), including sexual abuse (61). In such cases, it appears that the patient has been unaware of the relationship between these nonepileptic events, stressors, and inadequate coping ability. However, patients with nonepileptic events are no different from any other sample of patients in that a subset may be intentionally producing or exaggerating neurologic deficits for primary or secondary gain. One investigation specifically examined the effect of insufficient effort on cognitive tests in a sample of patients with nonepileptic events. Binder et al. (56) administered a battery of tests, including a measure of effort or malingering, the Portland Digit Recognition Test, to samples of patients with either epileptic or nonepileptic events. They found that patients with nonepileptic events scored significantly lower on the Portland test compared to patients with epilepsy. However, only one of the 30 patients with nonepileptic events performed below chance performance, and another two patients scored below the cutoffs for motivational impairment. Binder et al. (56) concluded that it was likely that a small subset of some NES patients were frank malingerers.

Investigations of the prevalence and assessment of malingering among various patient populations have flourished in recent years. Recent reviews of this literature describe the many methods and tests by which effort can be measured and analyzed (62,63). An important conclusion derived from these reviews is that insufficient effort is not uncommon. More importantly, studies indicate that the clinician must formally, deliberately, and prospectively assess the effort or motivation of patients. However, it appears that many clinicians, while acknowledging that formal assessment is required to measure patient characteristics such as intelligence or naming ability, have instead assumed that they can rely on their subjective impressions to judge patients' effort and motivation. Research has demonstrated the need for a formal assessment of malingering (64). Forced-choice recognition tests, such as the Victoria Symptom Validity Test (65) and

the Test of Memory Malingering (66), are effective means of measuring effort and take only about 20 minutes to administer.

At least two DSM-IV diagnoses need to be considered when a patient is suspected of not making his or her best effort on tests or otherwise appears to be feigning or exaggerating deficits. Malingering (V65.2) is the *intentional* production of false or grossly exaggerated physical or psychological symptoms, motivated by external incentives, such as obtaining financial compensation. Similarly, the diagnosis of factitious disorders (300.16 or 300.19) is characterized by physical or psychological symptoms that are *intentionally* produced or feigned in order to assume the sick role (51). It is important to note that both of these diagnoses depend on the clinician's judgment that the patient is intentionally presenting himself or herself in a way the patient knows is not true. Accordingly, the clinician first must attempt to determine if the patient's poor performance or production of nonphysiologically derived symptoms is or is not intentional. As reviewed earlier, tests of effort may be useful in determining this, but situations may still arise in which the clinician cannot make a meaningful inference about the patient's intentions. Second, even when sufficient evidence exists to suggest that a patient is intentionally producing or exaggerating symptoms, the clinician needs to consider that the patient's motivation may be something other than financial compensation. Consideration of diagnoses other than malingering, such as one of the somatoform disorders, will not only increase diagnostic accuracy, but also potentially avoid incorrectly "labeling" the patient with a diagnosis that may be unfairly pejorative.

Personality Assessment of the Nonepileptic Seizure Patient

Several investigations have used MMPI or MMPI-2 to examine psychopathology among patients with nonepileptic events and to determine if these profiles could be differentiated from those produced by patients with epilepsy. An early investigation noted that mean MMPI scores did not differ significantly between pseudoseizure and epileptic patients (67). MMPI abnormalities of pseudoseizure patients were diverse and seldom characteristic of hysteria. In contrast, Wilkus and Dodrill (68) found MMPI differences when the type of NES was examined. As measured by the MMPI, patients whose psychogenic seizures had limited motor activity or major emotional components proved to have more emotional disturbance than patients with partial epileptic seizures. In contrast, patients whose psychogenic seizures had major motor features or lacked emotional expression did not differ significantly in emotional adjustment from individuals with generalized convulsive seizures. Another study found results that at least partially support the conclusions of Wilkus and Dodrill (68). Brown et al. (69) found that nonepileptic patients showed an increased sensitivity to somatic concerns, and "conversion V" profiles were more frequent among these patients. That pseudoseizure patients might attribute their symptoms to physical rather than psychological explanations was found in a more recent study (70), which used both the Quality of Life in Epilepsy Inventory-89 and the MMPI-2 Depression subscale.

A previous review of the MMPI as a diagnostic tool led to the conclusion that the MMPI is useful for differentiating patients with epilepsy from patients with NES but should be used cautiously because of a high error rate (71). The same conclusion appears to hold several years after this review was written; the MMPI-2 is useful in allowing the clinician to generate hypotheses about a patient's personality and behavior, but there are no profiles that are specific to one group of patients. It is well known, for example, that because patients with well-diagnosed epilepsy are at risk of various types of psychopathology, significant elevations on the MMPI-2 may result (72).

Assessment of Psychosocial Stressors and Patient Concerns

Psychologists sometimes have additional training or skill in eliciting relevant information in clinical interviews. It is commonly believed that patients with NES sometimes possess "secrets" or otherwise have "unconscious" conflicts that are not immediately apparent. Some have advocated the use of intravenous barbiturates, such as sodium amytal, to access these events or memories (73). It is not known if medication-assisted interviews result in the revelation of greater amounts of relevant information than nonmedicated interviews. Regardless, careful assessment of the patient's life and concerns remains critical. As this typically cannot be accomplished with psychometric instruments, the clinician must possess a sufficient amount of skill and tact to effectively investigate the sensitive issues that may underlie the apparent etiology and maintenance of nonepileptic events. Assuming the patient authorizes the clinician to do so, interviews with the patient's relatives, friends, or co-workers may contribute further to diagnosis and treatment.

Whereas a clinical interview is a standard component of any neuropsychological evaluation, additional time and effort should be expended in the case of a patient who may have NES, with particular attention given to the patient's interpersonal relationships. For instance, does the patient perceive family members as caring and supportive? How does the patient resolve conflicts or disagreements with friends and relatives? How did the patient's parents interact? How did they resolve conflicts? As already mentioned, many patients with NES have been sexually abused. Therefore, it is important to inquire about any experiences of this type or any other type of physical or emotional abuse. Although some patients may deny a history of sexual abuse, they may have current concerns about sexuality, including issues of orientation, lack of desire, unavailability of partners, or even sexual practices or impulses that result in conflicted feelings.

Summary of the Neuropsychological Evaluation of the Nonepileptic Seizure Patient

This review demonstrated that NES patients often perform poorly on neuropsychological tests, but that the etiology of this dysfunction is either unknown or is debatable. Although it seems that only a minority of NES patients intentionally produce or exaggerate psychological or neurologic deficits, formal and prospective assessment of effort or motivation should be a routine component of evaluation. NES patients outscore patients with epilepsy on some measures of psychopathology, particularly those related to somatic preoccupation, but currently there are no "cut scores" or configural rules that will allow the clinician to reliably differentiate a patient with NES from a patient with epilepsy. Finally, the neuropsychologist should remember that the most important psychiatrically or psychologically related information to NES patients may not come from the electroencephalogram or psychometric instruments, but from the patient in clinical interview.

Neuropsychological evaluation cannot reliably differentiate patients with epileptic seizures from those with NES. Instead, data from testing and interview can assist the patient and others by providing information about the patient's cognitive abilities, personality, effort and motivation, and current concerns. In our experience with NES patients, we often find evidence of disturbance of mood, self-esteem, and relationships with others. In such cases, it is sometimes emphasized to the patient that, to some degree, it does not matter whether their seizures are ultimately judged to be in response to an electrographic disturbance. Instead, we suggest to many of these patients that they are in need of, and can benefit from, psychotherapy regardless of the origin of their seizure disorder.

NEUROPSYCHOLOGICAL EVALUATION OF THE CHILD WITH EPILEPSY

Epilepsy is not an uncommon disorder in childhood; 2% to 4% of all children in Europe and the United States experience at least one convulsion associated with a febrile illness before the age of 5 years (74). Between 0.5% and 1% of all children have recurrent seizures, and most of them have an excellent prognosis (75). However, the etiologies and associated prognoses of epilepsy in childhood are diverse. Some diagnoses, particularly those arising during infancy or early childhood (e.g., West's syndrome, Lennox-Gastaut syndrome), typically are associated with significant and permanent impairments in cognitive function (76). Additionally, some epilepsies of childhood are associated with other medical problems, including autism and cerebral palsy, so that seizures represent only a portion of the child's difficulties. In contrast, some of the seizure disorders that develop in late childhood or adolescence have benign or favorable courses and may disappear after a few years without any obvious sequela. Examples of these disorders include nonlesional disorders such as the idiopathic generalized and benign partial epilepsies, which include typical absence epilepsy (77). In some epileptic disorders of childhood, such as the acquired epileptic aphasia of childhood or Landau-Kleffner syndrome, the role of neuropsychological testing has been pivotal in demonstrating response to surgical therapies with novel techniques, such as multiple subpial transection (78).

Relatively little has been published regarding neuropsychological evaluation or postoperative outcome in the child undergoing epilepsy surgery. The largest and most recent study on this topic was from the Bozeman Epilepsy Consortium, which studied preoperative and postoperative intellectual functioning in a sample of 82 children who underwent temporal lobectomy for treatment of medication-resistant seizures (79). For the entire sample, there were no significant declines in IQ scores following surgery. There were some differences in outcome, depending on the side of surgery, and it was noted that risk factors for significant decline of intellectual ability included older patient age at the time of surgery and the presence of a structural lesion other than mesial temporal lobe sclerosis on magnetic resonance imaging. Memory functioning was not examined in this study. A study of nine children who underwent temporal lobectomy failed to find marked changes in cognitive functioning after surgery, although decreases in delayed verbal memory were evident (80). Some postoperative improvements in quality of life were noted. A third investigation also found some postoperative improvement of quality of life among 33 children who underwent epilepsy surgery, but cognitive outcome was not discussed (81).

Normal preoperative intelligence is predictive of good postoperative seizure outcome following an anterotemporal lobectomy (82), but in another study there was not a significant relationship between these variables (83). Investigation of 25 children who underwent corpus callosotomy found significant postoperative improvements in social adjustment (84). Neuropsychological outcome generally paralleled that of neurologic outcome, with younger patients making greater postoperative gains than older patients.

Children with epilepsy are at risk of poor performance in school. One investigation found that children with epilepsy demonstrate significant levels of academic underachievement in four academic areas: word recognition, reading comprehension, spelling, and arithmetic (85). Seidenberg et al. (86) identified a number of factors that put children with epilepsy at risk of learning disorders, including seizure correlates, neuropsychological correlates, medication effects, and psychosocial correlates. The importance of each risk factor varies from case to case, and neuropsychological testing can serve as an important source of information about the impact of these risk factors and aids in establishing effective rehabilitation and individual educational plans (87). However, one study stressed that many studies of children and adults with epilepsy were conducted at teaching centers that serve disadvantaged populations to a disproportionate degree (88). Results from investigations at such centers may inappropriately link cognitive deficits and academic difficulties to epilepsy, rather than to low socioeconomic levels and cultural differences. Mitchell et al. (88) noted no relationship between severity or duration of seizure disorder or total exposure to anticonvulsant drugs and academic underachievement, but instead found that the academic underachievement noted in their sample of children with epilepsy was more properly ascribed to cultural/socioeconomic factors.

Neuropsychological evaluation of children with epilepsy typically will assess functioning of the same abilities already detailed in Table 4.1. A description of available tests for assessment of children's cognitive and academic abilities was provided in a recent review (89). As with adults, particular attention should be given to measures of memory and attention, given that these abilities are especially likely to be impacted by epilepsy or its treatment. However, it is not clear whether particular memory deficits have the same lateralizing value. One study noted that 12 children with left temporal lobe epilepsy demonstrated significantly lower performance than controls on verbal memory tests, whereas another 12 children with right temporal lobe epilepsy scored lower than controls on visual memory tests (90). However, the left and right temporal lobe patients did not evidence material-specific memory deficits. Similar results were found in another study (91). A third study also noted that children with epilepsy were at risk of memory difficulties, as evidenced by their significantly lower scores than children diagnosed with substance abuse or psychiatric disorders (92). Although laterality and material-specific differences are not consistently found in children with temporal lobe epilepsy (89), documentation of memory and other cognitive skills using contemporary instruments such as the Wide Range Assessment of Memory and Learning (93) or the Children's Memory Scale (94) is an important component in the assessment of children with epilepsy.

SUMMARY AND CONCLUSIONS

This review demonstrated the substantial progress made in the last decade regarding how neuropsychological evaluations can be used in the diagnosis and care of patients with epilepsy and illustrated those issues that neuropsychologists should be aware of when conducting such evaluations. Just as there is no "typical" patient with epilepsy, the referral questions and goals for the neuropsychologist may vary from case to case. Awareness of the issues and problems associated with different types of patients with epilepsy will enhance the utility of data provided by the neuropsychologist.

REFERENCES

1. Novelly R. The debt of neuropsychology to the epilepsies. *Am Psychologist* 1992;47:1126–1129.
2. Hamberger MJ, Walczak TJ. The Wada test: a critical review. In: Pedley T, Meldrum B, eds. *Recent advances in epilepsy.* New York: Churchill Livingstone, 1995:57–78.
3. French JA, Wallace SJ. Clinical trials of antiepileptic drugs in adults and children. In: Engel J, Pedley TA, eds. *Epilepsy:* a comprehensive textbook. Philadelphia: Lippincott-Raven Publishers, 1997:1435–1444.
4. Aarts JH, Binnie CD, Smith AM, et al. Selective cognitive impairment during focal and generalized epileptiform EEG activity. *Brain* 1984;107:293–308.
5. Aldenkamp AP, Overweg JG, Gutter T, et al. Effect of epilepsy, seizures and epileptiform EEG discharges on cognitive function. *Acta Neurol Scand* 1996;93:253–259.
6. Hauser WA. The natural history of seizures. In: Wyllie E, ed. *The treatment of epilepsy:* principles and practices. Philadelphia: Lea & Febiger 1993:165–170.
7. Spencer DD. The surgical treatment of temporal lobe epilepsy. In: Kotagal P, Luders HO, eds. *The epilepsies:* etiologies and prevention. New York: Academic Press, 1999:259–263.
8. Chelune GJ. The role of neuropsychological assessment in the presurgical evaluation of the epilepsy candidate. In: Wyler AR, Hermann BP, eds. *The surgical management of epilepsy.* Stoneham, MA: Butterworth-Heinemann, 1994:78–89.
9. Bell BD, Davies KG. Anterior temporal lobectomy, hippocampal sclerosis, and memory: recent neuropsychological findings. *Neuropsychol Rev* 1998;8:25–41.
10. Chelune GJ, Naugle RI, Luders H, et al. Individual change after epilepsy surgery: practice effects and base rate information. *Neuropsychol* 1993;1:41–52.
11. Fenwick PC, Blumer DP, Caplan R, et al. Presurgical psychiatric assessment. In: Engel J, ed. *Surgical treatment of the epilepsies.* New York: Raven Press, 1993: 279–290.
12. Koch-Weser M, Garron DC, Gilley DW, et al. Prevalence of psychologic disorders after surgical treatment of seizures. *Arch Neurol* 1988;45:1308–1311.
13. Wheelock I, Peterson C, Buchtel HA. Presurgery expectations, postsurgery satisfaction, and psychosocial adjustment after epilepsy surgery. *Epilepsia* 1998;39: 487–494.
14. Derry PA, Harnadek MC, McLachlan RS, et al. Influence of seizure content on interpreting psychopathology on the MMPI-2 in patients with epilepsy. *J Clin Exp Neuropsychol* 1996;19:396–404.
15. Dikmen S, Hermann BP, Wilensky AJ, et al. Validity of the Minnesota Multiphasic Personality Inventory (MMPI) to psychopathology in patients with epilepsy. *J Nerv Ment Dis* 1983;171:114–122.
16. Halgren E, Stapleton J, Domalski P. Memory dysfunc-

17. tion in epilepsy patients as a derangement of normal physiology. *Adv Neurol* 1991;55:385–410.
17. Bornstein RA, Pakalnis A, Drake ME, et al. Effects of seizure type and waveform abnormality on memory and attention. *Arch Neurol* 1988;45:884–887.
18. Mirsky AF, Primac DW, Marson D. A comparison of the psychological test performance on patients with focal and nonfocal epilepsy. *Exp Neurol* 1960;2:75–89.
19. Hermann BP, Seidenberg M, Schoenfeld J, et al. Neuropsychological characteristics of the syndrome of mesial temporal lobe epilepsy. *Arch Neurol* 1997;54:369–376.
20. Hermann BP, Wyler AR, Richey ET, et al. Memory function and verbal learning ability in patients with complex partial seizures of temporal lobe origin. *Epilepsia* 1987;28:547–554.
21. Glosser G, Deutsch GK, Cole LC, et al. Differential lateralization of memory discrimination and response bias in temporal lobe epilepsy patients. *J Int Neuropsychol Soc* 1998;4:502–511.
22. Loring DW, Lee GP, Meador KJ. Material-specific learning in patients with partial complex seizures of temporal lobe origin: convergent validation of memory constructs. *J Epilepsy* 1988;1:53–59.
23. Barr WB, Consortium BE. The right temporal lobe and memory: a critical reexamination. *J Int Neuropsychol Soc* 1995;1:139–149.
24. Giovagnoli AR, Avanzini G. Learning and memory impairment in patients with temporal lobe epilepsy: relation to the presence, type, and location of brain lesion. *Epilepsia* 1999;40:904–911.
25. Perrine K, Kiolbasa T. Cognitive deficits in epilepsy and contribution to psychopathology. *Neurology* 1999; 53[Suppl 2]:S39–S48.
26. Fuster JM. *The prefrontal cortex: anatomy, physiology, and neuropsychology of the frontal lobe,* 3rd ed. New York: Lippincott-Raven Publishers, 1997.
27. Mesulam MM. Large-scale neurocognitive networks and distributed processing for attention, language, and memory. *Ann Neurol* 1990;28:597–613.
28. Fowler PC, Richards HC, Boll TJ, et al. A factor model of an extended Halstead Battery and its relationship to an EEG lateralization index for epileptic adults. *Arch Clin Neuropsychol* 1987;2:81–92.
29. Heilman KM, Valenstein E, eds. *Clinical neuropsychology,* 3rd ed. New York: Oxford University Press, 1993.
30. Helmstaedter C, Kemper B, Elger CE. Neuropsychological aspects of frontal lobe epilepsy. *Neuropsychologia* 1996;34:399–406.
31. Upton D, Thompson PJ. General neuropsychological characteristics of frontal lobe epilepsy. *Epilepsy Res* 1996;23:169–177.
32. Lezak M. *Neuropsychological assessment,* 3rd ed. New York: Oxford University Press, 1995.
33. Aykut-Bingol C, Spencer SS. Nontumoral occipitotemporal epilepsy: localizing findings and surgical outcome. *Ann Neurol* 1999;46:894–900.
34. Loring DW. Neuropsychological evaluation in epilepsy surgery. *Epilepsia* 1997;38:S18–S23.
35. Holmes MD, Dodrill CB, Wilkus RJ, et al. Is partial epilepsy progressive? Ten-year follow-up of EEG and neuropsychological changes in adults with partial seizures. *Epilepsia* 1998;39:1189–1193.
36. Dikmen S, Matthews CG. Effect of major motor seizure frequency upon cognitive intellectual function in adults. *Epilepsia* 1977;18:21–30.

37. Bennett TL. Cognitive effects of epilepsy and anticonvulsant medications. In: Bennett TL, ed. *The neuropsychology of epilepsy.* New York: Plenum Press, 1992:73–95.

38. Dodrill CB, Wilkus RJ, Ojemann GA, et al. Multidisciplinary prediction of seizure relief from cortical resection surgery. *Ann Neurol* 1986;20:2–12.

39. Sawrie SM, Martin RC, Gilliam FG, et al. Contribution of neuropsychological data to the prediction of temporal lobe epilepsy surgery outcome. *Epilepsia* 1998;39:319–325.

40. Chelune GJ, Najm I. Risk factors associated with post-surgery decrements in memory. In: Luders HO, Comair W, eds. *Epilepsy surgery,* 2nd ed. Philadelphia: Lippincott Williams & Wilkins, (*in press*).

41. Olivier A. Risk and benefit in the surgery of epilepsy: complications and positive results on seizure tendency and intellectual function. *Acta Neurol Scand* 1988;78:114–121.

42. Chelune GJ. Hippocampal adequacy versus functional reserve: predicting memory functions following temporal lobectomy. *Arch Clin Neuropsychol* 1995;10:413–432.

43. Hermann BP, Chelune GJ, Loring DW, et al. Visual confrontation naming following left anterior temporal lobectomy: a comparison of surgical approaches. *Neuropsychology* 1999;13:3–9.

44. Seidenberg M, O'Leary DS, Giordani B, et al. Test-retest IQ changes of epilepsy patients: assessing the influence of practice effects. *J Clin Exp Neuropsychol* 1981;3:237–255.

45. Sawrie SM, Chelune GJ, Naugle RI, et al. Empirical methods for assessing clinically meaningful change following epilepsy surgery. *J Int Neuropsychol Soc* 1996;2:556–564.

46. Bear DM, Fedio P. Quantitative analysis of interictal behavior in temporal lobe epilepsy. *Arch Neurol* 1977;34:454–467.

47. Krahn LE, Rummans TA, Peterson GC. Psychiatric implications of surgical treatment of epilepsy. *Mayo Clin Proc* 1996;71:1201–1204.

48. Gumnit RJ. Psychogenic seizures. In: Wyllie E, ed. *The treatment of epilepsy: principles and practice.* Philadelphia: Lea & Febiger, 1993:692–695.

49. Krumholz A. Nonepileptic seizures: diagnosis and management. *Neurology* 1999;53[Suppl 2]:S76–S83.

50. Porter RJ. Epileptic and non-epileptic seizures. In: Rowan AJ, Gates JR, eds. *Non-epileptic seizures.* Boston: Butterworth-Heinemann, 1993:9–20.

51. American Psychiatric Association. *Diagnostic and statistical manual of mental disorders,* 4th ed. Washington, DC: American Psychiatric Press, 1994.

52. Bowman ES. Nonepileptic seizures: psychiatric framework, treatment and outcome. *Neurology* 1999;53[Suppl 2]:S84–S88.

53. Wilkus RJ, Dodrill CB, Thompson PM. Intensive EEG monitoring and psychological studies of patients with pseudoepileptic seizures. *Epilepsia* 1984;25:100–107.

54. Kalogjera-Sackellares D, Sackellares JC. Intellectual and neuropsychological features of patients with psychogenic pseudoseizures. *Psychiatry Res* 1999;86:73–84.

55. Jarvis PE, Barth JT. *The Halstead-Reitan Test Battery: an interpretive guide.* Odessa, FL: Psychological Assessment Resources, 1984.

56. Binder LM, Kindermann SS, Heaton RK, et al. Neuropsychological impairment in patients with nonepileptic seizures. *Arch Clin Neuropsychol* 1998;6:513–522.

57. Barry E, Krumholz A, Bergey C, et al. Nonepileptic posttraumatic seizures. *Epilepsia* 1998;39;427–431.

58. Westbrook LE, Devinsky O, Geocadin R. Nonepileptic seizures after head injury. *Epilepsia* 1998;39;978–982.

59. Griffith JL, Polles A, Griffith MA. Pseudoseizures, families and unspeakable dilemmas. *Psychosomatics* 1998;39:144–153.

60. Bowman ES, Markland ON. The contribution of life events to pseudoseizure occurrence in adults. *Bull Menninger Clin* 1999;63:70–88.

61. Slavney PR. Pseudoseizures, sexual abuse and hermeneutic reasoning. *Compr Psychiatry* 1994;35:471–477.

62. Nies K, Sweet J. Neuropsychological assessment and malingering: a critical review of past and present strategies. *Arch Clin Neuropsychol* 1994;9:501–522.

63. Sweet J. Malingering: differential diagnosis. In: Sweet J, ed. *Forensic neuropsychology.* Lisse: Swets and Zeitlinger, 255–285.

64. Trueblood W, Binder L. Psychologists' accuracy in identifying neuropsychological test protocols of clinical malingerers. *Arch Clin Neuropsychol* 1997;12:13–27.

65. Slick D, Hopp G, Strauss E, et al. Victoria Symptom Validity Test: efficiency for detecting feigned memory impairment and relationship to neuropsychological tests and MMPI-2 validity scales. *J Clin Exp Neuropsychol* 1996;18:911–922.

66. Tombaugh T. The Test of Memory Malingering (TOMM): normative data from cognitively intact and cognitively impaired individuals. *Psychol Assess* 1997;9:260–268.

67. Vanderzant CW, Giordani B, Berent S, et al. Personality of patients with pseudoseizures. *Neurology* 1986;36:664–668.

68. Wilkus RJ, Dodrill CB. Factors affecting the outcome of MMPI and neuropsychological assessment of psychogenic and epileptic seizure patients. *Epilepsia* 1989;30:339–347.

69. Brown MC, Levin BE, Ramsay RE, et al. Characteristics of patients with nonepileptic seizures. *J Epilepsy* 1991;4:225–229.

70. Breier JI, Fuchs KL, Brookshire BL, et al. Quality of life perception in patients with intractable epilepsy or pseudoseizures. *Arch Neurol* 1998;55:660–665.

71. Dodrill CB, Wilkus RJ, Batzel LW. The MMPI as a diagnostic tool in non-epileptic seizures. In: Rowan AJ, Gates JR, eds. *Non-epileptic seizures.* Boston: Butterworth-Heinemann, 1993:211–219.

72. Blumer D, Montouris G, Hermann B. Psychiatric morbidity in seizure patients on a neurodiagnostic monitoring unit. *J Neuropsychiatry Clin Neurosci* 1995;7:445–456.

73. Fackler SM, Anfinson TJ, Rand JA. Serial sodium amytal interviews in the clinical setting. *Psychosomatics* 1997;38:558–564.

74. Hauser WA. The prevalence and incidence of convulsive disorders in children. *Epilepsia* 1994;35[Suppl 2]:S1–S6.

75. Hauser WA. Epidemiology of epilepsy in children. *Neurosurg Clin North Am* 1995;6:419–429.

76. Aicardi J. Overview: syndromes of infancy and early childhood. In: Engel J, Pedley TA, eds. *Epilepsy: A comprehensive textbook.* Philadelphia: Lippincott-Raven Publishers, 1997.

77. Aicardi J. Overview: syndromes of late childhood and adolescence. In: Engel J, Pedley TA, eds. *Epilepsy: a*

comprehensive textbook. Philadelphia: Lippincott-Raven Publishers, 1997:2303–2305.

78. Grote CL, Van Slyke P, Hoeppner J. Language outcome following multiple subpial transection for Landau-Kleffner syndrome. *Brain* 1999;122:561–566.

79. Westerveld M, Sass K, Chelune G. Temporal lobectomy in children: cognitive outcome. *J Neurosurg* 92:24–30.

80. Williams J, Griebel ML, Sharp GB, et al. Cognition and behavior after temporal lobectomy in pediatric patients with intractable epilepsy. *Pediatr Neurol* 1998;19: 189–194.

81. Maehara T, Shimizu H, Oda M, et al. Surgical treatment of children with medically intractable epilepsy outcome of various surgical procedures. *Neurol Med Chir* 1996;36:305–309.

82. Gashlan M, Loy-English I, Ventureyra EC, et al. Predictors of seizure outcome following cortical resection in pediatric and adolescent patients with medically refractory epilepsy. *Childs Nerv Syst* 1999;15:45–50.

83. Goldstein R, Harvey A, Duchowny M, et al. Preoperative clinical, EEG, and imaging findings do not predict seizure outcome following temporal lobectomy in childhood. *J Child Neurol* 1996;11:445–450.

84. Lassonde M, Sauerwein C. Neuropsychological outcome of corpus callosotomy in children and adolescents. *J Neurol Sci* 1997;41:67–73.

85. Seidenberg M, Beck N, Geisser M, et al. Neuropsychological correlates of academic achievement of children with epilepsy. *J Epilpesy* 1987;1:23–30.

86. Seidenberg M, Beck N, Geisser M, et al. Academic achievement of children with epilpesy. *Epilepsia* 1986;27:753–759.

87. Seidenberg M, Clemmons DC. Maximizing school functioning and the school-to-work transition. In: Engel J, Pedley TA, eds. *Epilepsy: a comprehensive textbook.* Philadelphia: Lippincott-Raven Publishers, 1997: 2203–2209.

88. Mitchell WG, Chavez JM, Lee H, et al. Academic underachievement in children with epilepsy. *J Child Neurol* 1991;6:65–72.

89. Oxbury S. Neuropsychological evaluation-children. In: Engel J, Pedley TA, eds. *Epilepsy: a comprehensive textbook.* Philadelphia: Lippincott-Raven Publishers, 1997:989–999.

90. Cohen M. Auditory/verbal and visual/spatial memory in children with complex partial epilepsy of temporal lobe origin. *Brain Cogn* 1992;20:315–326.

91. Adams CB, Beardsworth E, Oxbury SM. Temporal lobectomy in 44 children: outcome and neuropsychological follow-up. *J Epilepsy* 1990;[Suppl]:151–168.

92. Williams J, Haut JS. Differential performances on the WRAML in children and adolescents diagnosed with epilepsy, head injury and substance abuse. *Dev Neuropsychol* 1995;11:201–213.

93. Sheslow D, Adams W. *Wide Range Assessment of Memory and Learning.* Wilmington, DE: Jastak, 1990.

94. Cohen M. *Children's Memory Scale: manual.* San Antonio, TX: The Psychological Corporation, 1997.

5

Affective Disorders in Epilepsy

John J. Barry, Anna Lembke, and *Nga Huynh

*Departments of Psychiatry and *Pharmacy, Stanford University Medical Center, Stanford, California 94305*

...we are not ourselves
When nature, being oppress'd, commands the mind
To suffer with the body.
King Lear, Shakespeare (1)

Hippocrates is credited with demystifying epilepsy, the "sacred disease," and proposing a direct relationship with "melancholia" (2). Aretaeus (ca. 100 AD) gave a description of epileptics as "languid and spiritless" (2), whereas Morel, like Kreaplin, focused on the "periodic alternation of depression and excitement" (3). Reynolds (1861) noted the interactions between seizures and mood states, and observed depression before an epileptic event and as a frequent hallmark of interictal complaints (4). The history of van Gogh, who possibly was epileptic from his consumption of the proconvulsant drink absinthe, illustrates many of the psychiatric features seen with epilepsy (5).

The link between epilepsy and dysfunctional mood states has been observed for more than 2,000 years, along with a concept of "epileptic deterioration" (6). Lennox (1944), however, challenged that view and attributed the higher prevalence of depression to sample selection, i.e., the fact that hospitalized epileptics may be more likely to display psychopathology, whereas nonhospitalized patients tend to function normally (7). This view was disputed by his colleague Gibbs (1948, 1952), who reported an incidence of psychiatric symptoms in 40% of epileptics with psychomotor epilepsy (6). The controversy between Lennox and Gibbs harbingers some of the conflicting views that have been reported on the psychopathology associated with epilepsy.

This chapter will attempt to critically review these issues and provide a practical approach to the evaluation and treatment of patients with epilepsy and an affective disorder.

AFFECTIVE DISORDERS IN NONEPILEPTIC AND EPILEPTIC PATIENTS

The fourth edition of the *Diagnostic and Statistical Manual of Mental Disorders* (DSM-IV) organizes the affective phenomena into "mood episodes" and "mood disorders" (8). Mood episodes include major depressive, manic, mixed, and hypomanic episodes. Mood disorders consist of depressive and bipolar disorders; mood disorders due to a general medical condition; and substance-induced mood disorders. Depressive disorders are classified into three types: major depressive disorder (MDD), dysthymic disorder, and depressive disorder not otherwise specified. The latter includes all forms of depression that do not meet any of the DSM-IV criteria for the suggested categories. In addition to the clinical semiology, depressive disorders can be classified into three types of disorders according to their temporal relation to the epileptic seizure: (i) interictal, (ii) periictal, and (iii) ictal. Interictal disorders refer to those identified when the patient is not having seizures. Periictal disorders include the cluster of affective symptoms that precede and/or follow the seizure by hours to days. Ictal disorders represent the seizure presenting with affective symptoms.

Interictal depressive disorders are the most frequently recognized psychiatric disorders in patients with epilepsy (9). However, the symptoms of depression frequently are not defined in the literature, and the scales used may not characterize the disorder. Using research diagnostic criteria (RDC), Robertson et al. (10) showed that patients with epilepsy can meet standard measures for what is described as an MDD (Table 5.1).

This observation was confirmed by Mendez et al. (11), who used DSM-III standards to compare epileptic and nonepileptic depressed inpatients. Although the epileptic patients met criteria for MDD, they presented atypical features with more paranoia and psychotic symptoms that were periictal and resolved with anticonvulsant adjustment. In addition, they tended to show a more chronic dysthymic course between MDD episodes. At these times, the epileptic patients demonstrated more irritability and emotionality (11). Psychotic features may be part of an MDD, representing a more severe form of the disorder (MDD with psychotic features). Psychosis also may occur separately from, but coexist with, affective complaints, leading to and presenting as a schizoaffective disorder.

TABLE 5.1. *Characteristics of a major depressive disorder[a]*

Depressed mood most of the day
Markedly diminished interest or pleasure in
    activities/people (anhedonia)
Weight loss or gain of more than 5% in 1 mo,
    decreased appetite
Insomnia/hypersomnia
Psychomotor agitation/retardation
Fatigue
Feelings of worthlessness or guilt
Diminished ability to concentrate, indecisiveness
Recurrent thoughts of death or suicide

[a]Five or more of the symptoms need to be present during at least a 2-week period.
From American Psychiatric Association. *Diagnostic and statistical manual of mental disorders*, 4th ed. Washington, DC: American Psychiatric Press, 1994, with permission.

Many studies found that depressive symptoms secondary to medical illnesses from causes other than epilepsy not only meet standard criteria for MDD (12), but also respond to medication in a similar fashion. This has also been our experience in patients with interictal depression, with the caveat that there may be unique mood changes surrounding the periictal period.

Dysthymic disorder is differentiated from MDD by a more chronic, persistent course, with less severe manifestation of the same symptoms (Table 5.2).

Blumer (13) emphasized the pleomorphic pattern of mood complaints in epilepsy consistent with the observations of Kreaplin, Gastaut, and others, and coined the term "interictal dysphoric disorder" (IDD). The symptoms have an intermittent course and can be categorized into depressive-somatoform and affective symptoms. The depressive- somatoform symptoms include (i) depressive mood, (ii) anergia, (iii) pain, and (iv) insomnia. The affective symptoms include (i) irritability, (ii) euphoric mood, (iii) fear, and (iv) anxiety. Unfortunately, there are no direct comparisons in the literature evaluating depression in epileptic patients using standard diagnostic techniques with those yielding a diagnosis of IDD. It is possible that a spectrum exists with a chronic dysthymic state characterized by the features of the IDD that may intermittently exacerbate and at that time meet criteria for MDD. This pattern may be similar to "double depression" seen in nonepileptic patients (8). Longitudinal studies are needed to clarify these issues.

Bipolar disorder is a cyclical disease characterized by the occurrence of manic and major depressive episodes. It is a chronic disease. Manic episodes last a week or longer and include symptoms of agitation, insomnia, hypersexuality, grandiosity, and occasionally psychosis (8,14). Florid depression may follow. When the severity of manic symptoms is milder, the bipolar disorder falls under the classification of a bipolar II disorder. Additional subtypes of bipolar disorder have been observed with more frequent cycling (more

TABLE 5.2. *Dysthymic disorder*

A. Depressed mood for most of the day, for more days than not, as indicated by either subjective account or observation by others, for at least 2 yr.[a]
B. Presence, while depressed, of two (or more) of the following:
    1. Poor appetite or overeating
    2. Insomnia or hypersomnia
    3. Low energy or fatigue
    4. Low self-esteem
    5. Poor concentration or difficulty making decisions
    6. Feelings of hopelessness
C. During the 2-yr period (1 yr for children or adolescents) of the disturbance, the person has never been without the symptoms in criteria A and B for more than 2 mo at a time.
D. No major depressive episode has been present during the first 2-yr of the disturbance (1 yr for children and adolescents), i.e., the disturbance is not better accounted for by chronic major depressive disorder, or major depressive disorder, in partial remission.[b]
E. The disturbance does not occur exclusively during the course of a chronic psychotic disorder, such as schizophrenia or delusional disorder.
F. The symptoms are not due to the direct physiologic effects of a substance (e.g., a drug of abuse, a medication) or a general medical condition (e.g., hypothyroidism).
G. The symptoms cause clinically significant distress or impairment in social, occupational, or other important areas of functioning.

[a]In children and adolescents, mood can be irritable and duration must be at least 1 yr.
[b]There may have been a previous major depressive episode provided there was a full remission (no significant signs or symptoms for 2 mo) before development of the dysthymic disorder. In addition, after the initial 2 yr (1 yr in children and adolescents) of dysthymic disorder, there may be superimposed episodes of major depressive disorder, in which case both diagnoses may be given when the criteria are met for a major depressive episode.
From American Psychiatric Association. *Diagnostic and statistical manual of mental disorders*, 4th ed. Washington, DC: American Psychiatric Press, 1994, with permission.

than four episodes a year), the so-called rapid cyclers. This type of mood variability can take place on a daily basis, and these patients are described as suffering from "ultrarapid" cycling (15). Patients with combined symptoms of mania/depression have been described as experiencing "mixed states" (15).

When evaluating a patient with epilepsy and symptoms of depression, we need to keep in mind the following two major issues. The first is to avoid the frequently quoted misconception that depression from a "good cause" is understandable and does not require treatment. This is a major fallacy and can lead to needless morbidity and potential mortality. The second results from the difficulty in determining the extent of depression in patients suffering from side effects, such as weight gain, lethargy, and poor concentration, caused by antiepileptic drugs (AEDs). The presence of anhedonia is an excellent marker for the presence of depression and often is impervious to physical complaints secondary to drugs or underlying illness. It is also a barometer of the intensity of the depression in the medically ill (12). The patient who is noted to display little interest in his or her surroundings or significant others needs to be assessed for depression and treated accordingly.

This is especially important because the depression seen in patients with epilepsy also has been associated with a significantly higher suicide rate than expected in the general population. This was noted by Barraclough (16), who reviewed eleven studies showing the overall rate in epileptic patients to be five times higher than in the general population. It was 25 times expected in those patients with complex partial seizures (CPS) of temporal lobe origin. Mendez et al. investigated this occurrence in two studies. The first study looked at causative factors in completed suicide in epileptic patients and found more psychotic symptoms in these patients (N = 4) (17). In a follow-up investigation, they reviewed the cases of 22 epileptic patients who had attempted suicide. They concluded that there was a relationship between interictal pathology such as borderline personality disorder and psychosis and none related directly to the periictal phenomenon (18). Of note, 54% of these patients were taking phenobarbital or primidone, a medication metabolized to phenobarbital.

Ictal and Periictal Affective Symptoms

The approach to depression or manic symptoms in patients with epilepsy must be evaluated in the context of their temporal relation to the ictal event. In 1828, Burrows wrote that "the epileptic attack may be preceded by a furious paroxysm, or merely by elevated ideas, by great depression...or the reverse" (3). In the 1860s, Falret crystallized these concepts by noting that psychiatric symptoms could be associated with the ictal event or the interval between attacks (3). Patients and their families frequently will note mood changes that herald the onset of an epileptic event. Blanchet and Frommer (19) evaluated this phenomenon in a study involving 27 patients over the course of 56 days. Thirteen patients experienced at least one seizure during this period. Mood ratings declined 3 days before the event and, most significantly, 24 hours before it. A return to baseline took place over the next 3 days, but most rapidly 1 day postictally. Interestingly, one patient noted the reverse, i.e., experienced elation instead of depression. More negative life events also were described prodromally (19).

Several reports examined the phenomena of manic and depression symptoms presenting as an ictal event. Williams (20) evaluated 2,000 epileptics "living normal lives." Of 100 patients who experienced ictal emotions, 65 noted ictal fear and 21 experienced a depression of varying severity (20). In eight patients, ictal depression persisted in the postictal period, lasting up to 3 days. Five patients developed suicidal ideation, with one suicide completion. Taylor and Lochery (21) evaluated simple partial seizures (auras) presenting as psychiatric symptoms in 88 patients and confirmed the frequency of fear, but not the complaints of depression. Ictal laughter (gelastic) and crying (dacrystic) also have been documented, with the former being more frequent than the latter (>100 cases reported in the literature) (22) and both phenomena characteristically presenting in association with complex partial seizures. These events usually take place independent of the patients' surroundings and are nonprovoked and inappropriate (22).

Periictal mania is unusual, but isolated case reports exist. Williams (20) found nine patients who experienced "pleasure" periictally, three of whom noted "elation." Barczak (23) reported three cases of manic symptoms postictally, all following a flurry of seizure activity. This was followed by four other letter-to-the-editor case reports with similar descriptions (24–27). All instances followed increased seizure activity, with a "normal" period and then, hours later, the appearance of manic-type symptoms. A similar pattern is seen in patients experiencing postictal psychotic events (28). All of these case reports found seizure activity to be localized to the right temporal lobe. A detailed discussion of postictal symptoms of depression can be found in Chapter 11.

PREVALENCE

Many reviews have noted an increased incidence of affective disorders in patients with epilepsy. When reviewing this literature, it is imperative to be aware of several factors. Of utmost importance is the sample population being evaluated, i.e., is it representative of the entire population of epileptic patients? Second, what types of seizure disorders were identified in the patients of the group being studied? For example, are they all patients with a temporal lobe focus, and is there a comparison or control group? Finally, what types of measures of depression are being used? Are they a self-report or interview technique, and can these measures be compared? Also, are there descriptions of the severity, symptom pattern, and longevity of the depression?

It is important to note that the assessment techniques described in the following sections, except for the Bear-Fedio Inventory, have been designed for the general population. As stated earlier, the affective disorder complaints of patients with epilepsy are unique, with fluctuating courses (13); therefore, any contemporary measure of depression might present an erroneous picture.

The actual incidence and prevalence of interictal depression in epilepsy remain uncertain, despite the numerous research studies addressing this issue. Comparing the results of one study to another is complicated by the diversity in methodologies and sample populations across studies. The ambiguity inherent in the diagnosis of epileptic subtypes is superimposed on the variability and ambiguity of depression measurement scales. Although the relevant literature is difficult to consolidate, the preponderance of evidence seems to favor a few basic conclusions. First, the incidence of depression in epilepsy is higher than in a matched population of healthy controls (range 11% to around 62%). Second, within a cohort of individuals with both epilepsy and depression, no specific subtype of epilepsy shows a higher incidence of depression than any other subtype, but a left-sided seizure focus may be important. Whether the incidence of depression in epilepsy is clearly elevated above those with other chronic illnesses, both neurologic and nonneurologic, has yet to be established (see below).

The diversity in methodologies in this body of work makes coherent synthesis of the data difficult. Assessment scales for depression range from self-reporting questionnaires (11,29–32), to objective measures of current but not past mood and anxiety states (32), to the use of the Clinical Interview Schedule (CIS) and/or DSM/RDC criteria, which incorporate both historical data and current mood states (10,32,33). Some investigators use "cutoff" scores to group depressed and nondepressed subjects. Others use the results of assessment scales as though they represent continued variables and compare mean scores, often with considerable variance, that might skew the data. The lack of uniformity in the assessment of depression across studies is complicated further by the wide spectrum of epilepsy subtypes. Whereas many investigators use single electroencephalographic (EEG) measurements to detect seizure focus, others rely on 24-hour EEG telemetry (30). Perhaps the biggest challenge to interpretation of the literature relates to the vast differences in sample populations. Most studies cull subjects from subspecialty neurology and epilepsy clinics, which in and of itself represents a skewed population. The variety of sample populations ranges from the community (34), to inpatient neurology units, female only (33), to psychiatric inpatient units (11), to medically intractable epileptic patients scheduled for surgery (3,35). Meaningful comparison of results across studies is not trivial given these vastly diverse sample populations.

According to the 1981 National Institute of Mental Health (NIMH) Epidemiological Catchment Area study, using DSM-III criteria the rate of depression in the general population was determined to be 4.9% for MDD, with a 3.3% incidence of dysthymia (lifetime prevalence). The National Comorbidity Study was completed in 1996 and showed a greater lifetime frequency of 17% for MDD (36). The rate of depression in patients with epilepsy reported in the literature ranges from a low of 11% with a current depression to around 62% with a lifetime-to-date depressive disorder (9,35). To clarify these findings, we have looked only at controlled studies that compare epilepsy to well-defined comparison populations (Table 5.3).

At least four controlled studies found that depression in patients with epilepsy is significantly increased as compared to healthy controls (29,37–39). In contrast, Fiordelli et al. (40), in a large, well-designed study, reported no increased risk of depression in patients with epilepsy as compared to a population of matched controls undergoing minor outpatient surgery. One might validly argue that the control population studied by Fiordelli et al. was not adequately screened for major illnesses and so does not represent a healthy control.

When patients with epilepsy are compared with patients who suffer from other neurologic diseases, including traumatic brain injury, neuromuscular diseases, and multiple sclerosis, several controlled studies suggest that there is no difference in the rates of depression (39,41–43) between these groups. For the most part, both groups seem to be at increased risk of depression compared to healthy controls. We know of only three controlled studies suggesting that epileptics have a higher rate of depression than patients with nonepileptic neurologic diseases (9,31,44).

TABLE 5.3. *Various studies on the prevalence of depressive disorders in epilepsy*

	Comparative studies finding significantly increased depression in (A)	Comparative studies finding no significantly increased depression in (A)
Epilepsy (A) vs. healthy controls (B)	Bear and Fedio (1977), Trimble and Perez (1980), Master et al. (1984), Dodrill and Batzel (1986)	Fiordelli et al. (40)
Epilepsy (A) vs. other neurologic disorders (B)	Bear and Fedio (1977), Mendez (1993) (44), Kogeorgos et al. (1982)	Klove and Doehring (1962), Matthews and Klove (1968), Standage and Fenton (1975), Mungas (1982), Dodrill and Batzel (1986)
Epilepsy (A) vs. other nonneurologic nonpsychiatric disorders (B)	Mendez et al. (1986), Dodrill and Batzel (1986)	Klove and Doehring (1962), Matthews and Klove (1968) (1969), Standage and Fenton (1975), Guerrant et al. (1962), Warren and Weiss (1969)
Epilepsy (A) vs. psychiatric disorders (B)		Klove and Doehring (1962), Warren and Weiss (1969), Perez and Trimble (1980), Mungas (1982), Master et al. (1984)
Temporal lobe epilepsy (A) vs. other types of epilepsy (B)	Shukla et al. (1979), Mendez et al. (1986), Perini and Mendius (1984), Altshuler et al. (1990)	Small et al. (1962), Guerrant et al. (1962), Matthews and Klove (1968), Standage and Fenton (1975), Kogeorgos et al. (1982), Master et al. (1984), Robertson et al. (1987), Mendez (1993) (44)
Left-sided seizure focus (A) vs. other foci (B)	Bear and Fedio (1977), Nielsen and Kristenson (1981), Perini and Mendius (1984), Brandt et al. (1985), Robertson et al. (1987), Altshuler et al. (1990), Mendez et al. (1986), Broomfield (1990) (55), Mendez (1993) (44), Victoroff et al. (1994) (35)	Mignone et al. (1970), Master et al. (1984), Hermann and Wyler (1989), Mendez et al. (1989), Robertson et al. (1987), Hermann et al. (1991) (30)
Frontal lobe hypometabolism (A) vs. no frontal lobe hypometabolism (B)	Broomfield et al. (1992) (55), Victoroff et al. (1994) (35)	

From Ring HA, Trimble MR. Depression in epilepsy. In: Starkstein SE, Robertson RG, eds. *Depression in neurologic disease.* Baltimore: Johns Hopkins University Press, 1993:63–83, and Altshuler L. Depression and epilepsy. In: Devinsky O, Theodore WH, eds. *Epilepsy and behavior.* New York: Wiley-Liss, 1991:47–65 unless specified by ( ), with permission.

Numerous studies compared depression in patients with epilepsy to depression in individuals with chronic illnesses that are not of neurologic origin. In support of psychosocial burden as a major risk factor for depression, most studies found equal rates of depression in these two groups (Table 5.3). There are few reports showing an increased incidence of depression in patients with epilepsy as compared with other chronic illnesses (11,39). Mendez et al. (11) compared 175 outpatient epileptics with 70 nonepileptic controls attending a vocational center for disabled people. They reported depression in 55% of the epilepsy group and 30%

of the control group. However, the study was based on a self-report questionnaire, which was returned by only 35% of the epilepsy group and 38% of the controls. Dodrill and Batzel (39) reviewed the literature and separated out neurologic and nonneurologic illness control groups for comparison. Interestingly, they found increased rates of depression in epileptics as compared with those having nonneurologic disorders, but equal rates of depression in epilepsy and neurologic disorders (39). In summary, depression occurs more commonly in the epilepsy population as compared to healthy populations, but whether there is something integral to the biology of epilepsy that predisposes to depression, or whether psychosocial factors play the dominant role, continues to elude investigation.

Prevalence of Manic Disorders

Mania and disinhibition have been reported in patients with orbitofrontal and basotemporal cortical lesions of the right hemisphere (45, 46). Manic symptoms in epilepsy frequently have been quoted as being rare (47,23). Epileptic patients presenting with psychotic symptoms often are described in the literature as schizophrenic rather than having an affective disorder (48). With newer views on the varied presentation of mania outlined earlier, underrecognition may have resulted in the past.

Wolf (49) reported nine cases of mania in his literature review and added six others, most related to the periictal state or improved seizure control. Robertson reported 42 cases in his literature search (22), and there have been many case reports noting this association (23–27), often periictal and frequently with an epileptic focus in the nondominant hemisphere. Lyketsos et al. (48) performed a retrospective review of epileptic patients seen at the psychiatric consult service over a 3-year period. They found that 25 patients were diagnosed with temporal lobe epilepsy (TLE) and five (20%) met DSM-III criteria for bipolar disorder. Even though a control group was provided, this study suffers from the same deficiency as many others because of the sample selection process, i.e., symptomatic inpatients were selected for review. Despite this caveat, this study used standardized diagnostic methodology and illustrates the point that manic illness in patients with TLE may be more frequent than expected in the general population, i.e., 1.5% (15).

RISK FACTORS

A handful of studies looked specifically at populations that meet criteria for both epilepsy and depression, in an effort to find specific risk factors within epilepsy that might contribute to depression. The risk factors can be grouped into three major categories: (i) neuro-

biologic factors, which include those factors associated with the neurophysiologic and neurochemical changes associated with the epileptic seizure disorder itself; (ii) psychosocial risks; and (iii) iatrogenic factors.

Neurobiologic Factors

Seizure-Related Factors

The evidence favors no association between depression and epilepsy with respect to seizure type, frequency, seizure duration, and age at onset (10,31,50–52). Much enthusiasm has focused on TLE as a possible risk factor for depression, because it topographically subsumes the limbic system that is intimately involved in affect and mood regulation. Bear and Fedio (29) distilled their epilepsy population into those with TLE and found an increased risk of depression in TLE when compared to nonepileptic neurologic diseases. However, more studies than not show no difference between TLE and other types of epilepsy (Table 5.3). It may be that the increased rate of psychiatric disorders seen in patients with TLE simply represents the increased frequency of TLE in contrast to other seizure types (53). In addition, TLE with secondary generalization often is miscategorized, which is a significant confounding variable (9).

Laterality of the seizure focus has been evaluated as a risk factor for depression in epilepsy. Using 24-hour EEG monitoring on a female subject with TLE and agitated depression, Hurwitz et al. (54) described left-sided EEG discharges with depressed affect and right-sided discharges with laughter and seductive behavior. It has been postulated that the dominant hemisphere is responsible for positive emotional states, with the nondominant hemisphere displaying the opposite effect. Seizure activity in one hemisphere might "release" the contralateral hemisphere (53). Another theory postulates that nondominant hemispheric activity may result in denial and neglect of negative emotions (53). Several controlled studies comparing seizure foci and rates of depression found increased rates of depression with left-sided foci, independent of seizure type, whereas other well-done studies found no correlation (Table 5.3). The most likely explanation argues for complex factors.

Some recent work suggests that clarifying the phenomenology of depression and epilepsy may have less to do with the risk factors just mentioned and more to do with finding a possible link between epilepsy and frontal lobe dysfunction and hypometabolism. Positron emission tomography (PET) in particular, but also single photon emission computed tomography (SPECT) in psychiatric patients with depression, showed decreased frontal hypometabolism, especially in the left prefrontal cortex (36).

Similarly, epileptic patients have been studied using these modalities. Both PET and SPECT have been utilized for localization of a seizure focus prior to anterior temporal lobectomy (ATL). Bromfield et al. (55) evaluated 23 patients with complex partial seizures and at least mild depressive features (Beck Depression Inventory >11) and those without symptoms compared to normal controls. Results of this study showed that patients with a left temporal lobe focus were associated with more depressive features and with bilateral inferior frontal hypometabolism. Of note are similar findings in Parkinson's patients with depression, which perhaps explains the uniformity in rates of depression between the two patient populations (36).

Victoroff et al. (35) looked at 53 medically intractable epileptic patients scheduled for surgery and used standardized measures to assess for lifetime history of depression as well as current mood states (DSM-III-R, Structured Clinical Interview for Diagnosis-P, Hamilton Depression Rating Scale). They then used EEG telemetry and ^{18}F PET scans to assess seizure laterality and frontal lobe hypometabolism. They found that left ictal onset was associated with greater frequency of depression: 79% versus 50% (nonsignificant). No correlation was found between current mood state and hypometabolism, but, interestingly, a history of depression was significantly correlated with left frontal lobe hypometabolism.

Along these same lines, Hermann et al. (30) used the Wisconsin Card Sorting Test as a cognitive measure of frontal lobe function. They found that, although there was no correlation with mood and laterality, a left-sided seizure focus was significantly correlated with degree of frontal lobe dysfunction and dysphoria. In contrast, a right-sided focus was nonsignificantly inversely related to frontal lobe dysfunction and dysphoria. These two studies, along with that of Bromfield et al. (55), suggest that the etiologic underpinnings of depression in epilepsy may be related to associated frontal lobe hypometabolism, analogous to that seen in patients with idiopathic depression. Certain types of seizures may induce frontal lobe dysfunction and hypometabolism directly, or they may ignite a kindling phenomenon that leads to subsequent depression when other risk factors for depression are present. Thus, the interplay between factors is complex.

Another possible etiologic factor concerns the observation of "paradoxical" or "forced" normalization. This phenomenon was first described in 1953 by Landolt, who was astonished to find that behavioral disturbance seemed to be associated with improvements on the patient's EEG. The behavioral changes originally were noted to be in the form of psychotic symptoms and hence were referred to as "alternative psychosis" (56). It should be noted that several of these patients were taking ethosuximide, which may have been responsible for the behavioral disturbances (57). Wolf (56) reported four cases presenting as affective disorders: two depressive and two manic. The pathogenesis of this phenomenon has focused on the interplay of dopamine (DA), glutamate, and γ-aminobutyric acid (GABA). Although more frequently associated with ethosuximide, other AEDs have been implicated, often in patients with temporal lobe, localization-related epilepsies (57). Forced normalization has been reviewed by Krishnamoorthy and Trimble (57) and Trimble et al. (58). This concept is a hotly debated issue. Clinically, affective symptoms directly related to the cessation of seizure activity is not seen frequently (also debated).

ATL for intractable TLE is highly effective in a select sample of patients, with up to 80% of patients being seizure-free and with less than 5% morbidity and mortality (59). However, a significant number of patients may develop postoperative psychosis, depression, and anxiety (60). Jensen and Larsen (61) noted that depressive symptoms usually occur acutely, with six of their patients (n = 72) committing suicide in the first postoperative month. Bruton (62) reviewed 249 ATL patients and noted that only one was depressed preoperatively (0.4%). After surgery, depression was found in 24 (10%) patients, with six committing suicide. This contrasts with several other studies that noted high frequencies of depression in patients being evaluated for ATL (63,64). One review noted a particular association with a right temporal lobe focus (64).

Neurochemical Risk Factors Associated with Depression in Epileptics

In the 1960s, Schildkraut et al. introduced the concept of biogenic amine depletion as a cause of depression (36). The major neurotransmitters that have been implicated are norepinephrine (NE), serotonin (5-hydroxytryptamine [5-HT]), and finally DA. Others that are important in epilepsy and possibly depression are GABA and changes in the neuroendocrine system and neuropeptides. Epilepsy may precipitate unique biologic changes modulating these endogenous factors, resulting in the features of an endogenous depression.

Depletion of NE, 5-HT, and DA with consequent up-regulation of the postsynaptic receptor is of interest in patients with epilepsy. Elevation of all three of these neurotransmitters has been noted to increase the seizure threshold (65). 5-HT depletion has been postulated to be involved in the pathophysiology of epilepsy, but the exact mechanism is uncertain (66).

It seems possible that the relationship between epilepsy and depression could hinge on these neurotransmitter changes. The observation of increased epileptogenesis with increasing dosages of antidepressants is an interesting one, considering the role of serotonin and NE in the generation of seizures. Except for the tottering mouse model, in all animal studies, NE attenuates seizure occurrence. Serotonin also appears to be responsible for increasing the seizure threshold (65). The expectation, therefore, would be a decrease in seizures with the use of antidepressants. In fact, this has been the case in the studies of Ojemann (described later in the chapter) and Favale et al. (67), who studied 17 epileptics who had fluoxetine 20 mg per day added to their AED regimen. Six patients had a complete remission of their seizure activity, and the remaining patients were noted to have a 30% reduction of seizure frequency (67). In a confirmatory animal study, monoamine depletion via reserpine had no effect on seizure incidence associated with increasing dosages of desipramine in rats (65). Serotonin depletion blocks the anticonvulsant properties of fluoxetine; conversely, the augmentation of fluoxetine with 5-hydroxytryptophan increases the seizure threshold (65).

The role of DA in epilepsy may be similar to the role of neurotransmitters noted earlier, but it is far from clear. DA antagonists, like the phenothiazines, lower the seizure threshold, whereas DA agonists frequently increase the threshold (65,66).

GABA is one of the most important neurotransmitters in the brain. It acts at two types of GABA receptors: A and B. One of the major modes of seizure control consists of pharmacologic augmentation of GABA at the A receptor site. Many antimanic agents increase GABA, and low GABA levels have been found in patients with depression (68). However, several drugs, such as phenobarbital and vigabatrin, which are GABA agonists, are the cause of significant affective symptoms. Thus, the actual pathogenic mechanisms of GABA-ergic effects are yet to be identified. A complex interplay may be operant, because different areas of the brain may react differently to GABA augmentation (4).

The hypothalamic pituitary axis (HPA) may be significantly affected by epilepsy. Interictal neurohormonal changes in epilepsy include alterations of prolactin and gonadotropins (69). Some of these effects may be the result of AEDs themselves either working directly on the brain or by secondary effects on sex hormone binding globulin (69). Depression likewise can cause a variety of neurohormonal aberrations, especially when associat-ed with psychotic features. In unipolar depression, increases of corticotropin-releasing factor, adrenocorticotropic hormone, and abnormal thyroid dysfunction, especially hypothyroidism, occur along with unclear changes in the hypothalamic-pituitary–gonadal system (36). Although the interplay here between epilepsy and depression is unclear, NE and 5-HT, as well as cortisol, may significantly modulate the HPA.

The role of excitatory neurotransmitters and the glutamate receptor in the genesis of epilepsy has been the focus of much research (70). This receptor site is an extremely complex macromolecule with an N-methyl-D-aspartate (NMDA) site, which also may be important in depression. NMDA antagonists have antiepileptogenic (i.e., they block "kindling" of epileptic activity in animals) and antiepileptic properties. Although there is sparse data on the interplay of glutamate in the pathogenesis of depression, NMDA antagonists also possess antidepressant qualities and can be mildly euphoric in nondepressed patients (71). In addition, adaptive changes in the NMDA receptor site are seen with chronic administration of most antidepressants and may predict antidepressant response (72). Thus, modulation of the NMDA receptor site may be yet another area where the presence of epilepsy may create an environment that predisposes to neurochemical changes that result in the phenomenon of depression (71).

Folic acid deficiency is yet another potential risk factor for the development of depression in epilepsy. Folate is involved in one-carbon transfer reactions important in the synthesis of biologic macromolecules, including neurotransmitters (4). The role of folic acid depletion in psychiatric disorders had been noted in many studies, with the gradual onset of depression, psychosis, and, finally, dementia (73,74). One review quoted an incidence of folate deficiency in 21% (75) of psychiatric inpatients. Epileptics are especially prone to folate deficiency. Phenobarbital and phenytoin, in particular, deplete red blood cell, serum, and cerebrospinal fluid folate levels. Whether associated depression with folate reduction is purely an epiphenomenon is unclear. Charney (75) and Froscher et al. (76) noted improvement in patient mood with folate replacement, as did Reynolds et al. (73) in an epilepsy group. Double-blind placebo-controlled studies with folic acid replacement, however, have not confirmed a direct association (34). This finding is in contrast to similar investigations with methylfolate, which showed clinical improvement (4). Thus, an association between folate deficiency and psychiatric dysfunction in epileptic patients is clear, but a causal link is uncertain (77).

Psychosocial Factors

The impact of seizure frequency on patients' quality of life is an important factor that mediates much of the psychopathology seen in patients with epilepsy (66,78). The psychopathogenic roles of psychosocial factors in epilepsy can be appreciated in patients undergoing epilepsy surgery. For example, levels of learned helplessness and depression prior to surgery have been shown to be associated with higher levels of dysfunction post-surgically (79). The relationship of locus of control and depression prior and subsequent to ATL was evaluated by Hermann and Wyler (80). They found a correlation preceding but not following surgery, with complete seizure cessation being the most pivotal factor in outcome. This finding is somewhat in conflict to our clinical observations. Patients who have never adjusted to having epilepsy, especially those who are overprotected and become socially agoraphobic, often are presented with a frightful period of postsurgical adjustment. These patients and their families require close psychiatric follow-up and are more prone to depression, divorce, etc. Unclear biologic factors also are important and require further investigation.

Lennox discussed several important social factors that he felt impacted the emotional well-being of patients with epilepsy, including secrecy, educational, and employment difficulty (7). Hermann and Whitman (7) reviewed a variety of neurobiologic, psychosocial, and medication variables to assess predictors of depression in epilepsy inpatients being evaluated for possible ATL. Interestingly, the only significantly associated elements were psychosocial. Increased perceived stigma, amount of social support, poor vocational adjustment, external locus of control, increased stressful life events, poor adjustment to epilepsy, less adequate financial status, and female gender all were associated with interictal depression. The last four factors remained statistically significant variables after a multiple regression analysis (7). There are several methodologic limitations of this study, but the results underscore the significance of psychosocial issues in the etiology of interictal depression.

Another important psychosocial issue concerns the patient's perception of seizure activity. The individual's sense of lack of control over his or her life may result in an overall fear of seizures. This may cause agorophobic behavior that may be discordant from the actual extent and control of seizure activity. These maladaptive fears may result in significant disability and depression (53).

Finally, sexual dysfunction has been reported in patients with epilepsy, with prevalence ranging from 14% to 66%. Patients with partial seizures were found to be at higher risk (69). Although biologic and medication factors are largely causative, further self-esteem and mood changes may result.

Iatrogenic Factors

Iatrogenic cause of depressive disorders, resulting from the side effects of AEDs, is an important factor in depressive disorders. These may result from the introduction of AEDs with negative psychotropic properties

(81) or the discontinuation of AEDs with mood-stabilizing properties in patients with an underlying affective disorder (82).

The association of AEDs used in monotherapy, and especially in polytherapy, with cognitive functions has been well documented (81). The barbiturates seem to be the most widely recognized culprits, but other drugs, such as carbamazepine and valproate, given in high dosages also have been implicated. Likewise, there is a significant incidence of affective disorders instigated by the use of AEDs. Robertson et al. (10) noted the association of depression with the use of phenobarbital. Brent et al. (83) evaluated 15 epileptic children taking phenobarbital and compared their levels of depression using DSM criteria with 24 patients taking carbamazepine. The rate of depression (40% vs. 4%) and suicidal ideation (47% vs. 4%) was significantly more elevated in the phenobarbital group. A family history of depression also was significantly more prevalent in this group. In a follow-up study, 28 of these patients were evaluated a median of 26.5 months later (84). A similar finding was observed, i.e., higher rates of depression were seen in those patients taking phenobarbital (38% vs. 0%). Those patients who were switched from phenobarbital to carbamazepine had a nonsignificant trend to a decrease in both the frequency and the severity of depressive symptoms.

Depression as a side effect of AEDs is certainly not confined to phenobarbital. Topiramate, tiagabine, and vigabatrin have rates in clinical trials from 5% to 15% (85,86). In one review, vigabatrin had an associated rate of depression and irritability of 24% (87). Lamotrigine, gabapentin, and felbamate have an incidence of around 4.2%, 1.8%, and 5.3% respectively (88). Hypomania has been reported with the use of AEDs, such as zonisamide (89).

Polypharmacy can be a contributing factor. In one study by Thompson and Trimble, reduction of anticonvulsants from a mean of 2.8 to 1.6 resulted in significant decreases in anxiety and depression scores 3 and 6 months later (4). Thus, the simplification of a complex AED regimen in itself may result in a positive clinical effect.

Not only can the addition of an AED have negative psychotropic effects, but the discontinuation of AEDs can be associated with a discontinuation phenomenon. Anxiety and depression have been noted with the termination of AEDs during presurgical evaluation (82). Restarting the original AED may have an ameliorating effect.

TREATMENT

Once the diagnosis of an affective disorder is made, an assessment of the severity of the patient's complaints is imperative, given the aforementioned prevalence of suicide in this population. The suicidal risk increases in the presence of psychotic features, whether periictal or interictal. If outpatient treatment seems appropriate, then either a nonpharmacologic or psychopharmacologic treatment or both might be instituted.

Nonpharmacologic Interventions

A nonpharmacologic treatment paradigm might include individual, couples, family, or group therapy and relaxation training via biofeedback. Fenwick (90) introduced the concept of group two neurons, damaged cells surrounding an epileptic epicenter of group one cells that are firing continuously. He postulated that influencing the group two neurons would influence seizure propagation. Secondary inhibition is a term used by Fenwick (90) to describe behavioral techniques that augment inhibition of these recruitment cells. In fact, behavioral treatments have been utilized with some success by epileptic patients to control their seizure frequency (90).

Cognitive, behavioral, and interpersonal therapy techniques have been utilized for the amelioration of depression in psychiatric patients with significant effectiveness (91). These techniques have been compared to medication administered in an NIMH Collaborative Research Program for Depression. All modalities were equally efficacious, with

medication more useful in patients with severe depression (91). Combining modalities generally has an augmentation effect. In patients with epilepsy, cognitive behavioral therapy has been used successfully for treatment of depression in a small controlled study (92) and for social phobia associated with "seizure fear" (93).

Epilepsy, especially when intractable, can have a major impact on the family. Siblings and mothers are at increased risk of psychological dysfunction. In the Isle of Wight study, one fifth of mothers with epileptic children had histories of experiencing a nervous breakdown (94). Concerns of injury and a history of status epilepticus were associated with anxiety and depression in families supporting patients with refractory epilepsy (94). Couples and family supportive counseling may be useful in this situation and also prior to and following ATL.

Pharmacologic Interventions

Antidepressant Drugs

An assessment of depression must take into account a potential complication from AEDs. A thorough search for a temporal relationship between the institution of an AED or a dosage increase implicates the AED as causative. If that is the case, a change to another AED should be made, if possible. In addition, depressive symptoms that are associated temporally with the prodromal or periictal interval require a reassessment of AEDs. Either an increase in the dose of a partially effective AED or a switch to another medication in the case of nonresponse is necessary. In the case where the AED armamentarium has been exhausted and no change is possible, then the patient's depression can be treated as if it were interictal, although no data are yet available to substantiate this approach.

Antidepressants are the mainstay of pharmacotherapy in epileptic patients with depressive symptoms. After making a diagnosis of dysthymia, MDD, or the presence of an IDD, attention shifts to the use of antidepressants in these patients. The following discussion will

TABLE 5.4. *Antidepressant-induced seizure incidence*

Drug	Incidence (%)	Reference(s)
Amitriptyline	<0.1–0.3	110, 117, 121, 122
Amoxapine (overdose)	24.5–36.4	119, 131
Bupropion	0.6–1.0	114, 121, 122
Bupropion 225–450 mg/d (bulimic patients)	5.8	115
Bupropion <300 mg/d	<0.1	114
Bupropion 300–450 mg/d	0.36	118, 127
Bupropion >450 mg/d[a]	0.60–2.19	110, 122
Bupropion 600 mg/d	2.3	118, 127
Bupropion 600–900 mg/d	2.8	118, 127
Bupropion SR ≤300 mg/d	0.1	128
Bupropion SR 400 mg/d	0.4	128
Citalopram	<0.1	120
Citalopram 600–1,900 mg	18.0	123
Citalopram 1,900–5,200 mg	47.0	123
Clomipramine	0.70–1.04	121, 133
Clomipramine ≤250 mg/d	0.5	110
Clomipramine >250 mg/d	1.10–1.66	110
Clomipramine >250 mg/d (Patients with obsessive-compulsive disorder)	3.0	110
Desipramine	<0.1	110, 117
Desipramine (overdose)	17.9	131
Doxepin	<0.1	110, 117
Fluoxetine	<0.1–0.2	121, 125, 132
Fluvoxamine	0.2	121
Imipramine	<0.1–0.9	110, 117, 121
Imipramine <200 mg/d[a]	0.1	110, 122
Imipramine >200 mg/d[a]	0.6–0.9	122
Maprotiline	0.4–15.6	110, 116
Maprotiline (overdose)	12.2	131
Mirtazepine	<0.1	126
Nefazodone	Limited data	
Nortriptyline	<0.1	110, 117
Nortripyline (overdose)	22%	103
Paroxetine	0.1	121
Protriptyline	<0.1	117
Sertraline	<0.1	110, 113
Trazodone	<0.1	130
Trazodone (overdose)	<1	131
Tricyclic antidepressants	0.1–4.0	104, 110
Tricyclic antidepressants (overdose)	3.0–41.0	110, 131
Venlafaxine	0.26	124
Venlafaxine (overdose)	5.0	129

[a]Predisposed patients excluded.
From references 103, 104, 110, 113–133, with permission.

focus on the efficacy, side effects, drug interactions, and overall recommendation for the use of antidepressants.

In 1958, Kuhn (95), in Switzerland, reported on the efficacy of the tricyclic antidepressant (TCA) imipramine. Since then, there has been an explosion of new TCAs and of other types of antidepressants. Today, there are eight different TCAs, two types of tetra-cyclic antidepressants, five different selective serotonin reuptake inhibitors (SSRIs), two serotonin-2 antagonist reuptake inhibitors (SARIs), and four different monoamine oxidase inhibitors (MAOIs). In recent years, we have witnessed the introduction of a selective serotonin-norepinephrine reuptake inhibitor (SNRI) and one with combined noradrenergic-dopaminergic (NDRI) properties. A list of

TABLE 5.5. *Isoenzymes involved in the metabolism of antidepressant and antiepileptic drugs*

Medication	Isoenzyme					Protein binding (%)
	1A2	2C9/10	2C19	2D6	3A4	
Amitriptyline	S	S	S	S, **INH**	S	90–95
Amoxapine				S		90
Bupropion	Primarily metabolized by 2B6 isoenzyme					82–88
Citalopram			S, INH	INH (low)	S	50
Clomipramine	S	S	S	S, **INH**	S	97
Desipramine	S			S, **INH**	S	
Doxepin				S	S	80–85
Fluoxetine	INH (low)	**INH**	INH (med)	S, **INH**	INH (med)	94.5
Fluvoxamine	S, **INH**	**INH**	**INH**	S, INH (low)	**INH**	77–80
Imipramine	S	S	S	S	S	89
Maprotiline				S		88
Mirtazepine	S, INH (low)	S		S, INH (low)	S, INH (low)	85
Nefazodone	INH (low)			INH (low)	S, **INH**	>99
Nortriptyline	S			S	S	86–95
Paroxetine	INH (low)			S, **INH**	INH (low)	93–95
Protriptyline				S	S	Highly bound[a]
Sertraline	INH (low)	INH	INH	S, INH (med)	S, INH (low)	98
Trazodone				S		95
Trimipramine				S	S	95
Venlafaxine	INH (low)			S, INH (low)		30
Carbamazepine		IND	?IND	IND	S, IND	75
Ethosuximide					S, IND	30 (children 7–9 yr), 40–60 (adults)
Felbamate	Minimally metabolized; most is excreted in the urine					22–25
Gabapentin	Not metabolized, only renally cleared					<3
Lamotrigine	Metabolized primarily by glucuronic acid conjugation (no involvement of cytochrome P-450)					55
Phenobarbital	IND	IND	IND	IND	IND	40–60
Phenytoin	IND	S, IND	IND	S, IND	IND	90
Primidone			?S	IND	IND	20–25
Tiagabine					S	96
Topiramate			S, INH			13–17
Valproate		INH				80–94
Zonisamide					S	

IND, inducer; INH, inhibitor; INH (low), low inhibition; INH (med), medium inhibition; **INH,** high inhibition; S, substrate.
[a]Degree of protein binding difficult to obtain.
From references 145–152, with permission.

commonly used antidepressants is presented in Tables 5.4 and 5.5.

Despite the large number of antidepressant agents available and the relatively high frequency and severity of depression in epilepsy, there is an incredibly sparse literature on the efficacy of antidepressants in this situation. There is only one reported double-blind trial in which patients meet the criteria for MDD (96). In this study by Robertson and Trimble (96), patients given amitriptyline and nomifensine were compared to a placebo control group. During the first 6 weeks, subtherapeutic dosages of amitriptyline were used and no differences emerged, although all patients improved. In the second 6 weeks, the placebo patients were withdrawn from the study and nonresponders in the active medication group had their dosage doubled. Sixty-five percent of patients were judged to be responders. Limitations to the study are obvious, but there was no significant change in seizure frequency between groups and, except for valproate, only a slight increase in anticonvulsant dosages were found while the patients were taking antidepressants.

Two retrospective studies were conducted by Ojemann et al. (97,98). In the first study, the effects of the TCA, doxepin, given in varying dosages were assessed for efficacy and impact on seizure frequency (97). Seizure frequency improved in 79%, with a greater than 50% improvement in more than one half of patients. Depressive symptoms decreased at least mildly in 89%, with a suggestion of a causal link. In the second investigation, Ojemann et al. (98) looked at a variety of psychotropic medications given to epileptic patients and evaluated the effect of these drugs on seizure control. The records of 59 patients (40 with an MDD) were reviewed; 58% improvement in seizure frequency and 86% amelioration of psychiatric complaints were noted. The implications from both of these reports are the effectiveness and safety of these medications, with possible benefit to seizure control.

Whereas TCAs were the first antidepressants available for treatment of depression, SSRIs have become the first-line treatment in depressed patients without and with epilepsy. Their efficacy in MDD is comparable to that of TCA. Some investigators have suggested that TCA may be more effective for MDD with melancholia (99), but this is yet to be established. SSRIs have a low seizure propensity, are well tolerated in overdose, and have a favorable adverse effects profile. Furthermore, their efficacy in dysthymic disorders and for treatment of symptoms such as irritability and poor frustration tolerance make this class of antidepressant drugs more attractive among patients with epilepsy. SSRIs have yielded therapeutic efficacy in panic and obsessive-compulsive disorders as well (100).

Citalopram and sertraline can be considered first-line SSRIs because of their minimal pharmacokinetic interactions with AEDs (see later). Sertraline can be started at a daily dose of 25 to 50 mg, with 50-mg dosage increments at 2- to 3-week intervals until the desired therapeutic effects are obtained, a maximal dose of 200 mg per day has been reached, or adverse events are reported. Citalopram can be started at a daily dose of 10 mg per day. That dosage may be followed by increments of 10 to 20 mg every 2 to 3 weeks, pausing at whatever level results in clinical response. Dosage increases then are made if the patient plateaus at an unsatisfactory point, to a maximal dose of 60 mg per day. Alternatively, paroxetine also may be used.

It has been the author's (JJB) clinical observation that epileptic patients often respond to low dosages of antidepressants. The recommendation, "start low and go slow," seems generally appropriate. However, in the rare nonresponsive depressed epileptic patient, high-dose antidepressants may be necessary.

The TCAs have been reported to yield a good clinical response in MDD, panic, and attention-deficit disorders. Clomipramine has been found to be effective in obsessive-compulsive disorders. Their cardiotoxic effects and severe complications when used in patients' suicide attempts, however, have made them second-line antidepressants. Blumer and Zielinski (101) had anecdotal reports of the utility of low-dose TCA in patients with a variety of psychiatric disorders in epilepsy, but with depression in particular. They commented on the utility of relatively low dosages of TCA, generally around 100 to 150 mg of imipramine. Blumer also commented on the effectiveness of "double antidepressants" in depressed epileptics refractory to TCAs (13). Even with low TCA dosages, he noted that refractory depression in epileptics is an unusual clinical situation, seen in about 15% of patients with an IDD (7). This contrasts with the 10% to 30% nonresponse rate seen in patients with idiopathic depressions after much more extensive antidepressant treatment interventions (102).

MAOIs are efficacious, well tolerated, and associated with a low incidence of seizures in patients with MDD (103). They also are very useful for treatment of dysthymic disorders and social phobia. The potential risk of hypertensive crisis resulting from their interactions with certain foods rich in tyramine and medications limits their use in clinical practice to psychiatrists with experience in their use.

Trazodone is the oldest 5-HT$_2$ antagonist antidepressant on the market. More recently, nefazodone has been added to our armamentarium; it works similarly as trazodone, with agonist activity on 5-HT$_{1A}$ receptor as well as weak inhibition of the 5-HT transporter (104). Their principal indication is for treatment of MDD. In our opinion, however, they do not yield any advantages over SSRIs. Because of its sedative effects, trazodone has been used for treatment of insomnia of depressed and nondepressed patients. Nefazodone interacts with cytochrome P-450 isoenzyme CYP3A3/4 and can increase levels of triazalobenzodiazepines (alprazolam and triazolam) as well as H1 antagonists and carbamazepine (104). M-chlorophenylpiperazine (MCPP) is a metabolite of nefazodone and is itself broken down by the 2D6 isoenzyme. MCPP has been associated with dysphoric agitation, and its levels can be increased by SSRIs (104). Therefore, some patients may not tolerate the combination and may have difficulty switching from an SSRI to nefazodone without a washout period or gradual introduction of the medication (50 to 100 mg per day) (104). Trazodone has been reported to be associated with priapism (incidence 1 per 6,000) (104). Thus, both of these drugs have potential drawbacks.

Two new antidepressants, venlafaxine and mirtazapine, recently have been added to our pharmacologic armamentarium. To date, however, there are little data on their impact on seizure threshold, interaction with AEDs, and use in epileptic patients (103). Venlafaxine is a selective SNRI that has been used successfully in depressed, nonepileptic patients who failed to respond to SSRI, and it also should be considered in patients with epilepsy who fail to respond to an SSRI. In a recent study involving depressed nonepileptic patients, venlafaxine sustained release preparation was compared to fluoxetine and a placebo control group. Both antidepressants were equally effective overall and superior to placebo. In addition, venlafaxine showed a faster response rate and was

more effective for symptoms of concomitant anxiety compared to fluoxetine (105). This has mirrored the author's (JJB) experience with the drug as well.

Mirtazapine (NaSSA) is a recently released partial norepinephrine agonist that also blocks 5-HT$_2$ and 5-HT$_3$, thus increasing serotonergic tone. It tends to be extremely sedating but lacks the sexual side effects and nausea seen with the SSRIs. There have been reports of agranulocytosis with this drug (1.1 per 1,000); thus, its use with carbamazepine would not be recommended (103).

Bupropion is an antidepressant with combined noradrenergic-dopaminergic effects (104). Because of these pharmacodynamic properties, it is an antidepressant with potential efficacy in more severe forms of depression, particularly in those patients who are nonresponsive to TCAs. It also is effective for treatment of attention-deficit disorder. Bupropion has the advantage that it may be less likely to cause mania in bipolar patients compared to other antidepressants, although other studies have not confirmed this finding (104). It appears to be safe in patients with cardiac disorders. It has several active metabolites that may be responsible for its therapeutic activity by increasing noradrenergic activity (104). However, in higher dosages, these metabolites may be responsible for the increased seizure potential seen with this drug (see below).

Reboxetine is a new antidepressant recently released in the United States and the United Kingdom. It is a nontricyclic, selective norepinephrine reuptake inhibitor that is more potent than desipramine and without significant effects on CYP3A4 or CYP2D6. It has been reported to have a seizure frequency of 0.13%, but more experience with its use in the epileptic population is needed (103).

Three additional caveats are important when using antidepressants. First, in patients with idiopathic MDD, the first episode will be followed by at least one more in up to 50% to 80% of cases (102). No data regarding recurrence rates are available for depressed epileptic patients, but in other central nervous system (CNS)-associated depressive disorders, e.g., strokes, a long-term course is frequent if left untreated (106). Therefore, patients should be maintained on whatever effective dose resulted in complete response for at least 6 to 12 months. Gradual discontinuation should be decided on an individual basis using the number of past depressive episodes, the seriousness of the depression, and residual symptoms as a major determinant (102).

Second, abrupt discontinuation of an SSRI may result in an acute reemergence of mood symptoms, plus dizziness, nausea, fatigue, insomnia, paresthesias, etc., and is believed to represent a withdrawal state. Symptoms may last for months but usually last for 7 to 14 days, and they are seen more frequently with SSRIs having a short half-life, e.g., paroxetine (21 hours) in contrast to fluoxetine (72 to 144 hours). Treatment is reintroduction of the SSRI with a more gradual taper (107).

Finally, patients who respond partially to an antidepressant may be candidates for augmentation with another agent. There are a wide variety of strategies that can be used. It is generally recommended to refer such a patient, as well as the nonresponsive and/or psychotic depressed epileptic, to a psychiatrist who is well versed in neuropsychopharmacology.

Side Effects

There are a variety of side effects that have been noted with antidepressants, including sedation, nausea, akathisia, and headaches (102). Depressed epileptic patients are not immune to these reactions. The most debilitating complaint with the use of SSRIs usually involves sexual dysfunction resulting in decrease interest and/or arousal in up to 50% to 70% of patients. Most SSRIs, with the possible exception of citalopram, cause dysfunction to the same degree (108). Tolerance may develop over time; dosage reduction or switching to another SSRI may help. The rates of sexual difficulties in patients taking bupropion, mirtazapine, and nefazodone are no greater than placebo, with the latter two drugs alternatives for patients with epilepsy.

The addition of a serotonin antagonist (cyproheptadine), a DA agonist (amantadine), or an α_2 blocker (yohimbine) may be alternatives, but the side effects of these drugs may themselves cause difficulties (109).

Despite these troublesome side effects, potential seizure induction and exacerbation are probably the most frequent reasons for the neglect of appropriate pharmacotherapy in the epileptic population. An understanding of this issue requires a review of several factors, including the rate of spontaneous seizure occurrence in the general population, predisposing risk factors, and the validity of methods for determining seizure frequency. The incidence and prevalence of seizures in the general population were examined by Rosenstein et al. (110) in a population-based study in Rochester, Minnesota. They found a first seizure frequency of 0.073% to 0.086% and an annual incidence of epilepsy of 0.028% to 0.053% (point prevalence of up to 0.64%) (110). Therefore, the determination of the role of antidepressants in the induction of seizures must factor in these statistics.

The sample sizes of patients included in studies that related seizure occurrence to antidepressants may be small and can therefore yield false-positive results. When attempting to evaluate the difference between two groups in which the dependent variable occurs infrequently, in this case a seizure, a large number of subjects would be required. It has been estimated that a group of 9,000 patients would be needed to provide enough information to display differences between antidepressant drugs and a control group (110).

Another confounding variable in attempting to estimate seizure frequencies is the inclusion of patients with risk factors. It is well known that patients with specific predisposing clinical findings are more susceptible to seizures. These factors include previous history of seizures, CNS trauma, neoplasia, cerebrovascular disease, mental retardation, dementia, drug abuse, and withdrawal states (103,110).

Psychiatric disease states themselves may predispose patients to seizure activity. For example, the original concern with bupropion may have been colored by the patient population being evaluated, e.g., those with bulimia. In addition, clomipramine-induced seizure rates seem to vary, from 3.0% in patients with obsessive-compulsive disorder to 1.1% in those without obsessive-compulsive disorder (110). Additionally, concurrent use of other psychoactive drugs can decrease the seizure threshold (103).

Another method of assessing seizure risk is from occurrence rates seen in patients who overdose. Obviously, extrapolating this data to usual clinical situations is fraught with potential error. The most that can be gleaned from this literature is relative risks. The overall risk from TCA overdose is around 8.4%. Elevated peak plasma levels often are associated with seizure induction, usually >1,000 ng/mL, although seizures at lower levels occur (110,111). The QRS duration of >0.10 has been reported as being predictive of seizure activity, but results between studies have been inconsistent (111).

From this literature, drug dosage appears to be the important pivotal factor in the prediction of seizure induction. Preskorn and Fast (111) reviewed their experience with TCA seizures and serum levels. Nine patients who had serum levels recorded were reviewed retrospectively. The only risk factor was an elevated TCA serum level. The authors also noted that there have been no reported cases of seizures in patients receiving TCAs where the serum level has not been above the therapeutic concentration (111). It is interesting to note from this review that the average dosage of the TCA was 250 mg per day, which is within the recommended dose range.

The metabolism of TCAs can have a 30- to 40-fold variation in patients on the same dosage (112). It appears that 7% to 9% of Caucasians and 1% of Asians meet criteria for being "slow hydroxylators" of TCAs, with the CYP2D6 isozyme of the P450 microsomal enzyme system being specifically responsible (113). This is particularly important because this enzyme is inhibited by SSRIs, especially fluoxetine and paroxetine, thus potentially increasing TCA levels and decreasing the seizure threshold. Note also that 5% of Caucasians and 20% of Asians are poor metabolizers at the 2C19 isoform (113).

In addition to dose, the rate of drug escalation seems important in the genesis of seizures. In one review, dosage escalation was believed to be an important factor in 62% of patients who had a seizure while taking bupropion (110). Duration of treatment also may be an important factor with cumulative risk increasing over time (110).

As discussed earlier, the etiology of the association of antidepressants and seizure induction is unclear, because increases in the primary neurotransmitters involved, i.e., 5-HT and NE, would cause the opposite effect. The TCAs have varying capacities of antimuscarinic, local anesthetic, and antihistaminic effects (66). Other medications with these effects can likewise cause seizures in overdose (66); therefore, it may be these other factors that are responsible for the increasing seizure potential of these drugs when they are used at higher dosages.

Antidepressant action on somatostatin, neuropeptides, and acute effects on excitatory amino acids, e.g., NMDA, may be other elements to be included in this complex picture (103). Regardless of the cause, the dose-dependent seizure induction effects of these drugs is factual and needs to be considered in their use. Although the literature may not provide an absolute marker of risk, a relative assessment can be made.

Table 5.4 summarizes the seizure induction potential of antidepressants at varying dosages and in overdose. These medications will be discussed in groups, from those drugs that are relatively contraindicated in patients with epilepsy, to those that are the authors' "drugs of choice."

Group 1: Amoxapine, Clomipramine, and Bupropion (Incidence ~0.1% to 36.4%)

Amoxapine, clomipramine, and bupropion are not recommended in patients with epilepsy, with some very significant caveats. Amoxapine is a unique compound that has a metabolite,

7-hydroxyamoxapine, that is a DA receptor blocker and similar in structure to loxapine, a neuroleptic. It is perhaps for this reason that amoxapine is so toxic in overdose, with a 15.2% mortality in one study and a seizure rate of 36.4% (134). There also are reports of status epilepticus (135). Clomipramine seems to be one of the more seizure inducing of the TCAs. In the worldwide literature, rates of 3.0% were found in obsessive-compulsive disorder patients receiving dosages greater than 250 mg (110) and 1.1% in patients without obsessive-compulsive disorder. A rate of 0.5% was reported with dosages below 250 mg per day, but patients often had predisposing factors (110). Status epilepticus also has been reported with clomipramine when it is used with valproic acid, possibly because of an increase in clomipramine serum levels (136).

Bupropion provides an excellent example of the complexity of determining seizure frequency with antidepressants. In early studies, bupropion appeared to be relatively safe, even in dosages above 450 mg and in overdose (103). In a study involving bulimic patients (n = 69), Horne et al. (115) noted that four patients experienced grand mal seizures. The manufacturer's reports showed a 2-year risk of 0.48% with dosages of 450 mg per day or less (110). In yet another review involving 3,341 patients, the cumulative rate over 8 weeks was 0.36%, with dosages ranging from 300 to 450 mg per day (118,128). The safety of the sustained release compound was evaluated in a multicenter study involving 3,100 patients with dosages of 300 mg per day or less. The seizure rate was 0.15% for both the acute and the chronic phase of treatment (118); thus, peak serum levels seem important. Bupropion now is frequently combined with SSRIs in refractory idiopathic depressions. Bupropion was found to be safe in one study in which no patients experienced seizure activity, but the number of patients was small (n = 27) (137). To extrapolate all this information to patients with a predisposing factor such as epilepsy is difficult at best. There does appear, however, to be a rapid increase of seizure induction potential with increasing dose, e.g., a low thera-peutic index (110). Because there are many other antidepressant alternatives, it seems prudent to avoid bupropion at this time.

Group 2: Maprotiline (Incidence ~0.4% to 15.6%)

Maprotiline, like amoxapine, causes more toxic side effects in overdose than standard TCAs. In a 2-year, retrospective review involving 1,313 patients who overdosed, maprotiline was associated with seizures in 12.2% (131). Although high drug levels are associated with more seizure activity, longevity of treatment also appears to be a factor, with 42% of seizures occurring after 6 weeks of treatment. It has been postulated that the accumulation of a long-acting metabolite might be responsible (110). This observation also underscores the need to follow patients for longer intervals or risk underestimating seizure potential (110). Jabbari et al. (166) observed a seizure rate of 15.6% in a study with dosages up to 300 mg per day, but may be lower as a function of dose (110). Thus, maprotiline is another drug that should be avoided in patients with epilepsy.

Group 3: Amitriptyline and Imipramine (Incidence ~0.1% to 0.9%)

In general, TCAs have an overall seizure induction rate ranging from 0.1% to 4% (101). For imipramine, Peck et al. (122) reviewed 98 studies and found the rate to be 0.1% at dosages below 200 mg per day, contrasting with 0.6% to 0.9% above this dosage. The same authors evaluated 50 studies using amitriptyline and discovered a lower frequency than imipramine, whereas others reported rates of about 0.3% or higher (103,110).

Group 4: Nortriptyline, Desipramine, and Doxepin (Incidence ~0.1%)

There are little data on the seizure induction potential of the secondary amines. Nortriptyline and desipramine can cause seizures in overdose of 22% and 17.9%, respectively (103,110,131). However, there are very little data on patients receiving therapeutic dosages. Rosenstein et al. (110) reviewed their experience with desipramine in 400 depressed inpatients. They noted one seizure-related side effect in a patient with an elevated desipramine level, who also received 20 mg per day of haloperidol (110). Therefore, it appears that TCAs are generally safe antidepressants when used in low dosages, with a seizure potential of about 0.1% with gradual dose escalation and with careful monitoring of serum levels (110). Doxepin was discussed earlier in the review by Ojemann et al. (97).

Group 5: Fluoxetine, Paroxetine, Sertraline, Venlafaxine, Citalopram, Fluvoxamine, Trazodone, Mirtazapine, Nefazodone, and MAOIs (Incidence ~0.1% to 0.26)

The SSRIs appear to be the drugs of choice for patients with comorbid depression and epilepsy, but seizure-related side effects have been reported. Fluoxetine in clinical trials was noted to have a seizure induction frequency of 0.2%. The sample included patients with epilepsy, overdose, and elevated dosages, i.e., 60 mg per day (110). In one review of 16 cases of fluoxetine overdose, there were no fatalities (138). Base rates of seizure induction for paroxetine has been about 0.1% (120). In a review of the use of sertraline in 3,852 patients, only three patients (0.078%) experienced seizure activity, and all had a predisposing factor (epilepsy or family history of epilepsy) (103). Other cases of seizure induction with sertraline have likewise been associated with other factors, e.g., SIADH and hyponatremia (139) or a possible drug interaction with concomitant use of amphetamine (140).

A rate of about 0.05% was found in initial clinical trials with fluvoxamine (n = 34,587 patients), along with safety in epileptic patients (103). Other investigators found higher rates of about 0.2% (121), possibly because of contributing factors (103). Citalopram is a new SSRI with a similar rate of possible seizure induction (0.1% to 0.2%), but an increased incidence was found in overdose (above 600 mg) (123). It may have the advantage of fewer interactions with AEDs (103). Finally, the selective SNRI venlafaxine appears to have a relatively similar profile as the SSRIs (0.1% to 0.26%), with isolated case reports of seizure activity in overdose (129).

Overall, it appears that SSRIs and SNRIs are relatively safe medications, with perhaps fluoxetine possessing more potential for seizure induction. One must remember the original caveat that 0.086% of the population can be expected to have a spontaneous seizure at any time. Statistically, it appears that there is very little difference between the quoted seizure-inducing potential of most SSRIs and SNRIs, from chance occurrence. However, only controlled studies with large numbers of patients can truly ascertain the answer to this important question.

The MAOIs, both type A and B, including moclobemide (not released in the United States) also appear to be "safe" drugs for use in epilepsy (103). Among the several other antidepressants that have come onto the market, such as trazodone, nefazodone, mirtazapine, and reboxetine, there are relatively little data available at present to judge their safety in patients with epilepsy.

DA agonists have been used for treatment of depression, alone or when it fails to respond to antidepressant agents. These include the CNS stimulants, such as dextroamphetamine and methylphenidate. The latter drug was studied in 25 children who have comorbid epilepsy and attention-deficit/hyperactivity disorder. In those children whose seizure disorder was under good control, no exacerbation of seizure activity was found (141). In contrast, three of five children with seizures had an increase in seizure frequency. In one study, a reduced incidence of seizures was found with the use of methylphenidate in patients with a seizure disorder secondary to brain injury (142). These studies seem to at least partially corroborate the minimal role of increased DA resulting in seizure genesis.

MOOD STABILIZERS FOR BIPOLAR DISORDER AND MAJOR DEPRESSIVE DISORDER

Lithium has been considered the first-line treatment for patients with bipolar affective disorders (BAD). In 1994, Bowden et al. (15) compared valproate, lithium, and placebo in patients with BAD and found equal efficacy. In addition, valproate seemed to be more effective than lithium for patients with rapid-cycling BAD (15). Since that time, a variety of AEDs have been found to be effective, especially in the manic phase of BAD. These AEDs include carbamazepine, gabapentin, and lamotrigine, with topiramate and tiagabine also emerging as possible agents for this disorder (15). In general, these drugs are considerably more effective for the manic phase of BAD and are more useful for depression in BAD than in unipolar depressive disorder.

Lithium generally has a secondary place in the treatment of patients with BAD, especially if they have a comorbid diagnosis of epilepsy. Lithium has been associated with encephalopathy, especially when it is used in combination with carbamazepine (141). Lithium has been considered to be proconvulsant but has been used safely in studies by Shukla et al. (144) and by Lyketsos et al. (48). Considering the vast array of proven and blossoming AED possibilities for the effective treatment of BAD, lithium should be considered a second-line treatment alternative. It may prove useful when part of an augmentation strategy.

DRUG INTERACTIONS

Before making a decision on an appropriate antidepressant for the epileptic patient, it is important to carefully consider potential drug interactions between antidepressants and AEDs. These pharmacokinetic interactions are mediated, in large part, through the CP-450 hepatic system of isoenzymes, a group of enzymes located in the hepatic endoplasmic reticulum. They are classified into several families, depending on their amino acid sequence (number) and subfamily (letter), and a number designation referring to a specific gene product. The major isoenzymes mediating the metabolism of AEDs and antidepressants with potential drug–drug interactions are listed in Table 5.5.

With the exception of gabapentin, every AED and all antidepressants are metabolized in the liver. AEDs and antidepressants can influence these enzymes by acting as either an inducer or an inhibitor of the cytochrome P-450 enzymes. If inhibition takes place, an increase in the serum concentration of drugs that act as substrates and are metabolized by this isoenzyme may occur. The converse is true if the enzyme is induced by the drug (153). The isoenzymes responsible for the overall metabolism of both antidepressants and AEDs include 1A2, 3A4, 2C9, 2C19, and 2D6. The 2B6 isoenzyme also may metabolize bupropion as well as other AEDs (154).

The AEDs that have the most likely possibility of influencing the level of antidepressants, particularly the TCAs, are phenobarbital, carbamazepine, and phenytoin. These effects are probably the result of induction of the 2D6 isoenzyme. On the other hand, SSRIs also may influence levels of AEDs (155–163). The frequency of reported cases mostly involve carbamazepine and phenytoin, but others including valproate have been reported.

Among the case reports of SSRIs interacting with AED, fluoxetine appears to be the most frequently cited, with more than 50 patients having resultant increased levels of carbamazepine or phenytoin (147–155). The interaction was clinically significant in more than 35 of these patients. This contrasts with the next most frequently cited SSRI, paroxetine, with less than half this number of reported patients (155–163). Even though some reviews show little interaction with carbamazepine and phenytoin, fluoxetine appears to be a drug that should be either avoided or used with caution in depressed epileptic patients on these AEDs.

Induction at the 2D6 isoenzyme by carbamazepine, phenytoin, or phenobarbital can cause a potential decrease in serum TCA levels. Conversely, when switching patients taking a TCA from an inducing to a noninducing AED, the TCA serum levels can increase. Such is the case, for example, if a patient is taking imipramine and carbamazepine and is being switched to lamotrigine or gabapentin (164). In addition, attention must be paid not only to the parent compound, but also to its metabolites. For example, when combining carbamazepine with a TCA, the levels of the parent TCA compound may be lowered, but its metabolically active hydroxy-TCA metabolite may be increased (165). Also, valproic acid may inhibit the metabolism of TCAs, resulting in increased serum levels (166).

Although most depressed epileptic patients will respond to a single antidepressant, occasionally "double" antidepressant treatments may be useful. As discussed previously, this strategy may have unique benefits. However, potential drug interactions may occur. Both fluoxetine and paroxetine may elevate TCA levels by a three-fold factor. Sertraline has a more modest effect, increasing TCA levels around 25%. Venlafaxine, fluvoxamine, and citalopram do not appreciably affect the site of TCA metabolism (2D6). Although little interaction should be expected (167), other authors have urged caution when using these drugs in combination (164). These observations underscore the need to monitor serum TCA levels.

A serious complication resulting from the interaction of several types of antidepressants is the serotonin syndrome, which results from serotonergic hyperstimulation. Symptoms include restlessness, myoclonus, diaphoresis, tremor, hyperthermia, convulsions, and possibly death (168,169). Symptoms usually occur within several hours of a drug change. Many reports have been with the combination of an SSRI or, less frequently, a TCA (especially clomipramine and imipramine) with an MAOI. Treatment is nonspecific and includes discontinuation of the offending agent and supportive therapy with resolution, usually in 24 hours (170). Because many of the AEDs have serotonin effects, a drug interaction with an antidepressant can, theoretically, take place. This has been reported with carbamazepine (156) but is uncommon. Although the serotonin syndrome is uncommon, serotonin stimulation, especially if augmented with another agent acting similarly, may result in manifestations of serotonin excess (171).

OTHER TREATMENT MODALITIES

Vagal Nerve Stimulation

Like preliminary observations with gabapentin and lamotrigine, epileptic patients who were treated with vagal nerve stimulation (VNS) noted improvement in their mood not attributable to a reduction in seizure frequency (172). A prospective study by Harden et al. (173) confirmed this observation. A recent study by Rush et al. (174) evaluating the efficacy of VNS in 30 patients with refractory MDD or bipolar I (depressed phase) found a response rate of 40% (defined as ≥50% reduction in baseline scores) on the 28-item Hamilton Depression Rating Scale and the Clinical Global Impressions-Improvement index and 50% for the Montgomery-Asberg Depression Rating Scale. VNS also appears to affect mood-regulating neurotransmitter systems, e.g., serotonin, NE, GABA, and glutamate (175). These effects probably are due to connections of the left vagus nerve to the locus caeruleus, nucleus raphe, as well as affecting the amygdala, cingulate, hippocampus, etc. It is too early to ascertain the role of VNS for treatment of depression in patients with epilepsy, but future studies may help clarify this issue.

Electroconvulsive Therapy

Electroconvulsive therapy (ECT) is considered one of the most effective treatments for patients with MDD, especially when coupled with psychotic features. It usually is reserved for patients who are either refractory to other antidepressants and/or in an acute crisis (176). The same criteria apply to patients who have epilepsy and are depressed. ECT can be a safe procedure in the epileptic, raising the seizure threshold considerably during the course of several procedures (103). The mechanism of action of ECT has been debated because a myriad of biochemical changes take place. Many effects of ECT are similar to those seen with antidepressants, but significant differences also exist. This may explain the utility of ECT with mania and delirium (177). Several case reports have documented the safe use of ECT in depressed epileptics, even after ATL (178,179). ECT has even been postulated to be useful in patients in status epilepticus (180) by acting as an AED in its own right.

The procedure itself should be initiated without any change in the patient's AED regimen and bilateral ECT is recommended (M. Fink, *personal communication,* 2000). However, others have recommended unilateral nondominant ECT with dose titration (103). Bilateral ECT also is recommended because the presence of AEDs will preclude the necessary 5× elevation above the seizure threshold needed for effective unilateral ECT (181) in nonepileptic patients. A gradual dose reduction of the AED usually is required as the seizure threshold increases from each procedure. AEDs should be held on the morning of the procedure except if there is a significant risk of status epilepticus (103).

CONCLUSION

Affective disorders frequently occur in patients with epilepsy, especially in the form of a depressive disorder. In this chapter, we attempted to define these disorders and outline an evaluation and treatment strategy focusing on a variety of options, including psychotherapy and pharmacotherapy. The safety and potential of antidepressant drug interactions were discussed in detail. The hope of the authors is a more thorough recognition and treatment of affective disorders in epilepsy, because very effective modalities are available if used properly.

A quote from Lennox and Markham provides an appropriate conclusion (66): "The good physician is concerned not only with turbulent brain waves but with disturbed emotions and with social justice, for the epileptic is not just a nerve-muscle preparation; he is a person, in health an integrated combination of the physical, the mental, the social, and the spiritual. Disruption of any part can cause or aggravate illness."

REFERENCES

1. Koran LM. Medical conditions associated with obsessive compulsive symptoms. In: Koran LM, ed. *Obsessive-compulsive and related disorders in adults: a comprehensive clinical guide.* UK: Cambridge University Press, 1999:119.
2. Robertson M. Mood disorders in epilepsy. In: McConnell HW, Snyder PJ, eds. *Psychiatric comorbidity in epilepsy.* Washington, DC: American Psychiatric Press, Inc., 1998:133–167.
3. Schmitz B, Trimble M. Epileptic equivalents in psychiatry: some 19th century views. *Acta Neurol Scand Suppl* 1992;140:122–126.
4. Ring HA, Trimble MR. Depression in epilepsy. In: Starkstein SE, Robertson RG, eds. *Depression in neurologic disease.* Baltimore: Johns Hopkins University Press, 1993:63–83.
5. Blumer D. *Vincent van Gogh's epilepsy.* (*unpublished data*).
6. Stevens JR. Psychiatric aspects of epilepsy. *J Clin Psychiatry* 1988;49:4[Suppl]:49–57.
7. Hermann BP, Whitman S. Neurobiological, psychosocial, and pharmacological factors underlying interictal psychopathology in epilepsy. In: Smith DB, Treiman DM, Trimble MR, eds. *Advances in neurology,* Volume 55. *Neurobehavioral problems in epilepsy.* New York: Raven Press, 1991:439–452.
8. American Psychiatric Association. *Diagnostic and Statistical Manual of Mental Disorders,* 4th ed. Washington, DC: American Psychiatric Press, 1994.
9. Altshuler L. Depression and epilepsy. In: Devinsky O, Theodore WH, eds. *Epilepsy and behavior.* New York: Wiley-Liss, 1991:47–65.
10. Robertson MM, Trimble MR, Townsend DRA. Phenomenology of depression in epilepsy. *Epilepsia* 1987;28:364–372.
11. Mendez MF, Cummings JF, Benson DF. Depression in epilepsy: significance and phenomenology. *Arch Neurol* 1986;43:766–770.
12. Cassem EH. Depression secondary to medical illness. In: Frances AJ, Hales RE, eds. *Review of psychiatry,* Volume 7. Washington, DC: American Psychiatric Press, 1988:256–273.
13. Blumer D. Antidepressant and double antidepressant treatment for the affective disorder of epilepsy. *J Clin Psychiatry* 1997;58:3–11.
14. Akiskal HS. Mood disorders: clinical features. In: Kaplan HI, Sadock BL, eds. *Comprehensive textbook of psychiatry/VI.* Baltimore: Williams & Wilkins, 1995.
15. Barry JJ. Psychiatric uses for anticonvulsants. *Merritt-Putnam Lectures-CME Monograph,* 1999:89–104.
16. Barraclough B. Suicide and epilepsy. In: Reynolds EH, Trimble MR, eds. *Epilepsy and psychiatry.* Edinburgh: Churchill Livingstone, 1981:72–76.
17. Mendez MF, Doss RC. Ictal and psychiatric aspects of suicide in epileptic patients. *Int J Psychiatry Med* 1992;22:231–237.
18. Mendez MF, Lanska DJ, Manon-Espaillat R, et al. Causative factors for suicide attempts by overdose in epileptics. *Arch Neurol* 1989;46:1065–1068.

19. Blanchet P, Frommer GP. Mood change preceding epileptic seizures. *J Nerv Ment Dis* 1986;174: 471–476.

20. Williams D. The structure of emotions reflected in epileptic experiences. *Brain* 1956;79:29–67.

21. Taylor DC, Lochery M. Temporal lobe epilepsy: origin and significance of simple and complex auras. *J Neurol Neurosurg Psychiatry* 1987;50:673–681.

22. Robertson MM. Affect and mood in epilepsy: an overview with a focus on depression. *Acta Neurol Scand* 1992;86:127–135.

23. Barczak P. Hypomania following complex partial seizures. *Br J Psychiatry* 1988;152:137–139.

24. O'Shea B. Hypomania and epilepsy. *Br J Psychiatry* 1988;152:571.

25. Humphries SR, Dickinson PS. Hypomania following complex partial seizures. *Br J Psychiatry* 1988;152:571–572.

26. Morphew JA. Hypomania following complex partial seizures. *Br J Psychiatry* 1988;152:572.

27. Byrne A. Hypomania following increased epileptic activity. *Br J Psychiatry* 1988;153:573–574.

28. Sachdev P. Schizophrenia-like psychosis and epilepsy: the status of the association. *Am J Psychiatry* 1998;155:325–336.

29. Bear D, Fedio P. Quantitative analysis of interictal behavior in temporal lobe epilepsy. *Arch Neurol* 1977;34:454–467.

30. Hermann BP, Seidenberg M, Haltiner A, et al. Mood state in unilateral temporal lobe epilepsy. *Biol Psychiatry* 1991;30:1205–1218.

31. Kogeorgos J, Fonagy P, Scott DF. Psychiatric symptom patterns of chronic epileptics attending a neurological clinic: a controlled investigation. *Br J Psychiatry* 1982;140:236–243.

32. Altshuler LL, Devinsky O, Post RM. Depression, anxiety and temporal lobe epilepsy. *Arch Neurol* 1990;47:284–288.

33. Metcalfe R, Firth D, Pollock S, et al. Psychiatric morbidity and illness behaviour in female neurologic inpatients. *J Neurol Neurosurg Psychiatry* 1988;51: 1387–1390.

34. Edeh J, Toone BK. Antiepileptic therapy, folate deficiency, and psychiatric morbidity: a general practice survey. *Epilepsia* 1985;26:434–440.

35. Victoroff JI, Benson F, Grafton ST, et al. Depression in complex partial seizures: electroencephalography and cerebral metabolic correlates. *Arch Neurol* 1994;51: 155–163.

36. Musselman DL, DeBattista C, Nathan KI, et al. Biology of mood disorders. In: Schatzberg AF, Nemeroff CB, eds. *Textbook of psychopharmacology,* 2nd ed. Washington, DC: American Psychiatric Press, 1998:549–589.

37. Trimble MR, Perez MR. Quantification of psychopathology in adult patients with epilepsy. In: Kulig BM, Meinard H, Stores G, eds. *Epilepsy and behavior.* Lisse: Swets and Zeitlinger, 1980:118–126.

38. Master DR, Toone BK, Scott DF. Interictal behavior in temporal lobe epilepsy. In: Porter RJ, Ward AA, Mattson RH, et al., eds. *Advances in Epilepsy: XVth Epilepsy International Symposium.* New York: Raven Press 1984:557–565.

39. Dodrill CB, Batzel W. Interictal behavioral features of patients with epilepsy. *Epilepsia* 1986;27:564–576.

40. Fiordelli E, Beghi E, Bogliun G, et al. Epilepsy and psychiatric disturbance: a cross-sectional study. *Br J Psychiatry* 1993;163:446–450.

41. Matthews CG, Kove H. MMPI performances in major motor, psychomotor and mixed seizure classifications of known and unknown etiology. *Epilepsia* 1968;9: 43–53.

42. Kove H, Doehring DG. MMPI in epileptic groups with differential etiology. *J Clin Psychol* 1962;18:149–153.

43. Standage KF, Fenton GW. Psychiatric symptom profiles of patients with epilepsy: a controlled investigation. *Psychol Med* 1975;5:152–160.

44. Mendez MF, Doss RC, Taylor JL, et al. Depression in epilepsy: relationship to seizures and anticonvulsant therapy. *J Nerv Ment Dis* 1993;181:444–447.

45. Starkstein SE, Robertson RG. Mechanisms of disinhibition after brain lesions. *J Nerv Ment Dis* 1997;185: 108–114.

46. Bakchine S, Lacomblez L, Benoit N, et al. Manic-like state after bilateral orbitofrontal and right temporoparietal injury: efficacy of clonidine. *Neurology* 1989;39:777–781.

47. Benson DF. The Geschwind syndrome. In: Smith DB, Treiman DM, Trimble MR, eds. *Advances in neurology,* Volume 55. *Neurobehavioral problems in epilepsy.* New York: Raven Press, 1991:411–421.

48. Lyketsos CG, Stoline AM, Longstreet P, et al. Mania in temporal lobe epilepsy. *Neuropsychiatry Neuropsychol Behav Neurol* 1993;6:19–25.

49. Wolf P. Manic episodes in epilepsy. In: Akimoto H, Kazamatsuri H, Seino M, et al., eds. *Advances in Epileptology: Thirteenth Epilepsy International Symposium.* New York: Raven Press, 1982:237–240.

50. Indaco A, Carrieri PB, Nappi C, et al. Interictal depression in epilepsy. *Epilepsy Res* 1992;12:45–50.

51. Robertson MM. Depression in patients with epilepsy: an overview and clinical study. In: Trimble MR, ed. *The psychopharmacology of epilepsy.* Chichester: John Wiley & Sons, 1988:65–82.

52. Perini G, Mendius R. Depression and anxiety in complex partial seizures. *J Nerv Ment Dis* 1984;172: 287–290.

53. Lambert MV, Robertson MM. Depression in epilepsy: etiology, phenomenology, and treatment. *Epilepsia* 1999;40:S21–S47.

54. Hurwitz TA, Wada JA, Kosaka BA, et al. Cerebral organization of affect suggested by temporal lobe seizures. *Neurology* 1985;35:1335–1337.

55. Bromfield EB, Altshuler L, Leiderman DB, et al. Cerebral metabolism and depression in patients with complex partial seizures. *Arch Neurol* 1992;49:617–623.

56. Wolf P. Acute behavioral symptomatology at disappearance of epileptiform EEG abnormality: paradoxical or "forced normalization." In: Smith DB, Treiman DM, Trimble MR, eds. *Advances in neurology,* Volume 55. *Neurobehavioral problems in epilepsy.* New York: Raven Press, 1991:127–142.

57. Krishnamoorthy ES, Trimble MR. Forced normalization: clinical and therapeutic relevance. *Epilepsia* 1999;40:S57–S64.

58. Trimble MR, Ring HA, Schmitz B. Neuropsychiatric aspects of epilepsy. In: Fogel BS, Schiffer RB, Rao SM, eds. *Neuropsychiatry.* Baltimore: Williams & Wilkins, 1996:771–803.

59. Consensus development panel. National Institute of

Health consensus development conference statement: surgery for epilepsy. *Epilepsia* 1990;31:806–812.

60. Baldin PF. Psychosocial difficulties and outcome after temporal lobectomy. *Epilepsia* 1992;33:898–907.

61. Jensen I, Larsen JK. Mental aspects of TLE. *J Neurol Neurosurg Psychiatry* 1979;42:948–954.

62. Bruton CJ. *The neuropathology of TLE. Maudsley Monograph 31.* Oxford: Oxford University Press, 1988.

63. Blumer D, Montouras G, Hermann B. Psychiatric morbidity in seizure patients on a neurodiagnostic monitoring unit. *J Neuropsychiatry* 1995;7:445–456.

64. Kohler C, Norstrand JA, Baltuch G, et al. Depression in temporal lobe epilepsy before epilepsy surgery. *Epilepsia* 1999;40:336–340.

65. Dailey JW, Naritoku DK. Antidepressants and seizures: clinical anecdotes overshadow neuroscience. *Biochem Pharmacol* 1996;52:1323–1329.

66. Robertson MM. The organic contribution to depressive illness in patients with epilepsy. *J Epilepsy* 1989;2:189–230.

67. Favale E, Rubino V, Mainardi P, et al. Anticonvulsant effect of fluoxetine in humans. *Neurology* 1995;45:1926–1927.

68. Shiah I-S, Yatham LN. GABA function in mood disorders: an update and critical review. *Life Sci* 1998;63:1289–1303.

69. Morrell MJ. Sexual dysfunction in epilepsy. *Epilepsia* 1991;32:S38–S45.

70. Fisher RS. Update on the mechanism of action of the new antiepileptic drugs. *Merritt-Putnam Lectures-CME Monograph,* March 1999.

71. Berman R, Charney DS. Models of antidepressant action. *J Clin Psychiatry* 1999;60[Suppl14]:16–35.

72. Skolnick P, Layer RT, Nowak G, et al. Adaptation of N-methyl-D-aspartate receptors following antidepressant treatment: implications for the pharmacotherapy of depression. *Pharmacopsychiatry* 1996;29:23–26.

73. Reynolds EH, Chanarin I, Milner G, et al. Anticonvulsant therapy, folic acid and vitamin B_{12} metabolism and mental symptoms. *Epilepsia* 1966;7:261–270.

74. Trimble MR, Corbett JA, Donaldson D. Folic acid and mental symptoms in children with epilepsy. *J Neurol Neurosurg Psychiatry* 1980;43:1030–1034.

75. Charney MN. Psychiatric aspects of folate deficiency. In: *Folic acid in neurology, psychiatry, and internal medicine.* New York: Raven Press, 1979:475–482.

76. Froscher W, Maier V, Laage M, et al. Folate deficiency, anticonvulsant drugs, and psychiatric morbidity. *Clin Neuropharmacol* 1995;18:165–182.

77. Lishman WA. Vitamin deficiencies. In: Lishman WA, ed. *Organic psychiatry: the psychological consequences of cerebral disorders.* Palo Alto, CA: Blackwell Scientific Publications, 1987:486–507.

78. Wheelock I, Peterson C, Buchel HA. Presugery expectations, postsurgery satisfaction, and psychosocial adjustment after epilepsy surgery. *Epilepsia* 1998;39:487–494.

79. Naylor AS, Rogvi-Hansen B, Kessing L, et al. Psychiatric morbidity after surgery for epilepsy: short-term follow up of patients undergoing amygdalohippocampectomy. *J Neurol Neurosurg Psychiatry* 1994;57:1375–1381.

80. Hermann BP, Wyler AR. Depression, locus of control, and the effects of epilepsy surgery. *Epilepsia* 1989;30:332–338.

81. Smith DB. Cognitive effects of antiepileptic drugs. In:

Smith DB, Treiman DM, Trimble MR, eds. *Advances in neurology,* Volume 55. *Neurobehavioral problems in epilepsy.* New York: Raven Press, 1991:197–212.

82. Ketter TA, Malow BA, Flamini R, et al. Felbamate monotherapy has stimulant-like effects in patients with epilepsy. *Epilepsy Res* 1996;23:129–137.

83. Brent DA, Crumrine PK, Varma RR, et al. Phenobarbital treatment and major depressive disorder in children with epilepsy. *Pediatrics* 1987;80:909–917.

84. Brent DA, Crumrine PK, Varma RR, et al. Phenobarbital treatment and major depressive disorder in children with epilepsy. *Pediatrics* 1990;85:1086–1091.

85. Trimble MR. Anticonvulsant-induced psychiatric disorders. *Drug Safety* 1996;15:159–166.

86. Trimble MR. New antiepileptic drugs and psychopathology. *Neuropsychobiology* 1998;38:149–151.

87. Reynolds EH, Ring HA, Farr IN, et al. Open, double-blind and long-term study of vigabatrin in chronic epilepsy. *Epilepsia* 1991;32:530–538.

88. *Physicians Desk Reference,* 53rd ed. Montvale, NJ: Medical Economics Co., 1999.

89. Charles CL, Stoesz L, Tollefson G. Zonisamide-induced mania. *Psychosomatics* 1990;31:214–217.

90. Fenwick P. Evocation and inhibition of seizures behavioral treatment. In: Smith DB, Treiman DM, Trimble MR, eds. *Advances in neurology,* Volume 55. *Neurobehavioral problems in epilepsy.* New York: Raven Press, 1991:163–183.

91. Agras WS. Behavioral therapy. In: Kaplan HI, Sadock BJ, eds. *Comprehensive textbook of psychiatry/VI.* Baltimore: Williams & Wilkins, 1995:1788–1807.

92. Davis GR, Armstrong HE, Donovan DM, et al. Cognitive-behavioral treatment of depressed affect among epileptics: preliminary findings. *J Clin Psychol* 1984;40:930–935.

93. Newsom-Davis I, Goldstein LH, Fitzpatrick D. Fear of seizures: an investigation and treatment. *Seizure* 1998;7:101–106.

94. Thompson PJ, Upton D. The impact of chronic epilepsy on the family. *Seizure* 1992;1:43–48.

95. Kuhn R. The treatment of depressive disorders with G22 355 (imipramine hydrochloride). *Am J Psychiatry* 1958;115:459–464.

96. Robertson MM, Trimble MR. The treatment of depression in patients with epilepsy. A double-blind trial. *J Affect Disord* 1985;9:127–136.

97. Ojemann LM, Friel PN, Trejo WJ, et al. Effect of doxepin on seizure frequency in depressed epileptic patients. *Neurology* 1982;33:646–648.

98. Ojemann LM, Baugh-Bookman C, Dudley DL. Effect of psychotropic medications on seizure control in patients with epilepsy. *Neurology* 1987;37:1525–1527.

99. Roose SP, Glassman AH, Attia E, et al. Selective serotonin reuptake inhibitor efficacy in melancholia and atypical depression. Paper presented at the 147th annual meeting of the American Psychiatric Association, Philadelphia, PA, May 21–26, 1994.

100. Schatzberg AF, Cole JO, Debattista C, eds. *Manual of clinical psychopharmacology,* 3rd ed. Washington, DC: American Psychiatric Press, 1997:70.

101. Blumer D, Zielinski JJ. Pharmacologic treatment of psychiatric disorders associated with epilepsy. *J Epilepsy* 1988;1:135–150.

102. Charney DS, Berman RM, Miller HL. Treatment of depression. In: Schatzberg AF, Nemeroff CB, eds.

Textbook of psychopharmacology, 2nd ed. Washington, DC: American Psychiatric Press, 1998:705–731.

103. McConnell H, Duncan D. Treatment of psychiatric comorbidity in epilepsy. In: McConnell H, Snyder PJ, eds. *Psychiatric comorbidity in epilepsy: basic mechanisms, diagnosis, and treatment.* Washington, DC: American Psychiatric Press, 1998:245–362.

104. Golden RN, Dawkins K, Nicholas L, et al. Trazodone, nefazodone, bupropion, and mirtazapine. In: Schatzberg AF, Nemeroff CB, eds. *Textbook of psychopharmacology,* 2nd ed. Washington, DC: American Psychiatric Press, 1998:251–269.

105. Silverstone PH, Ravindran A. Once-daily venlafaxine extended release (XR) compared with fluoxetine in outpatients with depression and anxiety. *J Clin Psychiatry* 1999;60:22–28.

106. Starkstein SE, Robinson RG. Depression in cerebrovascular disease. In: Starkstein SE, Robertson RG, eds. *Depression in neurologic disease.* Baltimore: Johns Hopkins University Press, 1993:28–49.

107. PCS Rx Review. *SSRIs: patient considerations and economic factors.* Scottsdale, AZ: PCS Health Systems, 1999.

108. Sussman N. The role of antidepressants in sexual dysfunction. *J Clin Psychiatry* 1999;17:9–14.

109. Delgado PL, McGahuey CA, Moreno FA, et al. Treatment strategies for depression and sexual dysfunction. *J Clin Psychiatry* 1999;17:15–22.

110. Rosenstein DL, Nelson JC, Jacobs SC. Seizures associated with antidepressants: a review. *J Clin Psychiatry* 1993;54:289–299.

111. Preskorn SH, Fast GA. Tricyclic antidepressant-induced seizures and plasma drug concentration. *J Clin Psychiatry* 1992;53:160–162.

112. Potter WZ, Manji HK, Rudorfer MV. Tricyclics and tetracyclics. In: Schatzberg AF, Nemeroff CB, eds. Textbook of psychopharmacology, 2nd ed. Washington, DC: American Psychiatric Press, 1998:199–218.

113. Levy RH. Cytochrome P450 isozymes and antiepileptic drug interactions. *Epilepsia* 1995;36:S8–S13.

114. Davidson J. Seizures and bupropion: a review. *J Clin Psychiatry* 1989;50:256–261.

115. Horne RL, Ferguson JM, Pope HG, et al. Treatment of bulimia with bupropion: a multicenter controlled trial. *J Clin Psychiatry* 1988;49:262–266.

116. Jabbari B, Bryan GE, Marsh EE, et al. Incidence of seizures with tricyclic and tetracyclic antidepressants. *Arch Neurol* 1985;42:480–481.

117. Jick SS, Jick H, Knauss TA, et al. Antidepressants and convulsions. *J Clin Psychopharmacol* 1992;12:241–245.

118. Johnston JA, Lineberry CG, Ascher JA, et al. A 102-center prospective study in association with bupropion. *J Clin Psychiatry* 1991;52:450–456.

119. Leonard BE. Safety of amoxapine. *Lancet* 1989;2:808.

120. Milne RJ, Goa KL. Citalopram: a review of its pharmacodynamic and pharmacokinetic properties, and therapeutic potential in depressive illness. *Drugs* 1991;41:450–477.

121. Montgomery SA. Novel selective serotonin reuptake inhibitors. Part 1. *J Clin Psychiatry* 1992;53:107–112.

122. Peck AW, Stern WC, Watkinson C. Incidence of seizures during treatment of tricyclic antidepressants and bupropion. *J Clin Psychiatry* 1983;44:197–201.

123. Personne M, Persson H, Sjoberg G. Citalopram toxicity. *Lancet* 1997;350:519.

124. Product information. Effexor, venlafaxine. Philadelphia: Wyeth-Ayerst Laboratories, 1997.

125. Product information. Prozac, fluoxetine. Indianapolis: Dista Products Company, 1997.

126. Product information. Remeron, mirtazapine. West Orange, NJ: Organon Inc., 1996.

127. Product information. Wellbutrin, bupropion. Research Triangle Park, NC: Burroughs Wellcome Co., 1999.

128. Product information. Wellbutrin SR, bupropion sustained release. Research Triangle Park, NC: Burroughs Wellcome Co., 1999.

129. Setz SC, Anderson DA, Lawler, et al. Acute venlafaxine overdose a multicenter study. *J Toxicol Clin Toxicol* 1995;33:496.

130. Tasini M. Complex partial seizures in a patient receiving trazodone. *J Clin Psychiatry* 1986;47:318–319.

131. Wedin GP, Oderda GM, Klein-Schwartz W, et al. Relative toxicity of cyclic antidepressants. *Ann Emerg Med* 1986;15:797–804.

132. Wernicke JF. The side effect profile and safety of fluoxetine. *J Clin Psychiatry* 1985;46:59–67.

133. Cardoni AA. *Clomipramine.* Englewood, CO: Micromedics electronic version, 1999.

134. Litovitz TL, Troutman WG. Amoxapine overdose. Seizures and fatalities. *JAMA* 1983;250:1069–1071.

135. Merigan KS, Browning RG, Leeper KV. Successful treatment of amoxapine-induced refractory status epilepticus with propofol. *Acad Emerg Med* 1995;2:12

136. DeToledo JC, Haddad H, Ramsay RE. Status epilepticus associated with the combination of valproic acid and clomipramine. *Ther Drug Monit* 1997;19:71–73.

137. Bodkin JA, Lasser RA, Wines JD, et al. Combining serotonin reuptake inhibitors and bupropion in partial responders to antidepressant monotherapy. *J Clin Psychiatry* 1997;58:137–145.

138. Phillips S, Brent J, Kulig K, et al. Fluoxetine versus tricyclic antidepressants: a prospective multicenter study of antidepressant drug overdoses. The Antidepressant Study Group. *J Emerg Med* 1997;15:439–445.

139. Goldstein L, Barker M, Segal F, et al. Seizure and transient SIADH associated with sertraline. *Am J Psychiatry* 1996;153:732.

140. Feeney DJ, Klykylo M. Medication-induced seizures. *Am Acad Child Adolesc Psychiatry* 1997;36:1018–1019.

141. Gross-Tsur V, Manor O, van der Meere J, et al. Epilepsy and attention deficit hyperactivity disorder: is methylphenidate safe and effective. *J Pediatr* 1997;130:670–674.

142. Wroblewski BA, Leary JM, Phelan AM, et al. Methylphenidate and seizure frequency in brain injured patients with seizure disorders. *J Clin Psychiatry* 1992;53:86–89.

143. Schatzberg AF, Cole JO, Debattista C, eds. *Manual of clinical psychopharmacology,* 3rd ed. Washington, DC: American Psychiatric Press, 1997:320–323.

144. Shukla S, Mukherjee S, Decina P. Lithium in the treatment of bipolar disorders associated with epilepsy: an open study. *J Clin Psychopharmacol* 1988;8:201–204.

145. Harvey AT, Preskorn SH. Cytochrome P450 enzymes: interpretation of their interactions with selective serotonin reuptake inhibitors. Part I. *J Clin Pscyhopharmacol* 1996;16:273–285.

146. Nemeroff CB, DeVane CL, Pollock BG. New antide-

pressants and the cytochrome P450 system. *Am J Psychiatry* 1996;153:311–320.

147. Michalets EL. Update: clinically significant cytochrome P-450 drug interaction. *Pharmacotherapy* 1998;18:84–112.

148. Mullen WJ, North DS, Weiss MA. Pharmaceuticals and the cytochrome P450 isoenzymes: a tool for decision making. *Pharm Pract News* 1998:21–23.

149. Pham Z, Anderson PO. Cytochrome P450 in drug metabolism and interactions. *Discourse* 1996;18:1–4.

150. Riesenman C. Antidepressant drug interactions and the cytochrome P450 system: a critical appraisal. *Pharmacotherapy* 1995;15:84S–99S.

151. Spina E, Pisani F, Perucca E. Clinically significant pharmacokinetic drug interactions with carbamazepine: an update. *Clin Pharmacokinet* 1996;31:198–214.

152. Keck PE, McElroy SL. Antiepileptic drugs. In: Schatzberg AF, Nemeroff CB, eds. *Textbook of psychopharmacology*, 2nd ed. Washington, DC: American Psychiatric Press, 1998:431–454.

153. Messina FS. Fluoxetine: adverse effects and drug–drug interactions. *Clin Toxicol* 1993;31:603–630.

154. Schroeder DH. Metabolism and kinetics of bupropion. *J Clin Psychiatry* 1983;44:79–81.

155. Droulers A, Bodak N, Oudjhani M, et al. Decrease of valproic acid concentration in the blood when coprescribed with fluoxetine. *J Clin Psychopharmacol* 1997;17:139.

156. Dursun SM, Mathew VM, Reveley MA. Toxic serotonin syndrome after fluoxetine plus carbamazepine. *Lancet* 1993;342:442–443.

157. Fritze J, Unsorg B, Lanczik M. Interaction between carbamazepine and fluvoxamine. *Acta Psychiatr Scand* 1991;84:583–584.

158. Gernaat HBPE, Van De Woude J, Touw DJ. Fluoxetine and parkinsonism in patients taking carbamazepine. *Am J Psychiatry* 1991;148:1604–1605.

159. Grimsley SR, Jann MW, Carter G, et al. Increased carbamazepine plasma concentrations after fluoxetine coadministration. *Clin Pharmacol Ther* 1991;50:10–15.

160. Haselberger MB, Freedman LS, Tolbert S. Elevated serum phenytoin concentrations associated with coadministration of sertraline. *J Clin Psychopharmacol* 1997;17:107–109.

161. Jalil P. Toxic reaction following the combined administration of fluoxetine and phenytoin: two case reports. *J Neurol Neurosurg Psychiatry* 1992;55:412–413.

162. Lucena MI, Blanco E, Corrales MA, et al. Interaction of fluoxetine and valproic acid. *Am J Psychiatry* 1998;155:575.

163. Pearson HJ. Interaction of fluoxetine with carbamazepine. *J Clin Psychiatry* 1990;51:126.

164. Weber SW. Drug interactions with antidepressants. *CNS Special Edition* 1999:47–55.

165. Baldessarini RJ, Teicher MH, Cassidy JW, et al. Anti-convulsant cotreatment may increase toxic metabolites of antidepressants and other psychotropic drugs. *J Clin Psychopharmacol* 1998;8:381–382.

166. Monaco F, Cicolin A. Interactions between anticonvulsants and psychoactive drugs. *Epilepsia* 1999;40:S71–S76.

167. Nelson JC. Augmentation strategies with serotonin-noradrenergic combinations. *J Clin Psychiatry* 1998;59[Suppl 5]:65–69.

168. Brown TM, Skop BP, Mareth TR. Pathophysiology and management of the serotonin syndrome. *Ann Pharmacother* 1996;30:527–533.

169. Steinbach H. The serotonin syndrome. *Am J Psychiatry* 1991;148:705–713.

170. Brown TM, Skop BP, Mareth TR. Pathophysiology and management of the serotonin syndrome. *Ann Pharmacother* 1996;30:527–533.

171. Schwartz CE. A surfeit of serotonin: sumatriptan and serotonergic antidepressants. *Arch Intern Med* 1999;159:1141–1142.

172. The Vagus Nerve Stimulation Study Group. A randomized controlled trial of chronic vagus nerve stimulation for treatment of medically intractable seizures. *Neurology* 1995;224:230.

173. Harden C. Effect of vagus nerve stimulation on mood in adult epilepsy patients. AAN Scientific Program Abstract, 1999.

174. Rush JA, George MS, Sackeim HA, et al. Vagus nerve stimulation for treatment-resistant depressions: a multicenter study. *Biol Psychiatry* 2000;47:276–286.

175. Ben-Menacham E, Hamberger A, Hedner T, et al. Effects of vagal nerve stimulation on amino acids and other metabolites in the CSF of patients with partial seizures. *Epilepsy Res* 1995;20:221–227.

176. Figiel GS, McDonald WM, McCall WV, et al. Electroconvulsive therapy. In: Schatzberg AF, Nemeroff CB, eds. *Textbook of psychopharmacology*, 2nd ed. Washington, DC: American Psychiatric Press, 1998:523–545.

177. Dubovsky SL. *Electroconvulsive therapy. In: Kaplan HI, Sadock BJ, eds.* Comprehensive textbook of psychiatry/VI. Baltimore: Williams & Wilkins, 1995:2129–2140.

178. Regenold WT, Weintraub D, Taller A. Electroconvulsive therapy for epilepsy and major depression. *Am J Geriatr Psychiatry* 1998;6:180–183.

179. Kaufman KR, Saucedo C, Schaeffer J, et al. Electroconvulsive therapy for intractable depression following epilepsy neurosurgery. *Seizure* 1996;5:307–312.

180. Fink M, Kellner C, Sackeim HA. Intractable seizures, status epilepticus, and ECT. *JECT Lett* 1999;15:282–4.

181. Sackheim HA, Prudic J, Devanand DP, et al. A prospective, randomized, double-blind comparison of bilateral and right unilateral electroconvulsive therapy at different stimulus intensities. *Arch Gen Psychiatry* 2000;57:425–434.

6

Psychosis of Epilepsy

An Integrated Approach

Mark Rayport and *Shirley M. Ferguson

*Departments of Neurological Surgery and *Psychiatry, Medical College of Ohio, Toledo, Ohio 43614*

In this chapter, we offer a critical evaluation of the prolonged debate regarding the relationship between seizures and psychosis and seek the areas of consensus. We will consider episodic and chronic epileptic psychosis separately and distinguish between correlative and direct observations, believing that the latter offer understanding of causal relationships. We will describe our experience with a prospective interdisciplinary approach that joins the insights of the clinical disciplines of neuropsychiatry, neurological surgery, and neurology, with laboratory data from neurodiagnostic electrophysiology and radiology.

The antecedents of the vast literature of the past 2 centuries on the compelling topic of behavior disturbances in epilepsy (BDE) extend back through two and a half millennia to the brilliant iatric conclusion of Hippocrates that epilepsy, not sacred, arose from the brain, as did all behavior. Mental aberration as a possible accompaniment or manifestation of epilepsy is an idea prominent in the history of epileptic theory since antiquity.

Temkin's masterful historical review traces ideas about insanity in epileptics from ancient times to the end of the nineteenth century (1). In each historical period, ideas about the nature of insanity in epilepsy reflected current social, cultural, biologic, and psychiatric understanding and beliefs. Pre-twentieth century observers had highly developed clinical skills and an impressive ability to communicate

their findings and theories. Many of the observations and some of the theories have been corroborated. Others have been extended or reinterpreted in light of twentieth century knowledge.

The focused study of epilepsy appears to have begun in the early nineteenth century in the new psychiatric institutions. Esquirol (1772–1840) stressed the close association between epilepsy and insanity. He observed that "epileptic mania" could occur before, after, or independently of classical seizures and might last several days. Delasiauve (1794–1870) collected cases of epileptics who had come to the attention of the courts. He mentioned a man who had been institutionalized because of mental derangement, who had escaped and killed his wife, and who, on returning to confinement, was observed over time to have periods when he would show "a peculiar change" when his speech was described as "irritated" and he would express a violent urge to strike out. It was later found that he had been suffering from nocturnal epileptic attacks for a long time. After 1860, the influential psychiatric voices were those of Morel (1809–1879) and Falret (1824–1902), who brought a psychologically oriented approach to epileptics. Morel's friend Lasègue wrote of him that "he was the first, or one of the first, to discern the epileptic within the epilepsy; and instead of limiting himself to the description of the attacks, he has recounted the biography of the patient" (Temkin, op. cit., p. 317). Morel affirmed that epilepsy could exist in a "masked or larval" form ("épilepsie larvée"), which was diagnosed by the "main symptoms of epileptic insanity." Épilepsie larvée could exist by itself without any customary attacks of epilepsy, although it was no less dangerous (2). Falret stated that epileptic insanity could precede or follow a convulsion and might occur unrelated to a seizure; in the latter circumstance, previously unnoticed nocturnal attacks were discovered later. Patients who later acquired ordinary seizures became less violent (3). Specialized institutional care for epileptics was provided in Europe and the United States during the later decades of the nineteenth century. The National Hospital for the Paralyzed and Epileptic was founded in London in 1860. An epileptic colony was established in Germany at Bielefeld in 1867. In the United States, a separate institution for epileptics opened in 1891 at Gallipolis, Ohio, followed in 1902 by Craig Colony at Sonyea, New York.

Hughlings Jackson (1835–1911), the giant of English neurology, made his great contributions to the understanding of epilepsy from 1861 to 1906. Jackson interpreted the effect of seizure discharge on observable behavioral changes in light of evolutionary theory. In a seizure, the highest centers are affected first and disabled by the epileptic discharge. Lower centers take over and automatic action results. Jackson explained the behavior of the insane person as might be expected of a person living on a lower evolutionary plane. He thought that insane behavior resulted from activity of part of the brain that is healthy but out of control (1). Of transient "epileptic insanity," Hughlings Jackson (4) wrote that it could result from frequent slight seizures: "The gravity of these cases is not because the paroxysms are slight, but because the 'discharging lesion,' in cases in which such slight fits often occur, is of the highest and most intellectual nervous arrangements (substrata of consciousness)."

With the spread of psychological psychiatry in the early twentieth century, the study and care of epileptic patients passed from psychiatry to neurology. Emphasis shifted from the study of the epileptic person to the study of epileptic seizures.

Outstanding landmarks in twentieth century epileptology should be noted. An epochal highlight occurred in 1929 with the discovery of scalp electroencephalography (EEG) by Hans Berger (1873–1941). His communications created the basis of the discipline of clinical EEG and, perhaps more importantly, opened floodgates to physiologic investigation and understanding of the physiopathology of the epileptic process. In 1938, Houston Merritt (1902–1979) and Tracy Putnam (1894–1975) launched phenytoin, the first nonsedative antiepileptic drug (AED). In the 1930s, in the course of his landmark work in the neurosurgical treatment of medically intractable partial seizures and cortical mapping, Wilder Penfield (1891–1976) by electrical stimulation (5) evoked "experiential responses," some of which corresponded to memories. In 1948, Frederic A. Gibbs (1903–1992) et al. (6) published interictal EEG evidence of epileptiform EEG disturbance over the temporal lobes in patients with "psychomotor seizures," a term introduced in 1907 by Turner. In 1951, Gibbs (7) reported that behavioral disturbances occurred in 25% of cases with epileptiform activity of the temporal lobes.

After World War II, major scientific, technologic, clinical, and social advances made it possible to demonstrate and clarify correlations between cerebral physiopathology and clinical seizures. In Paris, Jean Talairach created his highly precise multiprobe stereotactic methodology. With Jean Bancaud (1921–1993) and other associates, he developed intracerebral stereoelectroencephalography (SEEG) for epilepsy (8–10). Talairach and Tournoux (11,12) recently extended this biplanar stereotactic methodology to the three-dimensional level. This proportional grid system has been adopted by the human functional brain imaging community for recording and comparison of data between patients and between centers. In the 1970s, a sequence of new antiseizure medications began with carbamazepine and valproic acid. Ground-breaking basic research into seizure mechanisms led to the designing of new AEDs. Significant advances in the diagnosis and classification of seizures devolved from videoelectroencephalography (VEEG) monitoring of spontaneous seizures led by J. Kiffin Penry (1929–1996) at the National Institutes of Health. This methodology was extended to videostereoelectroencephalography (VSEEG) with chronically implanted intracerebral electrodes, further improving presurgical localization in medically intractable partial seizures. Air encephalography, angiography, computed axial tomography (CT), algorithms of magnetic resonance imaging (MRI), proton emission tomography (PET), and single photon emission computerized tomography (SPECT) of the brain have yielded unprecedented clinical and scientific insights into normal and epileptic brain functioning.

Psychiatric interest in psychosis of epilepsy was reinitiated in the 1950s by the articles of Hill (13) and Pond (14) describing "epileptic paranoid hallucinatory psychosis" in patients with temporal lobe epilepsy (TLE). They differentiated this psychosis from schizophrenia by the absence of schizoid tendencies in the previous personality, the warmth of affect, and the continuation of social interaction. In a group of influential papers, Slater et al. (15) concluded that the "schizophrenia-like psychoses of epilepsy" (SLPE) were "symptomatic epileptic psychoses." They concurred with Hill and Pond with regard to the differences from schizophrenia, adding that their cases had organic mental findings and a lack of genetic taint. In Slater's sense, the expression "schizophrenia-like psychosis" acknowledged a limited overlap of the symptomatology of chronic psychosis of epilepsy with schizophrenia, but Eliot Slater (1904–1983) explicitly articulated the differences from schizophrenia.

Research into BDE remained controversial during most of the twentieth century, characterized as the "era of normalcy" of personality in epilepsy (16). The reluctance of the epilepsy community to accept psychiatric research is now dissipating in response to the widening emphasis, beyond seizure control, on quality of life for the epileptic person, and to rational advocacy for research into BDE (17,18). A spate of books and new journals have appeared in the past few years with previously unthinkable titles linking research on epilepsy and behavior. Psychoanalysis, phenomenologic psychiatry, and the psychobiologic viewpoint of Adolph Meyer (1866–1950) evolved into the biopsychosocial model of George L. Engel, followed by the leadership of Eli Robbins (1921–1994) in biologic psychiatry. Neuropsychiatry has been formally revived with a national association, a new journal, and major textbooks that reestablish the clinical mind–brain discipline on a platform of contemporary neuroscience and psychiatry. At this time, the study of BDE has yet to be accepted into neuropsychiatry in a manner commensurate with the opportunities it offers in the study of mind–brain relationships in man. Neuropsychiatry is beginning to have a home in the productive stream of the modern neuroscientific epileptology.

The latter twentieth century has been named for a process as "the era of neuroscientific observation" (19), a necessary and hopeful phase on the road to the understanding of our patients. The task of the twenty-first century will be to expand and integrate the scientific and humanistic legacy it has received from the nineteenth century and from the unparalleled twentieth century.

DEFINITIONS OF PSYCHOSIS OF EPILEPSY

The definitions and classification of psychosis of epilepsy evolved over time. In 1949, a psychiatric dictionary divided psychotic syndromes into schizophrenic, manic-depressive, and organic, the latter to be applied when the psychosis was associated with brain disorder (20). In 1956, Henderson and Gillespie (21), following Adolph Meyer, spoke of different types of mental disorder as "reaction types" to concentrate on the study of the individual as a "psycho-biological organism perpetually called upon to adapt to a social environment." They proposed a classification that numbered nine reaction types, one of these being epilepsy as a separate diagnostic entity.

Slater and Roth (22) considered psychosis of epilepsy "an integral part of the epileptic development out of pre-existing physiological change and content derived from aural and semi-confusional epileptic experiences." They agreed with Pond (14) that psychosis of epilepsy was not schizophrenia. They brought attention to the effect of definition on the successful pursuit of understanding. Differentiation of epileptic psychosis from other symptomatic psychosis or from schizophrenia could be difficult at times. They cautioned against making a "double diagnosis" if epilepsy antedated the paranoid psychosis. Their apt remark, "If typical fits occur, there will probably be no difficulty in diagnosis," expresses reality and echoed nineteenth century writing before the availability of EEG. Bruens (23) reviewed Slater's cases and concluded that "none of the psychoses fulfilled the criteria for the diagnosis of schizophrenia." He described the delusions and hallucinations of psychotic epileptics as "empathizable—the patient remains in our world." In 1979, Kristensen and Sindrup (24) described psychosis in 45 patients with complex partial seizures (CPS). They listed symptoms as simple persecutory delusions and hallucinations; the delusions were "not far off from everyday life." They also stated that the patient would have appropriate affect and that autistic traits were uncommon. They emphasized the etiologic importance of organic cerebral damage.

In counterpoint, Perez and Trimble (25) approached the diagnosis of psychosis in epileptic patients with a quantitative methodology based on the Present State Examination (PSE), a structured interview oriented to symptoms present during the examination or in the past month. PSE questionnaire data were analyzed and classified into descriptive classes of diagnoses using the CATEGO computer program (26). The findings in 23 consecutive cases of unequivocal epilepsy who were "suffering from active psychosis in the setting of clear consciousness" were compared with ten control patients diagnosed by senior psychiatrists as process schizophrenics. Of the 23 epileptics, 16 had TLE and seven had generalized epilepsy. Among the TLE cases, they found eleven (68.8%) whose symptom profile was that of "nuclear schizophrenic syndrome" similar to the nonepileptic schizophrenic group. The authors acknowledged that the PSE, which uses Schneider's first rank symptoms, is not recommended for classification of patients with organic brain pathology. They noted further that the diagnosis of paranoid psychosis was rare in their sample and mainly was found in association with affective disorder. This feature of their small study population contrasts with the consensus in the literature with regard to the prominence of paranoid symptomatology in epileptic psychosis. Subsequent authors supported the report of Perez and Trimble, seemingly reversing Slater's conclusions that psychosis of epilepsy was "schizophrenia-like but not schizophrenia" to it being "process schizophrenia" (27,28).

Other authors who used clinical research methodology concurred with Slater et al. (15) "that the psychoses observed are etiologically different from ordinary forms of schizophrenia and constitute a special kind of epileptic psychosis." Toone et al. (29) supported the specificity of the psychosis of TLE, stating that "epileptic psychosis is a distinct nosological entity." Parnas and Korsgaard (30) pointed out that the clinical findings in epileptic psychosis seldom fulfilled the bleulerian concept of schizophrenia. They concluded that the term "schizophrenia-like" should be avoided, that "a unitary theory cannot be maintained," and proposed a multifactorial hypothesis, indicating that organic and psychosocial causes had to be considered. They also advocated prospective research in contrast to the usual retrospective analysis. Since 1969, the present writers have reported prospective multifactorial studies in which they implemented the need to know the person with epilepsy—"to discern the epileptic within the epilepsy"

(Lasègue, 1873) in order to understand the phenomenology of the psychosis (31–35). Their findings form the basis of the definition of psychosis of epilepsy proposed here.

In summary, this brief chronologic review has shown notable consensus throughout recorded history with regard to the occurrence and psychiatric symptomatology of psychosis in epilepsy. Challenge to this consensus has come from investigators utilizing questionnaire-based enumeration of symptoms, methodology that detaches psychiatric symptomatology from its setting in the clinical course of the epilepsy, the content of the subject's mind, and his or her life circumstances. We would draw attention again to the problem of coexistent, noninterchangeable methodologies of research into BDE (32,33,35).

Proposed Definitions of Psychosis of Epilepsy

Episodic psychosis of epilepsy (EPE) occurs predominantly in patients with temporolimbic epilepsy (TLmE) or in those with partial seizures that propagate to the temporal limbic structures from other lobes. EPE results from an increase in the frequency of partial seizures or from partial or generalized status epilepticus (SE). EPE usually occurs in clear consciousness. The psychiatric symptomatology is characterized by prominent paranoid delusions and hallucinations that tend to relate variously to intrusive ictal experiences, cognitive impairment, and the patient's psychodynamics. There may be a prominent affective component. Duration of the episodes ranges from days to weeks. Typically, EPE is followed by full recovery, with the patient's mental condition reverting to the prepsychotic state.

Chronic or *nonepisodic psychosis of epilepsy* (nonEPE) has similar psychiatric symptomatology, but not the recovery. NonEPE may result from the coalescence of psychotic episodes resulting from increased frequency of seizures or partial SE. The episodic exacerbations observed in nonEPE suggest a role of increased partial seizure discharge in the continuance of the psychotic state.

Psychosis of epilepsy is not process schizophrenia insofar as primary thought disorder, the hallmark of that diagnosis, is not present. Neither is it a delirium because the patient does not have a primary disorder of attention, as in the so-called twilight states (36,37).

PATHOGENESIS OF PSYCHOSIS OF EPILEPSY

Some of the current hypotheses for the development of psychosis in epileptic patients are examined in the following.

Anatomopathologic Data

Correlations of epileptic psychosis with structural brain pathology have been reported extensively from many sources. Kristensen and Sindrup (24) studied retrospectively the hospital or epilepsy center records (1964–1976) of 192 patients, 45 (23.4%) of whom had suffered from "interictal paranoid psychotic disorder." The psychoses were episodic, lasting several weeks, or permanent. Their data, which included clinical neurologic, otoneurologic, pneumoencephalographic, and psychological studies, indicated to them the presence of an organic brain lesion. They concluded that "epileptic psychoses are organic caused by structural cerebral damage in deep limbic parts of the temporal lobe responsible for epilepsy and psychosis." Bruton (38) reviewed the Maudsley cases of temporal lobectomy for seizure control (TLX) operated by Murray A. Falconer (1910–1977), summarizing a role for alien tissue lesions. Ten patients with epilepsy and SLPE had larger cerebral ventricles, excess periventricular gliosis, and more focal cerebral damage compared with epileptics who had no psychotic illness (39). Epileptic patients who develop psychosis had neurodevelopmental abnormalities involving the medial temporal lobe (40).

We wish to point out that anatomic alterations in a physiopathologic syndrome, particularly one that is usually or initially episodic, plausibly furnish etiologic correlations for the epilepsy but are not by themselves explanatory for the psychosis.

Biochemical Explanations

Reynolds (41) suggested that psychosis could represent a pharmacologically induced mental state due to folate deficiency in epileptic patients treated with phenytoin.

The discovery of altered dopamine metabolism in major mental illness in the 1970s was applied to an explanation of psychosis in epilepsy. Trimble (42) proposed a role for dopamine, which is inhibited during epileptic seizures and increased in psychosis. Ring et al. (43) observed significantly decreased D2 receptor binding in the basal ganglia of seven actively psychotic epileptics compared with seven nonpsychotic epileptics, and they proposed that periictally arising psychoses were associated with increased seizure-provoked release of dopamine. The decreased binding could be the result of anticonvulsant drug therapy (44). Increased metabolism of an exogenous dopa tracer in the neostriatum in TLmE patients with a history of psychosis and in patients with schizophrenia was regarded as consistent with the theory that a state of psychosis arises when episodic dopamine excess is superimposed on a trait of basic dopamine deficiency in the striatum (45). A recent review concluded that epilepsy and psychiatric disturbances may have a shared organic basis but that, at present, the neurochemical mechanisms by which such psychiatric disorders could be produced remain unclear (46).

Electrophysiologic Data

Studies with extracranial EEG tracings and seizure monitoring have been inconclusive or have failed to elucidate the relationship between seizures and psychosis. Kohler (47) found that the EEG in the psychotic patient most often was characterized by the "simultaneous appearance of sharp waves, paroxysmal discharges and abnormal rhythm formatics." Kristensen and Sindrup (24) found in the psychotic patient a preponderance of temporal medial-basal spike foci. Ramani and Gumnit (48), in an epilepsy unit, studied ten patients diagnosed as having an "interictal psychosis." The patients were observed behaviorally, with VEEG and serum AED monitoring. They concluded that "the emergence of psychosis could not be explained."

We present an illustrative case.

Case KOM: *Left TLX results in freedom from intractable CPS for 4.5 years. Recurrence of CPS is followed by partial SE of the left temporal lobe and episodic paranoid psychosis in clear consciousness.*

During neuropsychiatric presurgical evaluation, KOM, a single right-handed man with intractable CPS and secondary generalization, who had no history of previous psychosis, was found to have a schizoid personality with paranoid sensitivity. Seizure monitoring with VSEEG defined a primary epileptogenic zone in the left hippocampal formation. After left TLX at age 31 years, he became seizure-free. He had no modification of personality. He remained seizure-free for 4.5 years while taking preoperative doses of monitored serum-level AED during the first 2 years, then during a period of very gradual (at his request) tapering, and then for 7 months without medication. While visiting relatives in another state, over the course of several days his behavior changed to indolence, mutism, and periods of staring. He had a CPS with secondary generalization. After several more CPSs, he became psychotic. His family contacted our epilepsy unit on the sixth day of symptoms. His readmission was promptly implemented. While in the epilepsy unit, KOM had no clinical seizures. On neuropsychiatric examination, he was acutely paranoid in clear consciousness. Immediate EEG revealed continual focal discharge in the left posterior temporal derivations. Neuropsychiatric diagnosis was EPE due to partial SE of left posterior temporal lobe. AEDs and neuroleptic medication were prescribed. He recovered psychiatrically as his AED serum levels rose into the therapeutic range. A recurrence of left temporal SE was associated with recurrence of the psychosis. The AED regimen was adjusted. He was discharged after 22 days, seizure-free and psychosis-free. He has remained free of seizures and psychosis for 9 years while taking AEDs and (at his request) low doses of psychotropic medication.

Comment: Paranoid psychosis developed acutely in a patient who had attained a successful outcome after left TLX 5 years earlier. When readmitted to the epilepsy unit, he did not have observable seizures. Prompt EEG confirmed the clinical diagnosis of SPSE. Reinstated AED therapy was guided by determination of serum levels. Antipsychotic medication was initiated. When psychosis reappeared during his hospital course, repeat EEG showed recurrence of left temporal SPSE. Improvement of the AED regimen resulted in disappearance of the psychosis and normalization of the EEG.

Relationship between Psychosis and Seizures

Although there is some consensus that psychosis occurs more than coincidentally among patients with temporolimbic seizures (TLmS) (49,50), the chronologic relationships between seizure activity and psychosis have remained unsettled. Clinical observation prior to the possibility of recording electrical activity of the human brain had led to the hypothesis that psychosis occurred in relation to increased frequency of seizures (4). Since the introduction of EEG, opinion has ranged from a causal relationship between seizures and psychosis (13–15,31,32,39,51) to antagonism between seizures and psychosis (36,50,52,53).

Recurrence of Partial Seizures

A pathogenetic role for seizure recurrence in the development of psychosis in TLmE was recognized by Slater et al. (15). Seventeen of their 69 cases (24%) had "epileptic confusional episodes" that led to chronic psychosis in clear consciousness, and other cases had psychoses "complicated by recurrent confu-

sional episodes." Falconer (54) pointed out that amelioration of seizure control was accompanied by amelioration of psychosis.

The present writers have drawn attention to the role of increased frequency of TLmS in the genesis of epileptic psychosis and emphasized that these seizures could be clinically evident or subtle (31–33,35,55). Even slight seizures can be followed not only by prolonged cognitive deficits, but also by alteration of thinking (e.g., paranoid ideation) and/or shift of affect.

We previously described psychiatric outcome after TLX, directing our attention to patients who were seizure-free after TLX as persons whose brain has been relieved of the epileptogenic "discharging lesion" (34). Our results confirm those of Falconer and other previous reports of a correlation between the seizure-free state—whether achieved by AED therapy or TLX—and absence of EPE and improvement in nonEPE (15,35,38,56).

"Forced Normalization" of the Scalp Electroencephalogram

Controversy about an inverse relationship between epileptic seizures and behavioral disturbance came to the fore in 1953 when Landolt (36) introduced the concept of "forcierte Normalisation": "Forced normalization is the phenomenon characterized by the fact that, with the occurrence of psychotic states, the EEG becomes more normal or entirely normal as compared with previous and subsequent EEG findings" (p. 114). Thus, paradoxically, seizures and EEG were improved while behavior was seriously disrupted. The prevalent form of disruption was paranoid psychosis in clear consciousness. Landolt presented the relationship between seizures and psychosis as "antagonistic." The treatment of epilepsy henceforth was limited by an existential choice: "seizures or madness." A second paradox.

The concept of antagonism between epilepsy and psychosis was reviewed by Wolf and Trimble (57). Wolf (58) proposed the term "paradoxical normalization" because when "forcierte Normalisierung" is translated intuitively but perhaps not entirely accurately into English as "forced normalization," it does not convey the more relaxed meaning that the word "forcierte" has in German. Of note is that the literature on paradoxical normalization has mostly made only passing reference to the limitations of the EEG in the detection of epileptiform activity in the deeply situated epileptogenic structures of the temporal lobe. Gloor (59) discussed in detail the neuroanatomic and biophysical bases of the limitations of scalp EEG.

Correlations of ictal and periictal activity in the hippocampus and amygdala with episodic psychotic symptomatology became available through the SEEG methodology of the Talairach school (8,9). Simultaneous recordings from scalp or extradural electrodes were noteworthy for absence of ictal activity, confirming the limitations of the EEG with respect to detection of deep intracerebral electrophysiologic activity (31,56,60–63). Our experience has led us to hypothesize that a nonepileptic EEG during EPE (so-called forced normalization of the [scalp] EEG) may stem from the voltage drop in neocortical derivations ("suppression") that corresponds with seizure discharge in the hippocampus or amygdala. We agree in this regard with the conclusions of Wieser (60,62,63). Assent has been expressed more recently that EEG "normalization" during psychosis may be causally related to continuing subcortical limbic seizure activity (18,57,58).

If the relationship of increased frequency of simple partial seizures (SPSs) to psychosis has thus repeatedly received support, what has obstructed its acceptance? A perceptible source of the difficulty is that the definition of "interictal" continues to rely on the absence of epileptiform activity in the customary EEG.

Psychosis After Temporal Lobe Surgery for Seizure Control

Paranoid psychosis in clear consciousness occurring after TLX for seizure control has been known since the inception of neurosurgical treatment of "psychomotor" epilepsy between 1939 and 1950 in Montreal (Penfield), Chicago (Bailey), and London (Falconer). Attention has been drawn recently to *de novo* psychosis after TLX in patients psychiatrically well before surgery (64). For discussion and additional bibliographic references, the reader may consult a review of this topic by Rayport and Ferguson (35).

Briefly, retrospective studies, which are the major source of cases, do not contain sufficient preoperative psychiatric data for independent verification of case allocation to the category of *de novo* psychosis after TLX. Three prospective investigations, Bailey's series (65), Stevens's cases (except Case PE) (64), and Rayport's series (34) yielded 81 cases of TLmSs who had various levels of preoperative psychiatric health. Psychosis after TLX occurred in three cases (3.7%) of those psychiatrically well before surgery. Among these, Stevens's Case KL and our Case KOM recovered when restored to the seizure-free state. The EPE of Stevens's Case HM fluctuated in parallel with seizure occurrence and progressed to a fixed psychosis. Psychosis after TLX occurred in nine (11.8%) of the cases not psychiatrically well preoperatively (64). They continued to have seizures after TLX and became psychiatrically worse; however, two of these cases improved psychiatrically during seizure-free periods attained by adjustment of AEDs. We concluded that EPE after TLX occurred in TLmE patients who were psychiatrically well or not well before surgery. Of note is the prognostic difference with regard to psychosis between those cases who were and were not seizure-free after TLX (35).

We have raised the question as to whether *de novo* psychosis after TLX is a risk of temporal lobe ablation or one of failed seizure control after TLX. The general neurosurgical experience with unilateral anterior temporal lobectomy in nonepileptic persons who have a healthy lobe contralaterally is psychiatrically benign. Therefore, it seems that psychosis after TLX is a risk of failed seizure control, as it is during failed AED treatment, whether the patient is psychiatrically well or not well at the inception of the therapy.

Radiologic Data

Structural and functional neuroimaging has been used extensively in the study of cases of intractable TLmS. The essentials relevant to the present purposes are summarized briefly. In structural imaging with CT and MRI, the salient findings are unilateral or bilateral reduction of the volume of the medial temporal structures (66). Functional imaging with PET displays regional metabolic activity. In the interictal state, the epileptogenic region may or not be hypometabolic; it is hypermetabolic during ictus (67). SPECT images the levels of cerebral perfusion, from which metabolic activity may be inferred. Newer equipment provides image resolution approximating that of PET. Interictal scans show regional hypoperfusion; hyperperfusion is seen ictally in response to the increase of blood flow meeting the metabolic demand of seizure discharge (68).

In a CT study of 24 patients with epilepsy and psychosis, 17 had TLE with CPS and seven had generalized epilepsy. An association was noted between a CATEGO category of nuclear schizophrenia and a left-sided lesion. The psychotic cases showed higher than expected values on a number of variables, particularly the septum–caudate width of the lateral ventricles and the size of the third and fourth ventricles (69).

MRI findings in 12 epileptic patients with nuclear schizophrenia as determined by recently administered PSE were compared with epileptic cases who had no psychiatric history. There were no differences in T1 relaxation times in the limbic regions between the two groups, but patients who had hallucinations showed "a significantly higher T1 value in the left temporal lobe," indicating specific abnormalities in left limbic system structures related to the psychotic phenomenology (70).

Jibiki et al. (71) obtained SPECT scans in two left hemisphere dominant subjects with TLE and schizophrenia-like symptoms. Between psychotic stages, focal hypoperfusion in the left temporal lobe was regionally consistent with the EEG focus in both cases. During the psychotic state, hyperperfusion was noted in the left medial temporal lobe in one subject and normal perfusion without interlobar asymmetry in the other (71). Computerized search of the literature indicated this study to be the first in which the same patients were tested between and during psychotic episodes. The findings suggest that SPECT could be helpful when the surface EEG is uninformative in a case suspected of partial SE as a cause of EPE.

Perfusion magnetic resonance imaging (*p*MRI), which also displays blood flow, could be used under similar circumstances. A pilot study of five patients with nonepisodic SLPE and five epileptic controls led to the tentative conclusion that the SLPE cases showed significant reduction in the index of regional cerebral blood flow in the left medial temporal region (72). The SLPE cases were not psychotic and were taking psychotropic drugs when tested.

CLASSIFICATION OF PSYCHOSIS OF EPILEPSY

The classifications of psychosis in epilepsy in the twentieth century literature differ by the criteria on which they are based. Bruens (23) based his classification on the state of consciousness and duration of the psychosis. The classification of Betts (73) rested on psychopathology: (i) global disruption of personality, including the schizophrenias and schizophrenia-like states; (ii) primary disturbance of mood; and (iii) organic psychosyndromes, including changes of behavior associated with subictal epileptic activity, confusional states, and delirium. Toone (74) classified the psychotic states by the presence or absence of seizure activity: "(1) psychoses directly related to the occurrence of seizure activity"; and "(2) interictal psychoses including schizophrenia-like, paranoid and affective psychoses." Mendez and Grau (53) classified psychosis as chronic interictal, alternating, and ictal: the first implied an absence of seizure activity; the second, an antagonism between seizures and psychosis; and the third, a direct connection between seizures and psychosis.

We proposed a classification based on the relationship between seizures and psychosis (35) that avoids reliance on the "interictal" criterion for reasons presented earlier. The occurrence of epileptic psychosis in relation to increased seizure frequency has been discussed under "Electrophysiologic Data." Because the seizure discharge itself typically is of short duration, the observed clinical manifestations are predominantly postictal. This is well illustrated in the SEEG records reported by So et al. (75) of an isolated EPE in clear consciousness, which followed a 9-hour interval of mild confusion after the last of nine TLmSs with secondary generalization. When the interval between SPSs is short, or during partial SE, each of the recurrent seizures reestablishes an ensuing postictal state involving activation of neuronal inhibition and incomplete recovery before the next ictus. The psychotic state correlates with this sequence of ictal and postictal neuronal activity. Therefore, in the clinical setting, where termination of seizure recurrence is the goal, it appears diagnostically and therapeutically immaterial to differentiate the epileptic psychosis into ictal or postictal.

The classification "interictal," signifying absence of ictal activity, cannot be based primarily on the criterion of a nonepileptic extracranial EEG record, as discussed in the section on "Relationship Between Psychosis and Seizures." Highlighting "interictal" as misleading, Engel and Taylor (18) offered a unifying concept that would justify dismissal of that term and substitute the recognition that subtle ictal activity may be related to psychiatric symptoms. They stated that, "simple partial seizures of limbic origin can cause virtually any psychiatric sign or symptom in clear consciousness while scalp EEG is almost always normal." Further, they point out that sensory symptoms caused by SPSs of neocortical origin can give rise to bizarre experiences that are acted on in strange ways to cre-

ate a persistent "interictal" behavior disturbance. Their conclusions support the views of the present authors (31–33).

There currently is no internationally accepted syndromic classification of psychosis in epilepsy. In a tabulation of clinical characteristics of psychosis related to seizure activity, psychoses were listed in the following categories that did not imply a difference in physiopathology, but of time frame: ictal psychosis, postictal psychosis, periictal psychosis, alternative psychosis, and interictal psychosis (76). Although the significance of some of these categories has been questioned, there remain the successive evolving physiopathologic phases of an underlying ictal event.

The etiologic role of partial TLmS occurrence in EPE appears to meet the criterion of a definable physiopathology. Implementing that formulation, the authors modified the short operational classification directed at diagnosis and therapy that they proposed in 1996 (35) (Table 6.1).

In contrast to EPE, the etiology of nonEPE currently is obscure. Physiopathologic data are lacking except for some aspects that bear resemblance to EPE. The recurrence of partial seizures and ensuing BDE over a long enough period of time has been observed to result in a nonepisodic state of chronic psychosis (14) (vide infra Cases GAD and WHJ). In corroboration, subsidence of seizures has been asso-

TABLE 6.1. *Classification of psychosis of epilepsy*

1. Episodic psychosis of epilepsy (EPE) due to
    A. spontaneous partial seizures, breakthrough, or untreated
    B. partial seizures resulting from drug withdrawal
2. Nonepisodic (chronic) psychosis of epilepsy (nonEPE) due to
    A. coalescence of EPE
    B. drug toxicity
    C. coincidence of psychosis and seizures
3. Unclassifiable relationship between psychosis and seizures by available clinical and laboratory data

From Rayport M, Ferguson SM. Psychiatric evaluation for epilepsy surgery. In: Shorvon SD, Dreifuss FE, Fish DF, et al., eds. *The treatment of epilepsy.* Oxford: Blackwell, 1996:50, with permission.

ciated with amelioration of psychosis. Slater et al. (15) reported that, as seizures became fewer over the years, complete remission of the psychosis occurred in 20 of their 69 cases. Bruens (23) recorded similar outcomes.

FINDINGS AND HYPOTHESES OF THE EPILEPSY COMPREHENSIVE PROGRAM OF THE MEDICAL COLLEGE OF OHIO

The orientation of the group that worked at the Medical College of Ohio from 1970 to 1993 was unique. As far as we know, there are no other reports in the literature that comprise a longitudinal interdisciplinary clinical investigation with equally intensive simultaneous study of patients by neurologic, neuropsychiatric, neurosurgical, and nursing epileptologists over a prolonged period of time. Observations of patients were made during all phases: during the preoperative period while seizure control was sought through AED therapy over months or years in individual cases; during noninvasive presurgical VEEG seizure monitoring; when indicated, during remonitoring with VSEEG, which included electrical brain stimulation; during the neurosurgical phase; and during long-term postoperative follow-up by direct contact with most patients, ranging from 3 to over 25 years. The neuropsychiatric database proved to be essential to the understanding of the psychic dimensions of the patient: his/her epileptic experiences, cognitive abilities, psychodynamics and interpersonal relationships, life story, and psychiatric history, if any, in order to establish the nature of clinically significant psychiatric symptoms and, when applicable, the mental content of the psychosis. Neuropsychiatric management was guided by the specific factors precipitating or contributing to the psychopathology. Five illustrative cases follow.

Case GAD: *Recurring partial seizures with productive behavior during automatism with amnesia led to misinterpretation of reality and progressed to a paranoid psychosis.*

GAD, a 35-year-old woman with intractable posttraumatic TLmE, had SPS with a pleasant olfactory aura evolving to CPS with behavioral automatism during a prolonged amnesic period. During the CPS, she would carry on with activities that she had planned prior to the ictus. If she had been hungry, she might continue with the food preparation. On recovery from the seizure, she would find the food ready to eat and credit its preparation to her guardian spirit. If preparation for a bath coincided with her pleasant olfactory aura, she would, upon recovery from the CPS, presume that the guardian spirit had drawn a fragrant bath for her. The magical sense of a relationship with an extraterrestrial agency became very real to her. Her seizures remained refractory to full control by AED. Over time, she became chronically paranoid. She developed grandiose delusions that she had been selected to draw up plans for interplanetary space stations. In response to this ideation, she would create diagrams showing the different planets and would converse in varying neologistic monologues that she described as the languages of the individual planets.

Comment: Psychosis resulted from her becoming identified with the magical character of her unremembered constructive activities. This case illustrates progression from episodic to chronic psychosis of epilepsy on the basis of continued occurrence of seizures. This case also illustrates that nonEPE may be a complication of failed seizure control.

Case MIR: *AED-resistant seizures of bilateral medial frontal origin localized by VSEEG monitoring. Repeated episodes of SE without psychiatric complications. Postictal psychosis occurred when SE coincided with a period of significant emotional stress.*

MIR, a 16-year-old adopted boy, became epileptic at the age of 4 years. He was accustomed to frequent seizures. He suffered from one to two minor seizures each night, two to three major seizures each week, and monthly episodes of SE. His seizures involved head droop and tonic elevation of both arms, often followed by prolonged automatism during which he might wander outside, up to the altar of the church during worship, or progress to secondary generalization. Following control of an episode of SE in the emergency room of the local hospital, he regained consciousness. He was referred because of his bizarre behavior. In the epilepsy unit, neuropsychiatric examination found him to be fully oriented and able to recall recent events. He was markedly paranoid, expressing persecutory and grandiose delusions. Psychotic themes were religious and sexual. In his delusions, he was convinced that he was the transmitter of God's will and had to struggle with the devil, who was trying to gain control. He had auditory and visual hallucinations with content related to the delusional themes mentioned. He was sure that the physiologic monitors in various corners of the nursing unit were cameras taking pornographic pictures. With adjustment of antiepileptic medication and prescription of antipsychotic medication, MIR recovered from the psychosis after several days. Insight returned gradually, but the psychotic theme lingered as he felt that God had resumed proper control.

Some time after the psychotic episode, the patient's mother revealed that in the weeks before this episode of SE, the family, which was deeply devoted to a fundamentalist faith that accepts the reality of the devil, had relied more than usual on their church for help because of a sexual experience of the patient's younger sister. The patient had been very much involved in the family's uncompromising feelings. These feelings gradually resolved. He continued to have episodes of SE. Psychosis did not recur during 14 years of ingravescent severity of seizures.

Comment: The psychotic mentation reflected the patient's emotional preoccupation with a very stressful event in his and his family's life.

Case RUD: *Posttraumatic TLmS originating from the right hippocampus, secondary generalization. SE was followed by psychosis. His chronic emotional stress was expressed in the content of the psychosis.*

RUD, a 23-year-old right-handed single man, began to have posttraumatic seizures at the age of 10 years, 1 month after striking his head against a diving board and having to be pulled out of the water. As an infant, he had been dropped to the floor of the church during his baptism.

SPS began with an epigastric sensation with fear, associated with a feeling of guilt and a fear of dying. SPS evolved to CPS in which he went blank, became minimally responsive, and crumbled. Secondary generalization first involving the left arm and leg took place six to seven times per month, sometimes in clusters of four convulsions in 1 day. The mental content of the SPSs reflected an intense and prolonged traumatic life experience of parental strife that led to divorce despite strong Catholic affiliation when he was age 19 years. The patient felt guilty, thinking that he was responsible for his seizures and for the marital discord. He had sought solace in his religion, trusting that the Lord would prevent the disruption at home. Church ritual had been very supportive. As changes in church ritual were implemented, RUD felt abandoned. He was in considerable conflict over his religious practice and finally resolved this conflict by leaving the church. He had a first episode of psychosis at age 22 years after a sequence of generalized tonic-clonic seizures. A year later, his brother brought him to our hospital in a psychotic state after an apparent series of seizures. RUD was very vocal, declaring that he was threatened by hell fires around him and warned the staff, whom he clearly recognized, to keep their distance for their own safety. He felt that Satan was trying to get control of him. He experienced various illusions: his hands were melting, his feet were like rock, and sounds were "weird." Upon recovery after 5 days, he recognized the abnormality of his thinking but felt the experience could serve as a reminder that he should return to the church. Later, he continued to refer to elements of the psychotic episode. He said, "I thought I had been warned by God to straighten out my act or go to hell—Judgment Day was coming." During the half-year before surgery, he read the Bible assiduously and attended church services regularly. Presurgical evaluation with VSEEG showed that the primary epileptogenic zone of his spontaneous TLmS was the right hippocampus. Interictal activity was recorded from the left hippocampus. He underwent right TLX at age 24 years. He has been seizure-free while taking AEDs and has experienced no psychotic episodes during 19-year follow-up.

Comment: An epileptic individual whose intractable seizures curtailed meaningful activity had chronic guilt over his possible role in the dissolution of his family and over his failure to succeed. He also had lost the comfort of religion when church ritual had changed. He felt alone and deserted, angry, and guilty. These various elements were present in the content of the psychosis. Postoperative freedom from seizures resulted in absence of psychotic symptoms. Psychotherapy now was able to help him strengthen ego control and maintain reality-oriented thinking toward the resolution of his conflicts.

Case KRS: *Two bouts of psychosis after an increase in seizure frequency and an episode of generalized SE had been diagnosed elsewhere as schizophrenia. During presurgical EEG monitoring, psychosis developed when seizure frequency rose. Uncontrollable behavior resulted in psychiatric consultation and transfer to isolation on the psychiatry floor with a diagnosis of catatonic schizophrenia. The epilepsy team observed very frequent subtle TLmSs. Following left temporal lobectomy, partial seizure frequency was markedly reduced. He remained free of psychotic symptoms during 3-year follow-up.*

KRS, a 27-year-old single right-handed man with right hemisphere dominance for language, had a seizure disorder from childhood. He was viewed by his despairing family as nonfunctional, unable to adequately handle everyday situations. The family had been advised that he also had a chronic psychosis. On two occasions prior to coming under our care, he was reported to have had a schizophrenic psychosis, the first after an increase in seizure frequency and the second after SE. Six years before admission, he had undergone a very conservative left anterior temporal corticec-

tomy at another medical center in the belief that this was the language hemisphere; this surgery was without benefit.

His very frequent SPSs started with sudden inability to understand what he heard or read, and evolved to CPSs and prolonged behavioral automatism. Postictally, difficulty remembering ongoing material continued for a number of hours.

During presurgical evaluation, seizure frequency increased as AEDs were being withdrawn gradually. On a weekend, KRS was transferred from the neurosurgery unit to the psychiatry floor because of bizarre behavior. The first psychiatric symptoms consisted of his eating hallucinated food particles after he refused food offered to him by a nurse's aide. This behavior suggested misidentification of the nurse as his mother, with whom food had become a major area in the battle for control. His behavior became unmanageable because of overactive and destructive movements. A psychiatric consultant diagnosed catatonic excitement and had KRS transferred to an isolation room on the general psychiatry ward, where the chart stated that seizures were absent. A diagnosis of schizophrenia, catatonic type, had been entered. When the epilepsy group observed him closely in the psychiatry unit on Monday, he was having frequent subtle SPSs, during which his writing at examiners' request progressed to vigorous repetitive stabbing motions with the pencil. Between SPSs, he was found to have cognitive changes and psychotic symptoms. The content of the psychosis reflected misinterpretation of his environment and unresolved intrafamilial issues. His diagnosis was revised to EPE. Gradual recovery over several weeks was interrupted by resurgence of psychotic thinking when small SPSs recurred. After he recovered, KRS reported that, while he was in isolation, he had concluded that he had misbehaved: "I was separated from my family to keep me out of the way." Items in the environment had been incorporated into his disordered thinking: A Swiss travel poster on the wall of his isolation room made him feel that he was in Europe as a prisoner in a concentration camp. After left TLX, he had a marked reduction in seizure frequency and severity. He continued taking AEDs and was without psychotic or cognitive symptoms during 3 years of follow-up. For the first time in his life, he found employment at a bank.

Comment: This case illustrates the etiologic basis of EPE in TLmE in two related ways: (i) increase in partial seizure frequency led to episodic psychosis; (ii) left TLX resulted in marked reduction of frequency and severity of seizures and in absence of psychotic symptomatology (31).

Case WHJ: *Recurrent episodes of EPE coalesced over time and produced a nonEPE in an individual with uncontrolled TLmSs.*

WHJ was a 38-year-old man who had a chronic seizure disorder dating from infancy. He had seizures as frequently as three to four times a day. During the aura, he would have an epigastric sensation, feel afraid and strange, experience receptive aphasia ("I hear you but I don't hear anything you say"), and have auditory hallucinations. After a behavioral automatism, he could find himself in a distant location. Neurologically, he was diagnosed as having SPS evolving to CPS with automatism and a prolonged postictal state that often lasted from 24 to 48 hours and sometimes up to weeks. On neuropsychiatric examination during the postictal period, he was suspicious and aggressive. This mental state came to pervade a greater proportion of his days to the point of constituting a chronic paranoid psychosis. With increases in seizure frequency, he would have an exacerbation of the psychosis. When the latter was associated with self-neglect or aggressive behavior directed at his "enemies," so called because he thought that they had done something morally wrong, he required mental hospital admission. Religion became a central component of his thinking. He stated, "God's all through my body," as he pointed to his bilateral Dupuytren's contractures, which he believed to be stigmata. "The seizures help me in doing righteousness. I can live with them. I am one of the afflicted."

Comment: The frequency, vividness, and progressive prolongation of the intrusion of ictus-related experiences into his life formed the basis of the development of the psychosis.

DIAGNOSIS OF EPILEPTIC PSYCHOSIS

Insofar as psychosis in TLmE can be precipitated by an increase in the frequency of partial seizures (4,18,31,32,51), the first step in diagnosis is to seek the etiologic history of the psychotic state.

In the case of an established epileptic patient of a health care facility, the etiology of the seizure disorder, the details of the original diagnostic workup, the formerly and currently prescribed antiseizure drugs, the degree of achieved seizure control and compliance with the dosage schedule, and the nature and date of a neurosurgical intervention for seizure control, if applicable, would be available. If these data are not immediately accessible, the physician or the epileptologist caring for the patient should be contacted immediately to avert a "fresh start" approach that would delay effective treatment and undermine patient confidence. It is essential to obtain a careful history of the time parameters and description of seizures in relation to the appearance of psychosis from the patient if he or she is able to give information, and certainly from an eyewitness who can provide precise details about the onset of the psychosis and its antecedents. For instance, careful questioning may reveal that the patient had an increase in frequency of seizures prior to the appearance of psychosis. Seizures may have been readily observable or subtle, as in the case of so-called nonconvulsive SE. The latter may not have been detected, but the resulting changes in thinking, emotional reactivity, and interpersonal behavior would not escape lay perceptiveness. During the night preceding the onset of the psychosis, the patient may have been unusually restless or wet the bed. Or there may have been an episode of convulsive SE. The eyewitness may describe previous seizure episodes accompanied by transient paranoid thinking.

In short, the unexpected development of abnormal behavior or altered state of consciousness with or without observed seizure activity should trigger consideration of EPE in the differential diagnosis.

There is no high-priced modern laboratory test that can substitute for thorough clinical interviewing by a competent health professional propelled by the challenge of problem solving in an area of mind–brain relationship.

EPE is eminently treatable provided a current database has been achieved to confirm the working diagnosis and to guide therapy. AED blood levels and toxicologic screening should be obtained without delay. Blood levels may show that AEDs had been discontinued or decreased with or without medical supervision. Psychosis may appear as seizures increase in response to decreased AED coverage. On the other hand, if the patient has been compliant but has been given one of the new AEDs, the latter may be the precipitating agent for the psychosis by one of two mechanisms: (i) As a drug side effect. It is known that reversible paranoid psychosis may occur in patients taking ethosuximide (Zarontin), ethotoin (Peganone), methsuximide (Celontin), phenacemide (Phenurone), or primidone (Mysoline). EPE has been encountered in patients participating in clinical trials of new AEDs. (ii) As an effect of a newer AED that may not provide the same antiseizure protection as the established AED for which the newer drug was substituted. The present writers are unaware of evidence-oriented clinical trials of new AEDs in patients who have undergone TLX for seizure control. They are aware of restoration of freedom from seizures in post-TLX cases when the newer AED was replaced with established AEDs that had not controlled the seizures prior to surgery but on which the patient had been seizure-free after TLX.

Diagnostic EEG with T1-T2 leads may be decisive and should not be delayed. If behavior control is a problem, antipsychotic treatment, e.g., haloperidol (Haldol), would be initiated to obtain a technically satisfactory tracing. Recording during sleep improves the likelihood of an informative EEG for epileptic activity. Current tracings should be compared with previous records, if they exist. EEG seizure monitoring for 24 hours may be considered.

Structural radiologic studies are not an immediate concern in the absence of new head trauma or suspicion of an intracranial mass lesion. A role for SPECT or *p*MRI, if the EEG studies are nondiagnostic in a case of suspected EPE due to partial SE, has been mentioned under Radiologic Data. The on-going ictal activity of SE would ease the timing requirements for injection of the ligand or radioactive tracer.

If a psychotic seizure patient is not known to the personnel of the medical center, neurologic and neuropsychiatric consultations should be sought upon admission to create the necessary database for expeditious treatment and subsequent follow-up. Information from the patient's regular physician should be secured to expedite informed treatment planning.

When a psychotic patient not known to be epileptic is referred because of seizures, the treating physician would sort out whether he or she is dealing with an epileptic person who becomes psychotic after a period of unreported seizures, or a person with a psychosis whose seizures are related to psychotropic medication, or to an unrecognized seizure disorder. In parallel with reevaluation of the antipsychotic medication, a diagnostic workup for seizure disorder would clarify the situation.

Difficulty in diagnosis should be addressed through consultation with and between neurologic and psychiatric epileptologists.

TREATMENT AND PREVENTION OF EPILEPTIC PSYCHOSIS

The treatment of psychosis in an epileptic patient is founded on neurologic and neuropsychiatric epileptology. Based on information in preceding sections, the fundamental principle underlying the management of psychosis of epilepsy is diagnosis and treatment of the seizures. Rational implementation involves joint action of neurology and psychiatry and the emergency department if the patient presents there. The patient must not be assigned to only one of the disciplines, namely psychiatry, because psychiatric symptoms are present and the scalp EEG is "negative."

The first step in treatment of EPE is reassessment of AED therapy with updated AED blood levels. Epileptic psychosis subsides when seizures have been reduced to low frequency or, optimally, fully controlled. These ends generally are attained only after some days. If behavior control is a problem, the usual practice is to start neuroleptic medication at the beginning of AED treatment. (Neuroleptic drug [NLD] therapy is discussed later.) The time frame for recovery from a psychotic episode is one to several weeks. The patient should be closely monitored psychiatrically and neurologically because persistence or relapse of the psychosis is a likely indication of recurring ictal epileptic activity. Recurrence of EPE during apparently satisfactory progress is not uncommon with partial SE.

Attention to prevention of recurrence of EPE is the next goal, because a potential complication of EPE recurrences may be chronic psychosis. After resolution of the epileptic psychosis, psychiatric evaluation and psychotherapy will help to clarify the psychodynamic link between the psychosis and the patient's life, or between the psychosis and seizure experiences or cognitive deficits. In our epilepsy center, the insight of the neuropsychiatrist has been greatly aided by knowledge of the patient gained during previous longitudinal contact in an environment in which equally careful neurologic and psychiatric data are being gathered.

With education of the patient and the patient's support system with regard to his or her condition, future episodes of psychosis may be averted by reenergized compliance with AED therapy. Recurrent psychosis or its antecedents may be recognized earlier so that treatment can be more prompt and efficient. Communication between the neurologic, neuropsychiatric, and nursing disciplines and the primary physician is essential to avert future

episodes of psychosis. A nurse clinical specialist in epilepsy contributes greatly to this process by educating the patient, the patient's support persons, and relevant social agencies.

In the case of a patient who has a chronic psychosis of epilepsy, particularly in a case having exacerbations or a fluctuating course, the same active program should be followed with emphasis on adjustment of AED selection and dosage to obtain the best level of seizure control in the context of quality of life.

The management of chronic psychosis in patients with epilepsy may require the use of NLDs. Most, if not all, of the NLDs lower the seizure threshold. Clinicians often have hesitated to use these drugs in patients with epilepsy for fear of causing seizures. Although it is essential to bear in mind the risk of additional seizures when starting NLD administration in these patients, this risk should never be a reason not to treat a patient in need of antipsychotic medication.

Among nonepileptic patients receiving an NLD, seizure incidence has ranged between 0.5% and 1.2% (77). The risk is higher in the presence of the following factors: History of epilepsy, abnormal EEG recordings, and history of central nervous system disorder. Risk factors related to NLDs are rapid escalation of dose, high doses, NLD polytherapy, and presence of other drugs that lower the seizure threshold. Chlorpromazine and clozapine are regarded as the NLDs most likely to cause seizures (78). High–low dose ranges of incidence are 9% to 0.5% for the former and 4.4% to less than 1% for the latter (78,79). Although these drugs have been largely superseded, most NLDs have been associated with seizure occurrence in the presence of the risk factors cited earlier.

Seizure occurrence among patients with epilepsy treated with NLDs has not been widely studied. Pacia and Devinsky (80) reported that 16 patients who had epilepsy among 5,629 patients treated with clozapine all experienced worsening of seizures while taking the drug in doses ranging from less than 300 to more than 600 mg per day. It follows that this NLD should be avoided or used in exceptional circumstances with extreme caution in patients with epilepsy. NLDs with a lower seizure risk include haloperidol, molindone, fluphenazine, perfenazine, and trifluoperazine. More data are needed for the newer NLDs. Risperidone appears to have a lesser effect on lowering seizure threshold than the older NLDs. Nearly all NLDs can cause dose-related EEG changes, which consist of slowing of background activity and paroxysmal discharges (81). The latter are not predictive of seizure occurrence.

Three recommendations apply to minimizing the proconvulsant effect of NLDs. (i) Obtain AED blood plasma levels prior to initiating NLD therapy; repeat for subsequent monitoring. (ii) For NLD dosage, "start low, go slow." (iii) Avoid NLD polytherapy.

Combined treatment with AED and NLD requires that the clinician be aware of pharmacodynamic (e.g., at receptor sites) and pharmacokinetic (absorption, distribution including protein binding, metabolism, excretion) drug interactions. NLDs and AEDs may utilize the same isoenzymes in the hepatic cytochrome P-450 system, thereby altering plasma drug levels. AEDs with enzyme-inducing properties, such as carbamazepine, phenytoin, phenobarbital, and primidone, increase the clearance of most NLDs. This is the most frequent pharmacokinetic interaction encountered in clinical practice. Adjustment of psychotropic drug dose may be necessary with the addition or discontinuation of AEDs that inhibit or induce hepatic enzymes (81).

Adverse systemic consequences may result from combined administration of clozapine and carbamazepine, each of which can cause leukopenia. The combination of these two drugs has been reported to cause an increased risk of neuroleptic malignant syndrome (82).

Temporal lobe ablation for seizure control in patients with psychotic manifestations continues to be controversial in surgical epilepsy centers (83,84). Consensus continues to develop with regard to an etiologic relationship between EPE and partial TLmS frequency, based on reports of freedom from EPE after successful TLX (15,18,34–36,38,56). Recurrences of EPE may be a confirmatory indication for TLX (35,56).

Recognizing that the etiology of chronic psychosis of epilepsy is not fully understood, Fenwick (84) accepted psychosis as an indication for TLX in patients who were found otherwise suitable. Chronic psychosis did not prevent cooperation with presurgical evaluation. Although successful TLX may not lead to recovery from schizophrenia, the functional psychosis may no longer require NLDs or lead to psychiatric hospitalization; it lessens the burden of living with seizures for the mentally ill person, and it may allow employment (85). Rejection of patients with intractable TLmS and chronic psychosis from presurgical evaluation for TLX as a matter of standard procedure no longer appears to be justified. Psychiatric presurgical evaluation should include exploration as to whether a relationship exists between seizure occurrence and psychotic symptomatology in formulating the post-TLX prognosis (35,83). Recent research has shown that nonepileptic schizophrenics can dependably complete an informed consent procedure (86). The indications for vagal nerve stimulation in relation to EPE and nonEPE are currently unknown.

DISCUSSION

We presented an historical perspective on psychosis of epilepsy to draw attention to the long-standing awareness in medical history of a relationship between epilepsy and mental disturbance dating from classical times and earlier (1,87). In the nineteenth century, prior to AED therapy, there were well-documented cases of epileptic patients who became psychotic.

In the twentieth century, a scientific base was established for the relationship between seizures and BDE. The recognition of psychosis as a complication of a seizure disorder involving the temporal limbic structures was delineated in the 1950s and 1960s by Gibbs et al. (6,7), Hill (13), Pond (14), Falconer et al. (88), and Slater et al. (15). Electrophysiologic correlates of episodic behavior disturbances in TLmE were established by SEEG recording of seizures (9,10,35,43,60–63,75). Correlative hypotheses about brain–behavior relationships based on neuropathologic studies have been expanded through visualization of brain structure by brain imaging. Promising as these insights appeared, it seems unlikely that fixed anatomic conditions with origins remote in time could provide an explanation for the occurrence of an episodic condition such as psychosis, which disappears if seizures are stopped.

We emphasized that the mental state of the epileptic patient with psychosis has been neglected in these efforts to resolve the controversies about the cause of psychosis and its relation to seizures (31). The diagnostic process that addresses the interrelationships between psychosis and epilepsy is available in the methodology of neuropsychiatry. The person with seizures must be understood in his or her dimensions, including seizure experiences, his or her history, personality style, conflicts, and cognitive abilities. The psychiatrist, because of the relatively more prolonged contacts with the patient, has the opportunity to witness seizure manifestations and to explore and record the patient's seizure-related experiences. Longitudinal patient contacts build an appreciation of the varying impacts of seizures on thought content and mood. Memories or feelings that usually are repressed or suppressed under control by cortical, reality-oriented thinking when seizures are not occurring may be activated as control of thinking is impaired by the physiopathology of the ictus (31). Vivid auras followed by an amnesic period with automatism may induce misinterpretations leading to the development of delusions. Cognitive impairment associated with, or increased by, recurring seizures may alter reality testing. With his or her mind thus informed, the psychiatrist can assess the interaction of these many parameters and their effect on the patient's life, and relate them to additional information obtained from key witnesses and other staff members.

Diagnostic evidence of a causal relationship between psychosis and partial seizures was obtained from (i) longitudinal neuropsychiatric history and observations that identify a time relationship between increased seizure frequency and psychosis; (ii) psychotic thinking reproduced during SEEG by electrical stimulation of limbic structures (31,89); (iii) elimination of EPE after seizure-relieving TLX; and (iv) reappearance of EPE or emergence of *de novo* psychosis in a patient without preoperative psychotic episodes, both resulting from the recurrence of seizures after TLX.

We questioned certain explanations, repeated in the literature, about the temporal relationships between psychosis and seizures. Landolt (52) proposed the theory of "forced normalization," which held that psychosis and seizures alternated. We would conclude that Landolt's hypothesis has not withstood observations that a scalp EEG may be nonepileptic while seizure activity is ongoing in the temporal limbic structures. The psychosis does not alternate with seizures but coincides with them (9,18,31,57,58,60,62). We have unpublished data supporting the proposition that paradoxical normalization of the EEG is likely to be related to suppression of surface EEG activity when a seizure occurs in subcortical structures. The array of data cited above indicates that "forced normalization" was a hypothesis built on insufficient data. It may owe its durability to the seductiveness of the paradox.

"Interictal psychosis" may be a misnomer for lack of data about seizure activity in the depth. Use of the term "interictal" should henceforth be limited by awareness of this constraint. Minimally invasive functional scanning (SPECT, fMRI) could be used on current clinical populations with EPE and partial SE to assess this hypothesis. Each patient would be his or her own control during and after psychosis.

"Interictal" psychosis also may be a misnomer for prolonged postictal disturbance of cognitive function and behavior. After barely observable small seizures, we have seen disruptive mental effects beyond the seconds or minutes of paroxysmal electrical activity. Hughlings Jackson (4) wrote in 1875 "that cases of epilepsy in which there are the slightest attacks are the worst for the mind." Prolonged behavioral disruption of course also occurs after obvious TLmSs, but when such are so subtle as to be unobserved, the term "interictal" would be erroneously applied.

The bulk of the literature on chronic psychosis in epilepsy was produced before monitoring of seizures with EEG and SEEG (90) was widely used and before the introduction of the modern antiseizure drugs. Chronic epileptic psychosis can result from coalescence of partial seizures with mental content that eventually may distort the person's interpretation of reality (14,33) or from EPE in patients whose seizures are poorly controlled (cf. Cases GAD and WHJ). The pathogenesis of nonEPE must be evaluated further. However, because of deinstitutionalization of psychiatric patients, it may no longer be possible to access a research population to elucidate this question. Of course, it also may be that a sizable population of patients with chronic epileptic psychosis would no longer exist because of prevention of nonEPE by better seizure control using AEDs. Psychosis of epilepsy encountered today may be predominantly episodic.

Psychiatric and neurologic epileptologists should appreciate the unique opportunity provided by presurgical neurosurgical study and focal ablation that allows for direct observation and collection of data at the brain–mind interface, with each patient serving as his or her own control. Such scientific data eventually allay undocumented hypothesizing about the nature of psychosis in epilepsy. Findings in the therapeutic laboratory of man, obtained by careful longitudinal neuropsychiatric study before and after surgery, integrated with observation of physiologic and behavioral events during electrical brain stimulation, connect with and give value to keen clinical observations from the past and enlarge our understanding of the person afflicted with epilepsy.

A line in the writings of John Hughlings Jackson (91) attests to his engagement. It reads: "No better neurologic work can be done than the precise investigation of epileptic paroxysms." We would draw to attention that the advice of Hughlings Jackson made 112 years ago can be effectively implemented through interdisciplinary research and treatment that intellectually articulate neurologic surgery, neurology, and neuropsychiatry in the care of persons with epilepsy.

SUMMARY AND CONCLUSIONS

1. The historical record has associated behavior disorders with epilepsy. The behavioral consequences of slight seizures were described and confirmed by neuropsychiatric and neurologic epileptologists in the latter nineteenth century. These observations were reconfirmed in the twentieth century by clinical observations correlated with ictal and postictal intracerebral EEG recordings of partial seizures of temporolimbic origin.

2. There is a continuing consensus that psychosis of epilepsy is to be considered a distinct diagnostic entity. The descriptor "schizophrenia-like" should be accorded its original meaning of resembling but not being nuclear schizophrenia.

3. Consensus has appeared with regard to the psychotogenic role of increased frequency of TLmSs, which may vary in their clinical manifestations from very slight to SE.

4. Pathogenic factors in the literature of psychosis of epilepsy have been separated into *correlational,* involving fixed, longstanding, anatomopathologic alterations, and *dynamic,* from electrophysiologic and neuroimaging studies whose concurrence in time with clinical epileptologic events endow them with explanatory value.

5. The "forced normalization" syndrome—seizures are absent, scalp EEG is better, but EPE is present—has been challenged by SEEG evidence of epileptic discharge in medial temporal limbic structures. So-called normalization of the scalp EEG is most likely due to the drop of cortical EEG voltage or "sup-

pression" that accompanies seizure activity in the depth.

6. Psychosis after temporal lobe surgery for seizure control is EPE. It is associated with failure of TLX to relieve preoperative seizures, with partial SE, or with failure of postoperative AED management.

7. A classification of psychosis of epilepsy based on the pathogenic role of partial seizures is proposed.

8. The longitudinal interdisciplinary approach of a comprehensive epilepsy program comprising the concurrent input from the disciplines of neurological surgery, neurology and EEG, neuropsychiatry, neuropsychology, and neuroscience nursing was described and brought into the clinical realm with case histories. Clinical neuropsychiatric data are scientific data as valuable and as informative as the physiologic data with which they can be correlated.

DEDICATION

We dedicate this chapter to the memory(s) of Wilder Penfield, Herbert Jasper, Erwin Straus, and Jean Bancaud, with personal gratitude for lasting inspiration.

ACKNOWLEDGMENT

We thank Andres M. Kanner, M.D., for his collaboration on psychopharmacologic treatment of psychosis of epilepsy.

We take pleasure in acknowledging the outstanding epileptologic care and management skills of Carolyn A. Schell, B.S.N., R.N., C.N.R.N., nurse coordinator of the Epilepsy Comprehensive Program.

REFERENCES

1. Temkin O. *The falling sickness. A history of epilepsy from the Greeks to the beginnings of modern neurology,* 2nd ed., rev. Baltimore: The Johns Hopkins Press, 1971.
2. Morel BA. D'une forme de délire, suite d'une surexcitation nerveuse se rattachant à une variété non encore décrite de l'épilepsie (épilepsie larvée). *Gazette hebdomadaire de médecine et de chirurgie* 1860;7:819–821.
3. Falret J. De l'état mental des épileptiques. *Archives générales de médecine, Ve série* 1861;17:461–491.
4. Hughlings Jackson J. On temporary mental disorders after epileptic paroxysms. *West Riding Lunatic Asylum*

Med Rep 1875;5. In: Taylor J, ed. *Selected writings of John Hughlings Jackson.* New York: Basic Books, 1958;1:119–134.
5. Penfield W, Jasper H. *Epilepsy and the functional anatomy of the human brain.* Boston: Little, Brown and Company, 1954.
6. Gibbs EL, Gibbs FA, Fuster B. Psychomotor epilepsy. *Arch Neurol Psychiatry* 1948;60:331–339.
7. Gibbs FA. Ictal and non-ictal psychiatric disorder in temporal lobe epilepsy. *J Nerv Ment Dis* 1951;113:522–528.
8. Talairach J, de Ajuriaguerra J, David M. Etudes stéréotaxiques des structures encéphaliques profondes chez l'homme. *Presse Med* 1952;28:605–609.
9. Bancaud J, Talairach J, Bonis A, et al. *La stéréo-électroencéphalographie dans l'épilepsie. Informations neurophysiopathologiques apportées par l'investigation fonctionelle stéréotaxique.* Paris: Masson, 1965.
10. Talairach J, Bancaud J. Stereotaxic exploration and therapy in epilepsy. In: Vinken PJ, Bruyn GW, eds. *Clinical handbook of neurology.* Amsterdam: North-Holland Publishing Co., 1974:15:758–782.
11. Talairach J, Tournoux P. *Co-planar stereotaxic atlas of the human brain. 3-Dimensional proportional system: an approach to cerebral imaging.* Stuttgart: Thieme, 1988. Rayport M, translator.
12. Talairach J, Tournoux P. *Referentially oriented cerebral MRI anatomy. Atlas of stereotaxic anatomical correlations for gray and white matter.* Stuttgart: Thieme, 1993.
13. Hill D. Psychiatric disorders of epilepsy. *Med Press* 1953;229:473–475.
14. Pond DA. Psychiatric aspects of epilepsy. *J Indian Med Prof* 1957;3:1421–1451.
15. Slater E, Beard AW, Glithero E. The schizophrenia-like psychoses of epilepsy. *Br J Psychiatry* 1963;109:95–150.
16. Guerrant J, Anderson WA, Fischer A, et al. *Personality in epilepsy.* Springfield, IL: Charles C. Thomas, 1962.
17. Engel J Jr, Bandler R, Griffith NC, et al. Neurobiological evidence for epilepsy-induced interictal disturbances. In: Smith DB, Treiman DM, Trimble MR, eds. *Advances in Neurology,* Volume 55. *Neurobehavioral problems in epilepsy.* New York: Raven Press, 1991:97–111.
18. Engel J Jr, Taylor DC. Neurobiology of behavioral disorders. In: Engel J Jr, Pedley TA, Aicardi J, et al., eds. *Epilepsy: a comprehensive textbook.* Philadelphia: Lippincott-Raven Publishers, 1998:194.
19. Duffy JD. The shifting paradigm of epilepsy. In: McConnell HW, Snyder PJ, eds. *Psychiatric comorbidity in epilepsy.* Washington, DC: American Psychiatric Press, 1998:1.
20. Hinsie LE, Shatzky J. *Psychiatric dictionary with encyclopedic treatment of modern terms.* London: Oxford University Press, 1949:447.
21. Henderson D, Gillespie RD. *A textbook of psychiatry.* London: Oxford University Press, 1956:26–27.
22. Slater E, Roth M. *Clinical psychiatry,* 3rd ed. Baltimore: Williams & Wilkins, 1969.
23. Bruens JH. Psychoses in epilepsy. In: Vinken PJ, Bruyn GW, eds. *Clinical handbook of neurology.* Amsterdam: North-Holland Publishing Co., 1974:15:593–610.
24. Kristensen O, Sindrup EH. Psychomotor epilepsy and psychosis: III. Social and psychological correlates. *Acta Neurol Scand* 1979;59:1–9.
25. Perez MM, Trimble MR. Epileptic psychosis: diagnos-

tic comparison with process schizophrenia. *Br J Psychiatry* 1980;137:245–249.

26. Wing JK, Cooper JE, Sartorius N. *The measurement and classification of psychiatric symptoms.* London: Cambridge University Press, 1974.

27. Mace CJ. Epilepsy and schizophrenia. *Br J Psychiatry* 1993;163:439–445.

28. Tandon R, DeQuardo JR. Psychosis and epilepsy. In: Sackellares JC, Berent S, eds. *Psychological disturbance in epilepsy.* Boston: Butterworth-Heinemann, 1996:9.

29. Toone BK, Garralda ME, Ron MA. The psychoses of epilepsy and the functional psychoses: a clinical and phenomenological comparison. *Br J Psychiatry* 1982; 141:256–261.

30. Parnas J, Korsgaard S. Epilepsy and psychosis. *Acta Psychiatr Scand* 1982;66:89–99.

31. Ferguson SM, Rayport M, Gardner R, et al. Similarities in mental content of psychotic states, spontaneous seizures, dreams, and responses to electrical brain stimulation in patients with temporal lobe epilepsy. *Psychosom Med* 1969;31:479–498.

32. Ferguson SM, Rayport M. Psychosis in epilepsy. In: Blumer D, ed. *Psychiatric aspects of epilepsy.* Washington, DC: American Psychiatric Press, 1984:7.

33. Ferguson SM, Rayport M. A multidimensional approach to the understanding and management of behavior disturbance in epilepsy. In: Howells JG, ed. *Modern perspectives in clinical psychiatry.* New York: Brunner/Mazel, 1988:15.

34. Ferguson SM, Rayport M, Blumer DP, et al. Postoperative psychiatric changes. In: Engel J Jr, ed. *Surgical treatment of the epilepsies.* New York: Raven Press, 1993:55.

35. Rayport M, Ferguson SM. Psychiatric evaluation for epilepsy surgery. In: Shorvon SD, Dreifuss FE, Fish DF, et al., eds. *The treatment of epilepsy.* Oxford: Blackwell, 1996:50.

36. Landolt H. Serial EEG investigations during psychotic episodes in epileptic patients and during schizophrenic attacks. In: Lorentz de Haas AM, ed. *Lectures on epilepsy.* Amsterdam: Elsevier 1958:91–133.

37. Weisbrot DM, Ettinger AB. Epilepsy and behavior: controversies and caveats. *Neurologist* 1997;3:155–172.

38. Bruton CJ. *The neuropathology of temporal lobe epilepsy.* Oxford: Oxford University Press, 1988.

39. Bruton CJ, Stevens JR, Frith CD. Epilepsy, psychosis, and schizophrenia: clinical and pathological correlations. *Neurology* 1994;44:34–42.

40. Hyde TM, Weinberger DR. Seizures and schizophrenia. *Schizophr Bull* 1997;23:611–622.

41. Reynolds EH. Biological factors in psychological disorders associated with epilepsy. In: Reynolds EH, Trimble MR, eds. *Epilepsy and psychiatry.* Edinburgh: Churchill Livingstone, 1981:264–290.

42. Trimble M. The relationship between epilepsy and schizophrenia: a biochemical hypothesis. *Biol Psychiatry* 1977;12:299–304.

43. Ring HA, Trimble MR, Costa DC, et al. Striatal dopamine receptor binding in epileptic psychosis. *Biol Psychiatry* 1994;35:375–380.

44. Csernansky JG, Csernansky CA, Iqbal Z. Epileptic psychoses and dopamine receptor sensitivity. *Biol Psychiatry* 1995;37:64–65.

45. Reith J, Benkelfat C, Sherwin A, et al. Elevated dopa decarboxylase activity in living brain of patients with psychosis. *Proc Natl Acad Sci USA* 1994;91: 11651–11654.

46. Smith PF, Darlington CL. Neural mechanisms of psychiatric disturbances in patients with epilepsy. In: McConnell HW, Snyder PJ, eds. *Psychiatric comorbidity in epilepsy.* Washington, DC: American Psychiatric Press, 1998:2.

47. Kohler GK. Psychosis in epilepsy: classification and EEG studies. *Fortschr Neurol Psychiatr* 1975; 43:99–153.

48. Ramani V, Gumnit RJ. Intensive monitoring of interictal psychosis in epilepsy. *Ann Neurol* 1982;11:613–622.

49. Davison K, Bagley CR. Schizophrenia-like psychoses associated with organic disorders of the nervous system: review of the literature. In: Herrington RN, ed. *Current problems in neuropsychiatry. Schizophrenia, epilepsy and the temporal lobe. Br J Psychiatry,* Special Publication No. 4. Ashford, Kent: Royal Medico-Psychological Association, 1969:113–184.

50. Trimble MR. *The psychoses of epilepsy.* New York: Raven Press, 1991.

51. Glaser GH. The problem of psychosis in psychomotor temporal lobe epilepsy. *Epilepsia* 1964;5:271–278.

52. Landolt H. Some clinical electroencephalographical correlations in epileptic psychoses (twilight states). *Electroencephalogr Clin Neurophysiol* 1953;5:121.

53. Mendez MF, Grau R. The post-ictal psychosis of epilepsy: investigation in two patients. *Int J Psychiatry Med* 1991;21:85–92.

54. Falconer MA. Reversibility by temporal-lobe resection of the behavioral abnormalities of temporal-lobe epilepsy. *N Engl J Med* 1973;289:451–455.

55. Rayport M, Ferguson SM, Corrie WS. Contributions of cerebral depth recording and electrical stimulation to the clarification of seizure patterns and behavior disturbance in patients with temporal lobe epilepsy. In: Doane BK, Livingston KE, eds. *The limbic system: functional organization and clinical disorders.* New York: Raven Press, 1986:171–182.

56. Serafetinides EA, Falconer MA. The effects of temporal lobectomy in epileptic patients with psychosis. *J Ment Sci* 1962;108:584–593.

57. Wolf P, Trimble MR. Biological antagonism and epileptic psychosis. *Br J Psychiatry* 1985:146:272–276.

58. Wolf P. Acute behavioral symptomatology at disappearance of epileptiform EEG abnormality: paradoxical or "forced" normalization. In: Smith DB, Treiman DM, Trimble MR, eds. *Advances in Neurology,* Volume 55. *Neurobehavioral* problems in epilepsy. New York: Raven Press, 127–143.

59. Gloor P. Contributions of electroencephalography and electrocorticography to the neurosurgical treatment of the epilepsies. *Adv Neurol* 1975;8:59–105.

60. Wieser HG. Depth recorded limbic seizures and psychopathology. *Neurosci Biobehav Rev* 1983;7:427–440.

61. Brazier MAB. Electrical activity recorded simultaneously from the sdcalp and deep structures of the human brain. A computer study of their relationships. *J Nerv Ment Dis* 1968;147:31–39.

62. Wieser HG. "Psychische Anfälle" und deren stereoelektroenzephalographisches Korrelat. *Zeitschr EEG-EMG* 1979;10:197–206.

63. Wieser HG. Temporal lobe or psychomotor status epilepticus. *Electroencephalogr Clin Neurophysiol* 1980;48:558–572.

64. Stevens JR. Psychiatric consequences of temporal lobectomy for intractable seizures: a 20–30 year follow-up of 14 cases. *Psychol Med* 1990;20:529–545.
65. Simmel ML, Counts S. Clinical and psychological results of anterior temporal lobectomy in patients with temporal lobe epilepsy. In: Baldwin M, Bailey P, eds. *Temporal lobe epilepsy.* Springfield, IL: Charles C Thomas, 1958.
66. Theodore WH. Structural neuroimaging. In: Lüders HO, ed. *Epilepsy surgery.* New York: Raven Press, 1992:26.
67. Henry TR, Chugani HT, Abou-Khahil BW, et al. Positron emission tomography. In: Engel J Jr, ed. *Surgical treatment of the epilepsies,* 2nd ed. New York: Raven Press, 1993:18.
68. Berkovic SF, Newton MR, Chiron C, et al. Single photon emission tomography. In: Engel J Jr, ed. *Surgical treatment of the epilepsies,* 2nd ed. New York: Raven Press, 1993:19.
69. Perez MM, Trimble MR, Murray NM, et al. Epileptic psychosis: an evaluation of PSE profiles. *Br J Psychiatry* 1985;146:155–163.
70. Conlon P, Trimble MR, Rogers D. A study of epileptic psychosis using magnetic resonance imaging. *Br J Psychiatry* 1990;156:231–235.
71. Jibiki I, Maeda T, Kubota T, et al. 123I–IMP SPECT brain imaging in epileptic psychosis: a study of two cases of temporal lobe epilepsy with schizophrenia-like syndrome. *Neuropsychobiology* 1993;28:207–211.
72. Marshall EJ, Syed GMS, Fenwick PBC, et al. A pilot study of schizophrenia-like psychosis in epilepsy using single-photon emission computerised tomography. *Br J Psychiatry* 1993;163:32–36.
73. Betts TA. Depression, anxiety, epilepsy. In: Reynolds EH, Trimble MR, eds. *Epilepsy and psychiatry.* Edinburgh: Churchill Livingstone, 1981:60–71.
74. Toone BK. The psychoses of epilepsy. In: Reynolds EH, Trimble MR, eds. *Epilepsy and psychiatry.* Edinburgh: Churchill Livingstone, 1981:113–137.
75. So NK, Savard G, Andermann F, et al. Acute postictal psychosis: a stereo EEG study. *Epilepsia* 1990;31:188–193.
76. Trimble MR, Ring HA, Schmitz B. Neuropsychiatric aspects of epilepsy. In: Fogel BS, Schiffer RB, Rao SM, eds. *Neuropsychiatry.* Baltimore: Williams & Wilkins, 1996:771–803.
77. Whitworth AB, Fleischlacker WW. Adverse effects of antipsychotic drugs. *Int Clin Pyschopharmacol* 1995;9[Suppl 5]:21–27.
78. Logothetis J. Spontaneous epileptic seizures and EEG changes in the course of phenothiazine therapy. *Neurology* 1967;17:869–877.
79. Toone BK, Fenton GW. Epileptic seizures induced by psychotropic drugs. *Psychol Med* 1970;7:265–270.
80. Pacia SV, Devinsky O. Clozapine-related seizures. *Neurology* 1994;44:2247–2249.
81. McConnell H, Duncan D. Treatment of psychiatric comorbidity in epilepsy. In: McConnell HW, Snyder PJ, eds. *Psychiatric comorbidity in epilepsy: basic mechanisms, diagnosis, and treatment.* Washington, DC: American Psychiatric Press, 1998:10.
82. Toth P, Frankenburgh FR. Clozapine and seizures: a review. *Can J Psychiatry* 1994;39:236–238.
83. Savard G. Psychosis and surgery of epilepsy. In: Lüders HO, ed. *Epilepsy surgery.* New York: Raven Press, 1992:461–465.
84. Fenwick P. Psychiatric assessment and temporal lobectomy. In: Wyler AR, Hermann BP, eds. *The surgical management of epilepsy.* Boston: Butterworth-Heinemann, 1994:20.
85. Reutens DC, Savard G, Andermann F, et al. Results of surgical treatment of temporal lobe epilepsy with chronic psychosis. *Brain* 1997;120:1929–1936.
86. Anonymous. Tool identifies patients not competent to be research subjects. *Psychiatr News* 2000;35:14,32.
87. Manyam BV. Epilepsy in ancient India. *Epilepsia* 1992;33:473–475.
88. Falconer MA, Hill D, Meyer A, et al. Treatment of temporal lobe epilepsy by temporal lobectomy: a survey of findings and results. *Lancet* 1955;1:827–835.
89. Rayport M, Ferguson SM, Schell CA. Discrete depth stimulation of temporal lobe reproduces psychiatric symptoms of temporal lobe epilepsy. *J Neuropsychiatry Clin Neurosci* 2000;12:158(abst).
90. Talairach J, Bancaud J, Szikla G, et al. Approche nouvelle de la neurochirurgie de l'épilepsie. Méthdologie stéréotaxique et résultats thérapeutiques. *Neurochiurgie* 1974;20[Suppl 1]:3–240.
91. Hughlings Jackson J. A particular variety of epilepsy ("intellectual aura"), one case with symptoms of organic brain disease. *Brain* 1888;11:179. In: Taylor J, ed. *Selected writings of John Hughlings Jackson.* New York: Basic Books, 1958;1:385–405.

7

Anxiety Disorders in Epilepsy

Angela Scicutella

*Department of Geriatric Psychiatry, Long Island Jewish Medical Center,
New Hyde Park, New York 11040*

The link between anxiety and epilepsy can be traced back to antiquity, when people attributed illnesses to gods. In the book *The Falling Sickness,* in which Temkin (1) chronicles the history of epilepsy, it is reported that the Greeks believed that people who "fell down suddenly, had been twisted in their mind by Pan especially, and Hekate." Pan was the god of nature whose blood-curdling screams allegedly terrified people to death and from where our word "panic" originates (2), whereas Hekate, the goddess of darkness and the underworld, was blamed when people were seized with "nightly horrors (considered a form of epilepsy), fear, and derangement of mind..." (1). Throughout the centuries, this inextricable connection between anxiety and epilepsy has remained. As recently as the 1800s, some people still considered fright to be a cause of epilepsy (1). In this chapter, the focus will be on more current ideas about how these two entities are related.

Whereas anxiety and fear seem to be conceptually synonymous in the minds of the ancients, the modern definition of anxiety has evolved separately over time. Fear is a primitive alerting signal that arises in response to a clear and present danger. In contrast, anxiety refers to a state of apprehension, uneasiness, or dread that occurs in anticipation of either internal or external threats, which are perceived as unpredictable or uncontrollable. These subjective feelings of anxiety are accompanied by physical symptoms, such as chest pain, stomach discomfort, or shortness of breath. Anxiety can be healthy when it motivates the individual to take action to prevent the consequences of the potential danger, or pathologic when it is excessive in either duration or intensity and interferes with one's ability to function (3). The determination of whether the anxiety is normal or pathologic requires that there be a good doctor–patient rapport so that the signs and symptoms of anxiety can be elicited and further assessed.

ASSESSMENT OF ANXIETY

When a patient presents to his or her physician with a chief complaint of anxiety, the clinician must perform a thorough history and careful physical examination. During the interview, the patient should be questioned about the situations in which the apprehension is experienced, any pattern of avoidance behavior, and accompanying physical symptoms of anxiety, such as palpitations, headache, dizziness, sweating, gastrointestinal discomfort, or respiratory difficulties. Independent observations by the patient's family and friends can aid the clinician in his evaluation. Because there are many medical impostors of anxiety, the physician also should perform laboratory tests including routine chemistries, thyroid function tests, a complete blood count, electrocardiogram, an echocardiogram, and, if indicated, an electroencephalogram (EEG) or a brain imaging study. Although positron emission tomography, panic-provoking substances (sodium lactate), and measurement of neurotransmitter metabolites in cerebrospinal fluid have been used in research investigations of specific anxiety syndromes, they have not been standardized for routine clinical settings (4). With the completion of this evaluation, if a medical disorder cannot account for the anxiety, the clinician then turns to the *Diagnostic and Statistical Manual of Mental Disorders* (DSM) (5) to categorize the particular subtype of anxiety, as will be delineated later.

In addition to the DSM, objective and well-validated psychiatric scales can aid in the assessment of anxiety. The scales for anxiety utilized in studies of epileptic patients include (i) the Spielberger State-Trait Anxiety Inventory (6), which measures anxiety in general and at a particular point in time; (ii) the Beck Anxiety Inventory (7), which measures the severity of anxiety symptoms with the intent of avoiding overlap with depressive symptoms; and (iii) the Hospital Anxiety and Depression Scale (8), which assesses anxiety in outpatients with physical illness. The Minnesota Multiphasic Personality Inventory (9) is one of the most frequently used instruments in the psychological evaluation of patients with epilepsy. Among its 550 questions, there are a number of items designed to identify symptoms of psychasthenia (anxiety). Finally, the Washington Psychosocial Seizure Inventory (10) and the Quality of Life in Epilepsy Inventory (11) are examples of more recently designed scales that attempt to assess the impact of seizures on psychosocial function and include questions on anxiety.

TEMPORAL RELATIONSHIP BETWEEN THE SYMPTOMS OF ANXIETY AND THE ICTAL EVENT

The anxiety disorders can be classified according to the temporal relation to the ictal event into periictal, ictal, and interictal. Periictal anxiety refers to symptoms occurring preceding the onset of the seizure and/or during the postictal period, which can extend up to 7 days after the seizure. Preictal anxiety has been reported to occur several days preceding

an epileptic attack. For example, Betts (12) described a patient who would become agitated and irritable 1 week prior to his tonic-clonic seizures and 2 days before the event would develop a rash, anticipatory anxiety, and a disturbed sleep pattern. Others have noted an increase in anxiety as measured by mood rating scales in the days prior to a seizure in patients with both generalized and partial seizure types (13).

In temporal lobe epilepsy (TLE), it has long been recognized that fear and anxiety are common ictal affects (14) that have been anatomically localized to the anteromedial temporal lobe (15) or structures of the limbic system (16). Historically, Hughlings Jackson (17) usually has been credited as first person to recognize that the fear was a part of the ictus itself, rather than a reaction to the fact that a seizure was about to occur. Descriptions of the fear range from "feeling tense and apprehensive" to "dread, horror, anguish, and despair" (18); usually the emotion is brief, lasting seconds to about 2 minutes (19). Fear can occur in isolation from other ictal phenomena as the sole expression of a simple partial seizure or can be the "aura" of a complex partial seizure. Williams (14) described a 14-year-old boy who experienced sudden fear lasting up to a few minutes in which he remained conscious and had no other accompanying ictal sensations. In addition to ictal fear, in the course of a simple partial seizure, patients may experience a variety of autonomic symptoms, which include visceral symptoms (i.e., changes in heart rate or respiration, pallor or flushing, a rising epigastric sensation, or nausea). Psychic phenomena, including hallucinations and feelings of déja vu, jamais vu, and derealization and depersonalization, may be present (20). When the ictus evolves into a complex partial seizure, the patient typically presents automatisms such as masticatory movements and purposeless hand movements. In such cases, patients may be amnesic to the symptoms of anxiety. Ictal fear has been reported as complex partial status epilepticus in which the fear lasted up to 12 hours in one patient (21) and up to 3 months in another (22). Following a right temporal lobectomy, the symptoms of anxiety ceased in both patients.

During the postictal period, patients can experience fear and anxiety that may last for hours or days (19). In most patients, symptoms of anxiety occur during the interictal period, be it in the presence of a generalized seizure disorder or TLE (23,24). Patients experience feelings of apprehension or manifest clinical anxiety syndromes such as panic disorder (PD) or generalized anxiety disorder (GAD). Interictal anxiety disorders will be discussed in greater detail later.

PREVALENCE OF ANXIETY DISORDERS IN EPILEPSY

Over the course of the twentieth century, a debate has been waged on whether a higher prevalence of psychiatric morbidity exists among epileptic patients as compared to controls. The data are full of methodologic problems, which include (i) a lack of adequate patient and control populations, (ii) the failure to use uniform psychiatric and neurologic diagnostic criteria, and (iii) sample selection bias with hospital compared to community studies demonstrating more psychopathology (25). Assessment of the prevalence of anxiety disorders in epilepsy is confounded by its frequent comorbidity with depressive disorders (26). Despite these obstacles, there are enough data to suggest a higher prevalence of anxiety symptoms in patients with epilepsy in both community and hospital studies than in controls. We will highlight some of the relevant studies.

In one of the earlier community-based investigations, done in 1956, Williams (14) reported that about 3% of 2,000 epileptic patients reported ictal fear. Two other well-designed community studies performed in the 1960s, one by Pond and Bidwell (27) in Britain and the other by Gudmundsson (28) in Iceland, reported neurosis in 15% and 17.7% of their respective study populations. Using unselected community-based populations of epileptics, as did the two previously cited researchers, but using more rigorous diagnostic

criteria, Edeh and Toone (29) in 1987 and Jacoby et al. (30) in 1996 found that anxiety disorders were diagnosed in 14.8% and 25% of their respective general practices. Most studies have defined anxiety as a generic category, but two groups recently investigated the relationship between epilepsy and PD. In France, 21% of a subgroup of 1,630 epileptic patients in the general population had a history of panic attacks as compared to 3% of controls (31). On the other hand, in a large epidemiologic study in the United States (32), an adjusted odds ratio of 5.9-fold was found in patients with PD who reported a seizure history, compared to persons with no psychiatric disorder.

In hospital studies, Currie et al. (33) in 1971 found anxiety disorders in 19% of 666 temporal lobe epileptics, whereas Taylor (34) in 1972 diagnosed anxiety disorders, including phobias and obsessional features, in 18% of TLE patients. Mittan and Locke (35) in 1982 reported that about 50% of 147 epileptics who completed a clinic survey identified worrying about their seizures as their primary psychological problem. Within the past 10 years, in a small controlled clinic study in Italy, 16% of patients with partial and generalized epilepsy were found to have anxiety disorders (36), whereas the rate for anxiety syndromes in a larger uncontrolled study of epileptics in a Nigerian clinic was reported to be as high as 25% (37). Finally, in patients admitted to specialized epilepsy monitoring units to assess for surgical candidature, Victoroff (38) found 31.67% had anxiety symptoms that were independent of a mood disorder, whereas Manchanda et al. (39) recorded a 10.7% prevalence rate of anxiety disorders.

The prevalence rate of epilepsy in the general population is about 1% (40), whereas that of PD is 1.5% to 2% and obsessive-compulsive disorder (OCD) is reported as 2% to 3% (41). Thus, the studies cited earlier clearly reflect a significantly higher prevalence of anxiety disorders among patients with epilepsy than in the general population, placing them, without a doubt, among the leading psychiatric comorbidities in epilepsy. Nevertheless, the methodologic flaws of many of the outlined studies preclude us from being certain about the "actual" incidence and prevalence of anxiety disorders in epilepsy. The use of future epidemiologic studies designed with greater methodologic rigor will yield more accurate statistics.

RISK FACTORS AND ETIOLOGIES

The pathogenic mechanisms mediating the development of anxiety disorders in epilepsy are complex and dependent on the interactions of multiple factors that include neurologic, pharmacologic, and psychosocial factors (42). The type and severity of epileptic syndrome is one of the neurobiologic factors that may play a prominent role in this process. This is illustrated by the fact that ictal fear is the most common affect linked to TLE (14,43). In addition, seizure severity was found to be among the most significant predictors of anxiety in 100 patients with medication-refractory epilepsy (44). From a neuroanatomic perspective, there is a hypothesis suggesting that a nondominant hemispheric lateralization may be related to the apprehension experienced by epileptic patients. This is supported by case reports of patients with anxiety who were subsequently diagnosed with structural lesions in the right temporal or parahippocampal areas (45,46). Data from positron emission tomographic scans have provided additional evidence supporting the role of the right temporal structures in the pathogenesis of anxiety in epilepsy. These studies demonstrated an increased blood flow and O_2 metabolism in right parahippocampal regions (47) in susceptible patients who were administered intravenous sodium lactate. This solution caused respiratory stimulation and a shift in the metabolic acid/base balance, and it led to a panic attack.

Electrophysiologic data support these views as well. Using electrical stimulation of temporal lobe structures, Penfield and Jasper (15) evoked fear responses in patients undergoing presurgical evaluation for intractable seizures. Gloor et al. (16) showed that anxiety occurred only when the electrical stimulation specifically involved limbic structures such as the amygdala. Additional evidence for the role of the amygdala comes from experiments with animal models. It is believed that repetitive electrical stimulations (kindling) of amygdala may have resulted in neuronal hyperexcitability of that structure, leading to longer-lasting anxiogenic consequences for the organism. Hypothetically, this phenomenon may be analogous to repeated seizures causing interictal anxiety in humans (48). Finally, changes of neurotransmitters, such as norepinephrine, dopamine, and serotonin, as well as neuroendocrine substances such as γ-aminobutyric acid, adrenocorticotrophic hormone, and neuropeptide Y, have been linked to anxiety in patients with epilepsy (49). Anticonvulsant drugs also can be the culprit agents in the development of anxiety (50). This will be discussed in greater detail in the section on Iatrogenic Anxiety Disorder in Epilepsy.

In terms of psychosocial risk factors, the primary concern is the unpredictable nature of this illness, because the loss of control over when or where a seizure will occur can promote feelings of dread and fear. Because of the seizures, restrictions may be placed on driving and employment, which in turn can lead to a lack of financial security and the need to depend on family members who may become overprotective and deprive the patient of growing and developing on his or her own. This can lead to poor self-esteem, as well as stigmatization and social rejection by peers who are uneducated or misinformed about epilepsy.

IATROGENIC ANXIETY DISORDER IN EPILEPSY

Physicians can precipitate anxiety disorders iatrogenically pharmacologically, when certain antiepileptic drugs (AEDs) are withdrawn for therapeutic reasons (50), during video EEG monitoring studies in the course of a presurgical evaluation (51), or in preparation for clinical trials (52). For example, Malow et al. (52) reported that three of 12 patients experienced symptoms of anxiety while being tapered from carbamazepine at different rates. Others found that 22 of 32 inpatients withdrawn from all AEDs prior to an investigational drug study had increased scores on anxiety rating scales (53). Anxiety can occur as a side effect of AEDs, as demonstrated by recent case reports of patients treated with felbamate (54), vigabatrin (55), and topiramate (56).

Surgical treatment for intractable epilepsy also has been cited as a source of anxiety. Although the procedure can abolish or reduce the number of seizures, postoperative outcome studies have revealed the development of *de novo* anxiety disorders. In 1992, Bladin (57) reported that of 107 patients who had undergone an anterotemporal lobectomy, 54% suffered significant postoperative anxiety. In another study, a health-related quality of life instrument specific for epilepsy was administered to 103 patients who had undergone surgery within the prior decade. The authors found that in patients rendered seizure-free by surgery, the anxiety scores were low, whereas those who had experienced a less than 75% reduction in seizure rate had scores that exceeded the cutoff for diagnosis of probable clinical anxiety (58). In a recent study, 42 of 60 surgical patients were diagnosed with anxiety 6 weeks postoperatively, and about 20% continued to experience anxiety 3 months after surgery (59).

Possible explanations for the anxiety experienced postsurgically include (i) impact of the resection of certain temporal lobe structures and their limbic connections that play a role in the manifestation of emotion; (ii) fear of seizure recurrence despite a successful operative outcome; (iii) apprehension related to the increased responsibilities, now that the patient is no longer considered to be ill; and (iv) disappointment and frustration in those patients whose surgery fails to reduce their seizure frequency (57,59).

Increased awareness on the part of the physician of the potential side effects associated with the different treatment modalities, coupled with the education of patients prior to prescription of these treatments, should minimize the incidence of iatrogenic anxiety.

DOES ANXIETY FACILITATE THE OCCURRENCE OF SEIZURES?

It is generally accepted that stressors of either a physiologic or psychological nature can lead to the occurrence of symptoms of anxiety. On the other hand, the question of whether anxiety can worsen seizure activity is less well understood. Both case reports and studies of groups of patients with epilepsy have shown that emotional factors can act as precipitants for seizures in patients with epilepsy. Caveness (60) reported the case of a young boy whose first seizure occurred after a minor car accident. Over a period of time, he had three seizures, each after a seemingly stressful event: a horror movie, a tooth extraction, and his parents' argument. More recently, Feldman and Paul (61) studied five poorly controlled epileptics using a technique to stimulate recall of the stressors that would precipitate a seizure. In one example, a patient viewed a videotape of herself having an event after she had listened to an audiotape of a young runaway crying to her father and then made the association that conflicts with her own father served as a trigger for her seizures. In a combined prospective and retrospective study of 151 patients, stress was identified as a precipitant of seizures by 54% of patients with psychomotor epilepsy and by 51% of those with generalized seizures (62). Similarly, Aird (63) prospectively evaluated 500 adult and pediatric subjects with drug-resistant epilepsy and reported that intense emotional factors were cited frequently by these patients as triggers for seizures. However, the study was flawed because emotional stress was difficult to isolate from other factors such as alcohol use and sleep deprivation.

Despite the obstacles inherent in examining emotion as an entity, there are a few prospective studies that support the hypothesis that stress influences the activation of seizure activity. In one study by Temkin and Davis (64), 12 subjects with a seizure frequency of four or more attacks per month had their seizure occurrence and daily events monitored for at least 10 hours per week for 3 months. Using within-individual analysis in seven of the 12 subjects and controlling for other precipitants such as sleep deprivation, illness, menses, and alcohol, the authors concluded that significantly fewer seizures occurred on low-stress days compared to high-stress days. Furthermore, it appeared that negative events were a more potent influence on seizure frequency than positive stressors, and a seizure in the past 24 hours resulted in an increase in subsequent seizures. Blanchett and Frommer (13) reported that 13 of 27 epileptic patients who completed mood rating scales for 56 days had worse scores for depression, anger, and anxiety on days prior to seizures, with subsequent improvement in the days after the seizure. In several patients, an increase in negative life events also had been recorded on days preceding seizures.

The findings of two other studies argued against a stress-induced seizure hypothesis. Milton et al. (65) prospectively monitored the timing of seizure recurrence in 24 epileptic patients who kept diaries of the events over an average of 237 days. They found that in 19 of 22 patients with seizure recurrences, there was no evidence of seizure clustering associated with stressful events. It was concluded that the process appeared more random, rather than one where stress would have induced a series of seizures. In 1991, Mattson (66) studied 177 patients retrospectively over a 2-year period; 58% of those surveyed indicated that seizures occurred at the time of stressful periods. In a prospective study, a subgroup of six of these patients were asked to keep diaries of their daily events and were examined in the neurophysiology laboratory to record EEG data. Stress led to sleep deprivation in one patient, medication noncompliance in a second patient, and hyperventilation in the remaining four patients, suggesting that stress exacerbated the frequency of the seizures, but did not cause the seizures.

Given the methodologic difficulties encountered in the aforementioned clinical studies, there are currently no definitive answers about whether anxiety becomes self-reinforcing, such that a pattern of "fear begetting seizures and seizures begetting fear is set up" (67).

PANIC DISORDER IN EPILEPSY

In order to understand the complex nature of the relationship between PD and TLE, we need to review the current nosology of the anxiety syndrome. DSM-IV (5) defines PD as recurrent, unexpected panic attacks, which are discrete periods of intense fear that develop abruptly and reach a peak within 10 minutes. In addition, at least four of the following 13 symptoms must be present: (i) palpitations, (ii) sweating, (iii) trembling, (iv) shortness of breath, (v) sensation of choking, (vi) chest pain, (vii) abdominal discomfort, (viii) dizziness, (ix) derealization, (x) fear of either loss of control or (xi) death, (xii) paresthesias, or (xiii) chills. The patient also must have experienced persistent worry about having further episodes or be concerned about the consequences of an attack for at least 1 month after the initial panic attack. In some patients, the fear of having a panic attack in a situation or place from which they could not escape creates marked discomfort and avoidant behavior that is known as agoraphobia. PD can be diagnosed either with or without agoraphobia. However, some patients are extremely apprehensive about experiencing panic symptoms and can develop agoraphobia without ever having a panic attack.

Because of the symptom overlap between PD and partial seizures, certain key features should be highlighted to assist in differentiating the two entities. In PD, the age of onset typically is between 20 and 30 years. Consciousness is preserved during the event, which typically lasts several minutes to a few hours, in some cases. There is no postepisodic confusion. Anticipatory anxiety is more common in PD, and the sequence of symptoms can vary from one episode to the next. A strong family history of PD and agoraphobia, as well as a clinical response to antidepressants or anxiolytics, suggests the diagnosis of PD. In contrast, TLE, which can occur at any age, is marked by impaired consciousness during the event and postepisodic confusion or amnesia is related to the entire or to part of the event. Partial seizures tend to be stereotypic in nature and last from 30 seconds to about 2 minutes. The presence of atypical symptoms, such as hallucinations or aphasia, and improvement with AED favor a diagnosis of TLE (68). When there is doubt, it is important to perform a thorough neurologic evaluation to identify any central nervous system pathology that could be suggestive of a seizure disorder. In some cases, routine or video EEG monitoring may not be sufficient to document a diagnosis of epilepsy. For example, Devinsky et al. (69) reported a 13-year-old patient with episodes of ictal fear in whom epileptiform activity could only be demonstrated when subdural electrodes were placed.

An additional diagnostic dilemma arises in those patients who have been described by Edlund et al. (70) as having atypical panic attacks. The latter are characterized by feelings of severe derealization, unusually intense somatic symptoms such as sweating and shaking without loss of consciousness, and associated irritability and aggressiveness. Routine EEGs revealed nonspecific abnormalities, and most of the patients improved with carbamazepine. However, routine EEG may not be sufficient to reach the proper diagnosis in all patients. In a study of 15 atypical cases, Weilburg et al. (71) noted that several patients would not have been correctly diagnosed with partial seizures if ambulatory EEG monitoring with sphenoidal leads had not been used.

When a patient presents with symptoms characteristic of PD or seizures, the possibility of a structural lesion in the temporal or paralimbic areas must be considered. In a fascinating case, Nickell (72) described a 39-year-old woman in remission for 3 years after successful treatment of PD symptoms with imipramine. The investigation of recurrence of panic attacks revealed that the attacks were shorter in duration and were associated with the occurrence of automatisms. Magnetic resonance imaging of the brain demonstrated multiple meningiomas in the region of the right hippocampus. It was suspected that they were present from the time of the original panic attacks. Growth of the tumors may have generated a seizure focus in the right hippocampal formation. Whether the initial panic attacks were related to these lesions cannot be ascertained, but the coincidence is thought provoking.

Although anxiety has been linked to temporal lobe dysfunction (15), a recent report questions whether the generation of these symptoms is restricted to these brain structures. In two patients with panic attacks and partial seizures of right parietal origin, the ictal activity recorded with subdural electrodes did not spread to mesiotemporal structures (73).

Finally, clinicians need to be aware of the following two aspects of interictal anxiety. (i) PD and TLE can coexist. In some case reports (74), epileptic patients were presumed to have an exacerbation of seizures when panic symptoms developed. Amelioration of symptoms occurred only when it was recognized that two entities were present, each requiring a distinct treatment regimen. (ii) Epileptic patients without panic attacks can become extremely anxious in anticipation that a seizure will occur in public and thus become agoraphobic (75).

OBSESSIVE-COMPULSIVE DISORDER

OCD is another anxiety spectrum syndrome in which a potential link with epilepsy has been questioned. In DSM-IV (5), OCD is characterized by recurrent obsessions or compulsions that are excessive or unreasonable. Obsessions manifest as persistent impulses, thoughts, or images that are intrusive, inappropriate, and time consuming. Compulsions are repetitive behaviors (checking, ordering) or mental acts (praying, counting) that the patient feels driven to perform in order to reduce the distress of the obsession.

The connection between obsessions and epilepsy seems to have been recognized since the end of the last century. In his 1894 article, Tuke (76) reported the frequent occurrence of seizures in the families of patients with "imperative ideas" that were defined as "impulses or emotions that arise with painful frequency and vividness." Subsequent to these early observations, it was thought that EEG evidence could provide a neurologic explanation for these symptoms, but the data have been inconsistent. Some researchers found no abnormal EEG tracings in their study subjects (77), whereas others concluded that EEGs in these patients were abnormal (78).

As in PD, symptoms of OCD can occur during the different phases of a seizure. Auras manifesting as forced thinking about a particular subject have been reported (15). The association of OCD symptoms with ictal states was reported by Ward (79). He described three patients, two with a frontal glioblastoma and a third patient with an infarct in the basal ganglia. These patients experienced strong transient compulsive feelings to walk in a particular direction or to move a limb, which in each case was resisted by the individual. Brickner et al. (80) reported a patient with postictal presentation of OCD symptoms consisting of compulsive swallowing every few seconds for 5 minutes. A patient with TLE and ictal and interictal OCD symptomatology experienced an increase in the intensity of his obsessive thoughts to harm women and children during his auras. Interictally, he would attempt to neutralize these intrusive thoughts by debating philosophically about them (81).

A review of the literature shows that the comorbidity of OCD and epilepsy has been restricted to several case studies. The role of an epileptic process in causing OCD is doubtful. For example, one patient had obsessions about owing money to shopkeepers and displayed a compulsive checking of a locked gate; these symptoms developed 32 years after the seizure disorder was first diagnosed (82). A 5-year-old girl demonstrated TLE and an OCD related to a Tourette's syndrome (83). Several cases are noteworthy in that surgery impacted on both of these conditions. In addition to becoming seizure-free, a temporal lobectomy resulted in decreased compulsive reorganizing behavior and repetitive touching

in a 10-year-old girl and decreased obsessive thoughts to harm her children in a 30-year-old woman (84,85). In another pediatric case, an 11-year-old girl with absence seizures and obsessive-compulsive behaviors, such as checking rituals and excessive hand washing, underwent a right anterior cingulotomy with improvement in OCD symptoms and control of her seizures (86). These cases suggest a possible overlap in pathology with epilepsy via involvement of limbic structures (87). In summary, although OCD has been reported in patients with epilepsy, a relationship between the two conditions has yet to be demonstrated.

GENERALIZED ANXIETY DISORDER IN EPILEPSY

Patients with seizures may experience anxiety as an exaggerated response to stress, which in DSM-IV is referred to as generalized anxiety disorder (5). This entity is defined by excessive anxiety and worry about a number of issues that occur almost daily for at least 6 months. The patient is unable to control the worry and experiences at least three of six somatic symptoms, which include (i) restlessness, (ii) being easily fatigued, (iii) diminished concentration, (iv) irritability, (v) muscle tension, or (vi) sleep disturbance.

A neurobiologic relationship between GAD and epilepsy has not been established. The symptoms of anxiety experienced by patients with epilepsy have been attributed to a "normal reaction" to the unpredictable nature of epilepsy and the psychosocial difficulties associated with a chronic illness (12).

DIFFERENTIAL DIAGNOSIS

Symptoms of anxiety and panic occur in a variety of medical and psychiatric illnesses. We list here the symptoms common to anxiety and medical disorders: (i) palpitations, dyspnea, and diaphoresis, which can be seen in cardiac diseases such as mitral valve prolapse, idiopathic cardiomyopathy, and coronary artery disease; (ii) dyspnea, occurring in respiratory illnesses such as asthma; and (iii) abdominal pain and diarrhea, presenting in gastrointestinal diseases such as irritable bowel syndrome. Among the endocrine illnesses to be considered when patients complain of anxiety, we must include hypoglycemia, hypothyroidism, hyperthyroidism, hyperparathyroidism, and the adrenal gland tumor pheochromocytoma. Drug reactions such as central nervous system intoxication from caffeine or amphetamines, as well as withdrawal from central nervous system depressants such as benzodiazepines or barbiturates, also can manifest with panic symptoms (4).

Among the neurologic conditions that need to be differentiated from anxiety disorders, we must first consider TLE. One should not assume TLE in all patients with seizure disorders and anxiety symptoms. Several case reports have identified adult-onset absence seizures (88), juvenile myoclonic epilepsy (89), and frontal lobe epilepsy (90).

Brain tumors (91) and arteriovenous malformations (92) are two neurologic conditions included in the differential diagnosis of PD. The differential diagnosis of OCD should include movement disorders such as Tourette's syndrome and Huntington's disease (87).

Among the psychiatric disorders to consider in the differential diagnosis, we must include nonepileptic seizures, presenting as the expression of a conversion disorder, or of a dissociative disorder (93). One noteworthy example is that of a 13-year-old girl diagnosed with psychogenic nonepileptic seizures during a video EEG monitoring study that failed to revealed any EEG changes concurrent with episodes of sudden falls and unresponsiveness. This girl was later found to have OCD; her falls were compulsions that she needed to perform to neutralize her obsessive anxiety about being kidnapped or lost and separated from her mother (94). Parasomnias are another type of nonepileptic event to include in the differential diagnosis. They may present as sleep terrors characterized by a sudden arousal from slow wave (stage 4) sleep, which can be accompanied by anxiety symptoms and confused with PD (95).

PHARMACOLOGIC TREATMENT OF ANXIETY DISORDERS IN EPILEPSY

The pharmacologic options for anxiety disorders include several classes of medications. Before discussing the use of the specific psychotropic drugs, we will review some of the relevant pharmacokinetic interactions between the psychotropic medications and AED. In general, enzyme-inducing AEDs, such as carbamazepine, phenytoin, and the barbiturates, tend to lower the serum concentrations of other drugs metabolized in the liver, which include most psychotropic drugs. Among the AEDs, there are two drugs, valproic acid and felbamate, that inhibit the metabolism of other drugs. Valproic acid inhibits the process of hepatic glucuronidation (96); felbamate inhibits certain cytochrome P-450 (CYP-450) isoenzymes, a family of more than 30 related enzymes involved in the oxidative metabolism of many drugs (97).

With respect to the psychotropic drugs, clinicians should be aware of the selective serotonin reuptake inhibitors (SSRIs). This class of antidepressants has been shown to be inhibitors of various CYP-450 isoenzymes. These pharmacokinetic properties have been described *in vitro* in four of the five antidepressants (fluoxetine, sertraline, fluvoxamine, and paroxetine). However, only the first three have shown significant inhibition of AED metabolism. Citalopram is one SSRI that does not have this pharmacokinetic effect, both *in vitro* and *in vivo*. We will illustrate some of the relevant interactions with a few examples. The CYP2C system metabolizes phenytoin and diazepam; the CYP3A4 system is involved in the metabolism of carbamazepine, alprazolam, and other benzodiazepines. Plasma concentrations of these agents may be increased if they are administered concomitantly with fluvoxamine and fluoxetine, as these latter drugs are all inhibitors of these two systems. In contrast, paroxetine inhibits the CB2 system, which is not involved in the metabolism of these benzodiazepines or anticonvulsants and so no interactions would be expected when administering these combinations of medications (97). Finally, because the SSRIs tend to be highly protein bound, competition for protein binding sites should be considered, so as to prevent higher levels of unbound AED in the plasma (104). A more extensive review of this topic can be found in Chapter 5 on affective disorders.

From a therapeutic standpoint, imipramine is the only tricyclic antidepressant (TCA) shown to be effective, under double-blind placebo-controlled conditions, for treatment of PD (98). Some case reports suggested a potential benefit of other TCAs in PD and GAD (99,100). Patients can have difficulty tolerating TCAs due to cardiac arrhythmias, orthostatic hypotension, and anticholinergic side effects such as constipation or dry mouth. In addition, the potential exists for experiencing jitteriness with these drugs, so gradual titration of the medication is advised (101). TCAs can cause seizures at high doses, but not at therapeutic doses. For example, the risk of seizure occurrence with imipramine at therapeutic levels has been reported to range between 0.3% and 0.6%. On the other hand, the potential of lowering the seizure threshold increases significantly at higher doses (96). Double-blind placebo-controlled studies of clomipramine (102), a drug chemically similar to the TCAs, has been shown to successfully treat the symptoms of OCD. The main limitations of this medication are orthostatic hypotension, sedation, weight gain, anticholinergic side effects, and the incidence of seizures, which has been reported to be of 1% (96,101).

The monoamine oxidase inhibitors (MAOIs), which pharmacologically increase dopamine and norepinephrine in the synapse by an enzymatic inhibition of monoamine metabolism, are effective for treating panic symptoms, as shown in one placebo-controlled study with phenelzine (103). Common side effects include orthostatic hypotension, edema, weight gain, insomnia, and sexual dysfunction. Of particular concern in prescribing MAOIs is the potential for a hypertensive crisis, which can occur in the presence of the endogenous pressor tyramine. Patients taking this antidepressant need to follow strict dietary guidelines and avoid foods rich in tyramine. Another interaction to avoid is the administration of MAOIs with serotonergic agents such as clomipramine and SSRIs, because of the potential for the serotonergic syndrome, which is manifested by tremor, myoclonus, autonomic signs, hyperthermia, and even death. To avoid this complication, MAOIs need to be discontinued when switching to an SSRI or other serotonergic agent. MAOI levels do not immediately return to normal when the drug is stopped; therefore, it is recommended to wait 2 weeks before starting a TCA or an SSRI. Five weeks should elapse before starting the MAOI if a patient was taking the SSRI fluoxetine, because of fluoxetine's long half-life (101). On the other hand, concerns about seizure risk with MAOIs are low, as the MAOIs are considered to be among the least proconvulsive of the antidepressants (96). Due to issues with hepatic metabolism, MAOIs may potentiate the action of central nervous system depressants such as barbiturates, so dosages should be adjusted as necessary (104).

The SSRIs, which are pharmacologically selective in their inhibition of serotonin reuptake, have been shown to be efficacious in the treatment of both PD and OCD (105,106). Reported side effects include diarrhea, insomnia, headaches, and jittery feelings. The lack of cardiac arrhythmias and diminished anticholinergic side effects make this class of drugs a good option for treating these anxiety disorders (101). SSRIs also are reportedly less epileptogenic than other antidepressants. Paroxetine, for example, was reported to have a seizure incidence of 0.1% (96).

Drugs in the benzodiazepine (BZD) class of AEDs pharmacologically enhance γ-aminobutyric acid transmission and can be useful for PD as well as GAD. Clonazepam and alprazolam both have been shown to be effective agents for anxiety (107,108). Shorter-acting agents, such as alprazolam, should be avoided because of the potential for rebound anxiety (101). Side effects of the

BZD class include tolerance, dependence, sedation, ataxia, memory disturbances, and occasional paradoxical disinhibition. In addition, abrupt discontinuation of the benzodiazepines can cause withdrawal symptoms, such as increased anxiety, insomnia, and autonomic hyperactivity (101). Because BZDs can be used as AEDs, there is no issue regarding the risk of seizures with these medications other than if they are abruptly discontinued.

Other agents that may be useful for treatment of GAD include venlafaxine, a potent inhibitor of neuronal serotonin and norepinephrine reuptake (109); buspirone, a partial serotonin (1A) agonist (101); and propranolol, a β blocker (110). Side effects of venlafaxine include nausea, dizziness, dry mouth, and nervousness (109); side effects of buspirone are similar, but also include headache (101). Adverse reactions of propranolol include weakness, hypotension, nausea, and depression (101). The risk of seizures during clinical testing of venlafaxine was reported to be 0.3% (111), whereas buspirone and propranolol appear to be safe choices in epileptic patients (110). These two drugs are metabolised through the CYP-450 systems: CYP2D6 for venlafaxine and propranolol, as well as CYP1A2 and CYP2C19 for the latter, and CYP3A4 for buspirone. The potential for drug interactions exists if inhibitors of these systems are administered simultaneously (99,110).

AEDs have been used for treatment of anxiety disorders, but all the data are based on open trials or case reports. Therefore, these data must be interpreted as preliminary until double-blind placebo-controlled studies confirm these findings. Valproic acid was reported to improve symptoms of panic in a few case studies and open clinical trials (112,113). Carbamazepine was successful in treating two patients with OCD and epilepsy (114); its efficacy in PD was mixed (115), whereas oxcarbazepine, which is chemically similar to carbamazepine, relieved panic symptoms in one patient who also had grand mal seizures (116).

NONPHARMACOLOGIC TREATMENT OF ANXIETY IN EPILEPSY

Historically, people have sought treatments of a nonpharmacologic nature in an attempt to reduce seizure activity. Gowers (117) reported that a ligature placed above the elbow of a patient whose seizures began in the hand would arrest the propagation of the attack. After some months, even without placement of the ligature, the seizure would cease at that precise site of its own accord. Efron (118) described a patient with grand mal seizures who could abort her epileptic fits at a particular stage of her aura when she sniffed the odor of jasmine. Later, when a silver bracelet was coupled with the perfume stimulus, seizures could be halted at the sight of the jewelry alone; this is an example of classical conditioning.

In an analogous fashion, nonpharmacologic strategies have been used to reduce the neuropsychiatric sequelae of epilepsy such as anxiety. Different forms of psychotherapy have been reported to be beneficial in decreasing seizure frequency as well as the emotional stress experienced by patients with refractory epilepsy. These include family therapy, which focuses on the impact of the illness on the family unit, and supportive psychotherapy, where the goal is to restore the patient's ability to function using empathy, advice, and problem-solving techniques (119,120).

Patients have described diminished fear of their seizures and improved self-confidence with behavioral approaches such as hypnosis (121), biofeedback (122), and muscle relaxation (123). Although these methods have suggested some promise in decreasing seizure frequency, objective measurement of anxiety reduction using rating scales was not specifically performed in the investigations. In contrast, yoga as a behavioral technique has been reported to decrease not only seizure frequency but also anxiety. Panjwani and colleagues (124) found statistically significant differences relative to controls of physiologic parameters used to measure anxiety, such as decreased lactate levels, decreased vanillylmandelic acid levels, and increased galvanic skin resistance.

Cognitive behavior therapy (CBT) as a treatment modality for anxiety involves challenging the patient's false or exaggerated beliefs about the condition that are maladaptive to daily functioning. This cognitive restructuring then is coupled with a behavioral technique such as desensitization, in which a controlled graded hierarchy of anxiety-provoking stimuli is presented to the patient. With progressive relaxation of muscle groups or imaging of peaceful scenes, the patient is taught to cope with the anxiety. Reinforcement of this approach is accomplished through homework assignments in which patients monitor negative thoughts and their approaches to coping with them (125). The effective use of CBT was described in one case of a 26-year-old woman who developed agoraphobia following a 9-year history of epilepsy subsequent to having sustained a subarachnoid hemorrhage (126). Another patient with TLE and OCD who was treated with CBT had a 50% reduction in his cleaning and counting rituals (127).

Group CBT for epileptics has been less successful, and this has been attributed to the heterogeneity of patients in terms of their seizure disorders and the selection of subjects who were not suited for learning self-control skills (128). Further research using larger sample sizes would be helpful in confirming the benefit of CBT in the group setting.

Psychoeducational methods that can help patients to deal with their illness include seminars such as the Sepulveda Epilepsy Education Program (129). Statistically significant decreases in anxiety rating scales were found in those who attended a weekend conference. Epilepsy self-help groups have shown that their focus on the current clinical and social implications of the disease, coupled with discussions emphasizing coping strategies, can decrease psychiatric complications (130). An interesting educational approach was taken by Sanders et al. (131) when they allowed patients to review videotapes of their own seizures. They discovered that this exercise did not produce any increase in the anxiety

scores of the rating scales used in the study, but rather assisted patients in better understanding and managing their seizures.

The adjustment to a chronic illness is a complicated process that involves many elements in addition to the duration and severity of the disease. To assess the psychological factors involved, Upton and Thompson (132) in 1992 reviewed the coping style of patients with epilepsy via a questionnaire. They found that the unsatisfactory scores in the anxiety category were associated with the strategy known as "wish-fulfilling fantasy," which involves longing for what might have been and imagining that the illness will be cured. Hopefully, the pharmacologic and nonpharmacologic interventions discussed here can help these patients deal more realistically and effectively with their seizures and any associated anxiety.

REFERENCES

1. Temkin O. *The falling sickness,* 2nd ed. Baltimore: The Johns Hopkins Press, 1971.
2. Barlow DH. *Anxiety and its disorders.* New York: The Guilford Press, 1988:73–74.
3. Yager J, Gitlin MJ. Clinical manifestation of psychiatric disorders. In: Kaplan HI, Saddock BJ, eds. *Comprehensive textbook of psychiatry,* 6th ed. Baltimore: Williams & Wilkins, 1995:637–669.
4. Fyer AJ, Mannuzza S, Coplan JD. Panic disorders and agoraphobia. In: Kaplan HI, Saddock BJ, eds. *Comprehensive textbook of psychiatry,* 6th ed. Baltimore: Williams & Wilkins, 1995:1191–1204.
5. American Psychiatric Association. *Diagnostic and statistical manual of mental disorders,* 4th ed. Washington, DC: American Psychiatric Press, 1994.
6. Spielberger CD, Gorsuch RL, Lushene RE. *STAI manual for the state-trait anxiety inventory.* Palo Alto, CA: Consulting Psychologists Press, 1970.
7. Beck AT, Epstein N, Brown G, et al. An inventory for measuring clinical anxiety. *J Consult Clin Psychol* 1988;56:893–897.
8. Zigmond AS, Snaith RP. The hospital anxiety and depression scale. *Acta Psychiatr Scand* 1983;67:361–370.
9. Hathaway S, McKinley J. *The Minnesota multiphasic personality inventory manual, revised.* New York: Psychological Corp., 1951.
10. Dodrill CB, Batzell LW, Quiesser HR, et al. An objective method for the assessment of psychological and social problems among epileptics. *Epilepsia* 1980;21:123–135.
11. Devinsky O, Vickrey BG, Cramer J, et al. Development of the quality of life in epilepsy inventory. *Epilepsia* 1995;36:1089–1104.
12. Betts TA. Neuropsychiatry. In: Laidlow J, Richens A,

Chadwick D, eds. *A textbook of epilepsy,* 4th ed. New York: Churchill Livingstone, 1993:397–457.

13. Blanchet P, Frommer GP. Mood change preceding epileptic seizures. *J Nerv Ment Dis* 1986;174: 471–476.

14. Williams D. The structure of emotions reflected in epileptic experiences. *Brain* 1956;79:29–67.

15. Penfield W, Jasper H. *Epilepsy and the functional anatomy of the human brain.* Boston: Little Brown, 1954.

16. Gloor P, Olivier A, Quesney LF, et al. The role of the limbic system in experiential phenomena of temporal lobe epilepsy. *Ann Neurol* 1982;12:129–144.

17. Hughlings Jackson J. Lectures on the diagnosis of epilepsy. In: Taylor J, ed. *Selected writings of John Hughlings Jackson,* Volume 1. London: Hodder and Stoughton, 1931:276.

18. Daly D. Ictal affect. *Am J Psychiatry* 1958;115: 97–108.

19. Paraiso J, Devinsky O. Neurobehavioral aspects of epilepsy. In: Feinberg TE, Farah MJ, eds. *Behavioral neurology and neuropsychology.* New York: McGraw Hill, 1997:641–656.

20. Weiser HG. Ictal manifestations of temporal lobe seizures. In: Smith D, Treiman D, Trimble M, eds. *Advances in neurology.* New York: Raven Press, 1991: 301–315.

21. McLachlan RS, Blume WT. Isolated fear in complex partial status epilepticus. *Ann Neurol* 1980;8: 639–641.

22. Henriksen GF. Status epilepticus partialis with fear as clinical expression. *Epilepsia* 1973;14:39–46.

23. Strauss E, Risser A, Jones MW. Fear responses in patients with epilepsy. *Arch Neurol* 1982;39:626–630.

24. Hermann BP, Chhabria S. Interictal psychopathology in patients with ictal fear. Examples of sensory-limbic hyperconnection. *Arch Neurol* 1980;37:667–668.

25. Standage KF, Fenton GW. Psychiatric symptom profiles of patients with epilepsy: a controlled investigation. *Psychol Med* 1975;5:152–160.

26. Altschuler LL, Devinsky O, Post RM, et al. Depression, anxiety andtemporal lobe epilepsy: laterality of focus and symptomatology. *Arch Neurol* 1990;47: 284–288.

27. Pond DA, Bidwell BH. A survey of epilepsy in fourteen general practices. II. Social and psychological aspects. *Epilepsia* 1959/1960;1:285–299.

28. Gudmundsson G. Epilepsy in Iceland: a clinical and epidemiological investigation. *Acta Neurol Scand Suppl* 1966;43[Suppl 25]:64–90.

29. Edeh J, Toone B. Relationship between interictal psychopathology and the type of epilepsy. *Br J Psychiatry* 1987;151:95–101.

30. Jacoby A, Baker GA, Steen N, et al. The clinical course of epilepsy and its psychosocial correlates: findings from a U.K. community study. *Epilepsia* 1996;37:148–161.

31. Pariente PD, Lepine JP, Lellouch J. Lifetime history of panic attacks and epilepsy: an association from a general population survey. *J Clin Psychiatry* 1991;52: 88–89.

32. Neugebauer R, Weissman MW, Ouellette R, et al. Comorbidity of panic disorder and seizures: affinity or artifact? *J Anxiety Disord* 1993;7:21–35.

33. Currie S, Heathfield KWG, Henson RA, et al. Clinical course and prognosis of temporal lobe epilepsy a survey of 666 patients. *Brain* 1971;94:173–190.

34. Taylor DC. Mental state and temporal lobe epilepsy. A correlative account of 100 patients treated surgically. *Epilepsia* 1972;13:727–765.

35. Mittan RJ, Locke GE. Fear of seizures: epilepsy's forgotten problem. *Urban Health* 1982;1:40–41.

36. Perini GI, Tosin C, Curraro C, et al. Interictal mood and personality disorders in temporal lobe epilepsy and juvenile myoclonic epilepsy. *J Neurol Neurosurg Psychiatry* 1996;61:601–605.

37. Gureje O. Interictal psychopathology in epilepsy prevalence and pattern in a Nigerian clinic. *Br J Psychiatry* 1991;158:700–705.

38. Victoroff J. DSM-III-R psychiatric diagnoses in candidates for epilepsy surgery: lifetime prevalence. *Neuropsychiatry Neuropsychol Behav Neurol* 1994;7: 87–97.

39. Manchanda R, Schaefer B, McLachlan RS, et al. Psychiatric disorders in candidates for surgery for epilepsy. *J Neurol Neurosurg Psychiatry* 1996;61:82–89.

40. Haerer AF, Anderson DW, Schoenberg BS. Prevalence and clinical features of epilepsy in a biracial United States population. *Epilepsia* 1986;27:66–75.

41. Kessler RC, McGonagle KA, Shanyang Z, et al. Lifetime and 12 month prevalence of DSM-III-R psychiatric disorders in the United States. *Arch Gen Psychiatry* 1994;51:8–19.

42. Hermann BP. The relevance of social factors to adjustment in epilepsy. In: Devinsky O, Theodore WH, eds. *Epilepsy and behavior.* New York: Wiley-Liss, 1991:23–36.

43. Hermann BP, Dikmen S, Schwartz MS, et al. Interictal psychopathology in patients with ictal fear: a quantitative investigation. *Neurology* 1982;32:7–11.

44. Smith DF, Baker GA, Dewey M, et al. Seizure frequency, patient perceived seizure severity and the psychosocial consequences of intractable epilepsy. *Epilepsy Res* 1991;9:231–241.

45. George MS, McLeod-Bryant S, Lydiard RB, et al. Panic attacks and agoraphobia associated with a giant right cerebral arteriovenous malformation. *Neuropsychiatry Neuropsychol Behav Neurol* 1990;3:206–212.

46. Ghadirian AM, Gauthier S, Bertrand S. Anxiety attacks in a patient with right temporal lobe meningioma. *J Clin Psychiatry* 1986;47:270–271.

47. Reiman EM, Raichle ME, Robins E, et al. The application of positron emission tomography to the study of panic disorder. *Am J Psychiatry* 1986;143:469–477.

48. DePaulis A, Helfer V, Deransart C, et al. Anxiogeniclike consequences in animal models of complex partial seizures. *Neurosci Biobehav Rev* 1997;6:767–774.

49. Lai CW, Trimble MR. Stress and epilepsy. *Epilepsy* 1997;10:177–186.

50. Trimble MR. Neuropsychiatric consequences of pharmacotherapy. In: Engel J, Pedley TA, eds. *Epilepsy: a comprehensive textbook.* Philadelphia: Lippincott-Raven Publishers, 1997:2161–2170.

51. Theodore WH. Abrupt withdrawal of antiepileptic drugs for intensive video-EEG monitoring. In: Wyllie E, ed. *The treatment of epilepsy: principles and practices.* Philadelphia: Lea & Febiger, 1993:1009–1013.

52. Malow BA, Blaxton TA, Stertz B, et al. Carbamazepine withdrawal: effects of taper rate on seizure frequency. *Neurology* 1993;43:2280–2284.

53. Ketter TA, Malow BA, Flamini R, et al. Anticonvulsant withdrawal emergent psychopathology. *Neurology* 1994;44:55–61.

54. McConnell H, Snyder PJ, Duffy JD, et al. Neuropsychiatric side effects related to treatment with felbamate. *J Neuropsychiatry Clin Neurosci* 1996;8:341–346.

55. Ring HA, Crellin R, Kirker S, et al. Vigabatrin and depression. *J Neurol Neurosurg Psychiatry* 1993;56:925–928.

56. Doose DR, Walker SA, Gisclon LG, et al. Single-dose pharmacokinetics and effect of food on the bioavailability of topiramate, a novel antiepileptic drug. *J Clin Pharmacol* 1996;36:884–891.

57. Bladin PF. Psychosocial difficulties and outcome after temporal lobectomy. *Epilepsia* 1992;33:898–907.

58. Malmgren K, Sullivan M, Ekstedt G, et al. Health-related quality of life after epilepsy surgery: a Swedish multicenter study. *Epilepsia* 1997;38:830–838.

59. Ring HA, Moriarty J, Trimble MR. Psychiatric associations of epilepsy surgery. *J Neurol Neurosurg Psychiatry* 1998;64:601–604.

60. Caveness WF. Emotional and psychological factors in epilepsy. *Am J Psychiatry* 1955;112:190–193.

61. Feldman RG, Paul NL. Identity of emotional triggers in epilepsy. *J Nerv Ment Dis* 1976;162:345–353.

62. Mignone RJ, Donnelly EF, Sadowsky D. Psychological and neurological comparisons of psychomotor and non-psychomotor epileptic patients. *Epilepsia* 1970;11:345–359.

63. Aird RB. The importance of seizure-inducing factors in the control of refractory forms of epilepsy. *Epilepsia* 1983;24:567–583.

64. Temkin NR, Davis GR. Stress as a risk factor for seizures among adults with epilepsy. *Epilepsia* 1984;25:450–456.

65. Milton JG, Gotman J, Remillard GM, et al. Timing of seizure recurrence in adult epileptic patients: a statistical analysis. *Epilepsia* 1987;28:471–478.

66. Mattson RH. Emotional effects on seizure occurrence. In: Smith D, Treiman D, Trimble M, eds. *Advances in neurology.* New York: Raven Press, 1991:453–460.

67. Betts T. Epilepsy and stress. *BMJ* 1992;305:378–379.

68. Handal NM, Masand P, Weilburg JB. Panic disorder and complex partial seizures, a truly complex relationship. *Psychosomatics* 1995;36:498–502.

69. Devinsky O, Sato S, Theodore WH, et al. Fear episodes due to limbic seizures with normal ictal scalp EEG: a subdural electrographic study. *J Clin Psychiatry* 1989;50:28–30.

70. Edlund MJ, Swann AC, Clothier J. Patients with panic attacks and abnormal EEG results. *Am J Psychiatry* 1987;144:508–509.

71. Weilburg JB, Schachter S, Worth J, et al. EEG abnormalities in patients with atypical panic attacks. *J Clin Psychiatry* 1995;56:358–362.

72. Nickell PV. Panic attacks, complex seizures and multiple meningiomas. *Anxiety* 1994;1:40–42.

73. Alemayehu S, Bergey GK, Barry E, et al. Panic attacks as ictal manifestations of parietal lobe seizures. *Epilepsia* 1995;36:824–830.

74. Spitz MC. Panic disorder in seizure patients: a diagnostic pitfall. *Epilepsia* 1991;32:33–38.

75. Betts RA. Depression, anxiety and epilepsy. In: Reynold EH, Trimble MR, eds. *Epilepsy and psychiatry.* New York: Churchill Livingstone, 1981:60–71.

76. Tuke DH. Imperative ideas. *Brain* 1894;17:179–197.

77. Rockwell FV, Simons DJ. The electroencephalogram and personality organization in the obsessive compulsive reactions. *Arch Neurol Psychiatry* 1947;57:71–77.

78. Jenike MA, Brotman AW. The EEG in obsessive-compulsive disorder. *J Clin Psychiatry* 1984;45:122–124.

79. Ward CD. Transient feelings of compulsion caused by hemispheric lesions: three cases. *J Neurol Neurosurg Psychiatry* 1988;51:266–268.

80. Brickner RM, Rosner AA, Munro R. Physiological aspects of the obsessive state. *Psychosom Med* 1940;2:369–383.

81. Kroll L, Drummond LM. Temporal lobe epilepsy and obsessive-compulsive symptoms. *J Nerv Ment Dis* 1993;181:457–458.

82. Garmany G. Obsessional states in epileptics. *J Ment Sci* 1947;93:639–643.

83. Eapen V, Champion L, Zeitlin H. Tourette syndrome, epilepsy and emotional disorder, a case of triple comorbidity. *Psychol Rep* 1997;81:1239–1242.

84. Caplan R, Comair Y, Shewmon DA, et al. Intractable seizures, compulsions and coprolalia: a pediatric case study. *J Neuropsychiatry Clin Neurosci* 1992;4:315–319.

85. Kanner AM, Morris HH, Stagno S, et al. Remission of an obsessive-compulsive disorder following a right temporal lobectomy. *Neuropsychiatry Neuropsychol Behav Neurol* 1993;6:126–129.

86. Levin B, Duchowny M. Childhood obsessive-compulsive disorder and cingulate epilepsy. *Biol Psychiatry* 1991;30:1049–1055.

87. Modell JG, Mountz JM, Curtis GC, et al. Neurophysiologic dysfunction in basal ganglia/limbic striatal and thalamocortical circuits as a pathogenetic mechanism of obsessive compulsive disorder. *J Neuropsychiatry Clin Neurosci* 1989;1:27–36.

88. McNamara ME. Absence seizures associated with panic attacks initially misdiagnosed as temporal lobe epilepsy: the importance of prolonged EEG monitoring in diagnosis. *J Psychiatry Neurosci* 1993;18:46–48.

89. Vazquez B, Devinsky O, Luciano D, et al. Juvenile myoclonic epilepsy: clinical features and factors related to misdiagnosis. *J Epilepsy* 1993;6:233–238.

90. Aoshima K, Mutsuko N, Takeshige R, et al. Seizures and psychiatric symptoms of epileptics with frontally localized foci. II. The localization of the EEG abnormalities and psychiatric symptoms. *Psychiatry Clin Neurosci* 1995;49:S298–S300.

91. Drubach DA, Kelly MP. Panic disorder associated with a right paralimbic lesion. *Neuropsychiatry Neuropsychol Behav Neurol* 1989;4:282–289.

92. Wall M, Tuchman M, Mielke D. Panic attacks and temporal lobe seizures associated with a right temporal lobe arteriovenous malformation: case report. *J Clin Psychiatry* 1985;46:143–145.

93. Sivec HJ, Lynn SJ. Dissociative and neuropsychological symptoms: the question of differential diagnosis. *Clin Psychol Rev* 1995;15:297–316.

94. Wolanczyk T, Brynska A. Psychogenic seizures in obsessive compulsive disorder with poor insight: a case report. *Pediatr Neurol* 1998;18:85–86.

95. Dantendorfer K, Frey F, Maierhofer D, et al. Sudden arousals from slow wave sleep and panic disorder: successful treatment with anticonvulsants—a case report. *Sleep* 1996;19:744–746.

96. Curran S, dePauw K. Selecting an antidepressant for use in a patient with epilepsy. *Drug Safety* 1998;18:125–133.

97. Nemeroff CB, DeVane CL, Pollack BG. Newer antidepressants and the cytochrome P450 system. *Am J Psychiatry* 1996;153:311–320.

98. Zitrin CM, Klein DF, Woerner MG. Behavior therapy, supportive psychotherapy, imipramine and phobias. *Arch Gen Psychiatry* 1978;35:307–316.

99. Mavissakalian M, Michelson L. Tricyclic antidepressants in obsessive compulsive disorder. Anti-obsessional or antidepressant agents. *J Nerv Ment Dis* 1983;171:301–306.

100. Kahn RJ, McNair DM, Lipman RS, et al. Imipramine and chlordiazepoxide in depressive and anxiety disorders: efficacy in anxious outpatients. *Arch Gen Psychiatry* 1986;43:79–85.

101. Janicak PG, Davis JM, Preskorn SH, et al., eds. *Principles and practice of psychopharmacotherapy.* Baltimore: Williams & Wilkins, 1993.

102. Thoren P, Asberg M, Cronholm B, et al. Clomipramine treatment of obsessive compulsive disorder. *Arch Gen Psychiatry* 1980;37:1281–1285.

103. Sheehan DV, Ballenger J, Jacobsen G. Treatment of endogenous anxiety with phobic, hysterical, and hypochondriacal symptoms. *Arch Gen Psychiatry* 1980;37:51–59.

104. Weisbrot DM, Ettinger AB. Epilepsy and behavior: controversies and caveats. *Neurologist* 1997;3:155–172.

105. Jenike MA, Hyman S, Baer L, et al. A controlled trial of fluvoxamine in obsessive compulsive disorder: implications for a serotonergic theory. *Am J Psychiatry* 1990;147:1209–1215.

106. Michelson D, Lydiard RB, Pollack MH, et al. Outcome assessment and clinical improvement in panic disorder: evidence from a randomized controlled trial of fluoxetine and placebo. *Am J Psychiatry* 1998;155:1570–1577.

107. Spier SA, Tesar GE, Rosenbaum JF, et al. Treatment of panic disorder and agoraphobia with clonazepam. *J Clin Psychiatry* 1986;47:238–242.

108. Ballenger JC, Burrows GD, DuPont RL, et al. Alprazolam in panic disorder and agoraphobia: results from a multicenter trial. *Arch Gen Psychiatry* 1988;45:413–422.

109. Derivan A, Haskins T, Rudolph R, et al. Double-blind, placebo controlled study of once daily venlafaxine XR in outpatients with generalized anxiety disorder. Abstract presented at the American Psychiatric Association Annual Meeting, Toronto, Canada, June 1998.

110. McConnell HW, Duncan D. Treatment of psychiatric comorbidity in epilepsy. In: McConnell HW, Snyder PJ, eds. *Psychiatric comorbidity in epilepsy.* Washington, DC: American Psychiatric Press, 1998:245–362.

111. *Physician's desk reference,* 53rd ed. Montvale, NJ: Medical Economics Co., 1999:3299.

112. Primeau F, Fontaine R, Beauclair L. Valproic acid and panic disorder. *Can J Psychiatry* 1990;35:248–250.

113. Woodman CL, Noyes R. Panic disorder: treatment with valproate. *J Clin Psychiatry* 1994;55:134–136.

114. Koopowitz LF, Berk M. Response of obsessive compulsive disorder to carbamazepine in two patients with comorbid epilepsy. *Ann Clin Psychiatry* 1997;9:117–173.

115. Uhde TW, Stein MB, Post RM. Lack of efficacy of carbamazepine in the treatment of panic disorder. *Am J Psychiatry* 1988;145:1104–1109.

116. Windhaber J, Maierhofer D, Dantendorfer K. Oxcarbazepine for panic disorder occurring after two grand mal seizures: a case report. *J Clin Psychiatry* 1997;58:404–405.

117. Gowers WR. *Epilepsy and other chronic convulsive diseases.* London: Churchill, 1881.

118. Efron R. The conditioned inhibition of uncinate fits. *Brain* 1957;80:251–262.

119. Williams DT, Spiegel H, Mostofsky DI. Neurogenic and hysterical seizures in children and adolescents: differential diagnostic and therapeutic consideration. *Am J Psychiatry* 1978;135:82–86.

120. Williams DT, Gold AP, Shrout P, et al. The impact of psychiatric intervention on patients with uncontrolled seizures. *J Nerv Ment Dis* 1979;167:626–631.

121. Szupera Z, Rudisch T, Boncz I. The effect of the cue-controlled modification of the level of vigilance on the intentional inhibition of seizure in patients with partialepilepsy. *Aust J Clin Hypnother Hypno* 1995;16:35–45.

122. Cabral RJ, Scott DF. Effects of two desensitization techniques, biofeedback and relaxation on intractable epilepsy: follow-up study. *J Neurol Neurosurg Psychiatry* 1976;39:504–507.

123. Rousseau A, Hermann B, Whitman S. Effects of progressive relaxation on epilepsy: analysis of a series of cases. *Psychol Rep* 1985;57:1203–1212.

124. Panjwani U, Gupta HL, Singh SH, et al. Effect of Sahaja yoga practice on stress management in patients of epilepsy. *Indian J Physiol Pharamacol* 1995;39:111–116.

125. Beck AT, Rush AJ, Shaw BF, et al. *Cognitive therapy of depression.* New York: Guilford Press, 1979.

126. Newson-Davis I, Goldstein LH, Fitzpatrick D. Fear of seizures: an investigation and treatment. *Seizure* 1998;7:101–106.

127. Kettl PA, Marks IM. Neurological factors in obsessive compulsive disorder. Two case reports and a review of the literature. *Br J Psychiatry* 1986;149:315–319.

128. Tan SY, Bruni J. Cognitive-behavior therapy with adult patients with epilepsy: a controlled outcome study. *Epilepsia* 1986;27:225–233.

129. Helgeson DC, Mittan R, Tan SY, et al. Sepulveda Epilepsy Education: the efficacy of a psychoeducational treatment program in treating medical and psychosocial aspects of epilepsy. *Epilepsia* 1990;31:75–82.

130. Becu M, Becu N, Manzur G, et al. Self-help epilepsy groups: an evaluation of effect on depression and schizophrenia. *Epilepsia* 1993;34:841–845

131. Sanders PT, Bare MA, Lesser RP. It is not harmful for patients with epilepsy to view their own seizures. *Epilepsia* 1995;36:1138–1141.

132. Upton D, Thompson PJ. Effectiveness of coping strategies employed by people with chronic epilepsy. *J Epilepsy* 1992;5:119–127.

8

Attention-Deficit Hyperactivity Disorder, Oppositional Defiant Disorder, and Conduct Disorder

David W. Dunn

Department of Psychiatry and Neurology, Indiana University, Indianapolis, Indiana 46202

Behavior problems are common in children with epilepsy. Much of the available data refer to broad categories of emotional troubles and less often define specific psychiatric diagnoses. For children and adolescents, the disruptive behavior disorders are the most frequent reason for referral to a child and adolescent psychiatry outpatient clinic. The disruptive behavior disorders are attention-deficit hyperactivity disorder (ADHD), oppositional defiant disorder (ODD), and conduct disorder. In this chapter, we will review the definitions, frequency, and therapies for the disruptive behavior disorders. We will answer the following four questions. (i) Are these disruptive behavior disorders commonly found in children with epilepsy? (ii) What are the predictors of these disorders in children with epileptic seizures? (iii) Are the presentations or natural history of the disruptive behavior disorders any different in children with epilepsy? (iv) What mod-ifications in therapy should be made in treating these disorders in the child with epilepsy?

The current accepted definitions of the disruptive behavior disorders are found in the *Diagnostic and Statistical Manual of Mental Disorders, Fourth Edition* (DSM-IV) (1). The diagnosis of ADHD requires an onset of symptoms prior to 7 years of age and definite evidence of impairment in two or more settings. DSM-IV lists nine items as the inattentive cluster and nine as hyperactivity-impulsivity, with six hyperactivity criteria and three impulsivity criteria. Examples of inattentive criteria are distractibility, poor concentration, forgetfulness, poor organization, and difficulty completing tasks. Hyperactivity is defined by constant movement, inability to stay seated, excessive talking, and an inability to play quietly. The criteria for impulsivity are interrupting, answering questions before they are finished, and trouble waiting one's turn. At least six of the nine criteria for either subtype must be present for at least 6 months in order to make the diagnosis. A diagnosis of ADHD, combined type, can be made if criteria for both inattention and hyperactivity-impulsivity are met. A diagnosis of ADHD, predominantly inattentive type, is considered if only criteria for inattention are fulfilled. If only criteria for hyperactivity-impulsivity are met, a diagnosis of ADHD, predominantly hyperactive-impulsive type, should be made.

The criteria should be seen as evolving (for reviews of the history of ADHD, see references 2 and 3). Early descriptions of this disorder stressed an association with brain damage and thus the diagnosis of minimal brain dysfunction. Eventually the presence of symptoms of inattention, hyperactivity, and impulsivity were considered evidence of central nervous system damage even if there was no prior history or evidence on examination to corroborate the presence of cerebral dysfunction. The lack of consistent evidence of brain damage led to a change in label to the hyperkinetic reaction of childhood, emphasizing the motoric overactivity of the child. By the time of DSM-III, there was a major change, with more emphasis on inattention and impulsivity and less on the motoric hyperactivity. The DSM-III diagnostic label was listed as attention-deficit disorder (ADD), which then was subdivided into ADD with or without hyperactivity. Questions about the subtype ADD without hyperactivity were raised, so the subtypes were eliminated in DSM-III-R and the diagnosis became ADHD. The current DSM-IV criteria have some critics, but the recent National Institutes of Health (NIH) Consensus Conference on ADHD concluded that there was reasonable evidence for the validity of the diagnosis (4). They suggested that more research was needed to better define criteria for older adolescents and adults and to more clearly differentiate ADHD from coexisting conditions.

Current theory has begun to consider a deficit in inhibition as the primary problem for children with ADHD, combined type. Barkley (5) contends that these children have a defect in behavioral inhibition that limits their ability to delay a response, to interrupt an ongoing behavior, or to screen competing stimuli. This adversely affects the executive functions of working memory, self-regulation, and analysis and planning, resulting in the behaviors characteristic of ADHD. This theory seems consistent with recent neuroimaging studies showing a difference in prefrontal and striatal regions when comparing ADHD children and adults with normal control populations.

ODD is the diagnosis used for the angry, irritating, hard to discipline child who stresses the adults in his world. The child with ODD differs from the child with conduct disorder by the absence of serious violation of the rules of society. Diagnostic criteria in DSM-IV require the presence of at least four of eight criteria that have persisted for at least 6 months and have caused significant impairment (1). These children exhibit temper tantrums, anger, and vindictiveness. They refuse to obey adults, annoy others, and blame others for their own mistakes. Developmentally, ODD may be an early manifestation of conduct disorder.

Conduct disorder is more severe than ODD and involves serious violations of the rules of society. DSM-IV lists 15 criteria, of which three or more must have been present in the past year and one in the past 6 months (1). The criteria are divided into four categories. The first includes physical aggression, such as fighting, using a weapon, forced sexual activity, and cruelty to people or animals. The other categories are destruction of property, lying and theft, and truancy or running away from home. If the onset is prior to age 10 years, the disorder is defined as childhood-onset type; if the onset is later, it is defined as adolescent-onset type.

Just as seen with ADHD, the definitions of ODD and conduct disorder have changed (6). These children have been labeled delinquent, a term that now is more applicable to the legal system, implying arrests or incarceration. They also were listed under the adult diagnosis of sociopathic or antisocial personality. Specific categories for children did not appear until DSM-II, when the diagnoses of unsocialized aggressive reaction of childhood, group delinquent reaction, and runaway reaction were listed. In DSM-III, conduct disorder became the appropriate term. It was divided into aggressive and nonaggressive, and socialized and unsocialized forms. These subtypes were dropped in DSM-III-R, and in DSM-IV conduct disorder became subtyped by age of onset into childhood-onset and adolescent-onset forms. Oppositional disorder first appeared in DSM-III and was relabeled ODD in DSM-III-R.

FREQUENCY OF ATTENTION-DEFICIT HYPERACTIVITY DISORDER, OPPOSITIONAL DEFIANT DISORDER, AND CONDUCT DISORDER IN EPILEPSY

Are the disruptive behavior disorders more common in children with epilepsy than in children from the general population? Major difficulties in determining the prevalence of the disruptive behavior disorders in epilepsy are the paucity of epidemiologic studies, the changing definitions of these disorders, and the variability of measures used to diagnose disruptive behavior disorders. Rutter et al. (7) documented behavioral disorders in 28.6% of children with uncomplicated seizures and in 58.3% of children with both seizures and additional central nervous system dysfunction. They used a combination of parent and teacher questionnaires and interviews with both the child and the parent to establish a diagnosis. Behavioral diagnoses were divided into neurotic, antisocial or conduct disorder, mixed disorder, hyperkinetic syndrome, and psychosis. Half of the children with seizures and behavioral problems had either conduct or antisocial disorder or a mixed disorder. The hyperkinetic syndrome was more frequent than expected in the children with epilepsy, but the numbers (four of 34 children) were too small to be reliable. McDermott et al. (8) did a population-based analysis using the Behavior Problem Index. They compared children with seizures, children with cardiac disorders, and controls. In each category, the children with epilepsy had more problems than either the children with cardiac troubles or the controls. Although the overlap is not exact, the factors hyperactive, headstrong, and antisocial are equivalent to ADHD, ODD, and conduct disorder, respectively. In each category, children with epilepsy experienced more difficulties than the children with heart disease or the normal controls. Hyperactive behavior was found in 28.1% of the children with epilepsy (cardiac 12.6%, controls 4.9%), headstrong or oppositional behavior in 28.1% (cardiac 18.3%, controls 8.6%), and antisocial behavior in 18.2% (cardiac 11.6%, controls 8.8%). Compared to controls, the adjusted odds ratios in children with epilepsy were 2.3 for antisocial behavior, 4.0 headstrong, and 7.4 hyperactive. Carlton-Ford et al. (9) reviewed the data from the National Health Interview Survey of 1988. Data were available from 11,160 children ages 6 through 17 years. Within this sample, there were 32 children with active epilepsy and 86 children with a history of seizures but no episodes in the past year. They found that 11% of the children with no history of seizures and 39% of the children with current or past epilepsy were highly impulsive. Although impulsivity was more common in the group with active epilepsy, there

was no statistically significant difference between the active and inactive epilepsy samples. The more prominent occurrence of ADHD symptoms in these latter two studies as compared to the study by Rutter et al. probably reflects the more stringent criteria used in England in the 1960s for the diagnosis of hyperkinetic syndrome. The higher prevalence rates reported by McDermott et al. and Carlton-Ford et al. are more consistent with present-day diagnostic practice.

Additional information on the prevalence of disruptive behavior disorders in children with epilepsy comes from assessments of behavior problems in epilepsy clinic populations. One problem with these studies is a potential referral bias. There probably is a tendency for children with more complicated seizures and children with comorbid behavior disorders to be seen in university-based tertiary clinics. A second problem with many of these studies is the failure to use exact diagnostic criteria or varying measures of the disruptive behavior disorders. Often, symptoms of disruptive behaviors are reported without complete criteria as outlined in DSM-IV, the broad category of ADHD is not separated into the subtypes of predominantly inattentive, predominantly hyperactive-impulsive, or combined types, and a clear delineation of coexisting conditions is lacking.

We were able to find only three studies that utilized DSM criteria for the diagnosis of ADHD in children with epilepsy. Hempel et al. (10) described ADHD in 40 of 109 (37%) children with epilepsy. They found that the children with intractable generalized seizures had a higher incidence of ADHD. Williams et al. (11) did neuropsychological testing in 79 children with epilepsy. They noted that 11 of the 79 children (14%) had a diagnosis of ADHD. In addition, the children with seizures had significantly lower attention scores on formal testing as compared to controls, even when the children with ADHD were removed from analysis. Similarly, Semrud-Clikeman and Wical (12) evaluated 33 children with complex partial seizures and found that 12 (36%) had ADHD. The diagnosis of ADHD was based on DSM-III-R criteria, with additional information obtained from structured interviews with both the parent and the child's teacher. Semrud-Clikeman and Wical used a computerized continuous performance test to assess attention and found inattention in children with epilepsy regardless of the prior diagnosis of ADHD. We recently began a study of children with chronic seizures assessing behavior with the Child Behavior Checklist (CBCL) and the Child Symptom Inventory. This latter test divides ADHD into inattentive and hyperactive-impulsive subtypes. We found that 19 of 96 children with seizures had symptoms consistent with ADHD, predominantly inattentive type, ten had ADHD combined type, and two had ADHD hyperactive-impulsive type. The latter three studies suggest that the inattentive form of ADHD may be overrepresented and underdiagnosed in the population of children with epilepsy.

Several studies reported symptoms of ADHD in children with epilepsy without reference to DSM criteria. In these clinically derived series, the prevalence of ADHD symptoms has ranged from 8% to 77%, reflecting differences in sample and diagnostic classification of behavioral symptoms. The highest figure comes from the study of Ferrie et al. (13), who noted that at least one symptom of ADHD was reported by either parent or teacher in 17 of 22 (77%) of children with epileptic encephalopathies, including intractable myoclonic or myoclonic-astatic seizures and the Lennox-Gastaut syndrome. Most had significant cognitive handicaps and thus probably would be more likely to have major problems with attention. The lower prevalence figure of 8% comes from the early report of Ounsted (14), who described severe overactivity, distractibility, inattention, aggression, mood lability, a lack of shyness, fearlessness, an absence of spontaneous affection, and wide scatter on formal psychological testing in 70 of 830 children with epilepsy. These children had more difficulties than currently would be considered consistent with pure ADHD and probably would be classified as having ADHD with comorbid ODD, conduct disorder, or possibly childhood-onset bipolar disorder.

In other studies, the prevalence of ADHD symptoms in children with epilepsy was in the range of 20% to 60%, again depending on the sample and the type of measure used to determine the presence of ADHD. Holdsworth and Whitmore (15), in a sample of 85 children with epilepsy, found that teachers reported problems with attention in 36 of the 85 (42%) children. When Holdsworth and Whitmore divided the children into groups based on school achievement, they noted that inattention was seen in 20% of the children with average to above average school performance and 59% of the children with below average or severely delayed achievement. Hoare and Kerley (16) used the Rutter parent and teacher's scales to evaluate 108 children with epilepsy. The three items of the hyperactive subscale were endorsed as probably abnormal by parents of 21% to 31% of the children with epilepsy and by teachers of 9% to 45% of children. The teachers reported more inattention and the parents more restlessness. Hoare and Mann (17) compared children with epilepsy to children with diabetes mellitus using the CBCL. They found that 30% of the children with epilepsy scored in the at risk range for attention problems versus 10% of the children with diabetes. Sturniolo and Galletti (18) asked for teacher's impressions of behavior of 41 children with idiopathic epilepsy. The teachers mentioned inattention or hyperactivity in 58% of the children. In the sample described by Harvey et al. (19), parents reported hyperactivity in 14 (22%) of 63 children with new-onset temporal lobe epilepsy. None of these studies used DSM criteria, and only Hoare and Kerley (16) and Hoare and Mann (17) used standardized measures of behavior.

Similar figures for the prevalence of ODD and conduct disorder are harder to find. In their study of the psychological adjustment of 108 children with chronic epilepsy, Hoare and Kerley (16) found that 14% of parents and 9% of teachers endorsed probable disobedient, the item most consistent with possible ODD. In addition, 5% of parents and 4% of teachers endorsed at least one of six items consistent with conduct disorder (16). In a subsequent study, Hoare and Mann (17) used the CBCL and noted that 18% of the epileptic children had at-risk scores for aggression versus 10% of controls, and 10% of epileptic children versus 7% of controls had at-risk scores for delinquent behavior. Caplan et al. found that three of 24 children with primary generalized epilepsy had ODD and one had conduct disorder (20). They also found that three of 30 children with complex partial epilepsy had ODD and two had conduct disorder. Diagnoses were based on the Diagnostic Interview for Children and Adolescents and were consistent with DSM-III. Studies from the our group found no significant difference between the CBCL subscales of aggression or delinquent behavior in children with chronic seizures and control samples of asthma (21). We recently completed an analysis of CBCL scores of children with new-onset seizures compared to siblings, and found no significant difference in either the aggression or delinquent subscales (22). In a current study of children with chronic epilepsy, we found that 12 of 96 children with seizures met diagnostic criteria for ODD and 12 for conduct disorder.

The question of violence in epilepsy has interested a number of researchers. Aggression toward others and destruction of property are major features of conduct disorder and angry irritable behavior is a component of ODD; thus, reports of rage or violence might indicate one of these disruptive behavior disorders. This would be a more convincing association if it could be shown that there is an increased risk of violence in the interictal period. Early reports suggested an association between temporal lobe epilepsy and aggressive or violent behavior. In a sample of 120 children with temporal lobe epilepsy, Glaser (23) described aggression during a seizure in 37% of children and interictal aggression in 56%. Ounsted (24) noted rage outbursts in 36% of children with chronic temporal lobe seizures. The children with rage outbursts developed seizures at an earlier age, had a higher prevalence of the hyperkinetic syndrome, and came from more chaotic homes. Currie et al. (25) heard reports of aggressive behavior from 7% of their 666 patients with temporal lobe epilepsy. Harvey et al. (19) evaluated 63 children under the age of 15 years who had new-onset temporal lobe epilepsy. They reported aggressiveness in 13 and rage attacks in five (19). Lewis et al. (26) evaluated 97 incarcerated delinquent boys and noted psychomotor symptoms in 78%. Combining history with electroencephalographic (EEG) results, they concluded that 18 of the 97 adolescents had epilepsy. Other researchers questioned the sample bias of these studies and the definitions used for either epilepsy or aggressive behavior (27). Volavka (28) concluded that violence may be marginally associated with epilepsy, with more important factors being the locus and extent of brain damage, male gender, and lower socioeconomic status.

Are the disruptive behavior disorders more prevalent in children with epilepsy? Comparative prevalence figures for the general population indicate that 3% to 5% of school-age children have ADHD, 2% to 16% have ODD, and 6% to 16% of boys and 2% to 9% of girls have conduct disorder (1). From the studies reviewed, we conclude that children with epilepsy do have an increased risk of ADHD, although the prevalence figures vary by population and definition of ADHD, we estimate that one third of children with epilepsy are at risk of ADHD. They may be at particular risk of the inattentive form of ADHD. In contrast, it is more difficult to show that children with epilepsy are at increased risk of ODD or conduct disorder. Although children with epilepsy may have more aggressive outbursts than children in the general population, prevalence figures for ODD and conduct disorder do not consistently exceed the range seen in the general population.

RISK FACTORS AND ETIOLOGIES

Assuming the child with epilepsy is at risk of ADHD and may have an increase in aggressive behaviors, how does one determine which child is at increased risk? Because of limited resources, it may be difficult to screen all children with epilepsy for behavioral disturbances. Ideally, the subgroup of children with epilepsy more likely to have behavioral problems should receive a screening assessment for behavioral problems.

A number of risk factors have been determined for behavioral disorders in children with epilepsy and for the disruptive behavior disorders in children from the general population. Behavioral problems in children with epilepsy usually are due to multiple factors. Factors often considered include demographic variables, central nervous system function, seizure type and epileptic syndrome, antiepileptic medication, and psychosocial effects of seizures on the child and family (29). Current research in ADHD suggests a combination of genetic and neurophysiologic factors in the causation of ADHD. Central nervous system damage, toxins such as lead, and medications contribute less frequently to the etiology of ADHD. Theories of social causation of ADHD have mostly been discredited. In comparison, the etiology of ODD and conduct disorders seems to involve a combination of genetic and social or environmental factors (2).

Gender should predict disruptive behavior disorder in children with epilepsy. Studies of children from the general population have consistently shown that ADHD, ODD, and conduct disorder are more common in boys (1). Surprisingly, the data are inconsistent. In children with seizures, Stores et al. (30) showed that boys, but not girls, with epilepsy fare worse than controls in measures of attention. Ounsted (14,24) noted that boys with seizures were more likely to have the hyperkinetic syndrome, but found no difference by gender in the prevalence of rage outbursts. We compared 116 girls and 108 boys with new-onset seizures and found no statistically significant difference in CBCL scores for attention problems, aggression, or delinquency (31).

The combination of seizures and central nervous system damage appears to be associated with an increased risk of behavioral problems (7,32,33). The reported prevalence of disruptive behavior disorders in children with both seizures and brain damage has varied widely. Steffenburg et al. (34) found ADHD in 7% and conduct disorder in 1% of children with epilepsy and mental retardation. Riikonen and Amnell (35) noted hyperkinetic behavior in 29 of 192 (15%) children who had experienced infantile spasms. All the children in this sample were mentally handicapped (35). The relatively low number of children with disruptive disorders in these two studies may be explained by the high prevalence of autistic disorder, which usually precludes a diagnosis of ADHD, ODD, or conduct disorder. When asking only about symptoms and not excluding a diagnosis based on other conditions, Ferrie et al. (13) found symptoms of ADHD in 77% of children with an epileptic encephalopathy.

Seizure type or epileptic syndrome often is considered a potential risk factor for behavioral problems in children with epilepsy. However, there has not been a consistent association between these potential risk factors and disruptive behavior disorders in children with seizures. Bennett-Levy and Stores (36), Carlton-Ford et al. (9), McCarthy et al. (37), and Williams et al. (11) all found no effect of seizure type on ADHD or inattention. Piccirilli et al. (38) found that children with benign focal epilepsy of childhood had impairment of attention if there was a right-sided epileptic focus, but normal attention if the focus was left sided. The limbic system and thus temporal lobe seizures have been associated with violence in some studies but not others (23,28). Although aggression and violence have been reported in individuals with temporal lobe seizures, Stevens and Hermann (27) found violence more often associated with basal forebrain dysfunction than temporal lobe epilepsy.

The degree of seizure control may be a factor in behavioral problems. Hermann et al. (39) found that poor control of seizures was associated with hyperactivity in girls with epilepsy, and poor control was associated with aggression and delinquency in both boys and girls. Inattention was a prominent factor in children with epileptic encephalopathy, a seizure type that usually is intractable (13).

Medication may be a risk factor for disruptive behavior in children with epilepsy, although the frequency and impact of adverse effects are not clearly established. Williams et al. (40) were not able to show any adverse impact on cognitive or behavioral measures after 6 months of antiepileptic drug treatment. This may be in part due to medications used most often at the present time. Phenobarbital and the benzodiazepines, drugs that currently are used less often in the school-aged child, have been associated with both inattention and hyperactivity (41). The newer antiepileptic drugs seem to have less adverse effects on behavior and cognition. Of the newer antiepileptic drugs, topiramate has caused decrease in attention, whereas gabapentin or lamotrigine had no effect (42). There are case reports of an increase in hyperactivity, aggression, and oppositional behavior in children with epilepsy and preexisting behavior or learning problems after starting gabapentin (43–45). Vigabatrin, which is not yet available in the United States, has caused hyperactivity and aggressiveness in children (46). Studies of the discontinuation of antiepileptic drugs have found that the children feel less tired and the parents note improved alertness and activation (47).

Psychosocial factors are significant predictors of ODD and conduct disorder, but they have not been major predictors for ADHD. Ounsted (24) found that one of the associations for aggression in children with epilepsy was coming from a chaotic home. Hermann et al. (39) noted that having divorced or separated parents was a predictor for aggressive and cruel behaviors in girls with epilepsy. In their study, divorced or separated parents predicted depressed, withdrawn, and obsessive-compulsive behaviors but not delinquent or aggressive behaviors in boys with seizures. Although genetics may be important in the disruptive behavior disorders, we were not able to find studies that looked specifically at family history of psychiatric disorder as a pre-

dictor of ADHD, ODD, or conduct disorder in children with epilepsy.

ASSESSMENT

There appears to be reasonably clear data showing that children with epilepsy have increased risk of both behavioral and academic problems that adversely impact their quality of life (29). These problems affect children with new-onset and chronic epilepsy. Can we reduce the number of children who should be screened for behavior or school problems? Children with epilepsy at risk of behavioral problems are definitely those with additional neurologic impairment, significant cognitive delay, and difficult-to-control seizures. However, assessing only those children with definite risk factors will result in a significant number of children with behavior and cognitive dysfunction being missed. For this reason, we think questions about behavior and school performance should be as much a part of the initial and interval history as questions about seizure type, frequency, and medication. The examiner should address questions to both the child and the parents. Parents are more accurate in descriptions of disruptive behaviors, and children are more reliable for reports of depression, anxiety, and substance abuse. Any suggestion of problems at school or behavioral change should prompt further investigation. Because the frequency of behavioral and cognitive problems is so high, we believe that physicians and nurses should have a high index of suspicion and should often request formal assessment.

Standardized questionnaires are efficient, useful screens for behavioral disturbances. Relatively simple assessments could include the CBCL or the Child and Adolescent Symptom Inventories (48,49). The CBCL is a 118-item questionnaire that gives dimensional ratings of behavior problems. The scores are normed for age and gender and have established reliability and validity. There are separate questionnaires for teachers and children 11 to 18 years of age. The Child and Adolescent Symptom Inventories are available as both parent and teacher forms, and as a youth self-report form. These inventories have items similar to those found in DSM-IV and suggest initial categorical diagnoses. These questionnaires will detect major behavioral problems and can be completed quickly at the initial visit and repeated if there are major changes in the child's seizure condition.

Once a specific behavioral problem has been identified, more focused questionnaires can be used. As one example, should the child have symptoms of ADHD, a specific questionnaire such as the ADHD Rating Scale-IV can be utilized (50). This is an 18-item questionnaire based on DSM-IV criteria. This is a well-validated questionnaire with norms for both age and gender. It can be completed quickly by parents or clinic personnel and can be scored easily. Another questionnaire frequently used for ADHD is the Conners' Parent-Teacher Rating Scale (51). These measures should be obtained at baseline and at routine follow-up visits. They can be particularly useful in determining efficacy of therapy.

ODD and conduct disorder are assessed in the Child and Adolescent Symptom Inventories and are associated with elevated scores on the externalizing behavior scale of the CBCL. More focused scales, such as the Disruptive Behavior Rating Scale-Parent Form, can be given at each visit to monitor progress of therapy (52). This 41-item scale closely follows the criteria present in DSM-IV. A 26-item teacher form that covers ADHD and ODD also is available.

If the child is experiencing school difficulties not explained by behavioral problems, formal psychological assessment with measures of intelligence and academic achievement should be obtained. This will help determine a diagnosis of either mental handicap or learning disability. In addition, the Freedom from Distractibility Scale may provide evidence of problems with attention (53). Observations by the psychologist administering the test are an additional source of information that may lead to investigation of other behavioral problems such as depression, anxiety, or psychosis.

DIFFERENTIAL DIAGNOSIS AND SPECIFIC SUBTYPES

Are children with epilepsy more likely to have a specific subtype of ADHD? In DSM-IV, ADHD is subdivided into predominantly inattentive type, predominantly hyperactive-impulsive type, and combined type. Other subtypes have been considered based on co-morbidity of ADHD. Jensen et al. (54) found evidence of two additional subtypes, ADHD with anxiety and ADHD with aggression/conduct disorder. Because of the multiple cerebral processes and anatomic loci of systems involved in attention (55), it is possible that children with epilepsy are more likely to have inattention than other subtypes of ADHD. As noted earlier, we are finding that ADHD, inattention type, is twice as common as ADHD, combined type, and ten times as common as the hyperactive-impulsive type in children with chronic epilepsy.

Mitchell et al. (56) addressed this question of subcategories of attention problems by studying 112 children, ages 4.5 to 13 years, with epilepsy and comparing them to normal controls. They used a computerized test of reaction times and found that the children with epilepsy were slower, more variable, and made more errors of omission than controls. There was no increase in errors of commission, implying that the children with epilepsy were inattentive but not impulsive. This difference remained significant even when they compared children with unmedicated epilepsy to controls. This suggests that children with epilepsy are more likely to have ADHD, predominantly inattentive type. In this study, the presence of inattention was not associated with seizure duration, severity, or antiepileptic drug use.

Additional support for the occurrence of the inattentive form of ADHD in children with epilepsy comes from the report of Semrud-Clikeman and Wical (12). They utilized a computerized continuous performance task to assess symptoms of ADHD. The children were divided into groups based on diagnoses of ADHD and complex partial seizures, complex partial seizures without ADHD, ADHD without seizures, and a control group with neither diagnosis. The group with combined ADHD and epilepsy did worse than controls on all measures. There was no difference between the groups with ADHD alone and those with epilepsy without a diagnosis of ADHD. The children with complex partial seizures were significantly different from controls in errors of omission but not errors of commission, again suggesting that children with seizures may have a predominantly inattentive form of ADHD.

Some additional support for the more frequent occurrence of inattention but not hyperactivity and impulsivity comes from studies showing higher scores on the attention subscales of formal psychological testing in children with seizures. Neuropsychological assessments reported by Williams et al. (11) and Fastenau et al. (57) demonstrated more attentional problems in children with epilepsy. In the study by Williams et al. (11), this was present even after the children with a prior diagnosis of ADHD were removed for analysis. Both adults with epilepsy and mentally retarded individuals with epilepsy have been found to have more problems with the subtests of general intelligence scales that assess attention (58).

Other studies have not substantiated the increase in attentional problems alone in children with seizures. McCarthy et al. (37) found no difference between children with seizures and general population norms using a continuous performance task. They did not break the results down into errors of omission and errors of commission. Stores et al. (30) found that boys were significantly different from controls on both measures of attention and hyperactivity, but girls with seizures were no different from controls. Kinney et al. (59) found that children with ADHD and epilepsy were similar to children with ADHD on measures of attention, activity, impulsivity, and aggression.

We were not able to find a study that evaluated the potential subtypes of ADHD and anxiety or ADHD and aggression/conduct disorder in children with epilepsy. Ettinger et al. (60) reported anxiety problems in children with epilepsy but did not mention an overlap with symptoms of ADHD. Kinney et al. (59) found no increased rate of conduct disorder or aggressive symptoms in children with ADHD and seizures compared to children with ADHD alone.

Other possible diagnoses should be considered prior to making a diagnosis of ADHD in the child with epilepsy. Weinberg (61) described a primary disorder of vigilance characterized by difficulty maintaining alertness, inattention, and restlessness. The motor restlessness seems to be used to promote alertness. He found that children with epilepsy and children receiving sedative antiepileptic medications may have a similar disorder of vigilance.

Psychiatric disorders must be considered in the differential diagnosis of ADHD. Both inattention and hyperactivity are frequent components of the pervasive developmental disorders. The child with a pervasive developmental disorder usually has more severe impairment of social relationships and delayed or atypical language. They also have repetitive, stereotypic behaviors with an obsessive, compulsive quality. Children with bipolar disorder have an excess activity level and impaired concentration, but with more episodic dysfunction. The family history may help distinguish ADHD from bipolar disorder. Inattention is a nonspecific symptom found in several disorders and is a complaint heard from children with both anxiety and depression. The inattention of anxiety may be related to intrusive thoughts and does not seem to be due to detractions in the environment, as seen with ADHD. The inattention in depression often is associated with apathy, discouragement, and withdrawn behavior.

At present, there are no subtypes of ODD. In DSM-IV, the broad category of conduct disorder is subdivided by age of onset, and severity is defined as mild, moderate, or severe (1). Children with epilepsy do not seem to have distinctive time of onset or severity of conduct disorder in the few cases in which epilepsy and conduct disorder are comorbid.

The diagnosis of ODD or conduct disorder in children with epilepsy should be distinguished from that of seizure-induced aggression or violence (62). Behavioral disturbance in children with epilepsy may occur during the prodromal period, ictally, postictally, or interictally. During the prodromal period, parents have described irritability that might mimic the symptoms of ODD. Violence may occur rarely during a complex partial seizure. These episodes are stereotypic and associated with clouding or alteration of consciousness. Memory for the event is absent or confused. Aggressiveness can occur during the phase of postictal confusion and is seen most often as a response to attempts at restraint. The isolated repetitive episodic nature of these behavioral disturbances should allow differentiation from ODD and conduct disorder.

Delgado-Escueta et al. (63) addressed the question of ictal violence. They were able to find only seven patients from a population of approximately 5,400 that seemed to have aggression during seizures, suggesting that ictal violence is rare. Fire setting also has been reported as a rare possibly ictal event. Milrod and Urion (64) described three children with photoparoxymal responses to intermittent photic stimulation and temporal lobe EEG abnormalities whose fire setting stopped with therapeutic levels of antiepileptic medication. In these three cases, there was a history of staring spells to suggest possible seizures.

Aggressive behaviors can occur during the postictal state. Gerard et al. (65) reported subacute postictal aggression in six of 1,300 patients with chronic seizures. All affected patients were male, had intractable epilepsy, and were remorseful after the aggressive event. The aggression was stereotypic and occasionally associated with symptoms of postictal psychosis.

Distinguishing interictal behavioral disturbance from a psychiatric disorder may be difficult. The interictal behavioral disorders are uncommon, and usually there is a clear history of seizures occurring during the time of change in behavior. Boone et al. (66) described a 13-year-old girl with a 6-week history of inattention, declining academic performance, and conduct disorder symptoms including aggression and sexual promiscuity (66). She also had brief spells of staring, picking at her clothes, shaking, and incontinence occurring once or twice a week. EEG revealed frontal epileptiform discharges, and neuropsychological testing showed evidence of frontal dysfunction. Treatment with carbamazepine resulted in control of seizures that was associated with return of behavior to normal as well as normalization of frontal lobe function on neuropsychological testing. Manford et al. (67) described a somewhat similar case of a child with a history of aggression, lying, stealing, and alcohol abuse that began at age 8 years. Clear-cut seizures consisting of motor automatisms and confusion were noted at 11 years of age. At 13 years of age, he underwent a left temporal resection with subsequent marked improvement in behavior and resolution of seizures. In both cases, deterioration and episodes consistent with complex partial seizures led to the diagnosis of an interictal behavioral disturbance and appropriate therapy.

Interictal behavioral problems may be due to associated behavioral or cognitive disturbances and not primarily to the epileptic state. Mendez et al. (68) compared 44 patients with epilepsy and a history of violence to 88 patients with epilepsy but no episodes of violence. They found that schizophrenia and mental retardation were significantly associated with violence in the patients with epilepsy.

Other psychiatric disorders should be considered in the differential diagnosis of ODD and conduct disorder. The child with depression often is irritable, overly sensitive to criticism, and withdrawn. The presence of poor sleep, fatigue, and loss of pleasure in almost all activities should help distinguish the child with depression from the child with ODD. During the manic phase of bipolar disorder, the child may violate societal rules. The episodic character of bipolar disorder should help distinguish bipolar disorder form conduct disorder.

TREATMENT

Once any of the disruptive behavior disorders are identified in the child with epilepsy, what can be done? Occasionally there may be a correctable problem that can be reversed. Both barbiturates and benzodiazepines can cause inattention and hyperactivity. A first step for the child taking these medications is to switch to an alternate antiepileptic medication. Other antiepileptic drugs less often are the source of behavioral difficulties. If the change in behavior seems to follow the addition of a new medication, changing to another agent probably is warranted. If no specific precipitant can be identified, the child may need medication, psychosocial therapy, or a combination of the two for a disruptive behavior disorder.

Pharmacologic Therapy

The child with ADHD and epilepsy can be treated in almost the same fashion as the child with ADHD without seizures. Stimulant medication is considered the first choice for therapy of ADHD, combined type, and ADHD, predominantly inattentive type (69). Either methylphenidate or dextroamphetamine can be used. Both methylphenidate and dextroamphetamine appear to be equally effective in reducing symptoms of ADHD, although there may be marginally more side effects associated with the use of amphetamines (70). There is a suggestion that amphetamines might be considered a first choice for the child with epilepsy, as dextroamphetamine has been reported to reduce 3-cycles per second spike-and-wave discharges (71). We were not able to find any direct comparisons of these two agents for treatment of the child with seizures. Pemoline has been associated with rare hepatotoxicity and should be considered a third-line medication (72).

Trials of methylphenidate for treatment of ADHD in children with seizures have shown this agent to be effective without significantly lowering the seizure threshold. Feldman et al. (73) gave methylphenidate 0.3 mg per kg per dose given twice daily to children with both epilepsy and ADHD. Behavior improved with the addition of a stimulant, and there was no increase in seizure frequency. Gross-Tsur et al. (74) studied the effect of methylphenidate 0.3 mg per kg given once a day to 30 children with epilepsy. None of the 25 children who had experienced no seizures in the previous 2 months had seizures, two who had seizures in the prior 2 months had no change or fewer seizures, and three with prior seizures had more seizures. The change in seizure number was not statistically significant. There was no change in antiepileptic drug levels or EEG findings. The parents of 70% of the children reported benefit from methylphenidate, and performance on a continuous performance test was improved. Semrud-Clikeman and Wical (12) administered methylphenidate to children with ADHD and complex partial seizures and assessed results with a continuous performance task. They found that, with methylphenidate, the scores for children with ADHD and complex partial seizures (CPS) went from 3.5 standard deviations below the mean to within 1.5 standard deviations of normal. This study demonstrates the effectiveness of stimulant medication for children with seizures but did not comment on changes in seizure control. The one caution in adding stimulants to antiepileptic medication is the potential change in antiepileptic drug blood levels. Although not seen in the study by Feldman et al. (73), stimulants have caused an increase in blood levels of phenytoin and phenobarbital (73,75).

If the child with ADHD does not have improvement in attention or activity level with stimulants or develops intolerable side effects, other medications that may be helpful are antidepressants, α-adrenergic agonists, and antipsychotics. The tricyclic antidepressants are effective in children with ADHD and may be particularly useful in those children with comorbid ADHD and anxiety disorders (76). The usual starting dose for imipramine, desipramine, and nortriptyline is 0.5 mg per kg per day. Side effects from the anticholinergic effects of the tricyclic antidepressants include dry mouth, constipation, and blurred vision. Cardiac conduction disturbances are the most dangerous side effect. Most children treated with tricyclic antidepressants will have an increase in heart rate. Pulse, blood pressure, electrocardiogram, and antidepressant serum levels should be monitored, with a goal of keeping the resting heart rate below 130 beats/min, the PR interval less than 200 ms, and the QRS interval less than 120 ms. Cardiac toxicity can be avoided by using the newer agents bupropion and venlafaxine. Both are effective in improving symptoms of ADHD. The main side effects are nervousness, insomnia, nausea, and headache. Serotonin reuptake inhibitors have been somewhat effective in adolescents with both depression and ADHD but have only a limited effect on symptoms of ADHD (76).

For the child with both ADHD and epilepsy, the additional concerns with use of the antidepressants are lowering of the seizure threshold and drug interactions (77). Bupropion at levels above 450 mg per day has been associated with new-onset seizures in 1% to 5% of patients. Lower levels also may increase seizure risk, although probably less than 1%. The risk of seizures from tricyclic antidepressants may be as high as 1% but is probably a result of elevated plasma drug levels. In the limited reports to date, the incidence of seizures associated with venlafaxine was less than 1%. Serotonin reuptake inhibitors and, to a lesser extent, the tricyclic antidepressants may act as inhibitors of drug metabolism, leading to an increase in antiepileptic drug levels. Antiepileptic drugs may induce metabolism, reducing levels of bupropion and the tricyclic antidepressants.

Other agents used for treatment of ADHD include the α-adrenergic agonists, clonidine and guanfacine, and the antipsychotic agents (78). Both have limited usefulness in children with ADHD. Clonidine and guanfacine may help reduce hyperactivity, but they are less effective in improving attention, which is a major difficulty for the child with seizures. The main side effect of both clonidine and guanfacine is sedation, which could further reduce vigilance in the child with epilepsy. Antipsychotic agents have been used for the severely hyperactive impulsive preschool child with ADHD and to help reduce aggression in the child with comorbid ADHD and ODD or conduct disorder. These agents may lower seizure threshold (77). This has been a problem, particularly with high-dose chlorpromazine and with clozapine. The incidence is probably less than 1% for haloperidol or the atypical antipsychotic agents risperidone, olanzapine, and quetiapine. The main side effects for these latter three drugs are weight gain and sedation.

Pharmacologic therapy of ODD and conduct disorder should be considered only as an adjunct to behavioral treatments. There are few controlled studies available showing the effectiveness of psychopharmacology for these disorders. In a placebo-controlled trial of methylphenidate in children with conduct disorder with or without ADHD, Klein et al. (79) were able to show positive short-term effects of methylphenidate in reducing antisocial behaviors regardless of the presence of ADHD symptoms. As discussed earlier, the use of methylphenidate is not contraindicated in children with epilepsy. Antiepileptic medications have been used to reduce aggressive behaviors and would be preferred for the child with both epilepsy and severe aggression. In the only double-blind placebo-controlled trial, carbamazepine was not shown to be superior to placebo (80). An open-label trial of valproic acid did suggest effectiveness in reducing explosive outbursts in teenagers, and initial reports of a randomized trial in delinquents has indicated possible improvement in aggressive behaviors (81,82). Lamotrigine in open-label studies has reduced self-injurious behaviors in an adolescent with mental retardation, but in a larger study, lamotrigine was associated with improvement in irritability and hyperactivity in three and worsening behavior in three patients with epilepsy and mental retardation (83,84).

The other medications that may be effective for control of severe aggression include antipsychotics, β-adrenergic blockers, lithium, serotonin reuptake inhibitors, and buspirone (28). Propranolol and buspirone have been used for patients with central nervous system impairment and have reduced levels of aggression and violence. A reduction in anger and irritability was associated with fluoxetine treatment in one open trial (85). Improvement in aggression has been shown in a controlled study of haloperidol and in an open-label study of risperidone (86,87). Lithium increases the risk of seizures and probably should be avoided (75).

Nonpharmacologic Therapy

The child with ADHD may benefit from certain psychosocial interventions. Although there are no specific studies addressing the use of psychosocial intervention in children with both epilepsy and ADHD, it seems reasonable to use those treatments that have been effective for children with ADHD alone. The recent NIH Consensus Statement concluded that behavior therapy and parent training were effective (4). However, stimulant medication was judged more effective than these psychosocial therapies. Preliminary data from a large multicenter study of therapies for ADHD suggest an advantage of medication plus psychosocial therapies for the child with ADHD and comorbid problems such as ODD or conduct disorder (88).

A first step in any psychosocial intervention should be education. We found that children with epilepsy and their parents continue to have a number of fears and concerns that should be amenable to an educational approach (89,90). Lewis et al. (91) showed that group educational programs can be beneficial for parents and for children with epilepsy.

Parent management training has been effective in helping children with ADHD, ODD, and conduct disorder (92,93). The therapist works primarily with parents, focusing on assessment of problems and behavior modification using combinations of positive reinforcement for approved behaviors and either ignoring or punishments that include timeouts or loss of privileges for misbehaviors. Contin-

gency management techniques usually are taught. School-based programs use a similar approach for these problems, with an emphasis on providing structure and rapid feedback for the disruptive child.

Cognitive behavioral techniques have been somewhat effective for children with ODD and conduct disorder, but less effective for those with ADHD (92,93). The child is instructed to address distorted perceptions and to utilize problem-solving techniques. Social skills training is used to correct disrupted interpersonal relationships.

Where available, multisystemic therapy can be used to address problems at home, at school, and in the community. This can be effective in the more intractable cases that have failed to respond to prior more limited therapy (94).

SUMMARY

Children with epilepsy appear to have an increased risk of ADHD with a prevalence of approximately 30%. ADHD, predominantly inattentive type, may be associated more often with epilepsy than ADHD, combined type. There are multiple risk factors. Boys may be at higher risk, and children with intractable seizures or additional central nervous system damage seem to have more impaired attention. Stimulant medications for the child with epilepsy and ADHD are effective and safe. Combining medication and psychosocial therapies may be beneficial for the child with seizures, ADHD, and additional comorbid conditions.

Children with seizures do not seem to have an increased risk of ODD or conduct disorder. A distinction should be made between episodic aggressiveness associated with seizures or the postictal state and the disruptive behavior disorders. The children with epilepsy and frontal dysfunction or mental retardation may be at increased risk of disruptive behaviors. The psychosocial therapies are essential for children with seizures and ODD or conduct disorder. Medications such as the antiepileptic drugs, stimulants, antidepressants, and antipsychotic agents can be used as adjuvant treatment.

REFERENCES

1. American Psychiatric Association. *Diagnostic and statistical manual of mental disorders,* 4th ed. Washington, DC: American Psychiatric Press, 1994.
2. Barkley RA. *Attention-deficit hyperactivity disorder,* 2nd ed. New York: The Guilford Press, 1998.
3. Silver LB. *Attention-deficit hyperactivity disorder.* Washington, DC: American Psychiatric Press, 1992.
4. Diagnosis and treatment of attention deficit hyperactivity disorder (ADHD). NIH Consensus Statement, November 16–18, 1998;16:1–37.
5. Barkley RA. *ADHD and the nature of self-control.* New York: The Guilford Press, 1997.
6. Earls F. Oppositional-defiant and conduct disorders. In: Rutter M, Taylor E, Hersov L, eds. *Child and adolescent psychiatry,* 3rd ed. Oxford: Blackwell Scientific Publications, 1994:308–329.
7. Rutter M, Graham P, Yule W. *A neuropsychiatric study in childhood.* Philadelphia: JB Lippincott, 1970.
8. McDermott S, Mani S, Krishnaswami S. A population-based analysis of specific behavior problems associated with childhood seizures. *J Epilepsy* 1995;8:110–118.
9. Carlton-Ford S, Miller R, Brown M, et al. Epilepsy and children's social and psychological adjustment. *J Health Soc Behav* 1995;36:285–301.
10. Hempel AM, Frost MD, Ritter FJ, et al. Factors influencing the incidence of ADHD in pediatric epilepsy patients. *Epilepsia* 1995;36[Suppl 4]:122.
11. Williams J, Griebel ML, Dykman RA. Neuropsychological patterns in pediatric epilepsy. *Seizure* 1998;7: 223–228.
12. Semrud-Clikeman M, Wical B. Components of attention in children with complex partial seizures with and without ADHD. *Epilepsia* 1999;40:211–215.
13. Ferrie CD, Madigan C, Tilling K, et al. Adaptive and maladaptive behaviour in children with epileptic encephalopathies: correlation with cerebral glucose metabolism. *Dev Med Child Neurol* 1997;39:588–595.
14. Ounsted C. The hyperkinetic syndrome in epileptic children. *Lancet* 1955;2:303–311.
15. Holdsworth L, Whitmore K. A study of children with epilepsy attending ordinary schools. I: their seizure patterns, progress and behaviour in school. *Dev Med Child Neurol* 1974;16:746–758.
16. Hoare P, Kerley S. Psychosocial adjustment of children with chronic epilepsy and their families. *Dev Med Child Neurol* 1991;33:201–215.
17. Hoare P, Mann H. Self-esteem and behavioral adjustment in children with epilepsy and children with diabetes mellitus. *J Psychosom Res* 1994;38:859–869.
18. Sturniolo MG, Galletti F. Idiopathic epilepsy and school achievement. *Arch Dis Child* 1994;70:424–428.
19. Harvey AS, Berkovic SF, Wrennall JA, et al. Temporal lobe epilepsy in childhood: clinical, EEG, and neuroimaging findings and syndrome classification in a cohort with new-onset seizures. *Neurology* 1997;49: 960–968.
20. Caplan R, Arbelle S, Guthrie D, et al. Formal thought disorder and psychopathology in pediatric primary generalized and complex partial epilepsy. *J Am Acad Child Adolesc Psychiatry* 1997;36:1286–1294.
21. Austin JK, Huster GA, Dunn DW, et al. Adolescents with active or inactive epilepsy or asthma: a comparison of quality of life. *Epilepsia* 1996;37:1228–1238.
22. Dunn DW, Austin JK, Huster GA, et al. Which children with new-onset seizures are at risk for behavioral problems? *Epilepsia* 1999;40(Suppl 7):56.
23. Glaser GH. Limbic epilepsy in childhood. *J Nerv Ment Dis* 1967;144:391–397.
24. Ounsted C. Aggression and epilepsy: rage in children with temporal lobe epilepsy. *J Psychosom Res* 1969;13: 237–242.
25. Currie S, Heathfield KWG, Henson RA, et al. Clinical course and prognosis of temporal lobe epilepsy. *Brain* 1971;94:173–190.
26. Lewis DO, Pincus JH, Shanok SS, et al. Psychomotor epilepsy and violence in a group of incarcerated adolescent boys. *Am J Psychiatry* 1982;139:882–887.
27. Stevens JR, Hermann BP. Temporal lobe epilepsy, psychopathology, and violence: the state of the evidence. *Neurology* 1981;31:1127–1132.
28. Volavka J. *Neurobiology of violence.* Washington, DC: American Psychiatric Press, 1995.
29. Dunn DW, Austin JK. Behavioral issues in pediatric epilepsy. *Neurology* 1999;53[Suppl 2]:S96–S100.
30. Stores G, Hart J, Piran N. Inattentiveness in schoolchildren with epilepsy. *Epilepsia* 1978;19:169–175.
31. Austin JK, Harezlak J, Dunn DW, et al. Behavior problems in children before first recognized seizures. *Pediatrics* 2001 *(in press).*
32. Breslau N. Psychiatric disorder in children with physical disabilities. *J Am Acad Child Adolesc Psychiatry* 1985;24:87–94.
33. Caplan R, Arbelle S, Magharious W, et al. Psychopathology in pediatric complex partial and primary generalized epilepsy. *Dev Med Child Neurol* 1998;40: 805–811.
34. Steffenburg S, Gillberg C, Steffenburg U. Psychiatric disorder in children and adolescents with mental retardation and active epilepsy. *Arch Neurol* 1996;53: 904–912.
35. Riikonen R, Amnell G. Psychiatric disorders in children with earlier infantile spasms. *Dev Med Child Neurol* 1981;23:747–760.
36. Bennett-Levy J, Stores G. The nature of cognitive dysfunction in school children with epilepsy. *Acta Neurol Scand* 1984;69[Suppl 99]:79–82.
37. McCarthy AM, Richman LC, Yarbrough D. Memory, attention, and social problems in children with seizure disorders. *Dev Neuropsychology* 1995;11:71–86.
38. Piccirilli M, D'Alessandro P, Sciarma T, et al. Attention problems in epilepsy: possible significance of the epileptogenic focus. *Epilepsia* 1994;35:1091–1096.
39. Hermann BP, Whitman S, Dell J. Correlates of behavior problems and social competence in children with epilepsy, aged 6–11. In: Hermann B, Seidenberg M, eds. *Childhood epilepsies: neuropsychological, psychosocial and intervention aspects.* New York: John Wiley & Sons, 1989:143–157.
40. Williams J, Bates S, Griebel ML, et al. Does short-term antiepileptic drug treatment in children result in cognitive or behavioral changes? *Epilepsia* 1998;39:1064–1069.
41. Bourgeois EFD. Antiepileptic drugs, learning, and behavior in childhood epilepsy. *Epilepsia* 1998;39:913–921.

42. Marein R, Kuzniecky R, Ho S, et al. Cognitive effects of topiramate, gabapentin, and lamotrigine in healthy young adults. *Neurology* 1999;52:321–327.
43. Wolf SM, Shinnar S, Kang H, et al. Gabapentin toxicity in children manifesting as behavioral changes. *Epilepsia* 1995;36:1203–1205.
44. Lee DO, Steingard RJ, Cesena M, et al. Behavioral side effects of gabapentin in children. *Epilepsia* 1996;37: 87–90.
45. Tallian KB, Nahata MC, Lo W, et al. Gabapentin associated with aggressive behavior in pediatric patients with seizures. *Epilepsia* 1996;37:501–502.
46. Ferrie CD, Robinson RO, Panayiotopoulos CP. Psychotic and severe behavioural reactions with vigabatrin: a review. *Acta Neurol Scand* 1996;93:1–8.
47. Aldenkamp AP, Alpherts WCJ, Sandstedt P, et al. Antiepileptic drug-related cognitive complaints in seizure-free children with epilepsy before and after drug discontinuation. *Epilepsia* 1998;39:1070–1074.
48. Achenbach TM. *Manual for the child behavior checklist/4–18 and the 1991 profile.* Burlington, VT: University of Vermont, 1991.
49. Gadow KD, Sprafkin J. *Child symptom inventory 4 norms manual.* Stony Brook, NY: Checkmate Plus Ltd., 1997.
50. DuPaul GJ, Power TJ, Anastopoulos AD, et al. *ADHD rating scale-IV: checklists, norms, and clinical interpretation.* New York: The Guilford Press, 1998.
51. Conners CK. *Conners' rating scales manual.* North Tonawanda, NY: Multi-Health Systems, 1990.
52. Barkley RA, Murphy KR. *Attention-deficit hyperactivity disorder: a clinical workbook*, 2nd ed. New York: The Guilford Press, 1998.
53. Bornstein RA, Drake ME, Pakalnis A. WAIS-R factor structure in epileptic patients. *Epilepsia* 1988;29:14–18.
54. Jensen PS, Martin D, Cantwell DP. Comorbidity in ADHD: implications for research, practice, and DSM-V. *J Am Acad Child Adolesc Psychiatry* 1997;36:1065–1079.
55. Voeller KKS. Attention-deficit hyperactivity disorder 1: neurobiological and clinical aspects of attention and disorders of attention. In: Coffey CE, Brumback RA, eds. *Textbook of pediatric neuropsychiatry.* Washington, DC: American Psychiatric Press, 1998: 449–482.
56. Mitchell WG, Zhou Y, Chavez JM, et al. Reaction time, attention, and impulsivity in epilepsy. *Pediatr Neurol* 1992;8:19–24.
57. Fastenau PS, Austin JK, Dunn DW, et al. The role of neuropsychological dysfunction in academic underachievement among children with chronic epilepsy. *Epilepsia* 1999;40[Suppl 7]:43.
58. Forceville EJM, Dekker MJA, Aldenkamp AP, et al. Subtest profiles of the WISC-R and WAIS in mentally retarded patients with epilepsy. *J Intellect Disabil Res* 1992;36:45–59.
59. Kinney RO, Shaywitz BA, Shaywitz SE, et al. Epilepsy in children with attention deficit disorder: cognitive, behavioral, and neuroanatomic indices. *Pediatr Neurol* 1990;6:31–37.
60. Ettinger AB, Weisbrot DM, Nolan EE, et al. Symptoms of depression and anxiety in pediatric epilepsy patients. *Epilepsia* 1998;39:595–599.
61. Weinberg WA. Epilepsy and interictal behavioral disorders in children and adolescents. *Int Pediatr* 1987;2: 196–204.
62. Engel J. *Seizures and epilepsy.* Philadelphia: FA Davis Co., 1989.
63. Delgado-Escueta AV, Mattson RH, King L, et al. The nature of aggression during epileptic seizures. *N Engl J Med* 1981;305:711–716.
64. Milrod LM, Urion DK. Juvenile fire setting and photoparoxysmal response. *Ann Neurol* 1992;32:222–223.
65. Gerard EM, Spitz MC, Towbin JA, et al. Subacute postictal aggression. *Neurology* 1998;50:384–388.
66. Boone KB, Miller BL, Durazo A, et al. Neuropsychological and behavioral abnormalities in an adolescent with frontal lobe seizures. *Neurology* 1988;38:583–586.
67. Manford M, Cvejic H, Minde K, et al. Case study: neurological brain waves causing serious behavioral brainstorms. *J Am Acad Child Adolesc Psychiatry* 1998;37: 1085–1090.
68. Mendez MF, Doss RC, Taylor JL. Interictal violence in epilepsy: relationship to behavior and seizure variables. *J Nerv Ment Dis* 1993;181:566–569.
69. Greenhill LL, Halperin JM, Abikoff H. Stimulant medications. *J Am Acad Child Adolesc Psychiatry* 1999;38: 503–512.
70. Efron D, Jarman F, Barker M, et al. Side effects of methylphenidate and dexamphetamine in children with attention deficit hyperactivity disorder: a double-blind, crossover trial. *Pediatrics* 1997;100:662–666.
71. Green WH. *Child and adolescent clinical psychopharmacology*, 2nd ed. Baltimore: Williams & Wilkins, 1995:72–73.
72. McCurry L, Cronquist S. Pemoline and hepatotoxicity. *Am J Psychiatry* 1997;154:713–714.
73. Feldman H, Crumine P, Handen BL, et al. Methylphenidate in children with seizures and attention-deficit disorder. *Am J Dis Child* 1989;143: 1081–1086.
74. Gross-Tsur V, Manor O, van der Meere J, et al. Epilepsy and attention deficit hyperactivity disorder: is methylphenidate safe and effective? *J Pediatr* 1997; 130:670–674.
75. McConnell HW, Duncan D. Treatment of psychiatric comorbidity in epilepsy. In: McConnell HW, Snyder PJ, eds. *Psychiatric comorbidity in epilepsy.* Washington, DC: American Psychiatric Press, 1998:245–361.
76. Spencer TJ, Biederman J, Wilens T. Pharmacotherapy of ADHD with antidepressants. In: Barkley RA, ed. *Attention-deficit hyperactivity disorder: a handbook for diagnosis and treatment,* 2nd ed. New York: The Guilford Press, 1998:552–563.
77. Alldredge BK. Seizure risk associated with psychotropic drugs: clinical and pharmacokinetic considerations. *Neurology* 1999;53[Suppl 2]:S68–S75.
78. Green WH. The treatment of attention-deficit hyperactivity disorder with nonstimulant medications. *Child Adolesc Psychiatr Clin North Am* 1995;4:169–195.
79. Klein RG, Abikoff H, Klass E, et al. Clinical efficacy of methylphenidate in conduct disorder with and without attention deficit hyperactivity disorder. *Arch Gen Psychiatry* 1997;54:1073–1080.
80. Cueva JE, Overall JE, Small AM, et al. Carbamazepine in aggressive children with conduct disorder: a double-blind and placebo-controlled study. *J Am Acad Child Adolesc Psychiatry* 1996;35:480–490.
81. Donovan SJ, Susser ES, Nunes EV, et al. Divalproex treatment of disruptive adolescents: a report of 10 cases. *J Clin Psychiatry* 1997;58:12–78.

82. Steiner H, Matthews Z. Randomized clinical trial of De-pakote in delinquents. Scientific Proceedings of the Annual Meeting of the American Academy of Child and Adolescent Psychiatry, 1997:82.

83. Davazo PA, King BH. Open trial of lamotrigine in the treatment of self-injurious behavior in an adolescent with profound mental retardation. *J Child Adolesc Psychopharmacol* 1996;6:273–279.

84. Ettinger AB, Weisbrot DM, Saracco J, et al. Positive and negative effects of lamotrigine in patients with epilepsy and mental retardation. *Epilepsia* 1998;39:874–877.

85. Rubey RN, Johnson MR, Emmanuel N, et al. Fluoxetine in the treatment of anger: an open clinical trial. *J Clin Psychiatry* 1996;57:398–401.

86. Campbell M, Small AM, Green WH, et al. Behavioral efficacy of haloperidol and lithium carbonate: a comparison in hospitalized aggressive children with conduct disorder. *Arch Gen Psychiatry* 1984;41:650–656.

87. Schreier HA. Risperidone for young children with mood disorders and aggressive behavior. *J Child Adolesc Psychopharmacol* 1998;8:49–59.

88. Newcorn J, March J, Hechtman L, et al. How should patients be matched to treatments: lessons from the MTA study. Scientific Proceedings of the 46th Annual Meeting of the American Academy of Child and Adolescent Psychiatry, 1999;15:63.

89. Shore C, Austin J, Musick B, et al. Psychosocial care needs of parents of children with new-onset seizures. *J Neurosci Nurs* 1998;30:169–174.

90. McNelis A, Musick B, Austin J, et al. Psychosocial care needs of children with new-onset seizures. *J Neurosci Nurs* 1998;30:161–165.

91. Lewis MA, Salas I, de la Sota A, et al. Randomized trial of a program to enhance the competencies of children with epilepsy. *Epilepsia* 1990;31:101–109.

92. Practice parameters for the assessment and treatment of children, adolescents, and adults with attention-deficit/hyperactivity disorder. *J Am Acad Child Adolesc Psychiatry* 1997;36[Suppl]:85S–121S.

93. Practice parameters for the assessment and treatment of children and adolescents with conduct disorder. *J Am Acad Child Adolesc Psychiatr* 1997;36[Suppl 10]: 122S–139S.

94. Henggeler SW, Schoenwald SK, Borduin CM, et al. *Multisystemic treatment of antisocial behavior in children and adolescents.* New York: The Guilford Press, 1998.

9

Psychiatric Aspects of Pediatric Epilepsy

Deborah Weisbrot and *Alan B. Ettinger

*Department of Psychiatry and Behavioral Sciences, State University of New York at Stony Brook,
Stony Brook, New York 11794; and *Huntington Hospital Epilepsy Monitering Program,
Long Island Jewish Medical Center, New Hyde Park, New York 11040*

Physicians who treat children with epilepsy will encounter patients with depression, anxiety, and a variety of behavioral difficulties. Left unrecognized, these problems lead to persistent emotional distress and have a profound adverse effect on academic, social, and emotional functioning. Psychological maladjustment in adults who developed epilepsy earlier in life may relate, in part, to psychological difficulties originating in childhood (1,2). Assessment of psychiatric symptoms in children is a challenging and time-consuming task for a busy neurologist, and one that usually is deferred to a child and adolescent psychiatrist. Nevertheless, all clinicians need to be aware of the presentation and treatment of psychiatric disorders in children in order to make accurate initial assessment and provide necessary treatment.

This chapter highlights our current understanding of psychiatric symptoms and disorders (depression, anxiety, psychosis, and attention-deficit disorder) in pediatric epileptic patients. It also reviews treatment issues, including psychopharmacologic management, psychotropic effects of antiepileptic drugs (AEDs), drug interactions, and the risks of AED reduction of seizure threshold.

ARE PEDIATRIC EPILEPTIC PATIENTS AT HIGH RISK OF PSYCHOPATHOLOGY?

Epilepsy is a common disorder, occurring in approximately 1% of the population (3,4). In childhood, epilepsy occurs in four of 1,000 children (5); over a lifetime, as many as one of ten individuals will suffer from at least one seizure. Although a vast and controversial literature has examined and debated psychiatric issues in epileptic adults (6), relatively few studies have investigated psychiatric aspects of pediatric epilepsy. Nonetheless, recent reports suggest that psychological distress is common in children and adolescents with epilepsy and that this distress often is unrecognized by clinicians (7).

There is little argument that pediatric epileptic patients have higher rates of psychiatric disturbances compared to healthy children. What remains unclear is whether epilepsy, compared to other chronic disorders, is associated with a particular vulnerability for psychiatric difficulties. This is controversial, in part, due to the paucity of rigorously designed investigations required to answer this question. Such studies would need to compare epilepsy with other conditions, carefully matching patients to accommodate the numerous potential confounding variables (6).

A broad range of estimates exists regarding the psychiatric morbidity of children and adolescents with epilepsy. Studies of children with epilepsy attending pediatric neurology clinics report 36% to 56% of patients have significant behavioral problems (8,9). Among community samples, rates of behavior problems are lower (approximately 20%) (10,11). The often quoted Isle of Wight study, which involved interviews and administration of standardized question-

TABLE 9.1. *Stressors and consequences in childhood epilepsy*

Stressor	Consequences
Unpredictable nature of seizures	Feelings of lack of control, anxiety, dependence, helplessness, and poor self-esteem (145)
Uncontrolled limb movements or loss of consciousness	Feelings of lack of control, anxiety, and dependence
Pressure to deal with potential fear, horror, or other reactions from peers who observe seizures	Feelings of being different and rejected by others. Stigma.
Receipt of medications that affect the central nervous system and thereby may alter behavior and cognition	Feeling of lack of control, and inadequate social and academic functioning
Fear of dying during a seizure (146)	Increased anxiety and dependence (147)
Possibility of frequent absences from school	Difficulties maintaining academic performance
Normal appearance between episodes	Pressures to function completely normally
Underestimation by teachers of the child's intellectual potential	Poor self-esteem

From Caplan R, Gillberg C. Child psychiatric disorders. In: Engel J, Pedley TA, eds. *Epilepsy: a comprehensive textbook.* Philadelphia: Lippincott-Raven, 1997:2125–2139, with permission.

naires to parents and teachers of 12,000 school children, strongly supported the notion of special risk of epileptic patients for psychiatric comorbidity (12). This study found that psychiatric disorders occurred in 8% of the general population, 16% of chronic medical disorders, 29% of children with idiopathic epilepsy, and 58% of epilepsy cases associated with cerebral structural lesions. Another study found that psychiatric disturbances were more frequent in children with epilepsy than those with asthma (13). None of these studies compared epilepsy to other central nervous system (CNS) diseases, leaving open the question whether psychopathology is a result of the seizure disorder rather than associated underlying CNS conditions. A comparison of pediatric patients with epilepsy versus migraine found comparable rates of anxiety and depressive symptomatology between these two disorders (14); however, family functioning variables were more influential in the epilepsy group. In contrast, Kaminer et al. (15) found no significant differences in psychopathology rates between adolescents with temporal lobe epilepsy and those with asthma.

Even if overall rates of psychiatric disturbances are comparable to other conditions, a number of potential stressors are more specific to epilepsy than other medical conditions. These factors are listed in Table 9.1. Particularly prominent is the lack of predictability of seizures and the intense stigma

associated with a diagnosis of epilepsy. All these stress factors can promote feelings of poor self-esteem, anxiety, and dependence in children and adolescents with epilepsy.

Ultimately, it is less important to prove whether epilepsy exceeds other chronic disorders in psychopathology rates than to define the specific influences leading to psychopathology in epilepsy that merit the clinician's attention. These are discussed in the following section.

ETIOLOGIES OF PSYCHOPATHOLOGY IN EPILEPSY

The practitioner's immediate response to seeing a depressed or anxious young epileptic patient may be to assume that the child is understandably upset about having seizures, thereby "normalizing" a child's complaints. The authors have heard a clinician contend, "Of course this kid feels terrible, he has seizures." Such an assumption is an unfortunate and simplistic underestimation of the significance of depressive symptoms.

The clinician who evaluates a child with behavioral problems or symptoms of depression or anxiety must consider a wide variety of potential etiologies. For example, depressive symptoms in some patients may be acutely reactive to the diagnosis of a seizure disorder (16). The intensity of such symptoms may diminish with supportive interventions by family members. However, a study that found psychiatric symptoms precede seizure onset speculates that underlying CNS disturbance rather than reactive causes are largely responsible for behavioral difficulties in these patients (17). On the other hand, Norrby et al. (18) found no differences in psychosocial well-being in children with well-controlled epilepsy compared with nonepileptic controls. This may reflect the absence of significant underlying CNS disturbances, but alternatively it suggests that the stigma and complications of seizures may be very important. The review by Kokkonen et al. (19) of psychosocial outcome in young adults whose epilepsy developed in childhood found that only impaired mental capacity and learning disabilities, rather than epilepsy itself, predicted poor social adjustment.

In some patients, AEDs are major culprits for mood disturbance. For example, Brent et al. (20) found higher rates of depressive symptoms in pediatric epileptic patients receiving phenobarbital compared to those treated with carbamazepine. (Other examples of AED psychotropic effects are discussed in a subsequent section.) Adverse AED effects on cognition also may significantly influence mood.

A useful scheme for classifying these causes for psychopathology was developed by Hermann and Whitman (21) and is outlined in Table 9.2. Among the numerous variables associated with psychopathology in epilepsy, seizure control has the strongest correlation with social competence and freedom from behavior problems (22).

PERSONALITY AND EPILEPSY

The literature on adult epilepsy is replete with contentions about aberrant personality styles common to epileptic patients, particularly those with temporal lobe epilepsy. Well-known features ascribed to the temporal lobe personality include hyposexuality, hyperreligiosity, hypergraphia, viscosity in thinking, poor impulse control, aggressivity, and humorlessness (23,24). Although a raging debate continues over the existence of such a personality syndrome in adults, there is much less evidence for its existence in children.

A number of personality stereotypes have been incorrectly ascribed to children with epilepsy. This practice continues to be present in our society despite attempts by the epilepsy community, including social service societies such as the Epilepsy Foundation of America, to educate the public. Children with seizure disorders often experience prejudicial comments by teachers, children, and other parents. These comments typically are based on assumptions that children with epilepsy are more withdrawn, socially isolated, aggressive, tense, unpredictable, and mentally inferior (25,26). Some parents may even hold these beliefs about their own children. Social stigmas may play a major adverse role in a child's adjustment in school settings. Children may develop signs of school avoidance or school refusal. Others develop panic attacks or anxiety in social settings related to embarrassment about having seizures in school or other social settings. Children with epilepsy easily absorb

TABLE 9.2. *Factors that cause or influence psychopathology in epilepsy*

CNS variables	Medication variables	Psychosocial variables
Age of seizure onset	Antiepileptic drug type	Fear of seizures
Degree of seizure control	Polytherapy	Perceived stigma
Duration of epilepsy	Antiepileptic drug toxicity	Perceived discrimination
Seizure type		Adjustment to epilepsy
Etiology		Feeling of lack of control over one's life
Aura type		Social support
Neuropsychological status		Socioeconomic status
		Childhood home environment

CNS, central nervous system.

these false ideas about their disorder unless active attempts are made to educate them and their families. Pilot educational programs for families have been initiated at a number of sites, and the results of such efforts have been promising, although very difficult to implement on a widespread basis (27).

Conduct Disorders and Aggression in Children with Epilepsy

Children with epilepsy have been stereotyped as being more aggressive than other children. The notion of a strong correlation between aggressive behavior and epilepsy has been promoted by numerous misconceptions about activities that occur during the seizure itself and distorted interpretations of the literature surrounding interictal aggressive behavior. As in adults, aggressive behavior displayed during a seizure or during the postictal confusional state in children usually is nondirected and clumsy, with little risk of producing substantial injury, unless such patients are physically restrained (28,29). Postictal aggressive behavior is rare in adults and usually occurs in the context of a postictal psychosis (30).

Numerous studies have promoted the belief that children with epilepsy have high rates of conduct disorders and other behavioral abnormalities (12,31). However, disorders of conduct, such as attention-deficit/hyperactivity disorder (ADHD) and oppositional disorder, are frequent in the general population. To some degree, symptoms such as impulsivity or aggression may have been incorrectly ascribed to a concomitant epileptic disorder. Some investigations have suggested a relationship between temporal lobe seizures, the development of rage attacks, and the subsequent development of antisocial features in adulthood. These studies have been brought into question (32–34) due to their focus on institutionalized samples and their failure to distinguish effects of underlying CNS disorders from behavioral disturbances associated with the seizures themselves. For example, studies by Lewis et al. (35,36) found that epilepsy, especially complex partial seizure

disorders, was more prevalent in young offenders than in the general population. However, many of these children who were studied also had perinatal insults, CNS infections, or head trauma, all of which have been shown to be independent risk factors for psychiatric disturbances (37,38).

Affective Disorders in Children with Epilepsy

Making the diagnosis of a depressive disorder in pediatric patients can be challenging, even in the absence of a seizure disorder. A common mistake made by busy clinicians is to miss a diagnosis of a depressive disorder when no blatant behavioral difficulties are present. Symptoms that should alert the clinician include a decline in academic functioning, withdrawal from friends, or lack of pleasure from previously enjoyable activities. Children often deny such symptoms and may not express depressive ideas spontaneously; instead they may have multiple somatic complaints. Parents may be far less attuned to their child's internal mood state than overt conduct problems, and they may be preoccupied by worries about the child's epilepsy. Although childhood self-report measures, such as the Children's Depression Inventory (CDI) (39,40), can be valuable in identifying and tracking symptoms of depression over time, self-report measures are not, in themselves, reliable measures with which to diagnose a depressive disorder.

A complete psychiatric evaluation is required to establish a diagnosis of depression. It also is critical to obtain a detailed family history to elicit the presence of genetic factors, i.e., other family members who have been depressed. A complete medical examination is indicated to rule out underlying physical conditions that may present as depression. According to the *Diagnostic and Statistical Manual of Mental Disorders, Fourth Edition* (DSM-IV), specific diagnostic criteria must be present to make the diagnosis of major depression. However, these criteria emphasize symptoms noted in adults rather than children. For example, pediatric patients do not tend to present with the vegetative symptoms of depression, such as lack of appetite or sleep disturbance. Alternatively, children and adolescents are more likely to dwell on distorted, negative views of themselves, their life, friends, and family. Dysthymic disorder is a syndrome distinct from major depression, characterized by milder depressive symptoms persisting over a year's period. Dysthymia in childhood is associated with potentially significant psychiatric morbidity.

Major depressive disorder is uncommon in childhood and more frequent in the adolescent population. Reported rates of depression are contingent on whether symptoms or a syndrome of depression was measured and dependent on the specific subgroup examined. Overall, major depression is rare in preschool children, has a frequency of approximately 2% in children of elementary-school age, and about 5% in adolescents. Boys and girls have equal rates prior to puberty, but in adolescence, girls have higher rates of depression (41). Many investigations suggest that adult epileptic patients (especially those with intractable seizures) are at particularly high risk of developing symptoms of depression (42,43). For example, at one university-based epilepsy center, more than 50% of adult patients had elevated depressive symptom scores on self-report measures (44). Although such studies have heightened clinician awareness of the problem in adults, few investigations have examined this issue in pediatric age groups.

In our pediatric series (7), 26% of children and adolescents with epilepsy had significantly elevated depression scores on the CDI. None of these children previously had been identified to be depressed, and none had ever received a psychiatric evaluation or treatment, suggesting that depression and anxiety may be substantially underrecognized in this population. Similarly, Dunn et al. (17) found that 23% of adolescents with epilepsy had symptoms of depression (45). The strongest predictors of depression were a negative attitude toward illness, dissatisfaction with family relationships, and unknown or external locus of control (a feeling of lack of control over one's life and destiny) (45).

A child can have significant depression and display only symptoms of irritability. Furthermore, patients often carry more than one psychiatric diagnosis. For example, it is not uncommon to see a child who has diagnoses of ADHD, dysthymia, and a receptive/expressive language disorder.

As mentioned earlier, among the numerous potential etiologies for depression in childhood epilepsy, medication factors may be especially important. A study by Brent (46) found that children and adolescents receiving phenobarbital had significantly higher rates of depression and suicidal ideation than those receiving carbamazepine. Patients receiving phenobarbital who had a family history of affective disorders were at particularly high risk. These results should be kept in mind when using phenobarbital in current clinical practice. Antiepileptic agents notorious for promoting depression should be replaced by other agents in high-risk patients. Newer AEDs, such as topiramate (TPM), also may prove to be significantly correlated with depressive symptomatology (47).

It is incumbent on the physician who suspects a patient may be depressed to inquire about suicidal ideation. Suicide attempts among epileptic patients are estimated to occur at two to seven times the rate in the general population (48,49). Conversely, epilepsy was the most frequent medical condition found among a group of pediatric patients evaluated for suicide attempts at one center (46).

Symptoms of Mania and Bipolar Disorder in Pediatric Epilepsy

Making the diagnosis of bipolar disorder in children and adolescents is one of the most challenging tasks in child psychiatry. Bipolar disorder often is confused with ADHD, and its presentation may be complicated by a number of other comorbid conditions. Classic bipolar disorder is uncommon in childhood but does occur rarely. The epidemiology of bipolar disorder is not well studied. In the adolescent and adult population, bipolar disorder has been estimated to occur at a rate of about 0.6% to 1% (50). In children and adolescents with epilepsy, little is known about the frequency of manic symptoms. Symptoms of mania are reported to be quite rare in adults with epilepsy (51), although there has been speculation that manic symptoms may be underdiagnosed in seizure disorders (see Chapter 5 on Affective Disorders).

Treatment of Childhood Depressive Disorder in the Presence of Epilepsy

Treatment of childhood depression should include parental and teacher involvement, in addition to directing attention to the child. Psychotherapy, including family therapy as well as individual sessions for the child, should be strongly considered. Recently, much emphasis has been placed on cognitive-behavioral approaches (52) and interpersonal therapy for adolescents. Interventions related to the school environment, such as reducing academic pressures, may be crucial. Depending on symptom severity and the history of prior treatment attempts, a child psychiatrist will consider prescribing antidepressant medications. Inpatient psychiatric evaluation may be required in the presence of suicidal ideation or attempts, dangerous behaviors, or severe side effects from previous medication trials. Psychoeducation of patient and family is critical.

The use of antidepressants in children and adolescents is a current area of research. Surprisingly, some notable double-blind, placebo-controlled studies of tricyclic antidepressants failed to show a superior response of drug compared to placebo in child and adolescent depression (53,54). This may be due, in part, to high placebo response rates, limited study observation periods, and inclusion of patients with mild depressive symptoms. Alternatively, neurodevelopmental factors may lead prepubertal children to be less responsive than adults to agents that enhance norepinephrine. Concerns regarding potential cardiac complications, including several cases of sudden death in prepubertal children, have steered many psychiatrists away from the use of tricyclic antidepressants. Instead, the selective serotonin reuptake inhibitors (SSRIs) have become first-line antidepressants. As of yet, however, there are only a few controlled studies examining and demonstrating the efficacy of SSRIs such as fluoxetine and paroxetine (53,55). A number of other double-blind controlled studies of SSRIs, such as sertraline and citalopram, are now under way. Other agents, such as bupropion and venlafaxine, also may be considered.

General principles regarding the safe use of psychotropic agents in epileptic patients in lieu of concerns about reducing seizure threshold are listed in Table 9.3. Much of our knowledge of these risks is compromised by the limited numbers of rigorously studied patients, dependence on anecdotal reports, and overemphasis on seizures incurred during drug overdoses (56).

Excessive concern over the potential risk of antidepressant lowering of the seizure threshold may inhibit the necessary use of these agents. The morbidity of untreated depression may be far greater than the risk of potentiating seizures. Fortunately, the overall risk of antidepressant-associated seizures is quite

---

TABLE 9.3. *Principles in the administration of psychotropic agents in epileptic patients*

Psychotropic agents may be used safely in the majority of epileptic patients
Choose an agent with the least epileptogenic properties
Use conservative dose titration and the lowest effective dosage of psychotropic agents
For selected psychotropic agents, monitor serum level (to identify poor metabolizers) and adjust dose
When treatment with a highly epileptogenic agent is required, optimize antiepileptic drug therapy

Adapted from Alldredge BK. Risk of lowering seizure threshold with antiepileptic drugs. *Neurology* 1999;53:[5 Suppl 2]:S68–75, with permission.

low, ranging from 0.1% to 0.6% (57). Seizures associated with tricyclic antidepressant use are estimated to occur in less than 0.6% of cases (57,58). Some authors have suggested that specific tricyclic agents, such as imipramine and amitriptyline, carry higher risks, whereas doxepin has very low risk (59).

Monoamine oxidase inhibitors (MAOIs), which are used very infrequently in the pediatric population because of other side effects, carry a low risk of inducing seizures and may even have anticonvulsant properties (60). Other types of antidepressants, such as amoxapine and bupropion, may carry higher potential for seizures, although concerns associated with the latter may be related to the excessively high doses tested in premarketing trials rather than the true risk associated with more moderate therapeutic doses (61). Bupropion has been reported to be useful in ADHD, especially with comorbid depression, or in the face of stimulant intolerance.

Although direct comparative studies are not available, it is believed that SSRIs (e.g., fluoxetine, sertraline, and paroxetine) carry a relatively low risk of inducing seizures (62,63).

Anxiety and Epilepsy

As in depression, anxiety in the pediatric patient is more difficult to recognize than disorders with more overt behavioral difficulties, such as ADHD or conduct disorders. Children with anxiety may cause little problem in a classroom. Unless a child develops symptoms of school refusal, panic attacks, or obsessive-compulsive symptoms, it can take a long time for a patient with anxiety disorder to be referred to a child psychiatrist. This disorder requires an extensive review of symptoms and family history. When a child presents with anxiety symptoms, a family history of anxiety is not uncommon.

Surprisingly, few studies have specifically examined anxiety in children or even adults with epilepsy. More than 50% of adult patients attending our tertiary epilepsy clinic

had significant anxiety symptomatology as measured on a self-report inventory (64). Sixteen percent of pediatric epileptic patients in another series from our center scored high for anxiety symptoms on the Revised Children Manifest Anxiety Survey (7). It is likely that even higher numbers of patients experience episodic fear and anxiety related to numerous factors, including fears of death, brain damage, or mental deterioration (65). Social phobias may result from the extreme embarrassment of having seizures in public, particularly in school. This may be more common than is usually recognized in children or adolescents with seizure disorders. However, when symptoms of school refusal or social avoidance occur in children with epilepsy, it is important to remember this diagnostic possibility.

Parents of children with epilepsy have another set of anxieties different from their children's fears. These anxieties may lead them to be overprotective or overindulgent of their children. This can promote a transmission of anxieties to their children. It is as important to work with the parents of an anxious child as it is to work with the child.

Interictal anxiety needs to be distinguished from the occasionally encountered sensation of "fear" that occurs as a symptom of a seizure (66). Ictal fear offers a clue to its nature when it occurs in the context of a complex partial seizure or a seizure with secondary generalization (with loss of consciousness and/or convulsions). In response to anxiety, children with seizure disorders can experience an increase in seizure frequency or even demonstrate psychogenically determined nonphysiologic episodes, i.e., pseudoseizures.

Panic attacks (which occur more frequently in adolescents compared to those in younger age groups) (67) may be easily confused with seizures, because some seizure types have similar autonomic phenomena, such as palpitations and piloerection. Clues to an epileptic etiology are symptoms of altered awareness or generalized convulsive activity. Interictal and ictal epileptic patterns on electroencephalogram (EEG), when present, may suggest seizures. However, even if an episode of anxiety is captured during EEG recording, an epileptic event that is unassociated with altered awareness may not have an obvious correlate on scalp EEG (68).

Treatment of Anxiety in Pediatric Epileptic Patients

Epileptic patients and their families need frank and repeated discussion to address both appropriate and irrational fears about epilepsy. Peer support groups can be helpful. In situations where symptoms of anxiety do not respond rapidly to psychosocial and behavioral interventions, consideration should be given to the use of psychotropic medication in conjunction with these other modalities.

The medications used to treat anxiety disorders in children are similar to those used for adults, although few double-blind placebo-controlled studies have been performed in childhood anxiety disorders. As in depressive disorders, SSRI antidepressants and tricyclics may be helpful for anxiety. Although medications such as imipramine also may treat anxiety, concerns related to tricyclic-related cardiac and other side effects have caused them to fall out of favor with many practitioners.

Benzodiazepines, which are commonly used to treat anxiety in adults, also have anticonvulsant effects, although tolerance to the latter effects makes this class of drugs less than ideal for chronic antiepileptic therapy (69). In the presence of intense panic or disabling anxiety, agents such as lorazepam and clonazepam may be useful as primary or adjunctive therapy (70). Even in the absence of an established epileptic disorder, withdrawal seizures may result from abrupt discontinuation of these agents. Both patients and parents should be carefully warned about this (71).

PSYCHOTIC SYMPTOMS IN PEDIATRIC EPILEPSY

Psychosis is a condition characterized by delusions, hallucinations, and disorganized speech and behavior. In the adult population,

psychosis has been identified during the seizure (ictal psychosis), within hours to days of a seizure (postictal psychosis), and interictally. Other chapters in this text explore these issues in adults (see also Chapters 5 and 6). Psychosis is a rare phenomenon in children with epilepsy and, when present, may be associated with significant cerebral abnormalities as may be seen with mental retardation. However, sporadic cases of psychosis have been reported in children with complex partial seizures, perhaps more commonly with left temporal lobe foci (72–74).

The frequency of psychosis related to childhood epilepsy is controversial. Although Lindsay et al. (75) contended that 10% of children with temporal lobe epilepsy will develop psychosis by adulthood, other studies argue for lower rates. Caplan et al. (76) reported that young patients with complex partial seizures are prone to display more illogical thought patterns, hallucinations, and delusions compared to children with primary generalized epilepsy. However, these children did not have the loose associations or negative signs (apathy, flat affect) typically seen in patients with a formal diagnosis of schizophrenia (77,78). This interesting finding needs to be replicated in additional studies.

When psychotic symptoms are present during seizures, they tend to be stereotyped. In contrast, the form and content of hallucinations, illusions, and abnormal thoughts tend to vary in psychosis. Following a seizure, children may be amnestic to the actual content of the hallucinations. Children with schizophreniform psychosis typically are able to describe the content of their auditory hallucinations and may not be upset by the experience. Periictal auditory or visual hallucinations may be frightening but recognized as unreal.

Treatment of Psychotic Symptoms

As in the case of antidepressants, the risk of lowering seizure threshold or inducing seizures *de novo* is low, overall approximately 1% of cases, with the notable exception of a significantly higher risk with clozapine (79). With the considerable concern regarding the production of tardive dyskinesia and extrapyramidal side effects from older neuroleptic agents such as butyrophenones or phenothiazines, use of the newer, atypical antipsychotic agents, such as olanzapine and risperidone, has become more favored in pediatric patients because the frequency of these side effects is less. However, other adverse effects, such as significant weight gain, have been noted with these other agents, particularly olanzapine. At times, a combination of new and older antipsychotic agents appears necessary to reduce psychotic symptoms.

There is limited information available about the risk of lowering seizure threshold with atypical antipsychotic agents; however, the general impression is that these agents carry a very low risk of inducing seizures (56,80). In contrast, clozapine is associated with a substantial dose-related risk of producing generalized epileptiform abnormalities on EEG, and myoclonic and generalized tonic-clonic seizures clinically (79). If clozapine, which has an approximately 3% to 4% overall risk of inducing seizures, is indicated, supplementation with an AED, particularly valproate (or lamotrigine in the authors' experience) may be helpful.

Among the traditional antipsychotic agents, some authors suggest that butyrophenones (e.g., haloperidol) have a lower risk of seizures than the phenothiazines (particularly the aliphatic class, e.g., chlorpromazine) (81). On the other hand, a dihydroindolone subtype of phenothiazine, i.e., molindone, has demonstrated minimal neuronal excitability on animal hippocampal slice studies (82) and low risk of seizures anecdotally. Despite increased neuronal excitability, the high potency and therefore low-dose requirements of fluphenazine or haloperidol make these two agents alternative choices if a phenothiazine is indicated (83).

DEVELOPMENTAL PERSPECTIVES

Infancy and Early Childhood

From the perspective of infant development, epilepsy affects the child's earliest developing sense of identity. Parents may be understandably fearful of separating from their baby or toddler. These fears may promote problems with separation anxiety. During early childhood, parents may experience severe anxiety when a toddler exhibits normal climbing and exploratory behavior. The fears of both parent and child can inhibit a child's expressions of normal curiosity, which are essential elements of later learning.

Early onset epilepsies, e.g., Landau-Kleffner syndrome, infantile spasms, and Lennox-Gastaut syndrome, often are associated with compromised development. Because delays in cognition and language and behavioral difficulties are common to these forms of epileptic syndromes, underlying brain pathology or the seizures they engender may disrupt developmental processes.

Seizures are estimated to occur in approximately one third of children with pervasive developmental disorders such as autism and Asperger's syndrome (84) and can be a factor in behavioral regression (74). It may be difficult to sort out the relative contributions of the CNS pathology or associated seizures with behavioral difficulties (12).

Epilepsy in Middle Childhood

In later childhood, academic problems and an increased frequency of ADHD emerge in children with epilepsy (see Chapter 8 on Attention-Deficit Disorders in Pediatric Epilepsy). Disorders of attention (a major element of academic difficulty) are reported frequently in children with seizure disorders. In one study of children in regular school environments, 68.7% of children with epilepsy experienced academic problems (10). The Isle of Wight study found that more than twice as many children with epilepsy showed serious reading delay when compared with nonepileptic children (12).

Early-onset epilepsy, brain damage, severity of epilepsy, and anticonvulsant toxicity have all been reported to contribute to intellectual deterioration. This deterioration in IQ has been estimated to occur in about 10% of children with epilepsy. Subnormal intelligence is found in as many as one third of epileptic children, if one includes borderline intelligence (85). Alternatively, the frequency of epilepsy in mentally retarded children varies from 3% to 32%, depending on the degree of cognitive impairment (86). The association of mental retardation with epilepsy has led to the very powerful, stigmatizing assumption that all children with epilepsy are mentally inferior.

Anticonvulsant polytherapy may have an adverse impact on cognitive functioning, including attention, concentration, memory, motor and mental speed, and mental processing (87). In school-age children, subtle drug effects are easily overlooked but may cause substantial cognitive impairment. A clinician needs to be alert to the report of teachers or parents that a child is not achieving on an expected level. Cognitive functioning should be assessed routinely in pediatric epileptic patients; otherwise, subtle signs of cognitive impairment may be overlooked at a critical time of intellectual development. In such cases, neuropsychological testing is invaluable in identifying specific deficits.

If a stimulant such as methylphenidate is indicated to treat moderate-to-severe attention-deficit disorder, the presence of a seizure disorder is not a contraindication to its use (88). However, if attentional deficits are possibly due to antiepileptic therapy, it is more advisable to try revising seizure therapies first, rather than adding a stimulant drug (89).

Adolescence and Epilepsy: Interference with the Processes of Maturation, Identity, and Independence

As is commonly known, adolescence is a period of development of a sense of identity and movement toward independence from parents. Nonetheless, adolescents continue to vacillate between dependency needs and self-sufficiency. As is the case with other serious illnesses, the onset of a seizure disorder at this period of time can be highly disruptive for an adolescent. As a result, more intense family conflicts and acting out behaviors may occur.

In adolescence, temporal lobe epilepsy becomes more frequent among the different varieties of possible epilepsy syndromes. These seizures can disrupt the normal adolescent yearning for greater independence from the family. Because limbic structures, including mesiotemporal areas, are the site of origin of these seizures and are thought to be related to mood and emotions, it is intuitive that these seizures may have some effects on emotions. When compared to patients with other disorders, adolescents with epilepsy are speculated to have more adjustment problems, sexual identity issues, and body image distortions (90). In contrast, a study by Kaminer et al. (15) demonstrated no difference in the rate of psychopathology in adolescents with temporal lobe epilepsy compared to adolescents with asthma.

Certainly, medication side effects, such as weight gain and hair loss, can add to negative self-esteem. The restriction on driving (an activity that symbolizes independence) also is problematic for many teens with epilepsy, as it is for adults. Awareness of these issues should motivate the clinician to probe for these problems during clinical interviews with patients and parents.

Family Perspectives

Although much emphasis in the literature is placed on biologic and medication-related influences on psychopathology in epilepsy, a number of studies remind us of the importance of family dynamics (91,92). Children's psychological adjustment to chronic illness appears to be integrally linked to family functioning. Families of epileptic children with behavioral difficulties are observed to have poorer global functioning, less social support, and limited financial resources compared to families of well-functioning children. Hermann et al. (93) reported that having divorced or separated parents was a strong predictor of behavior problems and depression in pediatric epileptic patients. Such studies demonstrate association of variables but do not necessarily identify the direction of cause and effect.

Controversy exists whether parents (most studies focused on mothers) of epileptic patients have higher rates of psychopathology than parents of children with other chronic disorders (12,94,95). When present, parental psychopathology correlates with psychiatric disturbances and dependency in epileptic children (94). The association of family stress or parental psychopathology with childhood behavioral difficulties does not reveal whether family psychopathology results from the child having seizures (the stress of coping with an ill child) or whether behavioral problems in the child lead to psychosocial family difficulties. Nevertheless, the clinician needs to take into account family dynamics that may be related to the behavioral difficulties as well as family resources that can be utilized to bring about improvements in the child's problems. Parental tendency toward overprotective behavior and expressions of their own anxieties may have an adverse impact on the child with epilepsy.

EPILEPTIC SYNDROMES AND ASSOCIATED ABERRANT BEHAVIORS

Numerous reports ascribe behavioral and personality traits to specific epileptic syndromes. Many of these series are uncontrolled, with many associated confounding variables. Although the merits and deficits of individual studies are beyond the scope of this chapter, Table 9.4 summarizes a useful discussion by Caplan (96) on this topic.

TABLE 9.4. *Epilepsy type and reported behavioral correlates*

Epileptic syndrome	Behavioral trait
Partial (focal) epilepsies	
Temporal lobe epilepsy	Hyperactivity, antisocial behavior, aggression (12,72,75,94,142,154) Schizophrenia-like psychosis, formal thought disorder, communication deficits (75,76)
Frontal lobe epilepsy	Limited data in children. May have more thought (55). In adults, reports contingent on specific frontal localization. Increased aggression, dysfunction, social behavior, behavioral, disinhibition, and attention deficits (156,157).
Benign rolandic epilepsy	Limited data in children. Believed to have normal psychological functioning.
Benign occipital epilepsy	No information present
Rasmussen's syndrome (chronic progressive epilepsia partialis continua of childhood)	Impaired cognitive and linguistic function (158–160)
Generalized epilepsies	
Childhood absence epilepsy	Considered a benign epilepsy type, but reports of academic problems, poor sibling relationships, reduced social outings, and emotional difficulties (2). Memory and attention deficits (161).
Juvenile myoclonic epilepsy	Irresponsibility and impaired impulse control, neglect of duties, emotional instability, quick temper, distractability (162)
Cryptogenic or symptomatic epilepsies	
Infantile spasms (West's syndrome)	Severe cognitive impairments, developmental delay, and impaired social interactions. Worse with poor seizure control.
Lennox-Gastaut syndrome	Behavioral difficulties common to mental retardation (e.g., hyperactivity)
Symptomatic epilepsies	
Landau-Kleffner syndrome (acquired epileptic aphasia)	Behavioral disturbances (163) including hyperactivity, aggression, depression, and psychosis (163–118)
Continuous spike and wave in slow wave sleep syndrome	Inattention, hyperactivity, impulsiveness, loss of sense of danger, aggressiveness, mood changes, disinhibition, mouthing of objects, reduced play, and perseveration (169). Subtle cognitive changes may occur first (169,170).

From Caplan R. Epilepsy syndromes. In: Caffey E, Brumback RA, eds. *Textbook of pediatric neuropsychiatry.* Washington, DC: American Psychiatric Press, 1998:977–1010, with permission.

NONEPILEPTIC SEIZURES IN CHILDHOOD

Nonepileptic seizures (NES; pseudo-seizures) are clinical events that resemble epileptic attacks but are unassociated with physiologic CNS dysfunction (97,98) (see also Chapters 24 and 25). NES may arise in the context of a conversion disorder in which episodes occur on a nonvolitional basis and may represent expressions of hidden negative feelings or conflicts. NES are one of the most common conversion symptoms in childhood. Alternatively, NES may involve intentional production of symptoms, either to achieve a sick role (factitious disorder) or as a symptom of malingering (intentional production of symptoms motivated by external incentive such as avoidance of responsibilities) (99). Factitious disorders are more common in parents who induce genuine seizures in their children (Munchausen syndrome by proxy), rather than as a cause of NES in children (100).

Distinguishing epileptic seizures from NES can be challenging, particularly if NES occur in the presence of a concomitant genuine epileptic disorder (101). In young children, NES may take the form of hyperventilation, breath-holding spells, shudders, night terrors, masturbatory behavior, and day dreaming (102,103). In older children or adolescents, NES may be manifested by a wide assortment of behaviors ranging from motionless states to convulsive activity. Mentally retarded children and children with pervasive developmental disorders may have repetitive, stereotyped behaviors that can be confused with seizures.

A number of tools can aid the clinician in making the diagnosis of NES. These include a careful history, clinical observation of the episodes, and EEG evaluation (including, when indicated, continuous monitoring with simultaneous EEG and video monitoring; video EEG). Because the level of pituitary hormone prolactin typically rises after complex partial or generalized seizures (104), especially those involving mesial temporal structures (105), demonstration of prolactin elevation (maximally 20 minutes after an episode) suggests an event is epileptic. Surveys for psychopathology, such as the Minnesota Multiphasic Personality Inventory (106), neuropsychological testing (107), and intravenous saline placebo "spell-induction" procedures (108), may be helpful but do not conclusively distinguish epileptic seizures from NES. Other caveats in differentiating epileptic seizures from NES are highlighted in Table 9.5.

Making the proper diagnosis of NES is critical in order to avoid unnecessarily exposing

TABLE 9.5. *Caveats in distinguishing epileptic from nonepileptic seizures*

Clinical activity
  Clinical phenomena commonly associated with generalized epileptic seizures, such as tongue biting, self-injury, and incontinence, also may occur in pseudoseizures (148).
  Movements commonly considered to be functional, such as pelvic thrusting, unusual vocalizations, thrashing movements, and the absence of a postictal confusional state, may occur in epileptic seizures, particularly those with frontal lobe origin (149,150).
  Patients may embellish upon poorly identified genuine epileptic symptoms.
EEG
  Normal interictal EEG does not exclude epileptic seizures.
  Normal EEG does not confirm the diagnosis of NES.
  Epileptiform abnormalities on interictal EEG do not exclude NES.
Video EEG
  Less severe epileptic seizures (especially those unassociated with altered awareness; simple partial seizures) may be too deep to have an obvious correlate on scalp-recorded EEG.
  Muscle artifact caused by clinical motor activity associated with a generalized convulsive seizure may obscure epileptic activity (149).
Prolactin
  Not reliably increased after nongeneralized seizures (104).
  Not reliably increased after seizures occuring outside mesial temporal regions (105).

EEG, electroencephalogram; NES, nonepileptic seizures.

children to AEDs and their potentially serious side effects. Further, undiagnosed NES may lead to interference with daily activities, frequent school absences, and the label of a sick child. Unfortunately, even among diagnosed cases, there is often a delay of 3 to 4 years before these attacks are properly identified as nonepileptic (109). In some situations, an obvious stressor may provoke NES, but precipitants may not be readily apparent. In adults with NES, a history of physical or sexual abuse frequently is elicited; this is reported less frequently in children and adolescents with NES (110,111).

NES prognosis in children and adolescents is better than in adults, especially if the symptoms are detected early and the duration of the disorder is short (110,112). Teaching children alternative ways to express negative feelings and reducing attention to the episodes and its associated secondary gain are recommended treatment strategies (100).

PSYCHOTROPIC EFFECTS OF ANTIEPILEPTIC DRUGS IN CHILDHOOD

A wide assortment of behavioral effects have been ascribed to the AEDs commonly used to treat seizures in children. Much of our knowledge of these effects is based on older and often anecdotally based literature (69). When selecting an AED or when assessing behaviors on AEDs, clinicians need to consider the potential positive and negative psychotropic effects of these agents. Table 9.6 lists examples of adverse psychotropic effects of AEDs commonly used in children and adolescents. The rates of these effects are highly variable. Underlying cognitive disturbances and the use of polytherapy tend to increase the risk of these adverse events.

There are few reports of negative behavioral effects from carbamazepine or valproic acid, although anecdotally, individual adverse responses to these drugs probably do occur. Both of these agents are commonly utilized to treat bipolar affective disorder (113,114), and these "mood-stabilizing" properties may have advantages in select epileptic patients with behavioral difficulties.

In adults, lamotrigine has been reported to promote increased energy and higher levels of alertness (115). This, together with lamotrigine's recently reported mood-stabilizing properties in bipolar disorder (116), may promote an increased sense of well-being and improved mood in epileptic patients. However, behavioral improvements as well as severe behavioral deterioration have been demon-

TABLE 9.6. *Adverse psychotropic effects of antiepileptic drugs*

Antiepileptic drug	Negative effects
Barbiturates (phenobarbital, primidone) (20,60,151)	Depression
	Sedation or paradoxic hyperactivity
	Cognitive impairment
	Behavioral agitation in developmentally disabled
Phenytoin (69)	Depression
	Chronic cumulative encephalopathy
Benzodiazepines (69)	Sedation
	Hyperactivity
	Delirium and psychosis during acute withdrawal
Ethosuximide (151)	Confusion, psychosis
	Sleep disturbances
	Aggressive activity, hostility
	Depression
Valproic acid (152)	Acute toxic encephalopathy
Gabapentin (121,122)	Agitation in intellectually challenged
Lamotrigine (17,118)	Agitation in intellectually challenged
Tiagabine (124)	Anxiety and depressive symptoms
Topiramate (153)	Dullness in concentration and associated depression

strated in mentally retarded individuals (117,118).

Gabapentin frequently is utilized by psychiatrists to treat behavioral dyscontrol syndromes in nonepileptic patients. A number of case reports suggest that gabapentin may be useful for treatment of children with refractory mood disorders and aggression (119,120). It is possible that the positive psychotropic effects of these agents will be observed to impact favorably on certain types of epileptic patients, as well. However, several case reports of severe behavioral agitation have been reported in developmentally disabled children who received gabapentin (121,122).

There is little current information available about psychotropic effects in pediatric patients of other recently introduced AEDs, such as tiagabine and TPM. Adult studies of tiagabine have suggested both positive (123) and negative (124) potential psychotropic effects. TPM has gained recent notoriety in adult studies for inducing attentional disturbances and psychomotor slowing (125). However, slow escalation of TPM dose and reduction of polypharmacy may permit better tolerance of the drug (126,127). Anecdotal experience and several reports (128–131) suggest that TPM may cause symptoms of depression, although this may be due in part to a reaction to cognitive side effects. Anxiety, irritability, behavioral problems, and even symptoms of psychosis (132) have been noted in patients treated with TPM (133). In contrast, a few recent reports indicate that TPM may be useful in treating both the manic and depressive phases of bipolar disorder (134–136); therefore, it is conceivable that some epileptic patients may enjoy favorable mood-stabilizing effects when receiving this drug. Vagal nerve stimulation (VNS), a novel therapy for partial and generalized epilepsy, involves the repetitive stimulation of the left vagus nerve via connections from a programmable neurocybernetic prosthesis implanted in the left upper chest region (137). Further examination of VNS effects on mood in pediatric epileptic patients is needed. Preliminary evidence

from two recent series (138,139) suggests that VNS may reduce depressive symptomatology in adult epileptic patients. Current studies examining the potential role of VNS in treating primary depression in nonepileptic patients are under way.

DRUG INTERACTIONS

When psychotropic and antiepileptic agents are prescribed concomitantly, careful attention should be directed to potential drug interactions, both pharmacokinetic (relating to drug absorption, distribution, metabolism, or excretion) and pharmacodynamic (relating to biochemical and physiologic effects). Metabolic interactions involving one drug's induction or inhibition of the metabolism of another or competition for protein binding are examples of common pharmacokinetic interactions. Sedation is a frequent pharmacodynamic effect of combining different agents.

Among the AEDs, phenytoin, carbamazepine, phenobarbital, and primidone tend to induce hepatic metabolism and may result in reductions in some concomitant psychotropic agents. Valproic acid tends to inhibit hepatic metabolism. Gabapentin, lamotrigine, TPM, and tiagabine have little effect on other agents, but some of these agents themselves may be vulnerable to the effects of other drugs.

Among the psychotropic agents, SSRIs inhibit assorted specific isoenzymes of the cytochrome P-450 class of hepatic enzymes (140), leading to the potential for reduced metabolism of concomitant drugs.

Drug interactions are discussed in greater detail in other chapters (see also Chapters 5, 7, 12, and 16).

PSYCHIATRIC ISSUES IN PEDIATRIC EPILEPSY SURGERY

Epilepsy surgery (resection of epileptogenic brain tissue) is a potentially curative form of therapy for intractable seizures. In recent years, epilepsy surgery has increasingly involved the pediatric epilepsy population. Although surgery might be considered to be a drastic form of therapy for patients in young age groups, compelling cognitive and psychosocial issues argue for avoiding delays in instituting early interventions. For example, recurrent seizures may be detrimental to the developing brain. Uncontrolled seizures compromise the ability to be independent and may lead to exclusion from normal scholastic, social, and vocational opportunities (141). Several studies have documented severe psychosocial dysfunction in children with intractable temporal lobe seizures and marked improvement in patients who underwent temporal lobectomy (72,142).

QUALITY OF LIFE INVENTORIES FOR PEDIATRIC EPILEPSY

The recent development of self-report quality-of-life inventories for adult epileptic patients has provided the clinician with an efficient tool to identify specific mood disturbances and psychosocial disability that otherwise may not be identified in the typical clinical interview. Information from these surveys may lead to further investigations and interventions, such as referral to psychiatric consultants or social services (143). An adolescent version of the quality of life in epilepsy inventories was developed recently (144).

CONCLUSION

The clinician treating children and adolescents with epilepsy needs to be aware of the wide range of presentations of psychiatric disorders in this population. Psychiatric disorders in childhood epilepsy, such as anxiety and depression, tend to be underrecognized and undertreated. The clinician should be familiar with the complex psychopharmacologic effects of AEDs and drug interactions. Further attention to these issues will lead to more effective and compassionate treatment for children and adolescents with epilepsy.

REFERENCES

1. Jalava M, Sillanpaa M, Camfield C, et al. Social adjustment and competence 35 years after onset of childhood epilepsy: a prospective controlled study. *Epilepsia* 1997;38:708–715.
2. Wirrell EC, Camfield CS, Camfield PR, et al. Long-term psychosocial outcome in typical absence epilepsy. *Arch Pediatr Adolesc Med* 1997;151:152–158.
3. Hauser W, Kurland L. The epidemiology of epilepsy in Rochester, Minnesota 1935 through 1967. *Epilepsia* 1975;16:1–66.
4. Hauser W. Incidence and prevalence. In: Hauser WA, Hesdorffer DC, eds. *Epilepsy: frequency, causes, and consequences.* New York: Demos Publications, 1990: 1–51.
5. Hauser WA, Kurland L. The epidemiology of epilepsy in Rochester, Minnesota, 1935 through 1967. *Epilepsia* 1975;16:1–66.
6. Weisbrot DM, Ettinger AB. Epilepsy and behavior: controversies and caveats. *Neurologist* 1997;3:155–172.
7. Ettinger AB, Weisbrot DM, Nolan EE, et al. Symptoms of depression and anxiety in pediatric epilepsy patients. *Epilepsia* 1998;39:595–599.
8. Hinton GG, Knights RM. Neurological and psychological characteristics of 100 children with seizures. In: Richard B, ed. *Proceedings of the First Congress for the International Association for the Scientific Study of Mental Deficiency.* London: Michael Jackson Publishing, 1969:351–356.
9. Whitehouse D. Psychological and neurological correlates of seizure disorder. *Johns Hopkins Med J* 1971; 129:36–42.
10. Holdsworth L, Whitmore K. A study of children with epilepsy attending ordinary schools. I. Their seizure patterns, progress, and behavior in school. *Dev Med Child Neurol* 1974;16:746–755.
11. Cavazzuti GB. Epidemiology of different types of epilepsy in school age children of Modena, Italy. *Epilepsia* 1980;21:57–62.
12. Rutter M, Graham P, Yule WA. *A neuropsychiatric study in childhood.* Philadelphia: JB Lippincott, 1970.
13. Hoare P. The development of psychiatric disorder among schoolchildren with epilepsy. *Dev Med Child Neurol* 1984;26:3–13.
14. Ettinger AB, Weisbrot DM, Vitale SV, et al. Relation of anxiety and depression symptoms with family functioning in pediatric patients with epilepsy vs. migraine. *Epilepsia* 1998;39[Suppl 16]:187–188.
15. Kaminer Y, Apter A, Aviv A, et al. Psychopathology and temporal lobe epilepsy in adolescents. *Acta Psychiatr Scand* 1988;77:640–644.
16. Taylor DC. Psychosocial components of childhood epilepsy. In: Hermann BP, Seidenberg M, eds. *Childhood epilepsies: neuropsychological, psychosocial and intervention aspects.* Chichester, England: John Wiley & Sons, 1989.
17. Dunn DW, Austin JK, Huster GA. Behavior problems in children with new-onset epilepsy. *Seizure* 1997;6: 283–287.
18. Norrby U, Carlsson J, Beckung E, et al. Self-assessment of well-being in a group of children with epilepsy. *Seizure* 1999;8:228–234.
19. Kokkonen J, Kokkonen ER, Saukkonen AL, et al. Psychosocial outcome of young adults with epilepsy in

childhood. *J Neurol Neurosurg Psychiatry* 1997;62: 265–268.

20. Brent DA, Crumrine PK, Varma R, et al. Phenobarbital treatment and major depressive disorder in children with epilepsy. *Pediatrics* 1987;80:909–917.

21. Hermann BP, Whitman S. Psychopathology in epilepsy: a multietiologic model. In: Hermann BP, Whitman S, eds. *Psychopathology in epilepsy. Social dimensions.* New York: Oxford University Press, 1986.

22. Hermann BP, Whitman S, Hughes JR, et al. Multietiological determinants of psychopathology and social competence in children with epilepsy. *Epilepsy Res* 1988;2:51–60.

23. Waxman S, Geschwind N. The interictal behavior syndrome in temporal lobe epilepsy. *Arch Gen Psychiatry* 1975;32:1580–1586.

24. Bear DM, Fedio P. Quantitative analysis of interictal behavior in temporal lobe epilepsy. *Arch Neurol* 1977; 34:454–467.

25. Stores G. School children with epilepsy at risk for learning and behavior problems. *Dev Med Child Neurol* 1978;20:502–508.

26. Hartlage CC, Green JB. The relation of parental attitudes to academic and social achievement in epileptic children. *Epilepsia* 1972;13:21–26.

27. Torrestad A, Hakanson M, Axelli T. Development of a program for the treatment of chronic pain and anxiety. A learning process leading from unsound to sound assessment. *Int J Technol Assess Health Care* 1992;8: 85–92.

28. Niedermeyer E. *Psychological-psychiatric aspects. The epilepsies, diagnosis and management.* Baltimore: Urban and Schwarzenberg, 1990:213–218.

29. Delgado-Escueta AV, Mattson RH, King L, et al. The nature of aggression during epileptic seizures. *N Engl J Med* 1981;305:711.

30. Gerad ME, Spitz MC, Towbin JA, et al. Subacute post-ictal aggression. *Neurology* 1998;50:384–388.

31. Pond DA, Bidwell BH. A survey of epilepsy in 14 general practices: II. Social and psychological aspects. *Epilepsia* 1959;60:285–299.

32. Hermann BP, Black RB, Chabria S. Behavioral problems and social competence in children with epilepsy. *Epilepsia* 1981;22:703–710.

33. Keating LE. Epilepsy and behavior disorder in school children. *J Ment Sci* 1961;107:161–180.

34. Lindsay J. The long-term outcome of temporal lobe epilepsy in childhood. In: Reynolds E, Trimble M, eds. *Epilepsy and psychiatry.* London: Churchill Livingstone, 1981:185–215.

35. Lewis DO, Pincus J, Shanok S, et al. Psychomotor epilepsy and violence in a group of incarcerated adolescent boys. *Am J Psychiatry* 1982;139:882–887.

36. Lewis DO. Neuropsychiatric vulnerabilities and violent juvenile delinquency. *Psychiatr Clin North Am* 1983;6:707–714.

37. Rutter M. Psychological sequelae of brain damage in childhood. *Am J Psychiatry* 1981;138:1533–1544.

38. Brown G, Chadwick O, Shaffer D, et al. A prospective study of children with head injuries. III. Psychiatric sequelae. *Psychol Med* 1981;11:63–78.

39. Kovacs M. The children's depression inventory (CDI). *Psychopharmacol Bull* 1985;21:995–998.

40. Kovacs M. *CDI.* North Tonawanda, NY: Multi-Health Systems, Inc., 1992.

41. Kashani JH, Carlson GA, Beck NC, et al. Depression, depressive symptoms, and depressed mood among a community sample of adolescents. *Am J Psychiatry* 1987;144:931–934.

42. Mendez MF, Cummings JL, Benson DF. Depression in epilepsy. *Arch Neurol* 1986;43:766–770.

43. Robertson MM, Trimble MR. Depressive illness in patients with epilepsy: a review. *Epilepsia* 1983;22: 515–524.

44. Ettinger AB, Weisbrot DM, Krupp LB, et al. Fatigue and depression in epilepsy. *J Epilepsy* 1998;11:105–109.

45. Dunn DW, Austin JK. Symptoms of depression in adolescents with epilepsy. *J Am Acad Child Adolesc Psychiatry* 1999;38:1132–1138.

46. Brent DA. Overrepresentation of epileptics in a consecutive series of suicide attempters seen at a Children's Hospital, 1978–1983. *J Acad Child Psychiatry* 1986;25:242–246.

47. Glauser TA. Topiramate. *Epilepsia* 1999;40[Suppl 5]:S71–S80.

48. Zielinski JJ. Epilepsy and mortality rate and cause of death. *Epilepsia* 1974;15:191–201.

49. Hawton K, Fagg J, Marsack P. Association between epilepsy and attempted suicide. *J Neurol Neurosurg Psychiatry* 1980;43:168–170.

50. Carlson GA, Abbott SF. Mood disorders and suicide. In: Kaplan HI, Sadock BJ, eds. *Comprehensive textbook of psychiatry.* Baltimore: Williams & Wilkins, 1995:2367–2391.

51. Barczak P, Edmunds E, Betts T. Hypomania following complex partial seizures. A report of three cases. *Br J Psychiatry* 1988;152:137–139.

52. Persons JB, Bostrom A, Bertagnolli A. Results of randomized controlled trials of cognitive therapy for depression generalize to private practice. *Cogn Ther Res* 1999;23:535–548.

53. Bostic JQ, Wilens TE, Spencer T, et al. Antidepressant treatment of juvenile depression. *Int J Psychiatry Clin Pract* 1999;3:171–179.

54. Geller B, Reising D, Leonard HL, et al. Critical review of tricyclic antidepressant use in children and adolescents. *J Am Acad Child Adolesc Psychiatry* 1999; 38:513–516.

55. York A, Hill P. Treating depression in children and adolescents. *Curr Opin Psychiatry* 1999;12:77–80.

56. Alldredge BK. Risk of lowering seizure threshold with antiepileptic drugs. Neurology 1999;53[5 Suppl 2]: S68–75.

57. Rosenstein DL, Nelson JC, Jacobs SC. Seizures associated with antidepressants: a review. *J Clin Psychiatry* 1993;54:289–299.

58. Edwards. Antidepressants and seizures: epidemiological and clinical aspects. In: Trimble MR, ed. *The psychopharmacology of epilepsy.* Chichester, England: John Wiley & Sons, 1985:119–139.

59. Ettinger AB, Perrine K. Psychiatric/psychosocial issues in epilepsy. In: French J, Shields WD, Sutula TT, et al., eds. *Epilepsy update.* Norwalk, CT: GEM Communications, 1996:13–24.

60. Stoudemire A, Fogel BS. *Psychiatric care of the medical patient.* New York: Oxford University Press, 1993.

61. Alldredge BK, Simon RP. Drugs that can precipitate seizures. In: Resor SR, Kutt H, eds. *The medical treatment of epilepsy.* New York: Marcel Dekker, 1992: 497–523.

62. Favale E, Rubino V, Mainardi P, et al. Anticonvulsant effect of fluoxetine in humans. *Neurology* 1995;45: 1926–1927.
63. Prediville S, Gale K. Anticonvulsant effect of fluoxetine on focally evoked limbic motor seizures in rats. *Epilepsia* 1993;34:381–384.
64. Francis S, Weisbrot DM, Jandorf L, et al. Anxiety in epilepsy. *Epilepsia* 1996;37:3(abst).
65. Mittan RJ, Locke GE. Fear of seizures: epilepsy's forgotten problem. *Urban Health* 1982;40:38–39.
66. Devinsky O, Sato S, Theodore WH, et al. Fear episodes due to limbic seizures with normal scalp EEG. A subdural electrographic study. *J Clin Psychiatry* 1989;50:28–30.
67. Mattison R. Separation anxiety disorder and anxiety in children. In: Kaplan HI, Sadock BJ, eds. *Comprehensive textbook of psychiatry.* Baltimore: Williams & Wilkins, 1997:2345–2351.
68. Devinsky O, Kelley K, Porter RJ, et al. Clinical and electroencephalographic features of simple partial seizures. *Neurology* 1988;38:1347–1352.
69. Rivinus TM. Psychiatric effects of the anticonvulsant regimens. *J Clin Psychopharmacol* 1982;2: 165–192.
70. Kutcher SP. Potentiating the anti-panic response when beginning treatment with a serotonin specific reuptake inhibitor (SSRI). *Child Adolesc Psychopharmacol News* 1999;4:10.
71. Hauser P, Devinsky O, DeBellis M, et al. Benzodiazepine withdrawal delirium with catatonic features. *Arch Neurol* 1989;46:696–699.
72. Lindsay J, Ounsted C, Richards P. Longterm outcome in children with temporal lobe seizures I: social outcome and childhood factors. *Dev Med Child Neurol* 1979;21:630–636.
73. Lindsay J, Ounsted C, Richards P. Longterm outcome in children with temporal lobe seizures II: marriage, parenthood, and sexual differences. *Dev Med Child Neurol* 1979;21:433–440.
74. Dunn DW, Austin JK. Behavioral aspects of pediatric epilepsy. In: Ettinger AB, Hermann BP, eds. *Psychiatric issues in epilepsy.* New York: Lippincott Williams & Wilkins, 1998.
75. Lindsay J, Ounsted C, Richards P. Longterm outcome in children with temporal lobe seizures: III: psychiatric aspects in childhood and adult life. *Dev Med Child Neurol* 1979;21:630–636.
76. Caplan R, Arbelle S, Guthrie D, et al. Formal thought disorder and psychopathology in pediatric primary generalized and complex partial epilepsy. *J Am Acad Child Adolesc Psychiatry* 1997;36:1286–1294.
77. Caplan R, Shields WD, Mori L, et al. Middle childhood onset of interictal psychoses: case studies. *J Am Acad Child Adolesc Psychiatry* 1991;30:893–896.
78. Caplan R, Guthrie D, Shields WD, et al. Formal thought disorder in pediatric complex partial seizure disorder. *J Child Psychiatry Psychol* 1992;33: 1399–1412.
79. Devinsky O, Pacia SV. Seizures during clozapine therapy. *J Clin Psychiatry* 1994;55:153–156.
80. Risperdal (risperidone tablets). Titusville, NJ: Janssen Pharmaceutica, 1996.
81. Trimble MR. *Treatment of epileptic psychoses. The psychoses of epilepsy.* New York: Raven Press, 1991: 150–163.
82. Remick PA, Fine SH. Antipsychotic drugs and seizures. *J Clin Psychiatry* 1979;40:78–80.
83. Markowitz JC, Brown RP. Seizures with neuroleptics and antidepressants. *Gen Hosp Psychiatry* 1987;9: 135–141.
84. Volkmar F, Nelson DSL. Seizure disorders in autism. *J Am Acad Child Adolesc Psychiatry* 1990;29:127–129.
85. Ellenberg JH, Hirts DG, Nelson KB. Do seizures in children cause intellectual deterioration? *N Engl J Med* 1986;314:1085–1088.
86. Corbet JA, Trimble MR, Nicol TC. Behavioral and cognitive impairment in children with epilepsy: the longterm effects of anticonvulsant toxicity. *J Am Acad Child Psychiatry* 1985;24:17–23.
87. Reynolds EH. Antiepileptic drugs and psychopathology. In: Trimble MR, ed. *The psychopharmacology of epilepsy.* Chichester, England: John Wiley & Sons, 1985.
88. Gross-Tsur V, Manor O, van der Meere J, et al. Epilepsy and attention deficit hyperactivity disorder: is methylphenidate safe and effective? *J Pediatr* 1997; 130:670–674.
89. Resnick TJ, Fenichel GM. Comorbidity and immunizations in children. In: Engel JJ, Pedley TA, eds. *Epilepsy: a comprehensive textbook.* Philadelphia: Lippincott-Raven Publishers, 1997:1971–1976.
90. Viberg M, Blennow G, Polski B. Epilepsy in adolescence; implications for the development of personality. *Epilepsia* 1987;28:542–546.
91. Austin JK. Childhood epilepsy: child adaptation and family resources. *J Child Adolesc Psychiatr Ment Health Nurs* 1988;1:18–24.
92. Hoare P, Kerley S. Helping parents and children with epilepsy cope successfully: the outcome of a group programme for parents. *J Psychosom Res* 1992;36: 759–767.
93. Hermann BP, Whitman S, Dell J. Correlates of behavior problems and social competence in children with epilepsy, aged 6–11. In: Hermann BP, Seidenberg M, eds. *Childhood epilepsies; neuropsychological, psychosocial and intervention aspects.* New York: John Wiley & Sons, 1989:143–157.
94. Hoare P, Kerley S. Psychosocial adjustment of children with chronic epilepsy and their families. *Dev Med Child Neurol* 1991;33:201–215.
95. Weisbrot DM, Gadow KD, Nolan EE, et al. Anxiety and depression in pediatric epilepsy patients: correlation with parental psychopathology. Abstract presented at the American Academy of Child and Adolescent Psychiatry, Toronto, Canada, October 1997.
96. Caplan R. Epilepsy syndromes. In: *Textbook of pediatric neuropsychiatry.* 1998:977–1010.
97. Ozkara C, Dreiffus FE. Differential diagnosis in pseudoepileptic seizures. *Epilepsia* 1993;34:294–298.
98. Bazil CW, Kothari M, Luciano D, et al. Provocation of nonepileptic seizures by suggestion in a general seizure population. *Epilepsia* 1994;34:768–770.
99. Mills MJ, Lipian MS. Malingering. In: Kaplan HI, Sadock BJ, eds. *Comprehensive textbook of psychiatry.* Baltimore: Williams & Wilkins, 1997:1614–1622.
100. Caplan R, Gillberg C. Child psychiatric disorders. In: Engel J, Pedley TA, eds. *Epilepsy: a comprehensive textbook.* Philadelphia: Lippincott-Raven Publishers, 1997:2125–2139.
101. Ramani V. Intensive monitoring of psychogenic

seizures, aggression, and dyscontrol syndromes. In: Gumnit RJ, ed. *Advances in neurology.* New York: Raven Press, 1986:203–217.

102. Metrick ME, Ritter FJ, Gates JR, et al. Nonepileptic events in childhood. *Epilepsia* 1991;32:322–328.

103. Duchowny MS, Resnic TJ, Deray MJ, et al. Video EEG diagnosis of repetitive behavior in early childhood and its relationship to seizures. *Pediatr Neurol* 1988;4:162–164.

104. Wyllie E, Luders H, MacMillan J, et al. Serum prolactin levels after epileptic seizures. *Neurology* 1984;34:1601–1604.

105. Sperling M, Pritchard P III, Engel J, et al. Prolactin in partial epilepsy: an indicator of limbic seizures. *Ann Neurol* 1986;20:716–722.

106. Dodrill CB, Wilkus RJ, Batzel LW. The MMPI as a diagnostic tool in non-epileptic seizures. In: Rowan AR, Gates JR, eds. *Non-epileptic seizures.* Boston: Butterworth-Heinemann, 1993:211–219.

107. Wilkus RJ, Dodrill CB, Thompson PM. Intensive EEG monitoring and psychological studies of patients with pseudoepileptic seizures. *Epilepsia* 1984;25:100–107.

108. Slater JD, Brown MC, Jacobs W, et al. Induction of pseudoseizures with intravenous saline placebo. *Epilepsia* 1995;36:580–585.

109. Lancman ME, Asconapé JJ, Graves S, et al. Psychogenic seizures in children: long-term analysis of 43 cases. *J Child Neurol* 1994;9:404–407.

110. Wyllie E, Friedman D, Luders H, et al. Outcome of psychogenic seizures in children and adolescents compared with adults. *Neurology* 1991;41:742–744.

111. Alper K, Devinsky O, Perrine K, et al. Nonepileptic seizures and childhood sexual and physical abuse. *Neurology* 1993;43:1950–1953.

112. Wyllie E, Friedman D, Rothner D, et al. Psychogenic seizures in children and adolescents: outcome after diagnosis by ictal video and electroencephalographic recording. *Pediatrics* 1990;85:480–484.

113. Small JG, Klapper MH, Milstein V, et al. Carbamazepine compared with lithium in the treatment of mania. *Arch Gen Psychiatry* 1991;48:915–921.

114. Calabrese JR, Delucchi GA. Spectrum of efficacy of valproate in 55 patients with rapid-cycling bipolar disorder. *Am J Psychiatry* 1990;147:431–434.

115. Brodie MJ, Richens A, Yuen A. Double-blind comparison of lamotrigine and carbamazepine in newly diagnosed epilepsy. *Lancet* 1995;345:468–476.

116. Fogelson D, Sternbach H. Lamotrigine treatment of refractory bipolar disorder. *J Clin Psychiatry* 1997;58:271–273.

117. Beran RG, Gibson RJ. Aggressive behaviour in intellectually challenged patients with epilepsy treated with lamotrigine. *Epilepsia* 1998;39:280–282.

118. Ettinger AB, Weisbrot DM, Saracco J, et al. Positive and negative psychotropic effects of lamotrigine in epilepsy patients with mental retardation. *Epilepsia* 1998;39:874–877.

119. McManaman J, Tam DA. Gabapentin for self-injurious behavior in Lesch-Nyhan syndrome. *Pediatr Neurol* 1999;20:381–382.

120. Ryback L. Gabapentin for behavioral dyscontrol [Letter]. *Am J Psychiatry* 1995;152:1399.

121. Wolf SM, Shinnar S, Kang H, et al. Gabapentin toxicity in children manifesting as behavioral changes. *Epilepsia* 1995;36:1203–1205.

122. Tallian KB, Nahata MC, Lo W, et al. Gabapentin associated with aggressive behavior in pediatric patients with seizures. *Epilepsia* 1996;37:501–502.

123. Dodrill CB, Arnett JL, Shu V, et al. Effects of tiagabine monotherapy on abilities, adjustment, and mood. *Epilepsia* 1998;39:33–42.

124. Leppik IE. Tiagabine: the safety landscape. *Epilepsia* 1995;36:S10–S13.

125. Crawford P. An audit of topiramate use in a general neurology clinic. *Seizure* 1998;7:207–211.

126. Faught E, French J, Harden C. Postmarketing Antiepileptic Drug Survery Group (PADS). Adverse effects of TPM: results from a large post-marketing survey. *Epilepsia* 1997;38[Suppl 8]:97(abst).

127. Faught E, Kuzniecky R, Gilliam F. Cognitive effects of TPM. *Neurology* 1997;48:336a(abst).

128. Shorvon SD. Safety of topiramate: adverse events and relationships to dosing. *Epilepsia* 1996;37[Suppl 2]:S18–S22.

129. Tassanari CA, Michelucci R, Chauvel P, et al. Double-blind, placebo-controlled trial of topiramate (600 mg daily) for the treatment of refractory partial epilepsy. *Epilepsia* 1996;37:763–768.

130. Abou-Khalil B, Fakhoury T. Neuropsychiatric profile of high-dose topiramate. *Epilepsia* 1997;38[Suppl 8]:207(abst).

131. Betts T, Smith K, Khan G. Severe psychiatric reactions to topiramate. *Epilepsia* 1997;38[Suppl 3]:64(abst).

132. Dohmeier C, Kay A, Greathouse N. Neuropsychiatric complications of topiramate therapy. *Epilepsia* 1998;39[Suppl 6]:189(abst).

133. Ketter TA, Post RM, Theodore WH. Positive and negative psychotropic effects of antiepileptic drugs in patients with seizure disorders. *Neurology* 1999;53[Suppl 1]:S52–S66.

134. Marcotte. Topiramate in the treatment of mood disorders. *151st Annual Meeting of the American Psychiatric Association*, Toronto, Canada, 1998, Abstract 115.

135. Calabrese JR, Shelton MD III, Keck PE Jr, et al. Pilot study of topiramate in acute severe treatment-refractory mania. *Proceedings of the 151st Annual Meeting of the American Psychiatric Association*, 1998:121–122.

136. Suppes T, Brown ES, McElroy SL, et al. A pilot trial of adjunctive topiramate in the treatment of bipolar disorder: application of the Stanley Foundation Bipolar Network (SFBN) prospective protocol. *Proceedings of the 37th Annual Meeting of the American College of Neuropsychopharmacology* 1998:306(abst).

137. Reid SA. Surgical technique for implantation of the neurocybernetic prosthesis. *Epilepsia* 1990;31[Suppl 2]:S38–S39.

138. Harden CL, Pulver MC, Nikolov B, et al. Effects of vagus nerve stimulation on mood in adult epilepsy patients. *Neurology* 1999;52[Suppl 2]:238a(abst).

139. Ettinger AB, Nolan E, Vitale S, et al. Changes in mood and quality of life in adult epilepsy patients treated with vagal nerve stimulation. *Epilepsia* 1999;40:62(abst).

140. Nemeroff CB, DeVane CL, Pollock BG. Newer antidepressants and the cytochrome P450 system. *Am J Psychiatry* 1996;153:311–320.

141. Duchowny MS, Harvey S, Sperling MR, et al. Indications and criteria for surgical intervention. In: Engel J, Pedley TA, eds. *Epilepsy: a comprehensive textbook.* Philadelphia: Lippincott-Raven Publishers, 1997:1677–1685.

142. Lindsay JJ, Glaser G, Richards P, et al. Developmental aspects of focal epilepsies of childhood treated by neurosurgery. *Dev Med Child Neurol* 1984;26: 574–587.

143. Cramer JA, Perrine K, Devinsky O, et al. A brief questionnaire to screen for quality of life in epilepsy: the QOLIE-10. *Epilepsia* 1996;37:577–582.

144. Devinsky O, Westbrook L, Cramer J, et al. Risk factors for poor health-related quality of life in adolescents with epilepsy. *Epilepsia* 1999;40:1715–1720.

145. Ziegler RG. Impairments of control and competence in epileptic children and their families. *Epilepsia* 1981; 22:339–346.

146. Austin JK, Dunn DW, Levstek DA. First seizures: concerns and needs of parents and children. *Epilepsia* 1993;34:24(abst).

147. Ziegler R. Risk factors in childhood epilepsy. *Psychother Psychosom* 1985;44:185–190.

148. Gates JR, Luciano D, Devinsky O. The classification and treatment of nonepileptic events. In: Devinsky O, Theodore W, eds. *Epilepsy and behavior.* New York: Wiley-Liss, 1991:251–263.

149. Leis AA, Ross MA, Summers AK. Psychogenic seizures: ictal characteristics and diagnostic pitfalls. *Neurology* 1992;42:95–99.

150. Saygi S, Katz A, Marks DA, et al. Frontal lobe partial seizures and psychogenic seizures: comparison of clinical and ictal characteristics. *Neurology* 1992;42: 1274–1277.

151. Stagno SJ. The epidemiology of epilepsy. In: Wyllie E, ed. *The treatment of epilepsy: principles and practice.* Philadelphia: Lea & Febiger, 1993:1149–1162.

152. Dreifuss FE. Valproate: toxicity. In: Levy RH, Mattson RH, Meldrum BS, et al., eds. *Antiepileptic drugs.* New York: Raven Press, 1989:643–651.

153. Curry WJ, Kulling DL. Newer antiepileptic drugs: gabapentin, lamotrigine, felbamate, topiramate and fosphenytoin. *Am Fam Physician* 1998;57:513–520.

154. Taylor DC. Aggression and epilepsy. *J Psychosom Res* 1975;13:229–236.

155. Caplan R, Guthrie D, Shields WD, et al. Communication deficits in pediatric complex partial seizure disorder and schizophrenia. *Dev Psychopathol* 1994;6: 499–517.

156. Devinsky O, Morrell M, Vogt B. Contribution of anterior cingulate cortex to behavior. *Brain* 1995;118: 279–306.

157. Powell AL, Yudd A, Zee P, et al. Attention deficit hyperactivity disorder associated with orbitofrontal epilepsy in a father and a son. *Neuropsychiatry Neuropsychol Behav Neurol* 1997;10:151–154.

158. Honavar M, Jonota I, Polkey CE. Rasmussen's encephalitis in surgery for epilepsy. *Dev Med Child Neurol* 1992;34:3–14.

159. Vargha-Khadem F, Isaacs EB, Papaleloudi H, et al. Development of language in six hemispherectomized patients. *Brain* 1991;11:473–495.

160. Caplan R, Curtiss S, Chugani HC, et al. Pediatric Rasmussen encephalitis: thought processes, language, PET, and pathology before and after surgery. *Brain Cogn* 1996;32:45–66.

161. Mirsky AF. Information processing in petit mal epilepsy. In: Hermann BP, Seidenberg M, eds. *Childhood epilepsies: neuropsychological, psychosocial, and intervention aspects.* New York: John Wiley & Sons, 1989:51–80.

162. Janz D. *Die Epilepsien.* Stuttgart: George Thieme, 1969.

163. Humphrey EL, Knopstein R, Bumpass ER. Gradually developing aphasia in children. *J Am Acad Child Psychiatry* 1975;14:652–665.

164. Sawhney IM, Suresh N, Dhand UK, et al. Acquired aphasia with epilepsy: Landau-Kleffner syndrome. *Epilepsia* 1988;29:283–287.

165. White J, Sreenivasan V. Epilepsy-aphasia syndrome in children: an unusual presentation to psychiatry. *Can J Psychiatry* 1987;32:599–601.

166. Dugas M, Masson M, Le Heuzey MF, et al. Aphasie "acquise" de l'enfant avec epilepsia (syndrome de Landau et Kleffner): douze observations personelles. *Rev Neurol* 1982;138:755–780.

167. Gordon B, Lesser R, Rance N, et al. Parameters for direct cortical stimulation in the human: histopathologic confirmation. *Electroencephalogr Clin Neurophysiol* 1990;75:371–377.

168. Zivi A, Broussaud G, Daymas S, et al. Syndrome aphasie acquise-epilepsie avec psychose: a propose d'une observation. *Ann Pediatr* 1990;37:391–394.

169. Perez ER, Davidoff V, Desplan PA, et al. Mental and behavioral deterioration of children with epilepsy and CSWS: acquired epileptic frontal syndrome. *Dev Med Child Neurol* 1993;35:661–674.

170. Boel M, Caesar P. Continuous spikes and waves during slow sleep: a 30-month follow-up study of neuropsychological recovery and EEG findings. *Neuropediatrics* 1989;20:176–180.

10

Personality Disorders in Epilepsy

Anthony L. Ritaccio and Orrin Devinsky

New York University–Mount Sinai Epilepsy Center, New York, New York 10016

Among the stereotypes that have surrounded epilepsy in both ancient and modern times is the idea that the epilepsy patient is in some way fundamentally changed by the disorder (1). Physicians and society at large in the nineteenth century and early parts of the twentieth century subscribed to the view that certain aberrant personality attributes were a common manifestation of the chronic epileptic condition. The concept of an epileptic personality, i.e., that there is an almost ubiquitous and characteristic negative set of behavioral changes in epileptic patients, evolved slowly, a collage formed by stigma, misunderstanding, and diverse behavioral changes that occur in epileptic patients who often have concurrent central nervous system disorder.

HISTORICAL PERSPECTIVE

The religious nature of epilepsy patients was stressed in the medical literature of the nineteenth century, much as it had been stressed as early as 2,000 years before in the period of the Hippocratic school. At the turn of the century, the pervasive understanding that epilepsy coincides with distinct personalities, personality pathologies, and psychoses was an artifact of observing a select number of chronically institutionalized epilepsy patients long before distinctions were made between specific epilepsy syndromes and their manifold etiologies. Modern views evolved during the nineteenth century. Based on extensive experience with a private outpatient population with idiopathic epilepsy, Reynolds (2) concluded that epilepsy does not necessarily involve any mental change at all, depletion of spirits and timidity are common in males, and excitability of temper occurs in both sexes. Gowers (3) also recognized that many epilepsy patients had normal personality and intellect, but that many others developed intraparoxysmal behavioral changes. He suggested that these changes resulted from many factors, but mainly from epilepsy per se. The early twentieth century brought diverse views concerning people with epilepsy and their behaviors. Kinnier Wilson (4) offered a progressive psychosocial view: "On epileptic temperament inordinate stress has been laid. Life is difficult for these patients, and much that is attributed to temperament can with greater reason be assigned to chronic invalidism and unlucky circumstance." Sjobring (5) professed the negative epileptic personality: "A mental change of a specific nature takes place in individuals suffering from epileptic seizures. They become torpid and circumstantial, sticky and adhesive, effectively tense and suffer from explosive outburst of rage, anxiety, etc." Kraepelin documented inevitable aggressiveness in a subset of outpatient epilepsy patients under his observation, "almost always an intensification of mental irritability occurs." The adhesive or viscous personality traits in which the patient has difficulty in disengaging from interpersonal exchanges was reviewed by many observers in the European literature under various terminologies such as the "enechetic constitution," "ixoid character," and "glischroid trait."

THE MODERN ERA

Two coincident developments in the modern era led to repopularization of the highly controversial concept of epileptic personality changes, namely, the elaboration of the role of the limbic system in emotion and behavior and the recognition that the majority of partial seizures had their origin in temporal lobe structures.

The association (if not fusing) of temporal lobe epilepsy (TLE) and behavioral changes had its origin in the 1951 report by Gibbs (6) of behavioral disturbances occurring in as many as 33% of his patients with "psychomotor seizures" of temporal lobe origin. Gastaut et al. (7) in 1954 reiterated common observations on the frequency of emotional viscosity, hyposexuality, hypoactivity, and hypoaggresiveness in epileptic patients, but were the first to suggest that the stereotype symptom complex appeared to be the antithesis of the Kluver-Bucy syndrome (KBS). The Kluver-Bucy syndrome is characterized by all exploratory behavior, increased sexual appetite, decreased aggressivity, and continuous environmental exploration as a consequence of bilateral temporal ablation (8).

Waxman and Geschwind (9) discerned a distinct subset of disrupted but nonpathologic behaviors believed to be associated with TLE, specifically, deepened emotions, circumstantiality, altered religious and sexual concerns, and hypergraphia. They coined the term "interictal behavior syndrome," often referred to as Geschwind syndrome or Gastaut-Geschwind syndrome. Bear and Fedio (10) expanded this syndrome to include the 18 traits based on the literature review. They found an increased frequency of all 18 traits in patients with TLE compared with normal neurologic controls. The interictal behavioral traits described by Bear and Fedio, together with several others reported in the literature, are summarized on Table 10.1. The purpose of this chapter is to at-

TABLE 10.1. *Interictal behavioral traits attributed to patients with epilepsy*

Trait	Clinical observation
Aggression	Overt hostility, rage attacks, violent crimes, murder
Altered sexual interest	Loss of libido, hyposexualism, fetishism, transvestism, exhibitionism, hypersexual episodes
Circumstantiality	Loquacious, pedantic, overly detailed, peripheral
Decreased emotionality	Emotional indifference, lack of initiative, dullness, hyperexcitability
Dependence, passivity	Helplessness, "at hand of fate," always requires assistance
Elation, euphoria	Grandiosity, exhilarated mood, diagnosis of biposal disorder
Emotional lability	Prominent mood changes with minor or no stimuli
Guilt	Tendency to self-scrutiny and self-recrimination
Humorlessness, sobriety	Overgeneralized ponderous concern, humor lacking or idiosyncratic
Hypergraphia	Keeping extensive diaries, detailed notes, writing
Hypermoralism	Attention to rules with inability to distinguish significant from minor infraction, desire to punish
Hypomoralism	Lack of attention to rules; lack of understanding or concern of "good" or "bad"
Increased emotionality	Deepening emotions; sustained intense affect; increased sensitivity, brooding
Irritability	Increased anger, temper
Obsessionalism	Ritualism, orderliness, compulsive attention to detail
Paranoia, jealousy	Suspicious, overinterpretation of motives and events; diagnosis of paranoid schizophrenia
Philosophical interest	Nascent metaphysical or moral speculations, cosmologic theories
Religiosity	Holding deep religious beliefs, often idiosyncratic, multiple conversations, mystical states
Sadness	Hopelessness, discouragement, self-deprecation; diagnosis of depression, suicide attempts
Sense of personal destiny	Egocentricity; personal events highly charged; divine guidance ascribed to many features of patient's life
Viscosity	Stickiness, tendency to repetition

tempt to review and critique evidence for the existence and specificity of characteristic behavioral syndromes among patients with temporal lobe onset epilepsy as well as other epilepsy syndromes.

PROBLEMS OF DEFINITION AND METHODOLOGY

Defining specific personality traits and aberrations in the population of patients with epilepsy is problematic and highly controversial. From a psychiatric standpoint, studies on interictal behavioral changes in epilepsy have not been "discipline neutral" (11). Over the past decades, stereotyped notions of personality attributes in patients with chronic seizures have been dominated by trait analysis within the psychometric tradition of writing scales, self-reporting methodologies, and multivariate statistics. Debates in the literature center on complex personality concepts (for example, hyperreligiosity) rather than attempt to integrate "first order" biologic variables that are undeniably implicated in the multivariate causality of complex behaviors *(vide infra)*.

Considering the variety of known epilepsy syndromes and their manifold etiologies, correlation of interictal behavior to a specific physiologic, anatomic locus is both difficult and primary in our understanding of epilepsy-behavioral correlates. Most studies on behavior and epilepsy were done without video electroencephalographic (EEG) confirmation of a specific ictal onset zone. Many authors simplistically approach "temporal lobe epilepsy" as a monolithic entity primarily involving mesiotemporal structures, thereby confining their analysis to broad generalizations about limbic-affective states. In contradistinction, current ictal analysis utilizing subdural grid electrode arrays frequently document presumed mesial temporal lobe onset epilepsies arising from neocortical extralimbic regions. Even when invasive monitoring documents a temporal lobe seizure "focus," there often is associated extratemporal glucose hypometabolism as defined by positron

emission tomography (12). In patients with TLE, as an illustration, prefrontal metabolic asymmetry is associated with cognitive impairment. Depression has been specifically correlated with left frontal hypometabolic changes in TLE patients (13).

The ability to analyze behavioral changes confined to the interictal period constitutes another methodologic deficiency. Preictal (premonitory), postictal, and interictal behavioral alterations are less well circumscribed temporally than ictal changes. In the extreme case of partial status epilepticus, it is readily apparent that cognitive impairments are observable as a continuum despite EEG evolution from discrete seizures to periodic discharges and finally reemergence of normal EEG background (14). For isolated seizures as well, transitions between ictal, preictal, postictal, and interictal behavioral states are fluid, and clinical distinctions made are potentially artificial. In addition, many studies were performed prior to the availability of magnetic resonance imaging (MRI), thus excluding identification of important anatomic contexts such as cortical dysplastic syndromes, vascular malformations, and low-grade neoplasms. Studies of TLE patients in the pre-MRI era no doubt included patients with erroneous localization/lateralization. Finally, past behavioral analysis of the population with epilepsy has centered around personality structure and not lifetime developmental or time-related variables. Methodologic issues are summarized in Table 10.2.

TABLE 10.2. *Methodologic issues confounding analysis of epilepsy-related behavioral syndromes*

Lack of adequate localization (electroencephalogram)
Lack of neuroanatomic correlate
Lack of differentiation of postictal from interictal symptoms
Lack of distinction between transient and sustained interictal symptomatology
Failure to address time-related variability in personality
Disparate epilepsy and comparison group populations
Lack of randomized controlled trials

ELABORATION, REPLICATION, AND CRITICISM OF THE INTERICTAL BEHAVIOR SYNDROME

The identification by Waxman and Geschwind (9) of a characteristic behavioral syndrome and the later expansion by Bear and Fedio (10) to include 18 specific traits have drawn criticism and incited controversy.

First, none of these traits are pathognomonic. All occur among patients with psychiatric and other neurologic disorders and in normals. Among the 18 self-rated traits, all were significantly higher in the TLE group. The most significant differences ($p <$ 0.0001) were humorlessness, circumstantiality, dependence, and sense of personal destiny. Proxy raters (i.e., family or friends) identified TLE patients as significantly different from controls on 14 traits, most strongly ($p < 0.0001$) for circumstantiality, obsessionalism, and dependence. Patients with right temporal foci reported more emotional traits and minimized their behavioral changes (i.e., polished their image), whereas patients with left temporal foci had more ideational traits and often tarnished their image on self-report relative to proxy reports. The previously reported associations of right hemisphere lesions causing denial and neglect syndromes whereas left hemisphere lesions more often cause depression (15–18) were consistent with the right/left:polish/tarnish correlation. However, subsequent studies did not support consistent lateralized personality changes in TLE (18–21).

There are several limitations to the study by Bear and Fedio (10). Groups were small; the two TLE and two control groups consisted of only 48 subjects. Patients were not consecutively studied. Also, the seizure disorder duration averaged 19 years, whereas seizure frequency averaged five per month; these were refractory patients. The number, type, dosage, and serum levels of antiepileptic drugs (AEDs) were not specified. Video EEG localization and MRI studies were not available at the time of study.

Replication studies using the Bear-Fedio inventory (BFI) have produced mixed results (Tables 10.3 and 10.4). In the study by Seidman (22), TLE patients rated themselves significantly higher than normal controls on eight of 18 traits (obsessiveness, viscosity, paranoia, circumstantiality, emotionality,

TABLE 10.3. *Literature summary of Bear-Fedio inventory: left–right temporal lobe epilepsy group comparisons*

Study	Self		Rater	
	Left	Right	Left	Right
Bear and Fedio (1977)	Dependence, anger, paranoia	Elation	Destiny	Obsessiveness
Seidman (1980)	Obsessiveness	0/18	Obsessiveness, humorlessness, altered sexuality	0/18
Nielson and Kristensen (1981)	Aggressiveness, depression, emotionality	0/18	ND	ND
Rodin and Schmaltz (1984)	0/18	0/18	0/18	0/18
Brandt et al. (1985)	Humorlessness	0/18	ND	ND
Weiser (1986)	Hypergraphia, altered sexuality, religiosity	Hypermoralism, sadness	ND	ND
Perini et al. (1996)	Depression, aggression, guilt			
Schmitz et al. (1997)	0/18	0/18		
Czernansky et al. (1990)	Religiosity			

ND, not done.

TABLE 10.4. *Literature summary of Bear-Fedio inventory: temporal lobe epilepsy versus other group comparisons*

Study	Self	Rater
Bear and Fedio (1977)[a]	All 18 traits	14 of 18 traits, except hypermoralism, hypergraphia, elation, and altered sexuality
Hermann and Reil (1981)		
TLE vs. *GE*	Sense of destiny, paranoia	ND
Seidman (1980)		
TLE vs. normal	Viscosity, obsessiveness, emotionality	Obsessiveness, viscosity, hypergraphia
Circumstantiality	Emotionality, paronoia, depression, anger, dependence, guilt	Circumstantial, aggressive
Rodin (1973)		
GE/TLE vs. normal	17/17[b]	
GE/TLE vs. psychiatric	0/18	
TLE vs. GE	Hypergraphia[c]	
Mungas (1982)		
TLE vs. neurobehavioral	0/18	0/18
TLE vs. psychiatric	0/18	0/18
Nielsen and Kristensen (1981)		
Medial vs. lateral TLE	Hypergraphia, elation, guilt, paranoia	ND
Brandt et al. (1985)		
L-TLE vs. normal	Circumstantiality, humorlessness, viscosity, sadness, obsessionalism	ND
R-TLE vs. normal	0/18	ND
GE vs. normal	Circumstantiality, viscosity, sadness, dependence, paranoia	ND
Swanson et al. (1995)		
PHI-CP vs. SP	Personal destiny, religiosity, philosophical interests	ND
PHI-CP vs. PHI-C	Total score, circumstantiality, religiosity, altered sexuality	ND
PHI-CP vs. UC	Total score, circumstantiality, religiosity, alter sexuality	ND
PHI-CP vs. SGTCS	0/18	ND
PHI-CP vs. TCS	0/18	ND

GE, primarily generalized epilepsy; ND, not done; PHI-CP, penetrating head-injured complex partial; SGTCS, secondarily generalized tonic-clonic seizures; TCS, tonic clonic seizures; TLE, temporal lobe epilepsy; UC, uninjured controls.
Underscore indicates group with increased scores.
[a]Normal controls and neuromuscular controls.
[b]Significance level not reported.
[c]Scores nonsignificantly increased in TLE for 12 of 17 traits.

anger, depression, and dependence) and were rated by others as higher on six of 18 traits (viscosity, obsessiveness, hypergraphia, emotionality, aggression, and circumstantiality). Seidman also found laterality effects in self-reports for obsessiveness (higher with left TLE) and rater reports for obsessiveness, humorlessness, and altered sexuality (higher in left TLE).

Nielsen and Kristensen (19) compared patients with medial (limbic) and lateral (neocortical) temporal lobe foci. Their localization technique, based on maximal amplitude in sphenoidal versus scalp electrodes, is not definitive. Patients with limbic foci had generally elevated traits throughout, but statistically significant increases were found only for hypergraphia, elation, guilt, and paranoia. Patients with left-sided foci had a nonsignificant increase in self-rating scores (i.e., tarnish).

Rodin and Schmaltz (18) compared normals, patients with pain or epilepsy (TLE and generalized epilepsy [GE]), and psychiatric inpatients. The combined epilepsy group scored higher on all 18 traits than the controls, and they scored higher on 16 traits than the pain patients. The TLE group scored higher than the GE group on 13 of 18 traits (significant by binomical probability); only hypergraphia was significantly different. There were no statistically significant differences between left and right TLE patients. Self- versus rater comparisons revealed that left TLE patients overreported for all 18 traits, but individual traits score differences were not significant. No tendency for underreporting was observed in the right TLE group. Trait scores were significantly correlated with mild intellectual impairment (higher humorless sobriety, circumstantiality, philosophical interest, guilt, religiosity) and carbamazepine level (lower elation, philosophical interests, sense of destiny, altered sexuality, and hypergraphia). Psychiatric inpatients scored higher on all 18 traits than epileptic patients, without any pattern (symptom cluster) differences between psychiatric and epilepsy groups. Similarly, Mungas (21) found no differences on any of the 18 BFI traits when he contrasted psychiatrically ill TLE patients with neurobehavioral and psychiatric controls. Bear et al. (23) used a standardized interview based on interictal characteristics to compare psychiatric inpatients with TLE or primary psychiatric disorders. The TLE group received significantly higher interview ratings on viscosity, circumstantiality, religiosity, philosophical interest, humorlessness, paranoia, and hypermoralism.

Hermann and Reil (24) compared TLE and GE patients and found significant elevations in TLE on four of 18 BFI scales: sense of personal destiny, dependence, paranoia, and philosophical interest. Brandt et al. (25) studied left and right TLE, GE, and normals with the BFI. Left TLE and GE patients endorsed significantly more items than controls; right TLE patients had only nonsignificantly elevated profiles compared with controls. The behavioral traits that best differentiated epilepsy and control subjects were circumstantiality, humorlessness, viscosity, sadness, and dependence.

Weiser (20) administered the self-rating questions of the BFI to 63 patients studied with frontal and temporal depth electrodes and found the following associations:

- Humorlessness increased in frontal
- Increase in all traits in frontal (trend level)
- Increased circumstantiality and hypermoralism in temporolimbic foci (trend level)
- Increased hypermoralism and humorlessness with right side (trend level)
- Increased religiosity, hypergraphia, and altered sexual content with left side (trend level)
- Female sex and emotionality
- Male sex and hypermoralism
- Unemployed and unskilled patients were more dependent and passive
- Left-handed patients had significantly increased altered sexuality
- Urban background correlated significantly with increased humorlessness
- Seizure onset before age 5 years correlated with increased sadness

Sorenson et al. (26) administered a modified BFI to patients with TLE, primary generalized epilepsy (PGE), patients with psoriasis, and healthy controls. The overall scores were highest for the combined epilepsy group, with psoriasis patients intermediate, and healthy controls lowest. TLE patients had more ideational traits than PGE patients. Csernansky et al. (27) used the BFI to study patients with limbic seizure foci. They found increased seizure frequency was associated with self-reported psychotic experiences (possibly postictal psychosis). Patients with left-sided foci had increased religiosity. Also, poorer neuropsychological functioning was associated with increased thought disorder, psychoticism, and affective disturbance.

The BFI reveals increased behavioral traits in patients with epilepsy (TLE and GE) in comparison to normal or nonbehavioral patient controls, but it does not distinguish epilepsy (TLE or GE) from psychiatric patients. Findings from TLE versus GE patient comparisons are inconsistent. When differences are present, the TLE group usually has higher scores than the GE group. Left–right differences in TLE are not strongly marked, although, in general, patients with left-sided foci endorse more items than those with right-sided foci, and they tend to tarnish their image (i.e., report more traits than raters). The complicating issue of frontal lobe seizure foci or involvement in patients with TLE is discussed later. Finally, personality traits are influenced by developmental and social environments, gender, intellectual status, AEDs, and other biologic and environmental factors. These factors have not been systematically studied.

The BFI has not defined a behavioral syndrome distinctive or specific for TLE. However, that was not its original intent. The BFI questions were not written to separate epilepsy and psychiatric patients or those with temporal versus frontal foci (28). The issue of selective temporal lobe seizure foci and specific behaviors is the crux of the controversy. The BFI consistently demonstrates that TLE patients have different behavioral traits than control subjects without epilepsy or behavioral disorders.

The BFI, although not providing a neat parcellation of trait clusters among different epilepsy and control groups, helped expand focus in epilepsy research and care from psychopathology to behavior change. Few investigators or clinicians doubt that some patients with temporolimbic and other epilepsies undergo personality changes. Most of the alleged behavioral traits occur more often or more intensely in epileptic patients than in normal subjects. What is the prevalence and form of these changes? In some instances, such as hypergraphia and religiosity, the frequency of intense behavioral change is low, but still appears to be higher among epileptic patients than in the general population. Other alterations, such as hyposexuality, are more common in epileptic patients. Studies utilizing more detailed evaluations (the BFI includes only five items per trait presented as true/false statements) can clarify the nature of the association between selected behavioral traits, epilepsy groups, and other variables.

OTHER CHALLENGES TO INTERICTAL BEHAVIORAL CHANGES IN EPILEPSY

Personality Changes in Primary Generalized Epilepsy

Personality changes in epilepsy are not restricted to patients with partial epilepsy, but also occur in patients with PGE syndromes such as juvenile myoclonic epilepsy (JME) (29) and absence epilepsy (30). In JME, reported traits included irresponsibility and impaired impulse control, neglect of duties, self-interest, emotional instability, exaggeration, inconsiderateness, quick temper, and distractibility. Janz (29) found that many JME patients repeatedly exposed themselves to sleep deprivation and often failed to comply with AEDs, taking their illness lightly. They denied problems and conflicts, or they often yielded to temptation against better judgment. There was limited support for Janz's clinical impression (31), although scientific evidence is sparse and some of these behaviors may reflect adolescence, not JME. Other studies found high rates of psychiatric disorders among patients with JME (32,33).

Absence epilepsy, long considered one of the most benign forms of epilepsy, recently has been associated with significant behavioral changes in a very well-controlled study. Wirrell et al. (34) compared all children in Nova Scotia with typical absence epilepsy or juvenile rheumatoid arthritis (JRA) diagnosed between 1986 and 1997, who were aged 18 years or older at follow-up (mean age 23 years). Remission occurred in 32 (57%) of the patients with typical absence epilepsy but in only 17 (28%) of the patients with JRA. Five categories of outcome were studied: academic-personal, behavioral, employment-financial, family relations, and social-personal relations. Patients with typical absence epilepsy had greater difficulties in the academic-personal and in the behavioral categories ($p < 0.001$) than those with JRA. Those with ongoing seizures had the least favorable outcome. Most seizure-related factors showed minimal correlation with psychosocial func-

TABLE 10.5. *Psychosocial and behavioral problems occurring more frequently in patients with a history of absence epilepsy versus juvenile rheumatoid arthritis*

Academic problems
  Requiring special education
  Below average academic performance
  Repeating a grade
  Failure to graduate high school or attend a university
  Being left behind in school
Psychosocial
  Poor sibling relationships
  Fewer regular social outings with friends or their partner
  Unwanted teenage pregnancy
Behavioral
  History of heavy alcohol use
  Behavioral problems reported by parents or teachers
  Psychiatric or emotional difficulties
Occupational
  Fewer months employed during the past 12 mo
  Higher rate of unskilled labor
  Poor job satisfaction

tioning. Problems that occurred more frequently among those with absence epilepsy are summarized in Table 10.5. Even patients whose epilepsy had remitted had significantly poorer outcome than the JRA patients in the academic-personal and behavioral domains. Another recent study found that 54% of pediatric patients with PGE had psychiatric disorders (35). Early age of onset and poor seizure control were significantly associated with the severity of illogical thinking in these children. Thus, the recent literature strongly supports prior research that PGE is a risk factor for cognitive and behavioral problems.

Personality Changes in Patients with Frontal Lobe Epilepsy (FLE)

The frontal lobes are important in personality, as highlighted by the effects of prefrontal surgeries. Thus, as limbic disorders can alter emotion- and drive-related behavior (e.g., sex and aggression), frontal dysfunction can alter personality, judgment, and executive functions. Further, the posterior orbitofrontal cortex and anterior cingulate gyrus, two critical limbic (paralimbic) areas, are located within the frontal lobe. Patients with anterior cingu-

late seizure foci can develop interictal psychosis, aggression, sociopathic behavior, sexual deviancy, irritability, obsessive-compulsive disorder, and poor impulse control (23,36–38). Orbitofrontal lesions can cause hyperphagia, failure to use autonomic cues to guide behavior, aberrant emotional responsiveness, increased aggression, dysfunctional social behavior (e.g., case of Phineas Gage [39]), behavioral disinhibition, and confabulation (40). Systematic studies on interictal behavior in patients with orbitofrontal seizure foci are lacking; however, behavioral disorders such as attention-deficit/hyperactivity disorder can occur (41). Given the critical role of this limbic cortex in social and emotional behavior, epileptic foci in this site could cause prominent interictal behavioral changes.

In the literature on the BFI, the study by Weiser (20), which is the only one to use invasive electrodes for localization and lateralization, failed to replicate any laterality effects found by Bear and Fedio (10). Interestingly, Weiser found a nonsignificant increase in all BFI behavioral traits in the group with TLE. In the Vietnam Head Injury Study, patients with tonic-clonic seizures had a higher frequency of psychiatric treatment than those with complex partial seizures (42), possibly reflecting greater frontal lobe involvement. The role of the frontal lobe in the personality and behavior of epileptic patients deserves greater attention. Functional imaging studies suggest that, even among patients with temporal lobe seizure foci, frontal dysfunction contributes to affective, personality, and cognitive disorders (12,13,43).

Selected Personality Traits

The current data do not clearly support or refute consistent or specific clustering of behavioral changes among TLE patients. Published studies lack adequate sample size and power, controls, neuroimaging, and video EEG localizing studies, as well as valid and reliable measures of behavior. We simply do not know if there is a TLE (or FLE or PGE) personality syndrome. Further, the answer may not be a simple yes or no. Because we are unable to define or refute a syndrome, it may be helpful to further explore evidence linking specific behavioral traits and TLE.

Viscosity

Viscosity is a tendency for prolonged interpersonal contacts talking repetitively, circumstantially, pedantically, and not ending conversations and visits after a socially appropriate interval. These individuals have a sticky (cohesive) social manner. Mayeux et al. (44) suggested that subtle interictal language impairment underlies viscosity, because circumstantiality correlated with impaired naming. Bear and Fedio (10) found viscosity significantly elevated in both right and left TLE compared to normal and neurologic controls. Brandt et al. (25) found increased viscosity among left TLE and GE patients, with no difference between right TLE and controls. Hoeppner et al. (45) showed a drawing of a boy stealing a cookie to TLE, GE, and control subjects. Taped responses were reviewed blindly. All four individuals with verbose responses, characterized by trivial, circumstantial, and subjective details, had left temporal foci. At the National Institutes of Health, a ten-item viscosity scale revealed significantly higher scores in the self-reports of patients with left TLE compared to right or bilateral TLE, absence seizures, panic disorder, or normal subjects (46). Proxy raters reported a trend for increased viscosity scores in the left TLE group, endorsing items such as "when I have a phone conversation with him/her, I always find I am the one who wants to get off first." Seizure duration and viscosity score were significantly correlated for patients with left TLE.

Viscosity may result from some combination of linguistic impairment, social cohesion, mental slowness, and psychological dependence. Language dysfunction associated with left temporal lobe seizure foci may contribute to a verbal style characterized by circumstantiality and excessive discourse. However, there may be independent effects of left temporal foci on social behavior. Viscosity, the personality trait, may largely be a desire for interpersonal closeness and a need for affiliation with another being. Discrete limbic lesions can profoundly alter how animals maintain contacts with other members of their own or other species (47–49). For example, rats with septal lesions will remain in contact with each other in an open field and, if left alone, will actively approach cats despite expressions of fear (47).

Hyposexuality

Various changes in interictal sexual behavior occur in patients with TLE. Hyposexuality frequently is reported (50–57), with anecdotal reports of hypersexuality (54,58), deviant sexual behavior including exhibitionism (52,59), transvestism (60,61), transsexualism (62), and fetishism (63,64). Hyposexuality, including decreased libido and impotence, occurs in approximately half of TLE patients without gender bias. In many cases, especially those with seizure onset before puberty, patients do not marry or regard their sexuality as a problem. Complaints are more likely to come from the spouse or parent who observes lack of interest in the opposite sex. Much of the original literature on hyposexuality from 1954 to 1985 was based on self-report (65) without detailed interviews to assess the relative roles of libido, arousal, erectile dysfunction, anorgasmia, and sexual satisfaction, as well as physiologic measures of endocrine and sexual function.

Most studies found higher rates of hyposexuality and sexual dysfunction in TLE than other epilepsy groups, although Fenwick et al. (56) did not observe any significant difference in sexual activity related to seizure type, type of epilepsy, or seizure frequency. A well-designed study of six men with erectile dysfunction found abnormal nocturnal penile tumescence and rigidity in five (66). The pattern of abnormality was consistent with neurogenic, not vasogenic, erectile dysfunction. In a self-report survey of 116 women with epilepsy, partial epilepsy patients experienced more dyspareunia, vaginismus, arousal insufficiency, and sexual dissatisfaction, whereas PGE patients experienced more anorgasmia and sexual dissatisfaction (67). Sexual symptoms were not associated with seizure frequency, AED exposure, sexual experience, depression, or prepubertal seizure onset.

The pathogenetic role of temporal lobe seizures in hyposexuality is supported by animal models (68) and observations that sexual activity can increase following successful seizure control with AEDs (69) and temporal lobectomy (52). In some postlobectomy subjects, marked hypersexuality similar to the Kluver-Bucy syndrome can develop occasionally (70). However, AEDs modulate hypothalamic-pituitary-gonadal axis hormone activity and can directly inhibit sexual behavior (65). Barbiturates may cause the greatest decrease in libido and sexual function (71). Valproic acid is associated with menstrual disorders, hyperandrogenism, and polycystic ovaries (72,73).

Religion

The ancient association between epilepsy and mystical/religious phenomena is paradigmatic of the difficulty reconciling dramatic anecdotes and long-standing medical opinion with limited clinical studies. Hippocrates began his monograph on the "sacred disease" by refuting the association between epilepsy and the divine: patients with epilepsy did not have prophetic or mystical powers; epilepsy is not a curse of the gods. Despite his modern insights, religious and magical treatments of epilepsy predominated throughout the Middle Ages and Renaissance (74). In the nineteenth century, psychiatrists stressed the religiosity of epileptic patients (75–77), whereas Siberian medicine men preferred epileptic pupils (77,78). Classic monographs on religious mysticism noted that "among the dread diseases that afflict humanity there is only one that interests us quite particularly; that disease is epilepsy" (78).

Intense religious experiences and strong religious beliefs are reported frequently by people with epilepsy. Many prominent religious figures allegedly had epilepsy, including prophets and founders of many religions (79). The evidence supporting epilepsy in these people varies. Intense religious experiences can occur in association with seizures (80–83), as Dostoyevsky (84) documented eloquently:

> The air was filled with a big noise, and I thought that it had engulfed me. I have really touched God. He came into me myself, yes, God exists, I cried, and I don't remember anything else. You all, healthy people, he said, can't imagine the happiness which we epileptics feel during the second before our attack. I don't know if this felicity lasts for seconds, hours, or months, but believe me, for all the joys that life may bring, I would not exchange this one... Such instants were characterized by a fulguration of the consciousness and by a supreme exaltation of emotional subjectivity.

Dewhurst and Beard (85) reported six TLE patients who underwent sudden religious conversions. There was a clear temporal relationship between conversion and increased seizure activity in five patients; one patient had a marked decrease in seizure frequency prior to conversion (she attributed her improved seizure disorder to the Almighty).

Increased religious conviction and practice is not a consistent behavioral feature in patients with epilepsy. There is little evidence that epilepsy or TLE patients as a group are hyperreligious, although a subgroup may have unusually strong religious beliefs. Two studies with questionnaires on religion failed to differentiate patients with right versus left TLE, TLE versus GE, or epileptic patients and controls (86,87).

Hypergraphia

Hypergraphia is not characteristic of interictal behavior among TLE or GE patients. However, several studies support that the subgroup manifesting this behavior most intensely are those with temporal lobe foci. Waxman and Geschwind (88) reported seven TLE patients with hypergraphia, which is a tendency toward extensive and sometimes compulsive writing. There was a striking pre-occupation with detail—words were defined and redefined and underlined, parentheses were used to make word meaning absolutely clear—the writers accorded great importance to their material. In four patients, the writings focused on moral and religious concerns. Hypergraphia was viewed as a component of the deepened emotions and especially viscosity of interictal behavioral changes.

Utilizing a mailed standard questionnaire, Sachdev and Waxman (89) demonstrated that TLE patients responded frequently and extensively (mean 1,301 words) as compared to other epileptic patients (mean 106 words). Hermann et al. (90) replicated the higher response rates and longest letters in the TLE group, but they did not find that the average response was longer in TLE patients compared to other seizure patients. Duration of epilepsy, hypomania, and number of significant life events during the past year positively correlated with hypergraphia (90,91). Hypergraphia occurs in 7% to 10% of TLE patients (90,91).

Dostoyevsky was the most famous hypergraphic TLE patient (92), although his prolific writing also reflected his pay per page and financial troubles. As a person, he was deeply emotional, irritable, angered over minor provocations, guilt ridden, depressed, and tortured over the question of God's existence. He described the relation between his writing and epilepsy in a letter to his brother (August 27, 1849): "whenever formerly I had such nervous disturbances, I made use of them for writing; in such a state I could write much more and much better than usual."

Aggression

Interictal violence and aggression is a highly contentious topic, especially the relationship between TLE and aggression. There appears to be a relatively elevated incidence of interictal violence and hostility in patients with epilepsy as compared to healthy controls. The neurosurgical series of Serafetinides (93) and of Taylor (94) demonstrated

rates of aggression approaching 30% in an analysis of preoperative behavior in TLE patients prior to temporal lobectomy. These studies have been criticized as being flawed because the data were obtained from a very select population (1%) of individuals chosen for surgical intervention. Rodin (95) identified 5% of patients presenting to his epilepsy center as manifesting aggressive behavior. Seizure type did not distinguish aggressive from nonaggressive patients. Gunn and Fenton (96) documented increased prevalence of epilepsy in British prisons relative to the general population. Study of the Illinois prison system documented a prevalence rate of epilepsy of 2.4%, elevated relative to the U.S. population at the time of the study. However, census of prisoners with epilepsy against matched nonepileptic controls did not reveal more serious violent crimes on the part of the epilepsy group (97).

Violence and hostility in epilepsy in all likelihood is a consequence of an interaction of neurophysiologic as well as social factors. Male sex is clearly higher risk of violence and epilepsy, and Serafetinides noted that aggressiveness as a personality trait in TLE patients was more likely in those with seizure onset prior to age 10 years. Other risk factors identified in the TLE group include premature interruption of formal schooling, lower intellectual quotient, and lower socioeconomic status. Ultimately, these risk factors are associated with a greater risk of aggression in nonepileptic patients as well.

PATHOPHYSIOLOLGY OF BEHAVIORAL CHANGES IN EPILEPSY

The pathogenesis of behavioral changes in epileptic patients is not well understood. Interictal behavioral disorders and changes have been associated with biologic, medication, and psychosocial variables. Multiple factors often coexist, and the relative contribution of each varies between individuals and for different behaviors. Because we cannot define an interictal behavioral syndrome of TLE (or

JME or FLE), identifying its mechanism is problematic. However, we may be more successful in elucidating the causes of specific behavioral changes such as hyposexuality and hypergraphia, or behavioral disorders such as depression and psychosis.

A behavioral change associated with a localization-related epilepsy suggests that specific structures are involved in the pathogenesis, but how? Structural lesions, such as mesial temporal sclerosis or dysplasia, may contribute but have not been associated with the frequency or intensity of behavioral changes. An insightful hypothesis was offered nearly 40 years ago by Sir Charles Symonds (98), "the epileptogenic disorder of function." While discussing the pathophysiology of interictal psychosis TLE patients, he suggested:

> If then neither the fits nor the temporal lobe damage can be held directly responsible for the psychosis, what is the link?...Epileptic seizures and epileptiform discharge in the EEG are epiphenomena. They may be regarded as occasional expressions of a fundamental and continuous disorder of neuronal function. The essence of this disorder is loss of the normal balance between excitation and inhibition at the synaptic junctions. From moment to moment there may be excess either of excitation or inhibition—or even both at the same time in different parts of the same neuronal system. The epileptogenic disorder of function may be assumed to be present continuously but with peaks at which seizures are likely to occur.

The epileptogenic disorder of function offers an overview, but it does not specify mechanisms. Changes in neurotransmitters, neuropeptides, neuroendocrine function, metabolism, synaptic connectivity, neuronal populations (e.g., loss of inhibitory interneurons), and other pathophysiologic changes associated with epilepsy can contribute to behavioral changes. Some personality traits in TLE patients are the opposite of KBS symptoms (7,51). Geschwind (99) suggested that KBS reflects sensory-limbic disconnection. Bear (100) posited that, in contrast to KBS, behavioral changes in temporolimbic epilepsy result from a sensory-limbic hyperconnection. Rarely, specific sensory stimuli are linked with powerful and persistent affective valence, such as one man with TLE who experienced sexual auras when he viewed a safety pin (63). Further support for hyperconnection or hyperactivity is provided by a cat model of TLE-induced hyposexuality in cats. Abnormal high-frequency neuronal activity in the temporal lobe but not motor cortex is associated a dramatic suppression of sexual behavior (68). However, the well-documented interictal hypometabolism and neuronal loss in TLE suggests that hypofunction underlies some cognitive (e.g., short-term memory) and behavioral (e.g., depression) changes (13). The diversity of mechanisms underlying behavioral changes in TLE may partly explain our frustrations in delineating a specific syndrome. It is likely that, in a given individual with epilepsy, behavioral changes may simultaneously result from hyperactivity in some systems, hypoactivity in some systems, and aberrant activity in other systems.

The tireless controversy encircling the association of TLE and specific behavioral changes must not obscure the documented high frequency of psychopathology among individuals with epilepsy. We must be vigilant to diagnose and treat significant problems such as depression, psychosis, and sexual dysfunction. Increased awareness of the range of behavioral changes and their risk factors, and increased understanding of the mechanisms, may lead to identification of patients at risk and preventive strategies, as well as earlier detection and more targeted, effective therapies.

TREATMENT

Interictal nonpathologic personality traits that disrupt the patient's functioning may be therapeutically addressed in numerous ways.

Unilateral anterior temporal lobectomy has been reported to eliminate marked irritability and global hyposexuality in some cases. Interictal episodic dyscontrol may respond to usage of β blockers and/or behaviorally oriented therapies. As a generalization, disruptive interictal personality traits are best referred for psychotherapy to a psychiatrist or psychologist with experience in epilepsy. The most pragmatic therapeutic advice is to consider the coexistence of a major affective disorder. Magnified personality disturbances are a common accompaniment of major affective disorders and may respond to appropriate treatment for the mood disorder. It is widely held that the estimated frequency of depressive syndromes encountered in epilepsy ranges from 20% to 60% and that affective disorders commonly are underrecognized and undertreated by neurologists. The current variety of selective serotonin reuptake inhibitors may be recommended in this instance. Some maladaptive personality traits (e.g., viscosity and hypergraphia) in epileptic patients share characteristics related to obsessive-compulsive disorders (101). Serotoninergic agents may be useful in this instance as well.

EPILEPSY AND BEHAVIOR: OVERVIEW AND TELEOLOGIC SPECULATION

Behavior in epilepsy is characterized by diversity. No specific or consistent behavioral syndrome occurs in epilepsy or specific epilepsy syndromes. Rather, clinical practice and an extensive literature are consistent with behavioral changes that defy traditional syndromic categorization. Epilepsy accentuates the variance (extremes) of behavior in one or both directions away from the mean. For example, changes in emotional state and affect are prominent. Yet a deepening or increase in emotionality (9,10) and a global decrease in emotional life and content (51), as well as emotional lability, occur more often in epileptic patients. Patients may be irritable and aggressive (53) or timid and apathetic (2,51). Epilepsy-related behavioral changes may be positive, including the many famous people with epilepsy in politics, religion, and the arts and sciences. The more frequent negative spectrum includes psychosis, depression, paranoia, and personality disorders. Teleologically, epilepsy (and other neurobehavioral disorders) may persist in our species partly because they diversify behavior. Even behavioral disorders such as paranoia or obsessive thinking can be beneficial at certain times. Diversity fuels natural selection. Although evolutionary biology focuses on morphologic diversity, mechanisms that enhance behavioral diversity also are critical. Thus, if there is a unifying theme to epilepsy-related behavioral changes, it may be deviation from the behavioral mean.

REFERENCES

1. Lishman WA. *Organic psychiatry*, 3rd ed. London: Blackwell Science Ltd., 1998:265–273.
2. Reynolds JR. *Epilepsy: its symptoms, treatment, and relation to other chronic convulsive disorders.* London: Churchill, 1861:39–77.
3. Gowers WR. *Epilepsy and other chronic convulsive disorders.* New York: William Wood & Co., 1885:101.
4. Wilson SAK. *Neurology.* Baltimore: Williams & Wilkins, 1940:1486.
5. Sjobring H. Ixophreni. In: *Psykologisk-pedagogisk uppslagsbok. Bd. 2.* Stockholm, 1944. Quoted and translated by Gudmundsson.
6. Gibbs FA. Ictal and non-ictal psychiatric disorders in temporal lobe epilepsy. *J Nerv Ment Dis* 1951;113: 522–528.
7. Gastaut H, Morin G, Leserve N. Etude du comportement des épileptiques psycho-moteurs dans l'intervalle de leurs crises. *Ann Medico-Psychol* 1955;113: 1–27.
8. Kluver H, Bray PC. Preliminary analysis of functions of the temporal lobe in monkeys. *Arch Neurol Psychiatry* 1939;42:979–1002.
9. Waxman SG, Geschwind N. The interictal behavior syndrome in temporal lobe epilepsy. *Arch Gen Psychiatry* 1975;32:1580–1586.
10. Bear DM, Fedio P. Quantitative analysis of interictal behavior in temporal lobe epilepsy. *Arch Neurol* 1977; 34:454–467.
11. Barratt ES, Kent T, Stanford MJ. Biologic variables defining and measuring personality. In: Rately JJ, ed. *Neuropsychiatry of personality disorders.* Oxford: Blackwell Science, 1995:36–37.
12. Jokeit H, Seitz RJ, Markowitsch HJ, et al. Prefrontal asymmetric interictal glucose hypometabolism and cognitive impairment in patients with temporal lobe epilepsy. *Brain* 1997;120:2283–2294.
13. Bromfield EB, Altshuler L, Leiderman DB, et al. Cerebral metabolism and depression in patients with complex partial seizures. *Epilepsia* 1990;31:625–626.
14. Ritaccio AL, March GR. The significance of BI-PLEDS in complex partial status epilepticus. *Am J Electroencephalogr Technol* 1993;33:27–34.
15. Galin D. Implications for psychiatry of left and right cerebral specialization. *Arch Gen Psychiatry* 1974; 31:572–583.
16. Gainotti G. Emotional behavior and hemispheric side of lesion. *Cortex* 1972;8:41–45.
17. Robertson MM, Trimble MR, Townsend HRA. The

phenomenology of depression in epilepsy. *Epilepsia* 1987;28:364–372.

18. Rodin E, Schmaltz S. The Bear-Fedio personality inventory and temporal lobe epilepsy. *Neurology* 1984;34:591–596.

19. Nielsen H, Kristensen O. Personality correlates of sphenoidal EEG foci in temporal lobe epilepsy. *Acta Neurol Scand* 1981;64:289–300.

20. Wieser HG. Selective amygdalohippocampectomy: indications, investigative technique and results. *Adv Tech Stand Neurosurg* 1986;13:39–133.

21. Mungas D. Interictal behavior abnormality in temporal lobe epilepsy: a specific syndrome or nonspecific psychopathology. *Arch Gen Psychiatry* 1982;39:108–111.

22. Seidman L. Lateralized cerebral dysfunction, personality, and cognition in temporal lobe epilepsy. Ph.D. thesis, University of Michigan, University Microfilms International, Ann Arbor, MI, 1980.

23. Bear D, Levin K, Blumer D, et al. Interictal behavior. I. Hospitalized temporal lobe epileptics: relationship to idiopathic psychiatric syndrome. *J Neurol Neurosurg Psychiatry* 1982;45:481–488.

24. Hermann BP, Reil P. Interictal personality and behavioral traits in temporal lobe and generalized epilepsy. *Cortex* 1981;17:125–128.

25. Brandt J, Seidman LJ, Kohl D. Personality characteristics of epileptic patients: a controlled study of generalized and temporal lobe cases. *J Clin Exp Neuropsychol* 1985;7:25–38.

26. Sorensen AS, Hansen H, Andersen R, et al. Personality characteristics and epilepsy. *Acta Psychiatr Scand* 1989;80:620–631.

27. Csernansky JG, Leiderman DB, Mandabach M, et al. Psychopathology and limbic epilepsy: relationship to seizure variables and neuropsychological function. *Epilepsia* 1990;31:275–280.

28. Bear D. Interictal behavior syndrome in temporal lobe epilepsy. *J Neuropsychiatry* 1989;1:308–311.

29. Janz D. *Die epilepsien.* Stuttgart: Georg Thieme, 1969.

30. Small JG, Milstein V, Stevens JR. Are psychomotor epileptics different? A controlled study. *Arch Neurol* 1962;7:187–194.

31. Bech P, Pedersen KK, Simonsen N, et al. Personality in epilepsy. *Acta Neurol Scand* 1976;54:348–358.

32. Perini GI, Tosin C, Carraro C, et al. Interictal mood and personality disorders in temporal lobe epilepsy and juvenile myoclonic epilepsy. *J Neurol Neurosurg Psychiatry* 1996;61:601–605.

33. Vazquez B, Devinsky O, Luciano D, et al. Juvenile myoclonic epilepsy: clinical features and factors related to misdiagnosis. *J Epilepsy* 1993;6:233–238.

34. Wirrell EC, Camfield CS, Camfield PR, et al. Long-term psychosocial outcome in typical absence epilepsy. Sometimes a wolf in sheep's clothing. *Arch Pediatr Adolesc Med* 1997;151:152–158.

35. Caplan R, Arbelle S, Guthrie D, et al. Formal thought disorder and psychopathology in pediatric primary generalized and complex partial epilepsy. *J Am Acad Child Adolesc Psychiatry* 1997;36:1286–1294.

36. Devinsky O, Abramson H, Alper K, et al. Postictal psychosis: a case control series of 20 patients and 150 controls. *Epilepsy Res* 1995;20:247–253.

37. Mazars G. Criteria for identifying cingulate epilepsies. *Epilepsia* 1970;11:41–47.

38. Devinsky O, Morrell M, Bogt B. Contribution of ante-

rior cingulate cortex to behavior. *Brain* 1995;118:279–306.

39. Damasio H, Grabowski T, Frank R, et al. The return of Phineas Gage: clues about the brain from the skull of a famous patient. *Science* 1994;264:1102–1105.

40. Devinsky O, D'Esposito M. *The neurology of cognition and behavior.* New York: Oxford University Press *(in press)*.

41. Powell AL, Yudd A, Zee P, et al. Attention deficit hyperactivity disorder associated with orbitofrontal epilepsy in a father and a son. *Neuropsychiatry Neuropsychol Behav Neurol* 1997;10:151–154.

42. Swanson SJ, Rao SM, Grafman J, et al. The relationship between seizure type and interictal personality. Results from the Vietnam Head Injury Study. *Brain* 1995;118:91–103.

43. Schmitz EB, Moriarty J, Costa DC, et al. Psychiatric profiles and patterns of cerebral blood flow in focal epilepsy: interactions between depression, obsessionality, and perfusion related to the laterality of the epilepsy. *J Neurol Neurosurg Psychiatry* 1997;62:458–463.

44. Mayeux R, Brandt J, Rosen J, et al. Interictal memory and language impairment in temporal lobe epilepsy. *Neurology* 1980;30:120–125.

45. Hoeppner JB, Garron DC, Wilson RS, et al. Epilepsy and verbosity. *Epilepsia* 1987;28:35–40.

46. Rao SM, Devinsky O, Grafman J, et al. Viscosity in complex partial seizures: relationship to cerebral laterality and seizure duration. *J Neurol Neurosurg Psychiatry* 1992;55:149–152.

47. Meyer DR, Ruth RA, Lavond DG. The septal social cohesiveness effect: its robustness and main determinants. *Physiol Behav* 1978;21:1027–1029.

48. Glendenning KK. Effects of septal and amygdaloid lesions on social behavior of the cat. *J Comp Physiol Psychol* 1972;80:199–207.

49. Kolb B, Nonneman AJ. Frontolimbic lesions and social behavior in the rat. *Physiol Behav* 1974;13:637–643.

50. Jensen I, Larsen JK. Mental aspects of temporal lobe epilepsy. *J Neurol Neurosurg Psychiatry* 1979;42:256–265.

51. Gastaut H, Collomb H. Etude du comportement sexuel chez les epileptiques psychomoteurs. *Ann Med Psychol (Paris)* 1954;112:657–696.

52. Blumer D, Walker EA. Sexual behavior in temporal lobe epilepsy. *Arch Neurol* 1967;16:37–43.

53. Saunders M, Rawson M. Sexuality in male epileptics. *J Neurol Sci* 1970;10:577–583.

54. Shukla GD, Hrivastava ON, Katiyar BC. Sexual disturbances in temporal lobe epilepsy: a controlled study. *Br J Psychiatry* 1979;134:288–292.

55. Taylor DC. Sexual behavior and temporal lobe epilepsy. *Arch Neurol* 1979;21:510–516.

56. Fenwick PBC, Toone BK, Wheeler MJ, et al. Sexual behavior in a centre for epilepsy. *Acta Neurol Scand* 1985;71:428–435.

57. Spark RF, Wills CA, Royal H. Hypogonadism, hyperprolactinemia, and temporal lobe epilepsy in hyposexual men. *Lancet* 1984;1:413–416.

58. Geschwind N, Shader RI, Bear D, et al. Behavioral changes with temporal lobe epilepsy: assessment and treatment. *J Clin Psychiatry* 1980;41:89–95.

59. Hooshmand H, Brawley BW. Temporal lobe seizures and exhibitionism. *Neurology* 1969;19:1119–1124.

60. Epstein AW. Relationship of fetishism and transvestism to brain and particularly to temporal lobe dysfunction. *J Nerv Ment Dis* 1961;133:247–253.

61. Petritzer BK, Foster J. A case study of a male transvestite with epilepsy and juvenile diabetes. *J Nerv Ment Dis* 1955;121:557–563.

62. Hoenig J, Kenna JC. EEG abnormalities and transsexualism. *Br J Psychiatry* 1979;134:293–300.

63. Mitchell W, Falconer MA, Hill D. Epilepsy with fetishism relieved by temporal lobectomy. *Lancet* 1954;2:626–630.

64. Epstein AW. Fetishism: a study of its psychopathology with particular reference to a proposed disorder in brain mechanisms as an etiologic factor. *J Nerv Ment Dis* 1960;23:247–249.

65. Morrell MJ. Sexual dysfunction in epilepsy. *Epilepsia* 1991;32[Suppl 6]:S38–S45.

66. Guldner GT, Morrell MJ. Nocturnal penile tumescence and rigidity evaluation in men with epilepsy. *Epilepsia* 1996;37:1211–1214.

67. Morrell MJ, Guldner GT. Self-reported sexual function and sexual arousability in women with epilepsy. *Epilepsia* 1996;37:1204–1210.

68. Feeney DM, Gullotta FP, Gilmore W. Hyposexuality produced by temporal lobe epilepsy in the cat. *Epilepsia* 1998;39:140–149.

69. Peters UH. Sexualstorungen bei psychomotorischer Epilepsie. *J Neurovis Relat* 1971;[Suppl 10]:491–497.

70. Blumer D. Hypersexual episodes in temporal lobe epilepsy. *Am J Psychiatry* 1970;126:1099–1106.

71. Mattson RH, Cramer JA, Collins JF, et al. Comparison of carbamazepine, phenobarbital, phenytoin, and primidone in partial and secondarily generalized tonicclonic seizures. *N Engl J Med* 1985;313:145–151.

72. Isojarvi JI, Laatikainen TJ, Pakarinen AJ, et al. Polycystic ovaries and hyperandrogenism in women taking valproate for epilepsy. *N Engl J Med* 1993;329: 1383–1388.

73. Murialdo G, Galimberti CA, Magri F, et al. Menstrual cycle and ovary alterations in women with epilepsy on antiepileptic therapy. *J Endocrinol Invest* 1997;20: 519–526.

74. Temkin O. *The falling sickness,* 2nd ed. Baltimore: Johns Hopkins University Press, 1971.

75. Esquirol JED. *Des maladies mentales.* Paris: Baillière, 1838.

76. Morel BA. D'une forme de delire, suite d'une surexcitation nerveuse se rattachant a une variete non encore decrite d'epilepsie (Epilepsie larvee). *Gazette habdomadaire de medecine et de chirurgie 7.* 1860:773–75, 819–821, 836–841.

77. Maudsley H. *The pathology of mind.* London: Macmillan and Co., 1879:446.

78. Leuba JH. *The psychology of religious mysticism.* London: Kegan Paul, Trench, Trubner & Co., 1925:204.

79. Devinsky O, Theodore WH, eds. *Epilepsy and behavior.* New York: Wiley-Liss, 1991.

80. Spratling WP. *Epilepsy and its treatment.* New York: WB Saunders 1904:473–474.

81. Howden JC. The religious sentiments in epileptics. *J Ment Sci* 1872–1873;18:491–497.

82. Mabille H. Hallucinations religieuses et delire religieux transitoire dans l'epilepsie. *Ann Medico-Psychol* 1899;9/10:76–81.

83. Cirignotta F, Todesco CV, Lugaresi E. Temporal lobe epilepsy with ecstatic seizures (so-called Dostoyevsky epilepsy). *Epilepsia* 1980;21:705–710.

84. Dostoyevsky FM. *The idiot.* London: Penguin Books, 1955. Magarshack D, translator.

85. Dewhurst K, Beard AW. Sudden religious conversions in temporal lobe epilepsy. *Br J Psychiatry* 1970;117: 497–507.

86. Willmore LJ, Heilman KM, Fennell E, et al. *Trans Am Neurol Assoc* 1980;105:85–87.

87. Tucker DM, Novelly RA, Walker PJ. Hyperreligiosity in temporal lobe epilepsy: redefining the relationship. *J Nerv Ment Dis* 1987;175:181–184.

88. Waxman SG, Geschwind N. Hypergraphia in temporal lobe epilepsy. *Neurology* 1974;24:629–631.

89. Sachdev HS, Waxman SG. Frequency of hypergraphia in temporal lobe epilepsy: an index of interictal behavior syndrome. *J Neurol Neurosurg Psychiatry* 1981;44:358–360.

90. Hermann BP, Whitman S, Arnston P. Hypergraphia in epilepsy: is there a specificity to temporal lobe epilepsy? *J Neurol Neurosurg Psychiatry* 1983;46:848–853.

91. Hermann BP, Whitman S, Wyler AR, et al. The neurological, psychosocial and demographic correlates of hypergraphia in patients with epilepsy. *J Neurol Neurosurg Psychiatry* 1988;51:203–208.

92. Geschwind N. Dostoyevsky's epilepsy. In: Blumer D, ed. *Psychiatric aspects of epilepsy.* Washington, DC: American Psychiatric Press, 1984:325–334.

93. Serafetinides EA. Aggressiveness in temporal lobe epileptics and its relation to cerebral dysfunction and environmental factors. *Epilepsia* 1965;6:33–42.

94. Taylor DC. Aggression and epilepsy. *J Psychosom Res* 1969;13:229–236.

95. Rodin EA. Psychomotor epilepsy and aggressive behavior. *Arch Gen Psychiatry* 1973;28:210–213.

96. Gunn J, Fenton G. Epilepsy in prisons: a diagnostic survey. *BMJ* 1969;4:326–328.

97. Whitman S, Coleman TE, Patmon C, et al. Epilepsy in prison: elevated prevalence and no relationship to violence. *Neurology* 1984;6:775–782.

98. Symonds C. Discussion. *Proc R Soc Med* 1962; 55:314–315.

99. Geschwind N. Disconnexion syndromes in animals and man. I. *Brain* 1965;88:237–294.

100. Bear DM. Temporal lobe epilepsy a syndrome of sensory-limbic hyperconnection. *Cortex* 1979;15:357–384.

101. Torta R, Keller R. Behavioral, psychotic and anxiety disorders in epilepsy. *Epilepsia* 1999;40[Suppl 10]: S2–S20.

11

Psychiatric Phenomena as an Expression of Postictal and Paraictal Events

Andres M. Kanner and *Ruben Kuzniecky

*Department of Neurological Sciences, Rush Presbyterian-Saint Luke's Medical Center, Chicago, Illinois 60612; and *Department of Neurology, University of Alabama at Birmingham, Birmingham, Alabama 35294*

The classification of psychiatric clinical phenomena in patients with epilepsy frequently is based on their temporal relation with seizure occurrence. Hence, we refer to *ictal* psychiatric symptoms when symptoms are the clinical expression of the actual seizure; *periictal* psychiatric symptoms refer to symptomatology preceding and/or following the ictus (i.e., *postictal*); and *interictal* symptoms are those that present independently of the seizure occurrence. A pathogenic role of the epileptic process on psychiatric phenomena is obvious in periictal disorders, but to a significantly lesser degree in interictal disorders. Yet, at some point in their practice all epileptologists have encountered cases of patients with florid "interictal" psychiatric and cognitive disturbances that become apparent around the beginning of a seizure disorder and remit and/or significantly improve upon its elimination. We use the term *paraictal* to refer to this type of psychiatric disorder.

The purpose of this chapter is to review the available data on postictal psychiatric phenomena and to illustrate examples of psychiatric and cognitive disturbances that are an expression of a paraictal process. Among the latter, we included the psychiatric and cognitive disturbances associated with the acquired epileptic aphasia of childhood (also known as Landau-Kleffner syndrome [LKS]), in which the "nonepileptic" clinical

disturbances are the major expression of the epileptic disorder and cure of the seizure disorder often is followed by recovery of language function (1). The second example is that of an intractable seizure disorder caused by hypothalamic hamartomas presenting characteristically with gelastic seizures, but also including complex partial, secondarily generalized tonic-clonic seizures, and at times atonic or tonic seizures. This seizure disorder is associated with severe psychiatric disturbances that remit or improve significantly with the cessation of the seizures following a successful surgical treatment (2).

POSTICTAL PSYCHIATRIC PHENOMENA

Postictal psychiatric symptoms (PPS) have been recognized for a long time, but in general they remain poorly understood, particularly with respect to their prevalence and pathogenic mechanisms. They may present as an individual symptom or as a cluster of symptoms, mimicking any type of psychiatric disorder, i.e., anxiety, depression, and psychosis. The advent of video electroencephalographic (VEEG) telemetry has been associated with an increased interest in postictal psychosis (PIP), but the other forms of PPS have remained unexplored. Most articles have consisted of small case series of PIP.

Postictal Psychiatric Symptoms

Periictal and postictal mood changes were described in the writings of Gowers (3) and Hughlings Jackson (4) in the nineteenth century and of Kraepelin (5) in the early twentieth century. More recently, Blanchet and Frommer (6) reported a decline in mood ratings 3 days prior to the seizure occurrence, with a return to baseline ratings noted 1 day postictally. Williams (7) noted the persistence of *ictal* symptoms of depression into the postictal period for as long as 3 days in eight patients.

We recently concluded an evaluation on the prevalence of PPS in 100 consecutive patients with pharmacoresistant partial epilepsy who underwent VEEG monitoring study, as part of a presurgical evaluation at the Rush Epilepsy Center (8). Every patient was asked to complete a 42-item questionnaire (The Rush Postictal Psychiatric Questionnaire) designed to identify 26 PPS and five cognitive symptoms. These included symptoms of depression and neurovegetative symptoms, symptoms of anxiety disorders (i.e., general anxiety, panic attacks, agoraphobia), obsessions and compulsions, and psychotic symptoms. All patients also underwent magnetic resonance imaging (MRI) of the brain using a protocol designed to do volumetric measurements of the hippocampal formation and a psychiatric evaluation to identify previous or concurrent *interictal* psychiatric disorders. Each question inquired about the frequency of occurrence of the symptom. Only symptoms that were identified after more than 50% of seizures were included in this study, so as to reflect an "habitual" phenomenon. For each symptom, we also inquired about its occurrence during the *interictal* period. For symptoms identified during both interictal and postictal periods, we only included symptoms reported to be *significantly more severe* during the postictal period. These were classified as *postictal exacerbation* of interictal psychiatric symptoms.

Among the 100 patients, 62 were women and 32 were men, with a mean age 34.1 ± 10 years and a mean seizure disorder duration of 21.1 ± 11.5 years. Seventy-nine patients had seizures of temporal lobe origin, and 21 patients had seizures of extratemporal origin. Half of the patients had only complex partial seizures (CPS), and the other half had CPS and secondarily generalized tonic-clonic seizures (GTC). Seventy-eight patients had more than one seizure, and 22 had less than one seizure per month. Fifty-two patients had a past psychiatric history, which consisted of depression, anxiety, and attention-deficit disorders.

Patients reported a median of 9.5 postictal symptoms (range 0 to 24), which included a median of 6.2 psychiatric symptoms (range 0 to 21), the majority of which were symptoms of depression (median 5; range 2 to 9), not including neurovegetative symptoms (median 1, range 0 to 1). Forty-three patients had postictal symptoms of depression, of whom 13 had a cluster of symptoms that mimicked a major depression (except for the shorter duration). Five additional patients experienced irritability and poor frustration tolerance without other dysphoric symptoms. Forty-two patients experienced symptoms of anxiety, nine had symptoms of obsessions and compulsions, eight patients had psychotic symptoms, and two patients experienced hypomanic symptoms. A postictal exacerbation of interictal symptoms was identified in 25 patients. The same observation applied to six of 42 patients with postictal symptoms of anxiety. Fourteen patients experienced only postictal cognitive symptoms, and eight patients did not experience any postictal symptoms. The median duration of psychiatric symptoms was 24 hours (range 1 to 148 hours). The frequency of each individual symptom and respective duration are listed in Table 11.1.

Psychiatric history (not necessarily of depression) and a seizure frequency of less than one per month were the variables that predicted postictal depression symptoms. Psychiatric history, seizure frequency less than one per month, and a long duration of seizure disorder were the variables that predicted postictal anxiety symptoms. A psychiatric

TABLE 11.1. *Frequency and median duration of postictal psychiatric symptoms in 100 patients with intractable partial epilepsy*

Symptom	Frequency (range)	Median duration (h)
Irritability	30	24 (0.5–108.0)
Poor frustration tolerance	36	24 (0.1–108.0)
Anhedonia	33	24 (0.1–148.0)
Hopelessness	25	24 (1.0–108.0)
Helplessness	31	24 (1.0–108.0)
Crying bouts	26	6 (0.1–108.0)
Suicide ideation	16	24 (1.0–240.0)
Active suicidal thoughts	11	—
Passive suicidal thoughts	16	—
Feelings of self-deprecation	27	24 (1.0–120.0)
Feelings of guilt	23	24 (0.1–240.0)
Early-night insomnia	11	—
Middle-night awakening	13	—
Early a.m. awakening	11	—
Excessive somnolence	43	24 (2.0–720.0)
Loss of appetite	36	24 (2.0–148.0)
Excessive appetite	10	15 (0.5–48.0)
Loss of sexual interest (not related to fatigue)	26	39 (6.0–148.0)
Constant worrying	33	24 (0.5–108.0)
Panicky feelings	10	6 (0.1–148.0)
Agoraphobic symptoms	31	24 (0.5–296.0)
Due to fear of seizure recurrence	20	—
Obsessions/compulsions	11	15 (0.1–72.0)
Self-consciousness	26	6 (0.05–108.0)
Psychotic symptoms	8	15 (0.1–108.0)
Excessive energy	9	2 (0.15–48.0)
Thought racing	15	2 (0.1–24.0)
Fatigue	56	24 (0.1–148.0)
Difficulty concentrating	71	6 (0.1–108.0)
Problems with memory	66	6 (0.1–108.0)
Confusion	65	2 (0.1–72.0)
Disorientation	46	1 (0.05–24.0)
Thought blockage	42	9 (0.1–98.0)
Only cognitive symptoms	14	—
No postictal symptoms	8	—

(nonpsychotic) history predicted the occurrence of postictal psychotic symptoms. The data from this study suggest that PPS can be a relatively frequent occurrence among patients with intractable partial epilepsy. These findings, however, cannot be generalized to all patients with epilepsy, as our sample was restricted to patients with partial refractory epilepsy. That a psychiatric history was a predictive variable for the occurrence of all types of PPS suggests that these PPS may reflect the equivalent of a Todd's paralysis phenomenon, in which the seizures unmask a latent or subclinical psychiatric processes. Unfortunately, a literature search failed to yield other studies on the prevalence of PPS.

Postictal Psychiatric Disorders

As previously mentioned, PPS may cluster and mimic discrete psychiatric disorders. The prevalence of postictal psychiatric disorders (PPD) in the general population of patients with epilepsy is yet to be established. The reported PPDs have focused almost exclusively on PIP identified in the course of VEEG. This is not surprising, because the circumstances around VEEG are optimal to facilitate the occurrence of PPD. These include the occurrence of frequent seizures over a short time period, following the discontinuation or dose reduction of antiepileptic drugs (AEDs). In a study published in

1996, we estimated the yearly incidence of PPD during VEEG to be 7.9% among patients with partial epilepsy (9). The majority, or 6.4%, presented as PIP.

Postictal Psychotic Disorders

In the study cited (9), we identified psychiatric symptomatology that mimicked a PIP in ten of 13 patients. It presented as a delusional psychosis in four patients; and it mimicked a mixed manic-depressive–like psychosis in one patient, a psychotic depression-like disorder in two, a hypomanic-like psychosis in one, and a manic-like psychosis in one. The tenth patient presented with bizarre behavior associated with a thought disorder. In every case, the onset of symptoms lagged by a mean period of 24 hours (range 12 to 72 hours) relative to the time of the last seizure. The mean duration of the PIP was 69.6 hours (range 24 to 144 hours). The psychotic episode remitted with low doses of neuroleptic medication (2 to 5 mg per day of haloperidol) in five patients; one patient required high doses (40 mg per day of haloperidol); and remission occurred without pharmacotherapy in four patients. Six of these ten patients had experienced an average of 2.4 PIP prior to VEEG; in the remaining four patients, the PIP was the first one ever experienced. Other authors have reported similar findings with respect to clinical characteristics, course, and response to pharmacotherapy (10–15). Kanemoto et al. (16) studied the clinical differences between PIP and acute and chronic interictal psychosis of epilepsy. They noted that patients with PIP are more likely to experience grandiose and religious delusions in the presence of elevated moods and a feeling of mystic fusion of the body with the universe. On the other hand, perceptual delusions or voices commenting were less frequent, and feelings of impending death were common among patients with PIP.

The different case series (9–16) reported the following characteristics of PIP. (i) Delay between the onset of psychiatric symptoms and the time of the last seizure. (ii) Relatively short duration. A shorter duration was noted among our patients, as only two patients had an episode lasting more than 5 days. This was true in five of nine patients in the series of Savard et al. (11) and in seven of 14 patients in the series of Logsdail and Toone (10). (iii) Affect-laden symptomatology. (iv) Clustering of symptoms into delusional and affective-like psychosis. (v) Increase in the frequency of secondarily generalized tonic-clonic seizures preceding the onset of PIP. (vi) Onset of PIP after having seizures for a mean period of more than 10 years.

Clinical phenomena during PIP have included cases of manic symptoms following CPS (17). Directed aggression has been reported to occur significantly more frequently during PIP than during interictal psychosis or during the postictal confusional state of CPS (18). PIP also has been reported with unusual presentations, including cases of Capgras' syndrome (19,20) and a case mimicking a Kluver-Bucey syndrome reported in a patient with persistent seizures following a left temporal lobectomy (21).

Various investigators have attempted to identify potential pathogenic mechanisms of PIP. In a study conducted at the Rush Epilepsy Center, we compared the neuropsychometric studies, brain MRI, and interictal and ictal data derived from VEEG and past psychiatric history from 17 patients with PIP, 20 patients with postictal depressive disorder (PID) and 20 controls (22; Kanner et al., *submitted*). A logistic regression model clearly demonstrated that bilateral independent *ictal* foci were strong predictors of PIP. By the same token, the presence of PIP predicted bilateral ictal foci with a probability of 89%. Umbricht et al. (14) reported similar findings in a study comparing eight patients with PIP, seven patients with interictal psychosis, and 29 controls. In addition, they found that patients with PIP and interictal psychosis had a lower verbal IQ and the absence of mesial temporal sclerosis. Devinsky et al. (13) reported a higher frequency of bilateral independent interictal foci in 20 patients with PIP compared to 150 controls.

Postictal Depression

PID is another expression of PPD. In contrast to PIP, PID remains practically unexplored. In the study of prevalence of postictal symptoms carried out at the Rush Epilepsy Center (8), 13 of 100 patients experienced a cluster of symptoms of depression that mimicked a major depression disorder with a duration exceeding 24 hours but significantly shorter than the 2 weeks required by the *Diagnostic and Statistical Manual of Mental Disorders,* Fourth Edition (DSM-IV) criteria (23). In a separate study carried out at the same center and cited earlier (22; Kanner et al., *submitted*), we identified 20 patients with PID lasting more than 24 hours and mimicking major depression.

Pathogenic mechanisms of PID also have been studied in a limited manner. In the study comparing 17 patients with PIP, 20 controls, and 20 patients with PID cited earlier, there were no differences in interictal and ictal data, MRI, and neuropsychometric testing with controls (22; Kanner et al., *submitted*). However, patients with PID were more likely to have a psychiatric history than controls.

Experimental Perspective of Postictal Psychiatric Symptoms

In a search for neurobiologic evidence of behavioral disturbances in animal models of epilepsy, Engel et al. (24) focused on the behavioral changes noted during the postictal period, specifically, on postictal aggression that presents as reactive biting in amygdaloid-kindled seizures in rats. Caldecott-Hazard et al. (25,26) identified the role of opioid involvement in postictal explosive motor behavior, noting that pretreatment with naloxone can exacerbate it, whereas pretreatment with morphine can suppress it. Engel et al. suggested that this hyperreactivity could reflect

endogenous opioid withdrawal phenomena. Indeed, endogenous opioids usually are released during seizures; therefore, the animal is exposed repeatedly to transient increments, creating a state of dependency.

Engel et al. (24) suggested that this model may reflect the pathogenic mechanisms mediating *interictal* depression, as endogenous opioids also may play the role of natural mood elevators and have been thought to mediate, at least in part, the therapeutic effects of electroconvulsive therapy (27,28). They support this hypothesis with data from positron emission tomographic studies that used the mu opioid receptor ligand [^{11}C] carfentanil. These studies revealed that temporal lobe hypometabolism is associated with enhanced opioid receptor binding (29,30). In support of a pathogenic role of endogenous opioids in *postictal affective disturbances,* Engel et al. cite the transient suppression of the multiple-squeak response in the rat, the duration of which can be shortened by pretreatment with naloxone. This reaction to pain has been considered to reflect a measure of affective function (31). Whether these theories are applicable to the occurrence of postictal depressive episodes in humans is yet to be established. In our opinion, however, such mechanisms could be responsible, at least in part, for the occurrence of *postictal* symptoms of depression in vulnerable patients (i.e., patients at risk of depressive disorders) in whom the biochemical transient changes can bring to the surface a latent process. This hypothesis may, in fact, be supported by our data suggesting that PPS may be the expression of a Todd's paralysis of a latent psychiatric disorder (see above).

Engel et al. (24) also reviewed the potential role of dopamine changes in mediating psychotic processes in epilepsy. They point out how amygdaloid kindling in cats can induce enhanced sensitivity of dopamine receptors (24). Because psychotic symptoms are dopamine mediated, postictal and interictal psychotic processes conceivably could result from such changes.

PARAICTAL PSYCHIATRIC DISORDERS

As mentioned earlier, psychiatric and cognitive phenomena resulting from a paraictal process include phenomena with a beginning and ending that approximate those of epileptic disorders. The psychiatric symptoms and cognitive deficits are quasicontinuous interictally with a waxing and waning course, with periictal exacerbations. As shown later, the severity of the actual seizures may range from very rare to intractable clinical seizures, but the electroencephalographic (EEG) recordings show abundant epileptiform activity.

The underlying pathogenic mechanisms are obviously suspected to be closely tied to the epileptic activity and its impact on brain structures that mediate specific cognitive, affective, and behavioral functions. To date, however, the responsible mechanisms have yet to be established. Some of the possible culprits include (i) the impact of interictal spikes on cognitive functions and (ii) neuronal changes triggered by continuous interictal bombardment, among others.

The impact of interictal epileptiform activity was studied extensively by Binnie et al. (32,33). Although it is still the source of much debate, there appears to be agreement that generalized and focal discharges often can be associated with disturbed cognition. Schwab (34) in 1939 was the first to demonstrate an absent or delayed response during a generalized epileptiform discharge using a simple reaction task test. Aarts et al. (35) coined the term "transient cognitive impairment" to reflect this phenomenon. Binnie et al. (33) demonstrated transient cognitive impairment in 50% of 91 patients during generalized or focal discharges. Right-sided discharges were associated with impairment in visual spatial tasks, whereas errors in verbal tasks were demonstrated during left-sided discharges. The authors observed that the error rates increased if the stimulus was presented in the midst of the discharge. If the epileptiform discharge occurred within 2 seconds before the stimulus, the degree of disruption was greater. Kasteleijn-Nolst Trenite et al. (36) reported similar findings with respect to the type of deficit in relation to side of discharge in 36% of a group of 69 children. The relationship between epileptiform discharge occurrence and cognitive functions is complex, as increased concentration on a task can result in a decrease in the rate of epileptiform discharges (37).

With respect to the second potential mechanism, Grigonis and Murphy (38) demonstrated disruption in the formation of normal synaptic connections by focal epileptic discharges in the brain of young animals. Much research still is necessary to begin understanding these complex issues.

In the next section we illustrate two examples of paraictal cognitive and psychiatric disorders. The first, acquired epileptic aphasia of childhood (or LKS), has gained much interest among epileptologists, pediatric neurologists, and child psychiatrists, despite its rare occurrence. This surge in interest resulted from attempts to relate LKS with one of the forms of the autistic spectrum disorder, mainly autistic regression (AR). The implications of this phenomenon will be discussed in some detail.

Acquired Epileptic Aphasia of Childhood

Acquired epileptic aphasia of childhood (or LKS) is an acquired epileptic aphasia or verbal auditory agnosia occurring in children who have already developed age-appropriate language function. It is thought to result from an epileptogenic lesion arising in the speech cortex during a critical period of development. It was first described in 1957 by Landau and Kleffner (1) in a report of six patients. In 1985, LKS was included in the International Classification of Epileptic Syndromes, giving it legitimacy as a recognized clinical entity.

LKS has a clearly defined set of clinical and electrographic characteristics. These include a receptive speech disturbance or verbal auditory agnosia (39), followed soon after by disturbances of expressive speech, which can evolve to a state of complete mutism. The onset of speech disturbance coincides with that of seizure activity (see below).

The symptoms of LKS appear between the ages of 2 and 8 years, characteristically with an acute or subacute presentation, although in some children the onset can have a stuttering course (40,41). The initial linguistic disturbances include problems with verbal comprehension (verbal auditory agnosia) that often can be mistaken for acquired deafness (42). Soon after, speech output is affected and paraphasias as well as phonologic errors appear. Symptoms may progress in a steady or fluctuating manner to a state of complete mutism, during which the child will fail to respond even to familiar nonverbal sounds, such as the ring of the door bell or the telephone, or the dog barking. The speech disturbances are associated with behavioral changes, which may include motor hyperactivity in up to 50% of children (40,41) and sleep disturbances. At the height of the auditory agnosia, some autistic-like features, such as self-stimulatory behavior, may be identified. However, the child with LKS never loses the ability to relate with family members and understand social cues. The onset of the language disorder is concurrent with that of seizures and/or electrographic evidence of epileptiform activity presenting characteristically, but not exclusively, as spike-wave discharges with a bilateral distribution, maximal in the posterior temporal regions of each hemisphere. This EEG pattern may occupy >80% of slow wave sleep, and it is known as continuous spike and slow wave of sleep (CSWS) (40). From 20% to 30% of children will never exhibit any evidence of clinical seizures (40). Seizures often are nocturnal; their clinical phenomena vary widely and often are very subtle. In our experience, seizures are identified for the first time in the course of prolonged VEEG monitoring study

in some patients. The clinical phenomena include brief clonic deviation of the eyes, at times associated with eye blinking, head dropping, and minor automatisms with occasional secondary generalization (43). Seizures, unlike the language disorder, respond readily to AED therapy (40,41) and generally subside by the age of 15 years (44). Another important diagnostic criterion of LKS is the relative isolation of the behavioral deficit to the linguistic and auditory perceptual spheres, that is, children show relatively normal performance on nonverbal cognitive tasks (43).

In some cases, spontaneous remission may occur weeks or months after onset (42). Mantovani and Landau (45) reported a considerable degree of recovery in four of nine patients reevaluated 10 to 28 years after the onset of their symptoms. Deonna et al. (46) followed seven patients diagnosed with LKS into their young adult years. Only one patient recovered completely; a second patient had normal language but was severely dyslexic; a third patient had only recovered comprehension; and the other four patients showed lack of comprehension and continued displaying severe expressive language problems. Review of the available data suggests that when symptoms persist unchanged for more than 1 year, spontaneous recovery is rare, and a severe lifelong linguistic handicap is the common result (41, 42,47–51).

Figure 11.1 illustrates the classic EEG tracing of CSWS recorded from a child with LKS. Despite the bilateral distribution of this epileptiform activity, a unilateral source can be identified in many of these children by using the methohexital suppression test (43) or with magnetoencephalography (MEG) (52). A rather consistent distribution of spikes can be identified with referential montages and field potential mapping, consisting of a frontal negativity and a temporal positivity (53) and reflects a generator source represented by a tangential dipole in the inferior bank of the sylvian fissure (on the superior

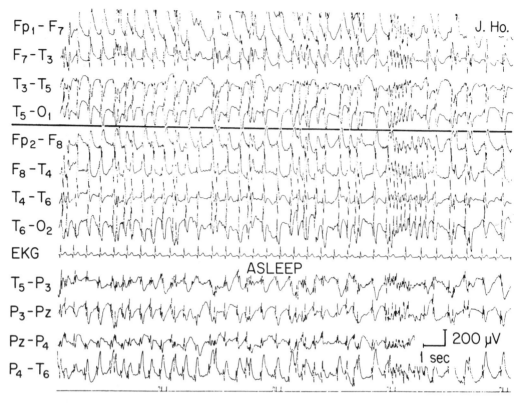

FIG. 11.1. Electrographic pattern of continuous spike and slow wave of sleep in a child with Landau-Kleffner syndrome prior to surgical treatment with multiple subpial transection.

surface of the temporal lobe). We refer to this pattern as the sylvian dipole. The presence of this sylvian dipole also has been demonstrated with MEG (52).

Several authors have suggested a possible relationship between the severity of linguistic deficits, behavioral abnormalities, and EEG abnormalities. This relationship is supported by the significant improvement in both domains with the normalization of EEG recordings during drug trials with steroids and by the recurrence of symptoms and epileptiform discharges on EEG following their discontinuation (54–58).

As stated earlier, LKS can remit spontaneously in a number of children. In those with persistent symptoms, pharmacologic treatment with AED has failed to yield encouraging results. Certain AEDs, such as carbamazepine, can worsen the severity of lan-

guage dysfunction and behavior. Valproic acid and clonazepam are the two AEDs most widely used in LKS, but their efficacy is limited at best when symptoms have taken a chronic course. Steroids can yield a significant improvement of language deficits, together with eradication of the epileptic pattern of CSWS in about 50% of children. It should be noted, however, that in other children, such eradication of epileptic activity fails to exert any impact on language deficits or behavioral problems. The lack of a consistent relationship between eradication of spikes and symptom remission in some of these children is puzzling and is yet to be understood. The acute and long-term side effects of steroids limit the duration of therapy.

Morrell et al. (43) suggested a surgical treatment for LKS with the use of multiple subpial transection (MST) and, in 1995, reported their results of the first 14 children treated surgically with this technique. This surgical technique was developed with the aim of eliminating epileptic activity from eloquent cortex without interfering with function (59). The technique interrupts intracortical horizontal fibers that are necessary for generation of epileptic discharges (60–63), while preserving the vertical columnar organization of the cortex, the basic functional unit of cortical physiology (64–66).

The 14 children who went on to have surgery were derived from a pool of 37 children with a CSWS pattern. At present, we require that children considered for surgery meet the following criteria. (i) Acute (or sometimes stuttering) onset of aphasia and auditory agnosia in an otherwise normal child who has already developed age-appropriate language. (ii) Failure to show any signs of improvement of linguistic functions for 2 years. (iii) Severe, clearly epileptiform, EEG abnormality characterized by bilateral spike-wave discharge in slow wave sleep. (iv) Electrophysiologic evidence of a unilateral origin of the bilateral epileptiform discharge. (v) Presence of clinical seizures was not mandatory. (vi) Neuropsychological test findings indicating relative preservation of nonverbal cognitive capacities in the presence of devastating loss of verbal skills. These inclusion criteria were rigorously met by 12 of the 14 patients who underwent MST. The two remaining cases differed from the other 12 children in that the methohexital suppression test revealed bilateral independent foci and their neuropsychological data indicated more widespread dysfunction than could be accounted for by loss of linguistic capacity alone. Surgery was performed on the side where preponderance of epileptic activity was identified.

Among these 14 children, ten were female; a left hemisphere focus was identified in ten patients. The mean age of onset of aphasic symptoms was 3.9 years (range 3 to 6.5 years); the mean age at surgery was 7 years (range 5 to 13 years). All but two children had clinical seizures that began contemporane-

ously with, or prior to, the onset of aphasia. The two children who never had clinical seizures nevertheless had the typical electrographic pattern of CSWS. The CSWS pattern was present in all but one patient; that patient had recurrent spike and wave activity in the right centrotemporal regions.

At the time of surgery, none of the 14 patients had been able to engage in useful linguistic communication for at least 2 years. After a mean follow-up period of 44 months (range 13 to 78 months), seven patients (50%) had recovered age-appropriate language, were taking regular classes, and no longer required speech therapy. Four patients (29%) displayed a marked improvement, as they could express themselves and understand verbal instructions, but they still were in need of speech therapy. Two patients failed to display any improvement, and one patient improved for 6 months and then declined.

A gradual recovery process of language function was observed in every one of these eleven patients. Every child received speech therapy after surgery. Most children were uttering the first words by 12 weeks after surgery, and substantial improvement was reported by 6 months. A steadily accelerating improvement continued to be reported in six children; in the remaining five, progress followed a slower pace. Interestingly enough, sign language returned before verbal skills in those children who had learned sign language before the complete loss of linguistic ability.

Nine of the 12 patients with clinical seizures became seizure-free; three continued to have seizures. Two patients had only a CSWS EEG pattern but no clinical seizures prior to surgery. Nine patients (64%) had normal EEG recordings (Fig. 11.2). In five children (36%), recurrent epileptiform activity was identified. The three patients who failed to sustain any change in language function continued to have clinical seizures and to display abnormal EEG recordings. The other two patients with persistent epileptic activity on EEG (but no clinical seizures) had the least improvement among the four patients in the "Marked Improvement" category. Of the remaining nine patients with

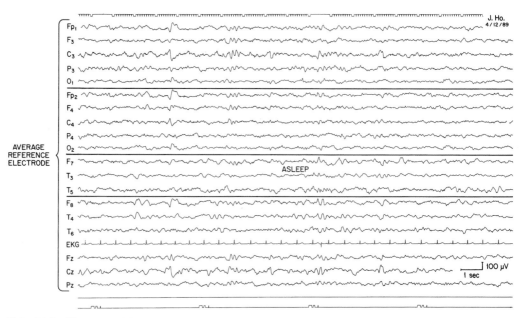

FIG. 11.2. Electrographic recordings during sleep of a child with Landau-Kleffner syndrome after surgical treatment with multiple subpial transection. Presurgical recordings of continuous spike and slow wave of sleep are shown in Fig. 11.1.

normal postsurgical EEG recordings, seven were classified in the "Normal Speech" and two in the "Marked Improvement" categories. These findings further support a relationship between disturbances of linguistic ability and epileptic activity.

Morrell et al. (67) believed that timing of the surgery is an important parameter in the outcome of this surgical intervention. They explained that different neural systems have critical periods in development during which the adult patterns of synaptic engagement are gradually established. At such times, there is first a superabundant outgrowth of axon terminals resulting in hyperinnervation of the synaptic target. This excessive outgrowth appears to be entirely under genetic control. Over the remainder of the critical period, the synaptic contacts are pruned extensively. Environmental inputs influence synaptic use, which, in turn, modulates the process of synaptic pruning. Synaptic contacts activated by use become cemented, whereas those that are not environmentally engaged whither away (68–73). Neural networks for linguistic

functions develop late, and their neural circuitry remains malleable during the first 8 to 10 years of life (74–77). Morrell et al. (67) hypothesized, then, that the impact of epileptic activity originating from this anlage of speech cortex may result in chaotic and behaviorally meaningless activation of synaptic contacts, which would have been "pruned" under normal circumstances and, in this manner, set up permanent inappropriate and nonfunctional linkages. If these epileptic discharges persist beyond the critical period for this particular system, then irreversible damage will have been caused to the circuit and normal speech will not develop. If, on the other hand, these epileptic discharges are eliminated during that period when the system still is malleable, there might be a chance that enough normal connections would be established to mediate reasonable linguistic behavior. Therefore, the impact of an epileptic lesion is more deleterious during synaptogenesis than when it arises in a mature and completely developed normal circuit. This explains why resolution of the epileptic activity in the middle teens is not associated with a recovery of speech, by which time the critical period for the development of the speech circuit is complete. Morrell et al. (67) concluded that a timely elimination of epileptic activity with MST is a permissive intervention that simply allows the normal process of selective synaptic pruning to take place.

Landau-Kleffner Syndrome and Autistic Regression: A Variation on the Theme?

As one of several syndromes with a CSWS pattern, LKS and the syndrome of continuous spike and wave of sleep, also known as electrical status epilepticus during sleep (ESES) (78), often are confused with each other. Additional diagnostic confusion has been compounded in recent years by a *"dilution"* of the original diagnostic criteria of LKS. A diagnosis of LKS often is made in children with failure to speak who have *any kind* of epileptiform activity on EEG (i.e., autistic children or children with developmental delay), or in children with a CSWS EEG pattern, irrespective of the clinical picture. This has been the source of ample debate, specifically as it pertains to children with AR. The diagnostic confusion between AR and LKS stems from the fact that some of these children may have seizures and by the parental reports of regression in language, sociability, and play, following "apparent" normal development (79). It has been suggested (without any scientific basis) that AR may be a variant of LKS; such a hypothesis was buttressed by the hope that the same treatment modalities that mediated the reversal of loss of language functions in LKS could yield the same therapeutic effects in children with AR. The focus of these children's diagnostic evaluation was suddenly shifted to the epileptic domain. Children with AR are being evaluated with VEEG monitoring studies to "rule out" LKS and to determine if they can be candidates for epilepsy surgery or corticosteroid therapy.

Careful analysis can demonstrate clear differences between LKS on the one hand and ESES and AR on the other. Children with AR

and ESES have more serious cognitive disturbances than those with LKS. For one, cognitive deficits are not only restricted to verbally mediated functions but show a multisystem decline that results in severe retardation and, in children with ESES, may reach a quasidementia (78), often with psychotic features, hyperactivity, and aggressive behavior. In ESES, clinical seizures may occur in sleep only, or in both the awake state as well as in sleep, and include absence seizures and drop attacks resulting from myoclonic and atonic seizures. Partial and generalized tonic-clonic seizures also can occur (78).

In children with AR, regression of cognitive functions occurs at an early age, often when the child has only acquired a few words in his or her vocabulary (79). The onset often is insidious. Rapin (79) questioned the "normal" development of cognitive milestones preceding the regressive process and pointed out the possibility that these children's cognitive delays may have gone unrecognized, becoming more obvious at the time of their regression.

As already stated, the onset of language disturbance in children with LKS parallels that of clinical seizures and/or electrographic evidence of epileptiform activity. On the other hand, there appears to be no association between the reported regression in AR and the presence of epileptic activity on EEG or seizure occurrence. Rapin (79) found that only 19% of children with AR had epilepsy and 25% had abnormal EEG. Kurita et al. (80) found no difference in the prevalence of paroxysmal EEG between children with autistic spectrum disorder with and without regression.

As mentioned earlier, the EEG pattern of CSWS is common to children with LKS and to those with ESES, but not so in AR. Guillioto and Morrell (81) carried out a retrospective analysis of 19 cases referred with a presumptive diagnosis of LKS and with the EEG pattern of CSWS, to determine whether detailed examination would reveal subtle electrophysiologic differences between children with "true" LKS and children with AR. Cases were divided into two groups on the basis of neuropsychological criteria. Group 1 (eight patients) exhibited a diffuse cognitive impairment that included both linguistic and nonlinguistic capacities. Group 2 (eleven patients) had a relatively isolated impairment of language function with sparing of other cognitive capacities. The latter group represented the "pure" LKS cases. Mapping of the distribution of electrical abnormality revealed that six of eight patients in group 1 had widespread, multifocal discharge. One of eight had bilateral high parietal disturbance, and one of eight had a primarily left-sided abnormality that became bilateral and multifocal during slow wave sleep. All of the eleven patients in group 2 showed discharges limited to the parietotemporal region of both hemispheres. Moreover, these discharges revealed the characteristic sylvian dipole. These observations were reproduced in a larger study by Lewine et al. (52), who used MEG in children with LKS and AR. All patients with LKS had a unilateral intrasylvian dipole while children with AR with epileptiform activity showed multiple generator sites and inconsistent orientation of spike dipoles. Thus, these data demonstrate that LKS and AR are clinically and electrographically different disorders. In children with LKS, there is concordance among clinical characteristics, neuropsychological deficits, and epileptic profile, all of which point to a dysfunction of language cortex. In contrast, children with a clinical diagnosis of AR have diffuse cognitive deficits and multifocal epileptogenic sources.

Of great concern is the ongoing use of therapies with significant potential morbidity (i.e., surgery and corticosteroids) in children with AR. Do we have the scientific data to support the prescription of such treatments in these children?

In children with AR, there currently are no published data with objective and valid outcome measures to suggest the efficacy of AED, corticosteroids, or surgery. A recent report by Nass et al. (82) supports these views. These authors treated seven children with AR with MST and observed only "temporary"

improvement during the postsurgical evaluation. These results are not surprising, given the experience of Morrell et al. (43) with MST in their LKS series: the children who failed to derive any benefit had diffuse cognitive deficits and more than one epileptic source. In their analysis of surgical failures, Morrell et al. (43) recognized that these children would not be considered for surgery today (and, in retrospect, that they probably did not meet criteria of LKS). Accordingly, we do not believe that surgery has a role in the treatment of children with AR.

Whereas LKS is associated with behavioral and cognitive changes that may parallel the presence of epileptic activity, the same conclusion cannot be reached in the case of AR. The role of epileptic activity in the pathogenesis of AR remains to be established. Until this relationship is clarified, we should avoid using treatment modalities with potential morbidity in children with AR.

SEIZURE DISORDER ASSOCIATED WITH HYPOTHALAMIC HAMARTOMA

Hypothalamic hamartoma and gelastic epilepsy (HHGE) is a congenital developmental epileptic syndrome occurring from early birth, often associated with precocious puberty and characterized by a poor response to AED treatment (2,83,84). This syndrome is thought to be a *subcortical epilepsy* and often is associated with behavioral changes and cognitive decline.

Patients with HHGE present with a number of symptoms, with epilepsy being the most prominent at first. There is a spectrum of seizures in patients with HHGE (85). Some patients may only have simple partial events, whereas others may have severe secondary generalized epileptic seizures such as drop attacks or tonic events (86). The seizures often begin in the newborn period, although many parents do not recognize these events early in the child's life. In most patients, gelastic events often are the only seizure manifestation during the first 5 to 10 years of life. However, most patients develop other seizure types before puberty. These consist of CPS, motor events, and at times secondary generalized GTC or drop attacks. The frequency of the gelastic seizures is astonishing; some patients may have up to 100 attacks per day. The frequency of other seizures is variable, but often they occur weekly.

The initial clinical epileptic syndrome is not a reliable indicator for ultimate prognosis. Although most patients present early on with gelastic events, some of them will continue having only gelastic seizures, whereas others will develop other seizure types as described earlier. However, the development of CPS or drop attacks often indicates an ominous sign, with changing seizure patterns and medical intractability.

Precocious puberty is seen in over half the patients with intractable epilepsy and gelastic seizures due to hypothalamic hamartoma (84,87). Precocious puberty often develops in those affected by age 7 years. Most often, significant signs of puberty are seen before the age of 2 years. Indeed, parents can often recognize the larger size of affected children (relative to their chronological age) during the first 2 years of age. These observations are made even before any signs of precocious puberty are apparent.

The behavioral and cognitive changes reported in these patients are quite variable. In most patients, behavioral difficulties are characterized by aggressive behavior, uninhibited tendencies, attention deficit with hyperactivity, and irritability. Up to 30% of patients may have autistic features. In those patients who appear to have normal cognition, insidious changes often develop before puberty (2). The association between seizures and behavioral changes is not clear; the number of seizures in this syndrome often is difficult to estimate. However, depth EEG recordings from the hamartoma often demonstrate almost continuous discharges with or without secondary spread. It is possible that this almost continuous epileptic activity causes considerable diffuse dysfunction. However, the factors determining the marked behavioral and cognitive

degeneration have not been established. We have been impressed by the fact that many patients who have frequent gelastic seizures do not deteriorate, whereas others with other types of epileptic seizures have worse outcome. For parents, the behavioral and cognitive problems often are more important than the seizures.

Results of electrophysiologic investigations often are either normal or unrevealing during the first few years of life. Patients may present with focal epileptogenic discharges, but most often multifocal epileptogenic abnormalities are recorded. With evolution, however, the EEG abnormalities have a tendency to evolve into two different patterns. The first is localized multifocal or focal epileptogenic discharges, often in the frontal or temporal lobes. The second consists of generalized spike and wave discharges. Clinical correlation suggests that patients with the second type of EEG pattern often have drop attacks or generalized tonic-clonic seizures.

Until 1995 to 1996, it was thought that patients with HHGE had seizures localized to the frontal or temporal regions. It was the failure of temporal or frontal lobectomy that gave impetus to investigate the possible origin of seizures in the syndrome. Two observations, one by the late Claudio Munari et al. (83) and the other by Kuzniecky et al. (2), suggested that the gelastic seizures in these patients originated from the hypothalamic hamartoma. Clinical observations suggest that the location of hamartoma is intimately related to the generation of gelastic attacks. Although ictal laugh has been reported in patients with temporal and extratemporal lobe epilepsy, it is rare. Munari's group reported on the ictal depth EEG recordings arising from a hypothalamic hamartoma in one patient with the syndrome (83,88). This was confirmed by Kuzniecky et al. (2) and has now been observed in over a dozen patients investigated at the University of Alabama at Birmingham Epilepsy Program. Another piece of evidence is the data from electrical stimulation studies using depth electrodes that have reproduced the gelastic events. Finally, indirect evidence for activation of hypothalamic hamartoma during seizures is suggested by the findings of ictal single photon emission computed tomographic activation during the gelastic attacks.

Even though recent data suggest that the source of seizures in these patients is the hypothalamic mass, the intrinsic mechanism of epileptogenesis in these patients is not clear. It is possible simply that the presence of a large mass of dysplastic neurons in the hamartoma gives rise to seizures. However, not all hamartomas in this area cause epilepsy. Clinical and experimental evidence suggests that the mamillary bodies and adjacent structures may be important subcortical pathways for seizure generation and propagation (89). It is known that sessile hamartomas attached to the mamillary bodies with displacement all the surrounding structures often are associated with seizures and behavioral disturbances. Alternatively, other mechanisms involving neuropeptide secretion or major displacement of the hypothalamus may be responsible for seizures in this syndrome (84).

Since the recognition that hamartomas are responsible for seizures and other symptoms, a number of surgical strategies have been revived. Three approaches have been utilized with relatively good results. The first one, proposed by Kuzniecky et al. (2), uses stereotactic radiofrequency lesion of the hamartoma. To date, this has been performed in eight patients with relatively no morbidity and good results in most patients. The second approach is removal of lesions using a ventricular endoscopic technique; this approach has been associated with good results and low morbidity. In the third approach, Regis et al. *(personal communication)* have utilized a gamma knife with good initial results. It is too early to say which technique will be most appropriate for these patients, but it is clear that it no longer is acceptable to be passive about the treatment of these children.

Our experience suggests that successful lesioning or removal of the hamartoma leads to major improvements in cognitive performance and behavior. Most astonishing is the rapid cognitive and behavioral changes observed in these patients. This is not totally surprising in view of the almost continuous interictal and ictal epileptogenic abnormalities. The abolition of this deleterious ictal and interictal activity produces significant improvements in behavior and cognition. These findings support early surgical intervention in HHGE.

CONCLUDING REMARKS

In this chapter, we reviewed two clinical expressions of psychopathology in epilepsy that remain poorly understood. In the case of individual PPS, or of clusters of symptoms mimicking psychiatric disorders, our studies suggest that they may be relatively frequent among patients with poorly controlled partial seizure disorders. The presence of postictal psychiatric phenomena carries practical clinical implications: the suggestion of underlying silent psychopathology is to be considered carefully. In case of postictal psychotic disorders, the presence of bilateral independent ictal foci needs to be carefully investigated. More in-depth research into postictal psychiatric phenomena may shed light on potential pathogenic processes of psychiatric disorders.

Psychopathology as an expression of paraictal disorders is undoubtedly one of the more intriguing and fascinating areas of psychopathology of epilepsy that promises to yield explanations of potential pathogenic mechanisms of psychopathology of epilepsy. LKS is a disorder in which the temporal relationship between seizure and cognitive/psychiatric disorders often can be established, especially in cases with spontaneous remission and in about half of patients successfully treated with steroid therapy and surgery. Failure to see an improvement in cognitive and psychiatric domains despite cessation of the epileptic activity remains an unanswered question but may result from structural changes at the synaptic and cellular levels in the absence of timely interventions. In the case of HHGE, the close relationship between psychiatric and seizure disorder became apparent following the successful treatments of the seizure disorder that were associated with dramatic improvement in psychopathology. It is clear that we have just begun to understand some of the very complex questions of these disorders. It is, however, the very beginning of the long road in our quest for answers!

REFERENCES

1. Landau WM, Kleffner F. Syndrome of acquired aphasia with convulsive disorder in children. *Neurology* 1957;7: 523–530.
2. Kuzniecky R, Guthrie B, Mountz J, et al. Intrinsic epileptogenesis of hypothalamic hamartoma and gelastic epilepsy. *Ann Neurol* 1997;44:60–67.
3. Gowers WR. *Epilepsy and other chronic and convulsive diseases.* London: JA Churchill, 1881.
4. Hughlings Jackson J. In: Taylor J, Holmes G, Walshe FMR, eds. *Selected writings of John Hughlings Jackson.* London: Hodder and Stoughton, 1931:119–134.
5. Kraepelin E. *Psychiatrie. 7. Auflage.* Liepzig: JA Barth, 1903.
6. Blanchet P, Frommer GP. Mood change preceding epileptic seizures. *J Nerv Ment Dis* 1986;174:471–476.
7. Williams D. The structure of emotions reflected in epileptic experiences. *Brain* 1956;79:29–67.
8. Kanner AM, Soto A, Gross-Kanner HR. There is more to epilepsy than seizures: a reassessment of the postictal period. *Neurology* 2000;54[Suppl 3]:352A.
9. Kanner AM, Stagno S, Kotagal P, et al. Postictal psychiatric events during prolonged video-electroencephalographic monitoring studies. *Arch Neurol* 1996; 53:258–263.
10. Logsdail SJ, Toone BK. Postictal psychosis. A clinical and phenomenological description. *Br J Psychiatry* 1988;152:246–252.
11. Savard G, Andermann F, Olivier A, et al. Postictal psychosis after complex partial seizures: a multiple case study. *Epilepsia* 1991;32:225–231.
12. Lancman ME, Craven WJ, Asconape JJ, et al. Clinical management of recurrent postictal psychosis. *J Epilepsy* 1994;7:47–51.
13. Devinsky O, Abrahmson H, Alper K, et al. Postictal psychosis: a case control study of 20 patients and 150 controls. *Epilepsy Res* 1995;20:247–253.
14. Umbricht D, Degreef G, Barr WB, et al. Postictal and chronic psychosis in patients with temporal lobe epilepsy. *Am J Psychiatry* 1995;152:224–231.
15. Szabo CA, Lancman M, Stagno S. Postictal psychosis: a review. *Neuropsychiatry Neurosurg Behav Neurol* 1996;9:258–264.
16. Kanemoto K, Kawasaki J, Kawai J. Postictal psychosis: a comparison with acute interictal and chronic psychoses. *Epilepsia* 1996;37:551–556.
17. Barczak P, Edmunds E, Bettes T. Hypomania following complex partial seizures. A report of three cases. *Br J Psychiatry* 1988;152:137–139.
18. Steinert T, Froscher W. Differential diagnosis of aggressive behavior in epilepsy. *Psychiatr Prax* 1995;22:15–18.
19. Drake ME. Postictal Capgras syndrome. *Clin Neurol Neurosurg* 1987;89:271–274.
20. Kim E. A postictal variant of Capgras' syndrome in a patient with a frontal meningioma. A case report. *Psychosomatics* 1991;32:448–451.
21. Anson JA, Kuhlman DT. Postictal Kluver-Bucy syndrome after temporal lobectomy. *J Neurol Neurosurg Psychiatry* 1993;56:311–313.
22. Kanner AM, Soto A. Ictal recordings in postictal psychosis and postictal depression. *Neurology* 1998;50 [Suppl 50]:A397.
23. American Psychiatric Association. *Diagnostic and statistical manual of mental disorders,* 4th ed. Washington, DC: American Psychiatric Press, 1994.
24. Engel J Jr, Bandler R, Griffith NC, et al. Neurobiological evidence for epilepsy induced interictal disturbances. *Adv Neurol* 1991;55:97–111.
25. Caldecott-Hazard S, Ackermann RF, Engel J Jr. Opioid involvement in postictal and interictal changes in behavior. In: Fariello RG, Morselli PL, Lloyd K, et al., eds. *Neurotransmitters, seizures and epilepsy II.* New York: Raven Press 1984:305–314.
26. Caldecott-Hazard S, Engel J Jr. Limbic postictal events: anatomical substrates and opioid receptor involvement. *Prog Neuropsychopharmacol Biol Psychiatry* 1987;11: 389–418.
27. Holladay JW, Tortella FC, Long JB, et al. Endogenous opioids and their receptors: evidence for the involvement in the postictal effects of electroconvulsive shock. *Ann N Y Acad Sci* 1986;462:124–139.
28. Tortella FC, Long JB. Characterization of opioid peptide-like anticonvulsant activity in rat cerebrospinal fluid. *Brain Res* 1988;426:139–146.
29. Frost JJ, Mayberg HS, Fisher RS, et al. Mu-opiate receptors measured by positron emission tomography are increased in temporal lobe epilepsy. *Ann Neurol* 1988; 23:231–237.
30. Hitzemann JR, Hitzemann BA, Blatt S, et al. Repeated electroconvulsive shock: effect on sodium dependency and regional distribution of opioid-binding sites. *Mol Pharmacol* 1987;31:562–566.
31. Carroll MN, Lim RKS. Observations on the neuropharmacology of morphine and morphine-like analgesia. *Arch Int Pharmacodyn* 1960;75:383–403.
32. Binnie CD, Channon S, Marston DL. Behavioral correlates of interictal spikes. *Adv Neurol* 1991;55:113–126.
33. Binnie CD, Kasteleijn-Nolst Trenite DGA, Smit AM, et al. Interactions of epileptiform EEG discharges and cognition. *Epilepsy Res* 1987;1:239–245.
34. Schwab RS. A method of measuring consciousness in petit mal epilepsy. *J Nerv Ment Dis* 1939;98:690–691.
35. Aarts JHP, Binnie CD, Smit AM, et al. Selective cognitive impairment during focal and generalized epileptiform EEG activity. *Brain* 1984;107:293–308.
36. Kasteleijn-Nolst Trenite DGA, Smit AM, Velis DN, et al. On-line detection of transient neuropsychological disturbances during EEG discharges in children with epilepsy. *Dev Med Child Neurol* 1990;32:46–50.
37. Hutt SJ, Newton S, Fairweather H. Choice reaction time and EEG activity in children with epilepsy. *Neuropsychologia* 1977;15:257–267.
38. Grigonis AM, Murphy EH. The effects of epileptic cortical activity on the development of callosal projections. *Dev Brain Res* 1994;77:251–255.
39. Rapin I, Mattis S, Rowan AJ. et al. Verbal auditory agnosia in children. *Dev Med Child Neurol* 1977;19: 192–207.

40. Beaumanoir A. The Landau-Kleffner syndrome. In: Roger J, Dravet C, Bureau M, et al., eds. *Epileptic syndromes in infancy, childhood and adolescence.* London: John Libbey Eurotext Ltd., 1985:181–191.

41. Deonna T. Acquired epileptiform aphasia in children (Landau-Kleffner syndrome). *J Clin Neurophysiol* 1991;8:288–298.

42. Deonna T, Beaumanoir A, Gaillard F, et al. Acquired aphasia in childhood with seizure disorder: a heterogenous syndrome. *Neuropediatrics* 1977;8:263–273.

43. Morrell F, Whisler WW, Smith MC, et al. Landau-Kleffner syndrome: treatment with subpial intracortical transection. *Brain* 1995;118:1529–1546.

44. Deonna T, Roulet E. Epilepsy and language disorder in children. In: Fukuyama Y, Kamoshita S, Ohtsuka C, et al., eds. *Modern perspectives of child neurology.* Tokyo: The Japanese Society of Child Neurology, 1991: 259–266.

45. Mantovani JF, Landau WM. Acquired aphasia with convulsive disorder: course and prognosis. *Neurology* 1980;30:524–529.

46. Deonna T, Peter CL, Ziegler A-L. Adult follow-up of the acquired aphasia-epilepsy syndrome in childhood. Report of seven cases. *Neuropediatrics* 1989;20:132–138.

47. Van Harskamp F, Van Dongen HR, Loonen MCB. Acquired aphasia with convulsive disorder in children: a case study with a seven-year follow-up. *Brain Lang* 1978;6:141–148.

48. Dugas M, Masson M, Le Heuzey MF, et al. Aphasie "acquise" de l'enfant avec épilepsie (syndrome de Landau et Kleffner). Douze observations personnelles. *Rev Neurol* 1982;138:755–780.

49. Dulac O, Billard C, Arthuis M. Aspects électro-cliniques et évolutifs, de l'épilepsie dans le syndrome aphasie-épilepsie. *Arch Francaises Pediatr* 1983;40: 299–308.

50. Bishop DVM. Age of onset and outcome in acquired aphasia with convulsive disorder (Landau-Kleffner syndrome). *Dev Med Child Neurol* 1985;27:705–712.

51. Loonen MCB, Van Dongen HR. Acquired childhood aphasia. Outcome one year after onset. *Arch Neurol* 1990;47:1324–1328.

52. Lewine JD, Andrews R, Chez M, et al. Magnetoencephalography patterns of epileptiform activity in children with regressive autism spectrum disorders. *Pediatrics* 1999;104:405–418.

53. Hoeppner TJ, Morrell F, Smith MC, et al. The Landau-Kleffner syndrome: a perisylvian epilepsy. *Epilepsia* 1992;33[Suppl 3]:122.

54. Marescaux C, Hirsch E, Finck S, et al. Landau-Kleffner syndrome: a pharmacologic study of five cases. *Epilepsia* 1990;31:768–777.

55. McKinney W, McGreal DA. An aphasic syndrome in children. *Can Med Assoc J* 1974;110:637–639.

56. Hirsch E, Marescaux C, Maquet P, et al. Landau-Kleffner syndrome: a clinical and EEG study of five cases. *Epilepsia* 1990;31:756–767.

57. Deonna T, Roulet E. Acquired epileptic aphasia (AEA): definition of the syndrome and current problems. In: Beaumanoir A, Bureau M, Deonna T, et al., eds. *Continuous spike and wave during slow sleep, electrical status epilepticus during slow sleep.* London: John Libbey, 1995:37–46.

58. Lerman P, Lerman-Sagie T, Kivity S. Effect of early corticosteroid therapy for Landau-Kleffner syndrome. *Dev Med Child Neurol* 1991;33:257–266.

59. Morrell F, Whisler WW, Bleck T. Multiple subpial transection: a new approach to the surgical treatment of focal epilepsy. *J Neurosurg* 1989;70:231–239.

60. Morrell F. Secondary epileptogenic lesions. *Epilepsia* 1959/1960;1:538–560.

61. Morrell F. Microelectrode studies in chronic epileptic foci. *Epilepsia* 1961;2:81–88.

62. Morrell F. Cellular pathophysiology of focal epilepsy. *Epilepsia* 1969;10:495–505.

63. Tharp BR. The penicillin focus: a study of field characteristics using cross-correlation analysis. *Electroencephalogr Clin Neurophysiol* 1971;31:45–55.

64. Mountcastle VB. Modality and topographic properties of single neurons of cat's somatic sensory cortex. *J Neurophysiol* 1957;20:408–434.

65. Hubel DH, Wiesel TN. Receptive fields, binocular interaction and functional architecture in the cat's visual cortex. *J Physiol* 1962;160:106–154.

66. Asanuma H, Sakata H. Functional organization of a cortical efferent system examined with focal depth stimulation in cats. *J Neurophysiol* 1967;30:35–54.

67. Morrell F, Kanner AM, Hoeppner TJ, et al. Surgical treatment of Landau-Kleffner syndrome. In: Tuxhorn I, Holthausen H, Boenigk H, eds. *Pediatric epilepsy syndromes and their surgical treatments.* London: John Libbey, 1997:462–482.

68. Changeux JP, Danchin A. Selective stabilization of developing synapses as a mechanism for the specification of neuronal networks. *Nature* 1976;264::705–712.

69. Purves D, Lichtman JW. Elimination of synapses in the developing nervous system. *Science* 1980;210:153–157.

70. Purves D. *Body and brain.* Cambridge, MA: Harvard University Press, 1988:231.

71. Huttenlocher PR, de Courten C, Garey LJ, et al. Synaptogenesis in the human visual cortex evidence for synapse elimination during normal development. *Neurosci Lett* 1982;33:247–252.

72. Huttenlocher PR, de Courten C. The development of synapses in the striate cortex of man. *Hum Neurobiol* 1987;6:1–9.

73. Wiesel TN. Postnatal development of the visual cortex and the influence of environment. *Nature* 1982;299: 583–591.

74. Guttman E. Aphasia in children. *Brain* 1942;65: 205–219.

75. Alajouanine T, Lhermitte F. Acquired aphasia in children. *Brain* 1965;88:644–662.

76. Rasmussen T, Milner B. The role of early left-brain injury in determining lateralization of cerebral speech functions. *Ann N Y Acad Sci* 1977;299:355–369.

77. Vargha-Khadem F, O'Gorman AM, Watters GV. Aphasia and handedness in relation to hemispheric side, age at injury and severity of cerebral lesion during childhood. *Brain* 1985;108:677–696.

78. Tassinari A, Bureau M, Dravet C, et al. Epilepsy with continuous spikes and waves during slow sleep. In: Roger J, Bureau M, Darvet C, et al., eds. *Epileptic syndromes in infancy, childhood and adolescence,* 2nd ed. London: John Libbey, 1992:245–256.

79. Rapin I. Autistic regression and disintegrative disorder: how important the role of epilepsy? *Semin Pediatr Neurol* 1995;2:278–285.

80. Kurita H, Kita M, Miyake Y. A comparative study of development and symptoms among dysintegrative psychosis and infantile autism with and without speech loss. *J Autism Dev Disord* 1992;22:175–188.

81. Guillioto LMFF, Morrell F. Electropsychological differences between Landau-Kleffner syndrome and other conditions showing the CSWS electrical pattern. *Epilepsia* 1994;35[Suppl 8]:126.

82. Nass R, Gross A, Wisoff J, et al. Outcome of multiple subpial transection for autistic epileptiform regression. *Pediatr Neurol* 1999;21:464–470.

83. Munari C, Kahane P, Francione S. Role of the hypothalamic hamartoma in the genesis of gelastic fits. *Electroencephalogr Clin Neurophysiol* 1995;95:154–160.

84. Valdueza J, Cristante l, Dammann O, et al. Hypothalamic hamartomas. Special reference to gelastic epilepsy and surgery. *Neurosurgery* 1994;34:949–958.

85. Berkovic SF, Andermann F, Melanson D, et al. Hypothalamic hamartomas and ictal laughter: evolution of a characteristic epileptic syndrome and diagnostic value of magnetic resonance imaging. *Ann Neurol* 1988;23:429–439.

86. Ponsont G, Diebler C, Plouin P. Hamartomes hypothalamiques et crises de rise. *Arch Francaises Pediatr* 1983;40:757–761.

87. Breningstall G. Gelastic seizures, precocious puberty and hypothalamic hamartomas. *Neurology* 1983;35:1180–1183.

88. Kahane P, Tassi L, Hoffman D, et al. Crises dacrystiques et hemartome hypothalamique: a propos d'une observation video-stereo-EEG. *Epilepsies* 1994;6:259–279.

89. Mirski MA. Unravelling the neuroanatomy of epilepsy. *AJNR Am J Neuroradiol* 1993;14:1336–1342.

12

Psychiatric Issues in Patients with Epilepsy and Mental Retardation

Alan B. Ettinger and *Alan L. Steinberg

Huntington Hospital Epilepsy Monitoring Program, Long Island Jewish Medical Center, New Hyde Park, New York 11040; and Department of Geriatrics and Psychiatry, State University of New York at Stony Brook, Stony Brook, New York 11790

Psychiatric issues are an integral part of the care of patients with mental retardation (MR) and are of particular concern in the face of an established or suspected comorbid epileptic disorder. Diagnostic aspects include the common challenge of distinguishing aberrant behaviors from seizures. Treatment issues include concerns about reducing seizure threshold when administering psychotropic agents, minimizing medication-related side effects, and attempting to treat both behavioral difficulties and seizures. Few studies have focused on psychiatric aspects of epilepsy in MR patients; nevertheless, in this chapter we will try to highlight our current understanding of this topic.

According to the *Diagnostic and Statistical Manual of Mental Disorders,* Fourth Edition (DSM-IV), MR is defined by three criteria: (i) an IQ less than or equal to 70, (ii) limitations in adaptive function, and (iii) an onset of deficits prior to the age of 18 years (1). MR is common, occurring in 1% to 3% of the population of developed countries (2). Although advances in molecular genetics have led to the identification of 350 to 500 causes of MR (3,4), Down syndrome, fragile X, and fetal alcohol syndrome are the most common identifiable conditions. However, there is a diverse list of potential etiologies for seizures in MR patients, including genetic syndromes (e.g., tuberous sclerosis), cerebral malformations (e.g., heterotopias), perinatal asphyxia, con-

genital strokes, and infectious states (e.g., meningitis).

Depending on the definitions used and the populations examined, prevalence rates of psychiatric disorders in patients with MR vary from 10% (5) to greater than 60% (6). Behavioral problems are common and varied. As early as 1858, Bucknill and Tuke described the need for treatment of symptoms in patients with MR (termed "institutionalized idiots"). It was reported that restraint was necessary in 35% of the cases because of violence to others, 33% for destruction of objects, 10% for "maniacal excitement," and 10% for self-injurious behavior (7). In current times, Szymanski et al. (8) studied the reasons for psychiatric referral and noted behavioral problems, including bizarre behaviors, depression, sexual problems, pica, aggression, and self-injury. Quine (9) noted attention seeking, hyperactivity, tantrums, aggression, and self-injury at the mild or severe level in 45% of individuals with MR. In a study of 4,461 individuals with MR, Einfeld (10) reported 22% with behavioral problems.

Epilepsy occurs in approximately 1% of the general population, but in as many as 30% of patients with MR and in up to 50% of patients with MR and multiple handicaps (11,12). Increased prevalence of epilepsy in MR probably reflects the central nervous system (CNS) causes of MR, which often also are etiologies of the epileptic condition (13). There is a limited correlation of severity of cognitive impairment with the occurrence of epilepsy (12), whereas the severity of motor deficits appears to significantly raise the risk of chronic seizures (12,14).

Reports on rates of psychiatric disorders in patients with MR and epilepsy are conflicting, and it is unclear to what degree, if any, epilepsy raises the risk of psychiatric disturbances in this population. For example, Lund (15) found a significantly higher rate of psychiatric disorders among patients with MR who had experienced seizures within the previous 12 months, compared to seizure-free patients. Other investigators found little difference (16). Nevertheless, we would expect patients with MR to have *at least* the same risk of experiencing the various psychiatric disorders as do non-MR patients with epilepsy (17).

Specific types of psychopathology in patients with MR and epilepsy have not been well studied. The retrospective review by Pary (18) of a university hospital-based population found affective disorders to be the most common primary psychiatric disorder. It is likely, however, that virtually any psychological condition may occur in such patients (13).

SEIZURES AND ABERRANT BEHAVIORS

Patients with MR have a high prevalence of epileptic seizures and of aberrant behaviors; often, it is difficult to distinguish one type of event from the other. Differential diagnosis also includes psychiatric disorders, muscle spasms, movement disorders, vasovagal or cardiac syncope, sleep disorders, and migraine (13). However, the wide variety of seizure types, particular nonconvulsive episodes, can make the exclusion of seizures particularly challenging. Table 12.1 highlights examples of behavioral symptoms and seizure phenomena that may produce such symptoms.

A careful history, clinical observation of the episodes, and evaluation with various types of electroencephalographic (EEG) studies are essential to distinguishing nonepileptic behavioral events from epileptic episodes. That both nonepileptic and epileptic events can occur in the same patient can be a con-

TABLE 12.1. *Potential ictal correlates for behavioral symptoms*

Behavior[a]	Could be mistaken for
Aggressive behavior to self or others, temper tantrums/outbursts, irritability, tendency to disturb others	Ictal or postictal confusion; postictal aggression.
Listless, sluggish, or inactive behavior; appearing preoccupied, staring into space, demonstrating fixed facial expression, lacking emotional responsiveness; failure to pay attention to instructions; sitting or standing in one position for a long time	Medication toxicity, absence or partial complex seizures
Seeking isolation, appearing withdrawn, preferring solitary activities	Periictal behavioral changes.
Demonstrating meaningless, recurring body movements, stereotyped behaviors, abnormal repetitive movements, moving or rolling head back and forth repetitively, showing repetitive hand or body or head movements	Automatisms associated with partial complex seizures
Screaming or yelling inappropriately	Ictal vocalizations
Odd or bizarre in behaviors	Ictal or postictal manifestations
Repetitive speech	Partial complex seizures
Depressed mood	Prodrome or postictal
Resisting any form of physical contact	Ictal or postictal
Talking to self loudly	Confusional state of ictal or postictal state

[a]Adapted from Aman MG, Singh NN. *Aberrant behavior checklist.* East Aurora, NY: Slosson Educational Publications, Inc., 1994:1–29, with permission.

founding element in the evaluation of these patients (19–21). Coexistence of nonepileptic seizures (NES) and epileptic seizures has been reported in 10% to 40% of series of patients with NES. The highest occurrence was in MR (22). Although the clinical phenomena associated with nonepileptic phenomena in epileptic patients may be stereotyped, the behaviors associated with epileptic and nonepileptic events tend to be different in appearance (23). Patients also may embellish on poorly identified genuine epileptic symptoms. Video EEG monitoring study often is necessary to distinguish the two types of events (see later).

Autistic children with MR are a group of patients in whom the identification of epileptic seizures can pose a diagnostic challenge. Approximately 40% to 60% of children with autism have been found to have epileptiform activity on routine EEG studies (24). A recent study done with magnetoencephalography revealed epileptiform activity in 82% of patients with an autistic regression disorder (25). Yet, only 30% of autistic patients will go on to develop epileptic seizures. The very frequent stereotypic mannerisms, the detached withdrawn attitude of these patients, and the failure to respond when spoken to compound the confusion in distinguishing the nature of these events. Coupled with an EEG that shows interictal spikes, clinicians are forced to exclude the possibility that such phenomena may be of epileptic origin. Only video EEG monitoring study can solve the clinical dilemma in these patients.

Landau-Kleffner syndrome is an acquired aphasia or verbal auditory agnosia in children thought to result from an epileptogenic process of language cortex occurring during a critical period of language development. Reports that Landau-Kleffner language deficits may respond to steroids (26–29) has sparked controversy on the use of these therapies, particularly in the absence of features following the strict diagnostic criteria.

Although there is an abundance of studies citing the clinical features of NES in patients without MR (30,31), the clinical features of nonepileptic behavioral episodes in MR patients are not well described. However, it is likely that the clinical semiology observed in the former group is applicable to MR patients. For example, there are no uniform types of behavioral changes among MR patients that distinguish epileptic from nonepileptic events. Nonepileptic behavioral changes typically last longer than seizures, have more asymmetric or asynchronous movements, and have a "stop and start" quality (30,32). However, clinical activities (e.g., tongue biting, incontinence, self-injury) commonly associated with epileptic seizures also may occur in nonepileptic events (33). Frontal lobe seizures, which often are accompanied by pelvic thrusting, vocalizations, thrashing movements, and minimal postictal recovery times, are easily mistaken for nonepileptic events (34–36). Nonepileptic events are more likely to be provoked by emotional stimuli. Crying and weeping also are more common during nonepileptic events (37).

A normal interictal EEG does not exclude epileptic seizures, nor does it confirm the diagnosis of NES. Interictal epileptiform abnormalities do not exclude NES because epileptic seizures and NES may coexist (21).

Capturing episodes of concern on simultaneous video and EEG recording can by helpful in assessing aberrant behaviors in patients with MR. Patients with convulsive events usually have identifiable ictal correlates on EEG, whereas nonepileptic behavioral changes are not associated with electrographic seizure patterns. However, certain exceptions must be kept in mind: (i) simple partial seizures (focal seizures unassociated with altered awareness) usually lack correlation on EEG scalp recordings (38); and (ii) the ictal EEG pattern of complex partial seizures of mesial frontal origin may not be readily detected on scalp recordings, given the angle subtended by the recording electrodes to the epileptic source, a restricted epileptogenic area, the frequent violent and bizarre automatisms that cause significant muscle and movement artifact, or a combination of all these factors (36). The following clinical characteristics may help in the recognition of epileptic seizures of mesial frontal origin: (i) a short duration, (ii) stereotypic event, and (iii) occurrence in clusters out of sleep (36). Video EEG often is essential in documenting that an episode occurs out of physiologic sleep; in which case, genuine epileptic seizures are strongly suggested (39).

Certain laboratory tests, such as the documentation of a rise of prolactin level 20 minutes after an episode, support the diagnosis of seizures (40), but this test is not specific to this type of event, as it also can occur following syncopal episodes. On the other hand, the reverse is not true. That is, failure to see a raise in prolactin blood levels does not rule out a diagnosis of epilepsy. Furthermore, prolactin testing may be confounded in patients with MR who receive neuroleptic agents for behavioral control. Prolactin levels are not reliably increased after nongeneralized seizures or after seizures that do not involve limbic structures (41), and this includes the same seizures that often mimic nonepileptic events, such as frontal lobe seizures. Measurement of serum creatine phosphokinase is a second laboratory test that may be helpful in distinguishing epileptic from nonepileptic *convulsive events,* as an increase of its concentration can be identified 18 to 24 hours following a generalized tonic-clonic seizure in 25% of patients. As with prolactin, failure to identify an increase in creatine phosphokinase level does not rule out a diagnosis of epilepsy.

PSYCHIATRIC DISORDERS IN MENTAL RETARDATION: DIAGNOSTIC AND THERAPEUTIC CONSIDERATIONS

General Treatment Approaches

Psychotropic drugs frequently are prescribed to patients with MR to treat psychiatric symptoms and manage behavioral symptoms. Clinicians may try to take advantage of psychotropic properties of antiepileptic drugs (AEDs) in patients with concomitant epilepsy to treat both seizures and behavioral problems (see later discussion); however, other pharmacologic and nonpharmacologic approaches can be considered.

The use of psychotropic medication in MR has been estimated to range from 40% to 50% in institutions and from 25% to 35% in community-residing individuals (42). Another study showed that of 1,056 persons with MR living in nursing homes, 31.8% received antipsychotics, of which thioridazine was the most common. Sixteen percent of residents received anxiolytics, of which diazepam was the most prescribed; 6.1% were given antidepressants, of which amitriptyline was the most common; and 7% received anticonvulsants, with carbamazepine (CBZ) and valproate used most commonly (43). In this study, 92.7% of the antipsychotic prescriptions were for "behavioral control." These medication choices are themselves problematic, given the high risk of side effects, and particularly the anticholinergic side effects that they possess, with the propensity to cause more confusion and agitation (the very symptoms for which they may have initially been prescribed). In patients with MR and epilepsy, there may be theoretical concerns about psychotropic-induced lowering of the seizure threshold.

A unique challenge of treating MR patients is their inability to provide an accurate rendering of their internal mental life and experiences. This leads the clinician to rely on an assessment of observable events, and this makes the observations of multiple staff members especially crucial. Success of treatment is predicated on a good working relationship between the clinician and the interdisciplinary team. Accurate diagnosis requires the assistance of caregivers trained by clinicians to be effective observers. Psychologists and behavioral specialists are invaluable to examine the effects of learning and behavioral strategies.

Another challenge is that different psychiatric syndromes may present with very similar behavioral features. For example, agitation can be the major manifestation of mania, depression, delirium, anxiety, or schizophrenia. Therefore, the clinician needs to search for objective indicators supporting the likelihood of one diagnosis over another. In a case of suspected mania, one would search for changes in sleep, irritability, or hypersexuality; in anxiety, one would carefully examine somatic complaints, recently occurring environmental stressors, and hyperventilation episodes. In suspected delirium, attention focuses on the alterations in the level of consciousness. Unfortunately, many clinicians may immediately treat the most recognizable component of that behavior, such as agitation, without considering the broader differential diagnosis.

Behavioral techniques, such as operant conditioning, time-outs, extinction, and positive reinforcement, have all been amply documented to successfully reduce or eliminate problematic repetitive behaviors; therefore, they should be a part of most treatment plans. Environmental modification, such as reduced stimulation and sometimes changes of staff, can lead to a reduction in symptomatology. Group programs, such as exercise, social skills training, and structured activities, also should be considered.

When prescribing medication, it is best to start with the lowest possible dosage and increase dosages gradually. MR patients are exquisitely sensitive to side effects. Proper dosing should be maintained for a suitable period of time to adequately assess its effect (e.g., up to 12 weeks for antidepressants). If appropriate to the class of medications, drug levels should be measured, both to monitor for safety and to ensure compliance and absorption. Agents with significant anticholinergic properties are best avoided, because they can increase confusion, disinhibition, and behavioral symptoms. Potential lowering of the seizure threshold should lead the clinician to monitor for epileptic events. Finally, the clinician must remember that the primary goal of treatment is not to control symptoms that are disturbing to others, but rather to provide the patient with relief from distressing symptoms.

Delirium

Delirium is one of the most common syndromes seen in clinical practice and is the first diagnosis to be excluded before implementing treatments. It is characterized by relatively acute confusion with behavioral changes, agitation, waxing and waning level of consciousness, deficits in attention and concentration, sleep cycle disruptions, and possible hallucinations. The delirious patient may be hyperactive or hypoactive, and clinical manifestations can vary dramatically over a short time period (44–46). The diagnosis can be elusive, and a clinician can easily be misled by symptoms such as anxiety, hallucinations, depression, and apathy.

Postictal psychotic episodes are among the first causes of delirium to be excluded in patients with epilepsy and MR. These episodes often occur following clusters of generalized tonic-clonic seizures. A symptom-free period prior to the onset of psychiatric symptoms may last up to 5 days and may "mask" the temporal relationship with the seizure cluster. This topic is discussed in greater detail in Chapter 11. Other causes of delirium include infectious states (including seemingly innocuous illnesses such as urinary tract infections), metabolic abnormalities, and medication side effects.

The treatment of delirium begins with the attempt to identify the underlying etiology as rapidly as possible. Of note, even after identifying and removing the offending cause, it can take up to 3 to 4 weeks for patients to return to their baseline mental state. Investigations on the etiologies of delirium may include checking for urinary tract and other infections, reviewing the medication list (including over-the-counter and herbal remedies), ruling out metabolic abnormalities, excluding new central nervous system insults such subdural hematoma, and evaluating for new cardiac or respiratory events. Because substance abuse has been noted to occur in the developmentally disabled, attention should be paid to the possibility of either acute intoxication or withdrawal from substances, most commonly alcohol (47–49). Early-onset Alzheimer's disease should be suspected in patients with trisomy 21.

Impulse Control Disorders

In their survey of 251 patients with MR referred for psychiatric consultation, King et al.

(50) found that the most frequent diagnosis was impulse control disorders. Self-injurious behavior, often considered a variant of impulse control disorders, was reported to occur in as many as 40% of patients (51). Barring the possibility that a proportion of this group labeled as aggressive or impulsive were, in fact, suffering from delirium or depression, the likelihood remains that this is a frequent diagnosis in this group. Studies of the efficacy of treatment options in this group are limited. However, anecdotal experience supports the use of antidepressants. Cook et al. (52) noted a response to fluoxetine in six of 17 patients studied, and other investigators (53,54) reported on what may have been a partial response to methylphenidate (although the symptom cluster being treated was not as clear). Certainly, AEDs with positive psychotropic properties should be strongly considered in patients with both MR and epilepsy. For example, Kastner et al. (55) reported an improvement in self-injurious behavior and impulse-realm symptoms in nine of 12 patients treated with valproate. Psychotropic features of AEDs are highlighted in a subsequent section.

The use of the antipsychotics has been evaluated for impulse control problems. McDougle et al. (56) reported a 57% response rate with the use of risperidone to treat aggression, irritability, and impulsive behaviors in autistic adults. Other investigators reported on the efficacy of dopamine antagonists, such as haloperidol, in decreasing motor stereotypies, aggression, and self-injurious behaviors (57,58). Overall, antipsychotic agents carry an approximate 1% risk of seizures, with specific agents having notably higher rates. Some authors suggest that butyrophenones (e.g., haloperidol) have a lower risk of seizures than the phenothiazines (e.g., chlorpromazine) (59). Among the more recently marketed atypical antipsychotic agents, clozapine carries a dose-related higher risk of seizures and may produce generalized spike-and-wave discharges on EEG (60). The combination of clozapine with antiepileptic agents such as valproic acid (VPA) may substantially reduce the risk of seizures (61). Other recently introduced antipsychotic agents, such as risperidone and olanzapine, appear to carry a reduced risk of lowering seizure threshold.

Other medications studied include opioid antagonists (achieving mixed results) (62,63) and β blockers (64–66), with up to 83% of patients reporting decreased symptoms. There are few studies of lithium or buspirone in this population (67,68), but lithium should be used with great caution in these patients, as it is well known to cause EEG changes and delirium at therapeutic levels and to facilitate the occurrence of seizures (69).

Depression

Although DSM-IV serves as a useful guide to the diagnosis of depression in the non-MR population, literature on its features in this population is limited. Symptoms of depression include changes in behavior, decreased cognition, increased irritability, increased somatic symptoms, changes in sleep cycle, self-injurious actions, suspiciousness or paranoia, and changes in appetitive behavior.

In MR patients with or without epilepsy, agents with significant anticholinergic side effects should be avoided. Medications should be maintained at proper therapeutic levels for suitable periods of time, which may be up to 12 weeks, to assess full efficacy.

The treatment of depression has been poorly studied in epileptic patients and particularly among those with MR. Surprisingly, there is little evidence in the literature for tricyclic antidepressant (TCA)-induced seizures at therapeutic plasma concentration. Patients receiving therapeutic doses of TCA and presenting with drug-induced seizures have been found to be slow metabolizers of these drugs. Further, clinical experience suggests that depressive symptoms in epileptic patients can be treated with modest doses of antidepressants, equivalent to half of the doses required for depressive disorders in nonepileptic patients. Thus, starting patients at low doses and making small increments until the desired clinical response is reached minimizes the risk of causing and/or exacerbating seizures (70). TCAs carry a higher risk of inducing seizures than the selective monoamine oxidase A inhibitors (MAOIs) and the selective serotonin reuptake inhibitors (SSRIs) (71,72).

Antidepressant-related seizure risk factors consist of conditions common to MR, including brain damage and an abnormal EEG. Other factors include high doses or blood levels of antidepressants, drug overdoses, or rapid escalations in antidepressant dose (59). Bupropion, maprotiline, and amoxapine are the antidepressants with the strongest proconvulsant properties and should be avoided in epileptic patients (73).

Just as in epileptic patients without MR, in our opinion, SSRIs should be considered as the first-line treatment in depressed patients with epilepsy. They have a low seizure propensity, are well tolerated in overdose, and have a favorable adverse effects profile (74,75). TCAs yield a good clinical response, but their cardiotoxic effects and severe complications when used in patients with suicide attempts make them a second-line antidepressant. MAOIs are efficacious, well tolerated, and associated with a low incidence of seizures in patients with depression (76). Their potential risk of hypertensive crisis resulting from their interactions with certain foods rich in tyramine and with some medications make them less optimal agents.

Potential pharmacokinetic interactions between AEDs and antidepressants should be considered. Most antidepressants are metabolized in the liver, and their metabolism is increased in the presence of AEDs with cytochrome P-450 (CYP-450) enzyme-inducing properties. These AEDs are phenytoin (PHT), CBZ, phenobarbital, and primidone. Alternatively, several SSRIs inhibit several CYP-450 isoenzymes. These include fluoxetine, paroxetine, and fluvoxamine. Sertraline and citalopram are less likely to have pharmacokinetic interactions with AEDs (70).

Two new antidepressants (venlafaxine and mirtazapine) act on serotonin and norepinephrine neurotransmitters. Currently, there are little data on their impact on seizure threshold, interaction with AEDs, and their use in epileptic patients with or without MR.

Mania

Mania may occur in developmentally disabled patients. Impulse control can be difficult to distinguish from mania, because they both may present with irritability, sleep changes, disinhibition (both verbally and behaviorally), and agitation. Mood elevation may help distinguish these diagnoses, but classic manic presentations are unusual and the exception. Mania should be strongly considered in MR patients whose symptoms are triggered by the start of an antidepressant or the increment in its dose. The presence of a family history of bipolar disorder should help the clinician suspect the possibility of a manic episode.

Lithium was the first "mood-stabilizing drug" used in the treatment of patients with bipolar disorders. Its use in epileptic patients with affective disorders, however, has been fraught with several problems. These include changes in EEG recordings and proconvulsant properties at therapeutic serum concentrations in patients with or without MR (69), in nonepileptic and epileptic patients. Lithium's neurotoxicity and related seizure risks increase with the concurrent use of neuroleptic drugs, in the presence of EEG abnormalities, or with any history of CNS disorder. For these reasons, and given the comparable prophylactic efficacy of VPA and CBZ in bipolar disorders, the use of lithium should be considered only after these two AEDs have been attempted and failed to yield the desired therapeutic effects (77).

AEDs with mood-stabilizing properties (see subsequent discussion) are a natural choice to concomitantly treat epilepsy and behavioral problems. There are few studies of standard antiepileptic drug use in bipolar disorder in the context of MR and epilepsy, and there are even fewer randomized controlled trials of the newer anticonvulsants (e.g., gabapentin [GPN], lamotrigine [LTG], and topiramate [TPM]) in patients even without MR.

PSYCHOTROPIC PROPERTIES OF ANTIEPILEPTIC DRUGS IN PATIENTS WITH MENTAL RETARDATION

In a recent review of AED use in epileptic patients with MR, Coulter (78) summarized the typical selection of AEDs based on relative efficacy of the drug against specific seizure type. PHT and CBZ are commonly used to treat partial seizures; VPA, gabapentin (GPN), LTG, tiagabine (TGB), and TPM also are effective. Ethosuximide (ESM) is indicated in the treatment of absence seizures; VPA and LTG also may be considered. Generalized myoclonic, tonic, and atonic seizures (all features of the Lennox-Gastaut syndrome commonly encountered in this population) may be treated with VPA, LTG, felbamate (FBM), or TPM. Generalized tonic-clonic seizures can be treated with PHT, CBZ, FBM, LTG, or TPM. Use of barbiturates is discussed later.

Knowledge of potential favorable or adverse psychotropic effects of AEDs is an important consideration when treating epilepsy in the setting of MR. Although there are a paucity of studies that focus on these concerns in MR patients, lessons from our experience with AEDs in other populations can be applied to the management of epileptic MR patients. This literature must be interpreted with caution, however, because many reports are anecdotal, some fail to examine premorbid psychiatric status, and many are based on cases with very high anticonvulsant levels (79).

Other methodologic pitfalls in the literature include associating mood change with the introduction of a new AED and ignoring potential effects of discontinuing the current agent, disregarding the positive effects on mood achieved by reducing seizures, failure to address the complex relationship of drug-induced cognitive impairment with mood, poor recognition of important inequities in drug trial comparison groups (e.g., groups with noncomparable drug levels), analysis of limited samples, selection bias, the negative effect of polytherapy irrespective of the specific agent, and failure to apply correction methods in statistical analysis of large numbers of variables (80). Other confounding variables include reliance on retrospective data, focusing on transient acute drug effects, and inappropriate extrapolation of data on drug effects in normal volunteers to epileptic patients (81). There also may be significantly lower rates of psychotropic effects on mood and behavior noted in general drug trial reports compared to studies that specifically target these factors.

For most AEDs, numerous conflicting reports abound concerning both positive and negative psychotropic effects, and the reader of the medical literature needs to remember that mean tendencies may differ from individual patient experience.

Another challenge in analyzing psychotropic effects of AEDs relates to our inability to assess these effects as completely independent variables. Patients who experience a reduction or resolution of seizures as a result of AED therapy may experience associated elevations in mood and improvements in quality of life. Conversely, the stigma of taking AEDs or reactions to experiencing side effects (e.g., cosmetic effects, fatigue, cognitive impairments) may adversely affect mood and behavior (82).

Whereas this section focuses on the psychotropic effects of individual AEDs, clinicians are very likely to encounter developmentally disabled epileptic patients receiving more than one medication, including antiepileptic and psychotropic drugs. This confounds the clinician's attempt to determine which agent is specifically responsible for the positive or negative effects on behavior. Recent consensus among epileptologists on the value of striving for AED monotherapy in the treatment of the non-MR epileptic patient also should apply to the MR population. Numerous studies have demonstrated that reduction in AED polypharmacy does not necessarily lead to seizure exacerbation, and patients may enjoy improvements in cognition and behavior when they receive a smaller number of medications (83–85).

AED effects on behavior may relate to their variable effects on different groups of cortical neurons. AEDs may alter neurotransmitter levels (e.g., norepinephrine and γ-aminobutyric acid [GABA]) or ion channel function, which in turn may impact on both seizures and mood (79). For example, the mood instability of bipolar disorder has been theorized to occur on the basis of decreased GABA-ergic neurotransmission or by altered sodium channel function. Some AEDs may improve mood instability by increasing GABA and modifying sodium channels.

Ketter et al. (86) proposed classifying AEDs into two global categories based on their psychotropic properties and mechanisms of action. One group is considered to have "sedating" effects in association with fatigue, cognitive slowing, and possible anxiolytic and antimanic effects. These actions are speculated to be related to a predominance of potentiation of GABA inhibitory neurotransmission and occur with barbiturates, benzodiazepines, valproate, GPN, TGB, and vigabatrin (VGB). A second group is thought to have "activating" effects with possible anxiogenic and antidepressant effects. The second group is associated with attenuation of glutamate excitatory neurotransmission and includes FBM and LTG. TPM, which possesses both GABA-ergic and antiglutamatergic actions, is said to have a mixed profile. Animal models and evidence from clinical experience are used to support this classification.

Individual Antiepileptic Drugs

Benzodiazepines

Benzodiazepines, such as chlorazepate, clobazam, clonazepam, diazepam, lorazepam, and nitrazepam, may be used in epileptic patients with MR as an anxiolytic agent or sedative hypnotic (87). They also appear to have limited antidepressant (88) and antimanic (89) properties. Benzodiazepines also have broad-spectrum antiepileptic properties and have been used commonly to treat Lennox-Gastaut syndrome (an epileptic syndrome characterized by generalized seizures, typically tonic, atonic, myoclonic, and atypical absence, characteristic spike-and-wave complexes, and usually cognitive dysfunction) (90). Their ten-

dency to cause sedation, cognitive impairment, tolerance, and addiction limit their utility as chronic antiepileptic therapy (91). Further, intravenous benzodiazepines administered to patients with Lennox-Gastaut syndrome (common in the MR population with epilepsy) has been reported to rarely induce generalized status epilepticus (92) or to convert absence status to generalized tonic status epilepticus (93). Adverse psychotropic effects among patients with MR may include behavioral abnormalities characterized by hyperactivity, restlessness, reduced attention span, irritability, disruptiveness, and/or aggressiveness (79,87). Special care should be taken when withdrawing benzodiazepine therapy, as delirium, psychosis, and withdrawal seizures can result (94).

Barbiturates

Despite the current availability of many more AEDs than were available in the past, barbiturates, such as phenobarbital and primidone, continue to be prescribed frequently for MR epileptic patients, not necessarily because of superior drug efficacy but probably due to physician discomfort with the newer and less familiar AEDs. This is unfortunate, because the barbiturates may significantly impair cognition in patients with already compromised intellectual abilities (79). The risk of withdrawal seizures also makes barbiturates a less than optimal AED for use in this population. Cognitive impairment due to barbiturates may be subtle, occur in the absence of frank sedation, and anecdotally may not be obvious to the patient until the patient notices an improvement after the drug is withdrawn (95). Reduction in the use of barbiturates in MR patients may be accompanied by significant behavioral improvements (96).

Although barbiturates have been used in the past to treat anxiety and insomnia (97), and scattered reports even suggest modest efficacy against bipolar disorder (98), most attention has been placed on their adverse psychotropic profile. Barbiturates are associated with a significant risk of eliciting depressive symptomatology. The classic study by Brent et al. (99) of patients receiving phenobarbital compared to CBZ demonstrated a statistically significant increase in the risk of depression and suicidal ideation in the former group, particularly among those with a personal or family history of affective disorder. In patients with documented depression, it is advisable to avoid barbiturates (100).

Barbiturates may cause paradoxical hyperactivity (101–103), conduct problems (104), behavioral agitation, and irritability (105,106) in children, adolescents, and patients with MR (95). Identifying these potential side effects is crucial, because an optimal approach to their treatment would be to remove the responsible agent rather than adding a psychotropic drug to control these behaviors.

Phenytoin

PHT is commonly used in patients with partial and generalized tonic-clonic seizures but is not effective in absence seizures (107). There are variable reports about a relation between depressive symptoms and PHT, although some of this may relate reactive symptoms to experiencing the stigma associated with cosmetic side effects of the drug (17). Although a dose-related sedation may occur, a paradoxical excited delirium may be seen with either therapeutic or toxic PHT levels (108).

An older literature describes a chronic cumulative encephalopathy that impacts on both behavior and global cognition (79) as well as an acute reversible encephalopathy accompanying toxic PHT levels, manifested by increased seizures, drowsiness, and cognitive impairment, sometimes with ataxia (108). These encephalopathic syndromes should be considered when evaluating MR patients who have shown declines in cognition or coordination. Consideration toward switching AEDs should be made, if this potentially reversible syndrome is suspected.

Ethosuximide

ESM is commonly used as a first-line therapy for typical absence seizures occurring in primary generalized epilepsy syndromes; however, atypical absence is more common in a population with MR. Although ESM may be effective against atypical absence, the common association with other seizures (e.g., atonic, myoclonic, generalized tonic-clonic) that do not respond to ESM makes it a less than optimal choice in these patients. ESM usually is considered to be a benign treatment for absence seizures in primary generalized epilepsies, but it can cause confusion, sleep disturbances, and a wide assortment of behavioral changes, such as aggressive activity, depression, hostility, and even psychosis (100). The controversial entity of "forced normalization" (109) has been invoked as a potential explanation for ESM-related behavioral abnormalities, in which ESM-induced "normalization" of the EEG results in a paradoxical behavioral abnormality (110).

Valproic Acid

VPA has broad-spectrum anticonvulsant properties that include antiepileptic effects against many seizure types common to the MR population, including atonic, myoclonic, atypical absence, and generalized tonic-clonic seizures (111). In one recent series, VPA was the most commonly prescribed AED in a population-based cohort of adults with learning disability and epilepsy (112). Like CBZ, VPA now is commonly used to treat bipolar affective disorder, particularly in patients who do not respond adequately to lithium; therefore, it is thought to have "mood-stabilizing" properties in epileptic patients as well (113,114). VPA also may have utility in the treatment of panic and possibly in obsessive-compulsive disorder (115). Agitation and mood problems in association with CNS neurologic abnormalities, such as head trauma or seizures, may be particularly responsive to VPA therapy (116). VPA also has been suggested to improve irritability and aggressive or self-injurious behavior among nonepileptic MR patients, including patients with dementia (55,117).

VPA may cause somnolence and rare acute toxic encephalopathies (118,119). In children with learning disabilities and complex partial seizures, VPA has been reported to induce or exacerbate hyperactivity and aggressive behavior (120). However, similar reports have been noted with other AEDs, such as GPN, described later (121).

Carbamazepine

CBZ is a widely prescribed AED for both partial and generalized tonic-clonic seizures that has some structural similarities to the TCA, imipramine. There are few reports of negative behavioral effects associated with CBZ, although one notable retrospective study of patients with MR treated with CBZ for mood disorders found adverse behavioral reactions in nearly 10% of cases (122).

Numerous reports suggest that CBZ may have utility in treating impulse control disorders, including borderline personality traits and aggression and dyscontrol syndromes (123). Based on antimanic and mood-stabilizing properties similar to those described with VPA, CBZ also may be considered for use in epileptic patients who demonstrate both behavioral difficulties and seizures.

However, absence, myoclonic, and atonic seizures that may occur commonly among patients with MR do not respond to CBZ and may actually worsen in severity (124,125). Conceivably, other drugs with similar spectra of action, such as PHT and phenobarbital, may have similar effects on these seizure types. Therefore, CBZ may be useful for patients with MR, epilepsy, and behavioral disturbances, but careful consideration should be given to seizure type.

Gabapentin

A number of reports from the epilepsy literature suggest that GPN may promote an improved sense of well-being independent of seizure reduction (126–130). However, separating these two effects may be difficult.

Open-label and case reports suggest that GPN has efficacy in treating mania (131–134) and the depressive phase of bipolar disorder (135,136). Anecdotally, it has been reported to reduce agitation and improve sleep patterns in manic patients. It is being evaluated in behavioral dyscontrol (137), agitation in senile dementia (138), anxiety states (139), social phobia (140), and self-injurious behaviors in neurologic syndromes (141). If further validated with clinical experience and more rigorous studies, these reports may have important relevance for treatment of MR epileptic patients with comorbid psychiatric syndromes. The absence of protein binding or serious metabolic interactions gives GPN an excellent safety profile when used in combination therapy.

In this population, GPN may not be the optimal AED for treating some common seizure types encountered, such as absence, myoclonic seizures, and atonic seizures. Further, anecdotal experience in MR adults suggests that some patients may develop agitation. There are several reports of the development or exacerbation of aggressive and agitated behaviors in epileptic children, most of whom had some degree of intellectual impairment (121,142).

Lamotrigine

LTG is a broad-spectrum AED with efficacy against both partial and generalized seizures. Anecdotal experience in epileptic patients suggests that LTG may enhance alertness. After the discovery of serious adverse effects, including bone marrow dyscrasias and hepatitis associated with the use of FBM, many considered LTG to be an important alternative treatment for refractory generalized epilepsies in MR epileptic patients. In a double-blind, placebo-controlled trial of LTG in the Lennox-Gastaut syndrome (143), 33% of patients receiving LTG experienced a 50% or greater reduction in seizure frequency. This study noted minimal behavioral effects, whereas two subsequent series found significant effects, both positive and negative, among MR epileptic patients treated with LTG. Beran and Gibson (144) noted the development of aggressive and/or violent behavior in 14 of 19 patients who received LTG; one patient demonstrated improvement in behavior. Ettinger et al. (145) reported three of 20 mentally retarded epileptic patients receiving LTG who developed new or worsened hyperactivity, irritability, and stereotypy. However, another four patients exhibited positive psychotropic effects, including reduction in irritability and hyperactivity, decreased lethargy, diminished perseverative speech, and/or improvement in cooperation and better social engagement. The reasons for these disparate effects were unclear, and serum LTG levels did not predict who developed positive versus negative symptoms. Behavioral improvements may have been a "mood-stabilizing" effect of LTG. LTG now is being used for treatment-resistant bipolar disorder (146–148). Although there are more published double-blind trials of CBZ and VPA than the newer AEDs in the treatment of bipolar disorder, the arguably more favorable side-effect profiles of GPN and LTG may make the latter two drugs more optimal choices for mood stabilization in bipolar disorder than the former two agents. A positive psychotropic effect of LTG is supported by the observation that several epileptic patients entered in a randomized double-blind study of LTG who experienced only slight reductions in seizure severity still elected to remain in the drug trial and demonstrated elevated mood on quality-of-life measures (149).

MR patients receiving LTG should be observed for development of allergic reactions, including pruritus and rash, which can progress to potentially life-threatening Stevens-Johnson syndrome (150).

Tiagabine

TGB (approved as adjunctive therapy for partial seizures) is a generally well-tolerated AED with a CNS side-effect spectrum similar to that of most AEDs, including dizziness, headache, ataxia, and nervousness (151). One study in intractable epileptic patients demonstrated improvements in mood among patients converted to TGB monotherapy. Mood elevation was not correlated with seizure reduc-

tion, suggesting that positive psychotropic benefits may be independent of antiepileptic effects (152). Limited case series also note potential benefits against bipolar disorder (153). TGB-induced absence status epilepticus recently was reported to be responsible for personality changes and behavioral abnormalities in patients with partial seizure disorders who received this drug (154). The literature on the use of TGB in the MR population is sparse, perhaps because of its limited utility in generalized seizure disorders.

Vigabatrin

VGB, which has been prescribed extensively outside the United States, appears to have a significant risk of inducing adverse psychiatric events, particularly psychosis (155). Risk factors may include severe epileptic disorders, a sudden reduction in seizure frequency, and a past history of psychosis. In children with static encephalopathies or hyperactive behavior, VGB (especially in high doses) may exacerbate hyperkinesia (156, 157); therefore, caution is advised when using VGB in patients with established psychopathology or static encephalopathies. Doses should be advanced slowly, and acute withdrawal of the drug should be avoided (158). Alternatively, there have been reports of favorable psychotropic effects of VGB, such as its utility in treating posttraumatic stress disorder (159). Recent evidence of potential constriction of visual fields also limits the current use of VGB.

Felbamate

The introduction of FBM several years ago was greeted with great enthusiasm as the first in a series of drugs termed "the new AEDs." FBM was particularly welcome for its potential contribution to the treatment of refractory epilepsy syndromes in the MR population, including Lennox-Gastaut syndrome. Subsequent discoveries about its association with fatal hepatitis and aplastic anemia have greatly restricted its use.

Anecdotal experience with FBM suggests that it has stimulant-like properties that may be experienced favorably or unfavorably by patients. Although some patients experienced increased alertness, improved attention, and enhanced concentration abilities as a welcome contrast to the sedation associated other AEDs, other patients complained of anorexia, insomnia, and anxiety (160–162). Numerous reports of mania, psychosis, and behavioral disturbances have been noted in association with use of FBM (163,164).

Topiramate

TPM is an AED with broad-spectrum antiepileptic properties recently approved by the Food and Drug Administration. Psychomotor slowing has been well reported with this AED. This adverse event is particularly common among patients on polytherapy and in those who have received rapidly advancing doses (165–167). In double-blind, placebo-controlled, and open-label trials of TPM administered to patients with partial-onset seizures, the most common adverse effects, observed in greater than 10% of subjects, included somnolence, psychomotor slowing, difficulty with memory, difficulty with concentration or attention, and speech or language problems (Natalie Addi, Ortho-McNeil Pharmaceuticals, *personal communication,* 2000) (168). Slow escalation of TPM dose and reduction of polypharmacy may permit better tolerance of the drug (169,170). Among healthy young adults randomized in blinded fashion to receive TPM, GPN, or LTG (171), only the TPM group demonstrated statistically significant declines on measures of attention and word fluency at both acute doses, and also persisting at 2- and 4-week intervals. Although TPM acute dosing was higher and chronic administration was escalated more rapidly than in current clinical practice, this study supports previous experience with TPM. Of note, self-reported ratings on the anger-hostility subscales of the Profile of Mood States Inventory also were elevated in the TPM group.

A recent double-blind, randomized trial of TPM in Lennox-Gastaut syndrome found 33% of patients experienced a 50% or greater reduction in seizures. In this study, 42% of patients experienced somnolence, 40% had anorexia, 21% experienced nervousness, and 21% demonstrated behavioral problems. Although no patients discontinued therapy because of an adverse event, one wonders whether this population may have been too cognitively impaired to communicate about the severity of their distress from side effects. For the clinician considering using TPM in this population, at this time it is unclear whether cognitive function is only mildly or severely compromised beyond baseline and how much this should impact on the risk-to-benefit ratio associated with this drug.

Anecdotal experience and several reports suggest that TPM may cause symptoms of depression, although this may be due in part to a reaction to the cognitive side effects (172–175). Anxiety, irritability, behavioral problems, and even symptoms of psychosis (176) have been noted in patients treated with TPM (86).

In contrast, a few recent reports indicate that TPM may be useful in treating both the manic and depressive phases of bipolar disorder (177–179). Because weight gain is often a serious side effect of the medications used to treat bipolar disorder, TPM's promotion of weight loss may be an advantage of this drug over other mood stabilizers (180). Patients using TPM should be advised to drink plenty of fluids, because TPM may be associated with a two- to four-fold increased risk of nephrolithiasis (172).

Vagal Nerve Stimulation

Vagal nerve stimulation (VNS), a novel therapy for partial and generalized epilepsy, involves the repetitive stimulation of the left vagus nerve via connections from a programmable neurocybernetic prosthesis (NCB) implanted in the left upper chest region (181). Intermittent VNS may be supplemented by additional activation of the NCB at the time of a seizure by holding a magnet over the left chest wall region. The mechanism of the antiepileptic effect of VNS is unclear, but animal studies suggest that stimulated vagal nerve afferent fibers terminating on the nucleus of the solitary tract (NTS) in the brainstem experience increased GABA transmission or decreased glutamate transmission at the NTS, resulting in inhibition of ascending outputs from the NTS upon numerous forebrain structures and other brainstem nuclei known to play a role in seizure control (182). Projections from the NTS upon limbic structures also may play a role in the potential mood-elevating effects of VNS.

VNS is a generally well-tolerated treatment. Adverse events include hoarseness, tingling sensations in the neck, and intermittent alterations in voice, all of which usually improve significantly over time. Although VNS is a more invasive therapy than the administration of AEDs, it also is associated with a number of advantages over typical AED treatment. Whereas most AEDs, particularly when used in polytherapy, are associated with CNS side effects such as sedation and impairment of cognition, VNS potentially offers antiepileptic effect in the absence of such adverse events.

Although VNS has been studied more extensively in the non-MR epilepsy population with seizures that are partial or partial with secondary generalization, VNS is a welcome addition to the options available to treat the refractory generalized epilepsy syndromes common to the MR population, such as Lennox-Gastaut (183). Preliminary reports of VNS experience in this population have been impressive, with reductions in seizures and increased attention and alertness reported (184). In another report of 15 children with Lennox-Gastaut syndrome or myoclonic epilepsies of infancy, over 25% of patients demonstrated a greater than 50% seizure reduction, although the methods for supporting the claim that behavioral improvements seen were independent of seizure reduction were not clarified (185).

Many clinicians may be concerned about implanting devices in MR patients, fearing that patients will pull at the operative site in the chest wall. Recent experience with VNS has defied these concerns. There has been good tolerance of the NCB implant by these patients; nevertheless, it is advisable to watch such patients carefully in the immediate postoperative period (Paul Devereaux, Cyberonics Corp., *personal communication,* 2000).

Animal models and recent human studies suggest that VNS may enhance memory. Electrical stimulation of the vagus nerve delivered after an aversive learning experience was shown to improve later retention performance in rats (186). In non-MR epileptic patients, a protocol administering electrical stimulation of the vagus nerve versus sham stimulation demonstrated statistically significant higher recognition memory in the former group (187). These studies offer hope for patients with cognitive impairments that are so common among epileptic patients and inherent to patients with MR.

Preliminary evidence from two recent studies suggest that VNS may reduce depressive symptomatology in adult epileptic patients (188,189). The former study found a trend toward statistically significant reduction of dysthymic symptoms on the Cornell Dysthymia Rating Scale (CDRS) compared to symptoms in control patients, although notably there were no significant differences on other mood inventories. There was no correlation between seizure reduction and mood improvements, but specifics of this analysis need to be clarified further. Results from a similar multicenter study are currently being analyzed (189). Current studies are under way examining the potential role of VNS in treating primary depression in nonepileptic patients.

There is little information available about psychotropic effects of VNS in epileptic patients with MR. However, studies in nonepileptic patients described earlier and the potential to reduce the dosage or number of AEDs administered in these patients offer optimism for improving mood and cognition in this population.

SUMMARY

Clinicians caring for epileptic patients with MR need to be well acquainted with psychiatric issues. A careful history and supplementary testing when warranted can help distinguish aberrant behaviors from seizure activity. Careful attention to psychotropic and pharmacokinetic considerations can minimize side effects and optimize patient treatment.

REFERENCES

1. American Psychiatric Association. *Diagnostic and statistical manual of mental disorders,* 4th ed. Washington, DC: American Psychiatric Press, 1994.
2. Hodapp RM, Dykens EM, Mash EJ, et al. Mental retardation. In: Steinberg AA, ed. *Child psychopathology.* New York: Guilford Press, 1996:362–389.
3. Luckasson R, Coulter D, Polloway EA, et al. *Definition, classification, and systems of supports.* Washington, DC: American Association on Mental Retardation, 1992.
4. Harris JC. *Developmental neuropsychiatry.* Oxford: Oxford University Press, 1995.
5. Borthwick-Duffy SA. Epidemiology and prevalence of psychopathology in people with mental retardation. *J Consult Clin Psychol* 1994;52:17–27.
6. Reiss S. Prevalence of dual diagnosis in community-based day programs in the Chicago metropolitan area. *Am J Ment Retard* 1990;94:578–585.
7. Bucknill JC, Tuke DH. *A manual of psychological medicine: containing the history, nosology, description, statistics, diagnosis, pathology, and treatment of insanity.* New York: Hafner, 1858 (1968).
8. Szymanski LS, Eissner BA, Rosefsky QB. *Mental health consultations to residential facilities for retarded persons.* Baltimore: University Park Press, 1980.
9. Quine L. Behavior problems in severely mentally handicapped children. *Psychol Med* 1986;16:895–907.
10. Einfeld SL. Clinical assessment of 4,500 developmentally delayed individuals. *J Ment Deficit Res* 1984;28:129–142.
11. Hauser WA, Hesdorffer DC. *Epilepsy: frequency, causes, and consequences.* New York: Demos Publications, 1990.
12. Sunder TR. Meeting the challenge of epilepsy in persons with multiple handicaps. *J Child Neurol* 1997;12 [Suppl 1]:S38–S43.
13. Coulter DL. Epilepsy and mental retardation: an overview. *Am J Ment Retard* 1993;98:1–11.
14. Goulden KJ, Shinnar S, Koller H, et al. Epilepsy in children with mental retardation: a cohort study. *Epilepsia* 1991;32:690–697.
15. Lund J. Epilepsy and psychiatric disorder in the mentally retarded adult. *Acta Psychiatr Scand* 1985;72:557–562.
16. Deb S, Hunter D. Psychopathology of people with mental handicap and epilepsy II: psychiatric illness. *Br J Psychiatry* 1991;159:26–30.
17. Weisbrot DM, Ettinger AB. Epilepsy and behavior: controversies and caveats. *Neurologist* 1997;3:155–172.
18. Pary RJ. Psychiatric hospitalization of persons with mental retardation, mental illness, and seizure diagnosis. *Am J Ment Retard* 1993;98:58–62.
19. Lesser RP, Lueders H, Dinner DS. Evidence for epilepsy is rare in patients with psychogenic seizures. *Neurology* 1983;33:502–504.
20. Ozkara C, Dreiffus FE. Differential diagnosis in pseudoepileptic seizures. *Epilepsia* 1993;34:294–298.
21. Ramani SV, Quesney LF, Olson D, et al. Diagnosis of hysterical seizures in epileptic patients. *Am J Psychiatry* 1980;137:705–709.
22. Neill JC, Alvarez N. Differential diagnosis of epileptic versus pseudoepileptic seizures in developmentally disabled persons. *Appl Res Ment Retard* 1986;7:285–298.
23. Devinsky O, Sanchez-Villasenor F, Vazques B, et al. Clinical profile of patients with epileptic and nonepileptic seizures. *Neurology* 1996;46:1530–1533.
24. Rapin I. Autistic regression and disintegrative disorder: how important is the role of epilepsy? *Semin Pediatr Neurol* 1995;2:278–285.
25. Lewine JD, Andrews R, Chez M, et al. Magnetoencephalography patterns of epileptiform activity in children with regressive autism spectrum disorders. *Pediatrics* 1999;104:405–418.
26. McKinney W, McGreal DA. An aphasic syndrome in children. *Can Med Assoc J* 1974;110:637–639.
27. Lerman P, Lerman-Sagie T, Kivity S. Effect of early corticosteroid therapy for Landau-Kleffner Syndrome. *Dev Med Child Neurol* 1991;33:257–266.
28. Marescaux C, Hirsch E, Finck S, et al. Landau-Kleffner Syndrome: pharmacologic study of five cases. *Epilepsia* 1990;31:768–777.
29. Morrell F, Whisler WW, Smith MC, et al. Landau-Kleffner syndrome: treatment with subpial intracortical transection. *Brain* 1995;18:1529–1546.
30. Gates JR, Ramani V, Whalen S, et al. Ictal characteristics of pseudoseizures. *Arch Neurol* 1985;42:1183–1187.
31. Gulick TA, Spinks IP, King DW. Pseudoseizures: ictal phenomena. *Neurology* 1982;32:24–30.
32. Krumholz A. Nonepileptic seizures: diagnosis and management. *Neurology* 1999;53:S76–S83.
33. Gates JR, Luciano D, Devinsky O. The classification and treatment of nonepileptic events. In: Devinsky O, Theodore W, eds. *Epilepsy and behavior.* New York: Wiley-Liss, 1991:251–263.
34. Leis AA, Ross MA, Summers AK. Psychogenic seizures: ictal characteristics and diagnostic pitfalls. *Neurology* 1992;42:95–99.
35. Saygi S, Katz A, Marks DA, et al. Frontal lobe partial seizures and psychogenic seizures: comparison of clinical and ictal characteristics. *Neurology* 1992;42:1274–1277.
36. Williamson PD, Spencer DD, Spencer SS, et al. Complex partial seizures of frontal lobe origin. *Ann Neurol* 1985;18:497–504.
37. Bergen D, Ristanovic R. Weeping is a common element during psychogenic nonepileptic seizures. *Arch Neurol* 1993;50:1059–1060.
38. Devinsky O, Kelley K, Porter RJ, et al. Clinical and electroencephalographic features of simple partial seizures. *Neurology* 1988;38:1347–1352.
39. Thacker K, Devinsky O, Perrine K, et al. Nonepileptic seizures during apparent sleep. *Ann Neurol* 1993;33:414–418.
40. Wyllie E, Luders H, MacMillan J, et al. Serum prolactin levels after epileptic seizures. *Neurology* 1984;34:1601–1064.

41. Sperling M, Pritchard P III, Engel J, et al. Prolactin in partial epilepsy: an indicator of limbic seizures. *Ann Neurol* 1986;20:716–722.

42. Aman M, Singh N. Patterns of drug use, methodological considerations, measurement techniques, and future trends. (*in preparation*).

43. Spreat S, Conroy J. Use of psychotropic medications for persons with mental retardation who live in Oklahoma nursing homes. *Psychiatr Serv* 1998;49:510–512.

44. Strub RL, Benson FD, Blumen D. *Acute confusional state.* New York: Grune & Stratton, 1982.

45. Daniel DG, Rabin PL. Disguise of delirium. *South Med J* 1985;78:666–671.

46. Dubin WR, Weiss KJ, Zeccardi JA. Organic brain syndrome: the psychiatric impostor. *JAMA* 1983;249: 60–62.

47. Krishef CH, DiNitto DM. Alcohol abuse among mentally retarded individuals. *Ment Retard* 1981;19: 151–155.

48. Krishef CH. Do the mentally retarded drink? A study of their alcohol usage. *J Alcohol Drug Educ* 1986;31: 64–70.

49. Westermeyer J, Kemp K, Nugent S. Substance disorder among persons with mild mental retardation. *Am J Addict* 1996;5:23–31.

50. King BH, DeAntonio C, McCracken JT, et al. Psychiatric consultation in severe and profound mental retardation. *Am J Psychol* 1994;151:1802–1808.

51. Griffin JC, Williams DE, Stark MT, et al. Injurious behavior: a state-wide prevalence survey of the extent and circumstances. *Appl Res Ment Retard* 1986;7:105–116.

52. Cook EH, Rowlett R, Jaselskis C, et al. Fluoxetine treatment of children and adults with autistic disorder and mental retardation. *J Am Acad Child Adolesc Psychiatry* 1992;31:739–745.

53. Handen BJ, Breaux AM, Jonosky J, et al. Effects and noneffects of methylphenidate in children with mental retardation and ADHD. *J Am Acad Child Adolesc Psychiatry* 1992;31:455–461.

54. Aman MG, Dern RA, McGhee DE, et al. Fenfluramine and methylphenidate in children with mental retardation and ADHD: laboratory effects. *J Am Acad Child Adolesc Psychiatry* 1993;32:851–859.

55. Kastner T, Finesmith R, Walsh K. Long-term administration of valproic acid in the treatment of affective symptoms in people with mental retardation. *J Clin Psychopharmacol* 1993;13:448–451.

56. McDougle CJ, Holmes, JP, Carlson DC, et al. A double-blind, placebo-controlled study of risperidone in adults with autistic disorder and other pervasive developmental disorders. *Arch Gen Psychiatry* 1998;55:633–641.

57. Anderson LT, Campbell M, Adams P, et al. The effects of haloperidol on discrimination learning and behavioral symptoms in autistic children. *J Autism Dev Disord* 1989;19:227–239.

58. Perry R, Campbell M, Adams P, et al. Long-term efficacy of haloperidol in autistic children: continuous versus discontinuous administration. *J Am Acad Child Adolesc Psychiatry* 1989;28:87–92.

59. Itil TM, Soldatos C. Epileptogenic side effects of psychotropic drugs: practical recommendations. *JAMA* 1980;244:1460–1463.

60. Denney D, Stevens JR. Clozapine and seizures. *Biol Psychiatry* 1995;37:427–433.

61. Kando JC, Tohen M, Castillo J, et al. Concurrent use of clozapine and valproate in affective and psychotic disorders. *J Clin Psychiatry* 1994;55:255–257.

62. Zingarelli G, Ellman G, Hom A, et al. Clinical effects of naltrexone on autistic behavior. *Am J Ment Retard* 1992;97:57–63.

63. Campbell M, Anderson LT, Small AM, et al. Naltrexone in autistic children: behavioral symptoms and attentional learning. *J Am Acad Child Adolesc Psychiatry* 1993;32:1283–1291.

64. Arnold LE, Aman MG. Beta blockers in mental retardation and developmental disorders. *J Child Adolesc Psychopharmacol* 1991;1:361–373.

65. Connor DF. Nadolol for self-injury, overactivity, inattention and aggression in a child with pervasive developmental disorder. *J Child Adolesc Psychopharmacol* 1994;4:101–111.

66. Connor DF, Ozbayrak KR, Sheldon B, et al. A pilot study of nadolol for overt aggression in developmentally delayed individuals. *Am Acad Child Adolesc Psychiatry* 1997;36:826–834.

67. Craft M, Ismail IA, Krishnamurti D, et al. Lithium in the treatment of aggression in mentally handicapped patients: a double-blind trial. *Br J Psychiatry* 1987; 150:685–689.

68. Ratey J, Sovner R, Parks A, et al. Buspirone treatment of aggression and anxiety in mentally retarded patients: a multiple baseline, placebo lead-in study. *J Clin Psychiatry* 1991;52:159–162.

69. McConnell H, Duncan D. Treatment of psychiatric comorbidity in epilepsy. In: McConnell H, Snyder P, eds. *Psychiatric comorbidity in epilepsy.* Washington, DC: American Psychiatric Press, 1998:245–361.

70. Kanner AM, Nieto JCR. Depressive disorders in epilepsy. *Neurology* 1999;53[Suppl]:S26–S32.

71. Blumer D. Antidepressant and double antidepressant treatment for the affective disorder of epilepsy. *J Clin Psychiatry* 1997;58:3–11.

72. Power B, Hackett L, Dusci L. Antidepressant toxicity and the need for identification and concentration monitoring in overdose. *Clin Pharmacokinet* 1995;29: 154–171.

73. Rasmussen J, Johnson A. Incidence of seizures during treatment with antidepressants, including the new selective serotonin re-uptake inhibitor paroxetine. *Proc 5th World Congr Biol Psychiatry* 1991:40–41.

74. Fromm G, Amores C, Thies W. Imipramine in epilepsy. *Arch Neurol* 1972;27:198–204.

75. Peck A, Stern W, Watkinson C. Incidence of seizures during treatment with tricyclic antidepressant drugs and bupropion. *J Clin Psychiatry* 1983;44:197–201.

76. Delucchi G, Calabrese J. Anticonvulsants for the treatment of manic depression. *Cleve Clin J Med* 1989;56: 756–761.

77. Bell AJ, Cole A, Eccleston D, et al. Lithium neurotoxicity at normal therapeutic levels. *Br J Psychiatry* 1993;162:688–692.

78. Coulter DL. Comprehensive management of epilepsy in persons with mental retardation. *Epilepsia* 1997;38 [Suppl 4]:S24–S31.

79. Rivinus TM. Psychiatric effects of the anticonvulsant regimens. *J Clin Psychopharmacol* 1982;2:165–192.

80. Devinsky O. Cognitive and behavioral effects of AEDs. Annual course of the American Epilepsy Society: new developments in antiepileptic drug therapy, New Orleans, Louisiana, 1994:E1–E50.

81. Bourgeois BFD. Antiepileptic drugs, learning, and behavior in childhood epilepsy. *Epilepsia* 1998;39: 913–921.
82. Ettinger AB, Weisbrot DM, Krupp LB, et al. Fatigue and depression in epilepsy. *J Epilepsy* 1998;11:105–109.
83. Bates ER, Wilder BJ, Brown R, et al. Antiepileptic drug reduction program at a center for the developmentally disabled. *Epilepsia* 1991;32[Suppl 3]:3(abst).
84. Schmidt D. Reduction of two-drug therapy in intractable epilepsy. *Epilepsia* 1983;24:368–376.
85. Bennet HS, Dunlop T, Ziring PR. Reduction of polypharmacy for epilepsy in an institution for the retarded. *Dev Med Child Neurol* 1983;25:735–737.
86. Ketter TA, Post RM, Theodore WH. Positive and negative psychotropic effects of antiepileptic drugs in patients with seizure disorders. *Neurology* 1999;53 [Suppl 1]:S52–S66.
87. Ko DY, Rho JM, DeGiorgio CM, et al. Benzodiazepines. In: Engel JJ, Pedley TA, eds. *Epilepsy: a comprehensive textbook.* Philadelphia: Lippincott-Raven Publishers, 1997:1475–1489.
88. Rickels K, Chung HR, Csanalosi IB, et al. Alprazolam, diazepam, imipramine, and placebo in outpatients with major depression. *Arch Gen Psychiatry* 1987;44: 862–866.
89. Bradwejn J, Shriqui C, Koszycki D, et al. Double-blind comparison of the effects of clonazepam and lorazepam in acute mania. *J Clin Psychopharmacol* 1990;10:403–408.
90. Farrell K. Symptomatic generalized epilepsy and Lennox-Gastaut syndrome. In: Wyllie E, ed. *The treatment of epilepsy*, 2nd ed. Baltimore: Williams & Wilkins, 1996:530–539.
91. Schoch P, Moreau JL, Martin JR, et al. Aspects of benzodiazepine receptor structure and function with relevance to drug tolerance and dependence. *Biochem Soc Symp* 1993;59:121–134.
92. Bittencourt PRM, Richens A. Anticonvulsant-induced status epilepticus in Lennox-Gastaut syndrome. *Epilepsia* 1981;22:129–134.
93. Prior PF, Maclaine GN, Scot DF, et al. Tonic status epilepticus precipitated by intravenous diazepam in a child with petit mal status. *Epilepsia* 1982;13: 467–472.
94. Hauser P, Devinsky O, DeBellis M, et al. Benzodiazepine withdrawal delirium with catatonic features. *Arch Neurol* 1989;46:696–699.
95. Stoudemire A, Fogel BS. *Psychiatric care of the medical patient.* New York: Oxford University Press, 1993.
96. Poindexter AR, Berglund JA, Kolstoe PD. Changes in antiepileptic drug prescribing patterns in large institutions: preliminary results of a five-year experience. *Am J Ment Retard* 1993;98:34–40.
97. Rickels K, Pereira-Ogan JA, Chung HR, et al. Bromazepam and phenobarbital in anxiety: a controlled study. *Curr Ther Res Clin Exp* 1973;15:679–690.
98. Schaffer LC, Schaffer CB, Caretto J. The use of primidone in treatment of refractory bipolar disorder. *Ann Clin Psychiatry* 1999;11:61–66.
99. Brent DA, Crumrine PK, Varma R, et al. Phenobarbital treatment and major depressive disorder in children with epilepsy. *Pediatrics* 1987;80:909–917.
100. Perrine K, Congett S. Neurobehavioral problems in epilepsy. In: Devinsky O, ed. *Neurologic clinics.* Philadelphia: WB Saunders, 1994:129–152.
101. Ounsted C. The hyperkinetic syndrome in epileptic children. *Lancet* 1955;2:203.
102. Wolf S, Forsythe A. Behavioral disturbance, phenobarbital and febrile seizures. *Pediatrics* 1978;61:728–731.
103. Thorn I. A controlled study of prophylactic long-term treatment of febrile convulsions with phenobarbital. *Acta Neurol Scand* 1975;60[Suppl]:67–73.
104. Corbett JA, Trimble MR, Nichol TC. Behavioral and cognitive impairments in children with epilepsy: the longterm effects of anticonvulsant therapy. *J Am Acad Child Psychiatry* 1985;24:17–23.
105. Camfield C, Chaplin S, Doyle AB, et al. Side effects of phenobarbital in toddlers: behavioral and cognitive aspects. *J Pediatr* 1979;95:361–365.
106. Ferrari M, Barabas G, Matthews W. Psychologic and behavioral disturbance among epileptic children treated with barbiturate anticonvulsants. *Am J Psychiatry* 1983;140:112–113.
107. Wilder BJ. Phenytoin: clinical use. In: Levy RH, Mattson RH, Meldrum BS, eds. *Antiepileptic drugs.* New York: Raven Press, 1995:334–344.
108. Dam M. *Phenytoin: toxicity.* New York: Raven Press, 1982.
109. Landolt H. Serial electroencephalographic investigations during psychotic episodes in epileptic patients and during schizophrenic attacks. In: deHass L, ed. *Lectures on epilepsy.* London: Elsevier, 1958.
110. Wolf P. Acute behavioral symptomatology at disappearance of epileptiform EEG abnormality: paradoxical or "forced" normalization. In: Smith D, Treiman D, Trimble M, eds. *Neurobehavioral problems in epilepsy. Advances in neurology.* New York: Raven Press, 1991:127–142.
111. Delgado-Escueta AV, Treiman DM, Walsh GO. The treatable epilepsies. *N Engl J Med* 1983;308: 1508–1514.
112. Deb S, Joyce J. The use of antiepileptic medication in a population-based cohort of adults with learning disability and epilepsy. *Int J Psychiatry Clin Pract* 1999; 3:129–133.
113. Small JG, Klapper MH, Milstein V, et al. Carbamazepine compared with lithium in the treatment of mania. *Arch Gen Psychiatry* 1991;48:915–921.
114. Freeman TW, Clothier JL, Pazzaglia P, et al. A double-blind comparison of valproate and lithium in the treatment of acute mania. *Am J Psychiatry* 1992;149: 108–111.
115. Post RM, Ketter TA, Denicoff K, et al. The place of anticonvulsant therapy in bipolar illness. *Psychopharmacology* 1996;128:115–129.
116. Stoll AL, Banov M, Kolbrener M, et al. Neurologic factors predict a favorable valproate response in bipolar and schizoaffective disorders. *J Clin Psychopharmacol* 1994;14:311–313.
117. Gupta S, O'Connell RO, Parekh A, et al. Efficacy of valproate for agitation and aggression in dementia: case reports. *Int J Geriatr Psychopharmacol* 1998;1: 244–248.
118. Zaret BS, Cohen RA. Reversible valproic acid-induced dementia: a case report. *Epilepsia* 1986;27:234–240.
119. Marescaux C, Warter JM, Micheletti G, et al. Stuporous episodes during treatment with sodium valproate: report of seven cases. *Epilepsia* 1982;23: 297–305.
120. Husain SB, Wical BS. Adverse behavioral effects of

valproate therapy in children with complex partial seizures. *Epilepsia* 1998;39[Suppl 6]:162(abst).

121. Wolf SM, Shinnar S, Kang H, et al. Gabapentin toxicity in children manifesting as behavioral changes. *Epilepsia* 1995;36:1203–1205.

122. Friedman DL, Kastner T, Plummer AT. Adverse behavioral effects in individuals with mental retardation and mood disorders treated with carbamazepine. *Am J Ment Retard* 1992;96:541–546.

123. Smith KR, Goulding PM, Wilderman D, et al. Neurobehavioral effects of phenytoin and carbamazepine in patients recovering from brain trauma: a comparative study. *Arch Neurol* 1994;51:653–660.

124. Snead OC. Exacerbation of seizures in children by carbamazepine. *N Engl J Med* 1985;313:916–921.

125. Shields WD, Saslow E. Myoclonic, atonic and absence seizures following institution of carbamazepine therapy in children. *Neurology* 1983;33:1487–1489.

126. Ojemann LM, Wilensky AJ, Temkin NR, et al. Long-term treatment with gabapentin for partial epilepsy. *Epilepsy Res* 1992;13:159–165.

127. Dimond KR, Pande AC, Lamoreaux L, et al. Effect of gabapentin (Neurontin) on mood and well being in patients with epilepsy. *Prog Neuropsychopharmacol Biol Psychiatry* 1996;20:407–417.

128. Harden C, Pick L. Alterations in mood and anxiety in epilepsy patients treated with gabapentin. *Epilepsia* 1996;37[Suppl 5]:137(abst).

129. Brodie MJ, Richens A, Yuen A. Double-blind comparison of lamotrigine and carbamazepine in newly diagnosed epilepsy. *Lancet* 1995;345:468–476.

130. Handforth A, Treiman DM. Efficacy and tolerance of long-term, high-dose gabapentin: additional observations. *Epilepsia* 1994;35:1032–1037.

131. McElroy SL, Soutullo CA, Keck PE, et al. A pilot trial of adjunctive gabapentin in the treatment of bipolar disease. *Ann Clin Psychiatry* 1997;6:99–103.

132. Ryback RS, Brodsky L, Manasifi F. Gabapentin in bipolar disorder [Letter]. *J Neuropsychiatry Clin Neurosci* 1997;9:301.

133. Knoll J, Stegman K, Suppes T. Clinical experience using gabapentin adjunctively in patients with a history of mania or hypomania. *J Affect Disord* 1998;49:229–233.

134. Schaffer CB, Schaffer LC. Gabapentin in the treatment of bipolar disorder. *Am J Psychiatry* 1997;154:291–292.

135. Young LT, Robb JC, Patelis-Siotis I, et al. Acute treatment of bipolar depression with gabapentin. *Biol Psychiatry* 1997;42:851–853.

136. Ghaemi SN, Katzow JJ, Desai SP, et al. Gabapentin treatment of mood disorders: a preliminary study. *J Clin Psychiatry* 1997;59:426–429.

137. Ryback RS, Ryback L. Gabapentin for behavioral dyscontrol [Letter]. *Am J Psychiatry* 1995;152:1399.

138. Sheldon LJ, Ancill RJ, Holliday SG. Gabapentin in geriatric psychiatry patients. *Can J Psychiatry* 1998;43:422–423.

139. Pollack MH, Matthews J, Scott EL. Gabapentin as a potential treatment for anxiety disorders [Letter]. *Am J Psychiatry* 1998;155:992.

140. Pande AC, Davidson JRT, Jefferson JW, et al. Treatment of social phobia with gabapentin: a placebo controlled study. *J Psychopharmacol* 1999;19:341–348.

141. McManaman J, Tam DA. Gabapentin for self-injurious behavior in Lesch-Nyhan syndrome. *Pediatr Neurol* 1999;20:381–382.

142. Lee DO, Steingard RJ, Cesena M, et al. Behavioral side effects of gabapentin in children. *Epilepsia* 1996;37:87–90.

143. Motte J, Trevathan E, Arvidsson JFV, et al. Lamotrigine for generalized seizures associated with the Lennox-Gastaut syndrome. *N Engl J Med* 1997;337:1807–1812.

144. Beran RG, Gibson RJ. Aggressive behaviour in intellectually challenged patients with epilepsy treated with lamotrigine. *Epilepsia* 1998;39:280–282.

145. Ettinger AB, Weisbrot DM, Saracco J, et al. Positive and negative psychotropic effects of lamotrigine in epilepsy patients with mental retardation. *Epilepsia* 1998;39:874–877.

146. Kotler M, Matar MA. Lamotrigine in the treatment of resistant bipolar disorder. *Clin Neuropharmacol* 1998;21:65–67.

147. Calabrese JR, Fatemi SH, Woyshville MJ. Antidepressant effects of lamotrigine in rapid cycling bipolar disorder [Letter]. *Am J Psychiatry* 1996;153:1236.

148. Kusumakar V, Yatham LN. An open study of lamotrigine in refractory bipolar depression. *Psychiatry Res* 1997;72:145–148.

149. Smith D, Davies G, Dewey M, et al. Outcomes of add-on treatment with lamotrigine in partial epilepsy. *Epilepsia* 1993;34:312–322.

150. Burstein AH. Lamotrigine. *Pharmacotherapy* 1995;15:129–143.

151. Rowan AJ, Uthman B, Ahmann P, et al. Safety and efficacy of three dose levels of tiagabine HCl versus placebo as adjunctive treatment for complex partial seizures. *Epilepsia* 1994;35[Suppl 8]:54.

152. Dodrill CB, Arnett JL, Shu V, et al. Effects of tiagabine monotherapy on abilities, adjustment, and mood. *Epilepsia* 1998;39:33–42.

153. Kaufman KR. Adjunctive tiagabine treatment of psychiatric disorders: three cases. *Ann Clin Psychiatry* 1998;10:181–184.

154. Ettinger AB, Bernal OG, Andriola MR, et al. Two cases of nonconvulsive status epilepticus in association with tiagabine therapy. *Epilepsia* 1999;40:1159–1162.

155. Sander JWAS, Hart YM, Trimble MR, et al. Vigabatrin and psychosis. *J Neurol Neurosurg Psychiatry* 1991;54:435–439.

156. Dulac O, Chiron C, Luna D, et al. Vigabatrin in childhood epilepsy. *J Child Neurol* 1991;6:2S30–2S37.

157. Appelton R. The role of vigabatrin in the management of infantile epileptic syndromes. *Neurology* 1993;43:S21–S23.

158. Ben-Menachem E, French J. Vigabatrin. In: Engel J, Pedley TA, eds. *Epilepsy: a comprehensive textbook.* Philadelphia: Lippincott-Raven Publishers, 1997:1609–1618.

159. Macleod AD. Vigabatrin and posttraumatic stress disorder. *J Clin Psychopharmacol* 1996;16:190–191.

160. Ketter TA, Malow BA, Flamini R, et al. Felbamate monotherapy has stimulant-like effects in patients with epilepsy. *Epilepsy Res* 1996;23:129–137.

161. Asconapé JJ, Brotherton TA, Lauve LM, et al. Felbamate: efficacy and tolerability in patients with refractory epilepsies. *Epilepsia* 1994;35[Suppl 8]:114(abst).

162. Ettinger AB, Jandorf L, Berdia A, et al. Felbamate-induced headache. *Epilepsia* 1996;37:503–505.

163. King JA. Increased incidence of adverse behavioral side effects associated with the addition of felbamate (FBM) to antiepileptic drug (AED) regimens in the mentally retarded (MR) population. *Epilepsia* 1994;35 [Suppl 8]:94(abst).

164. Woodhams KA, Bennett B, Bronstein KS, et al. Behavioral changes in individuals treated with felbamate. *Epilepsia* 1994;35[Suppl 8]:160(abst).

165. Katta PK, Crawford PM. Audit of topiramate use in a general neurology clinic. *Epilepsia* 1998;39:S3(abst).

166. Brodie MJ, Stephen LJ, Kilpatrick WS, et al. Prospective study of topiramate concentration monitoring in refractory epilepsy. *Epilepsia* 1998;39:66.

167. Biton V, Montouris G, Edwards K, et al. Comparison of two upward titration rates in initiation of therapy with topiramate. *Epilepsia* 1996;37:S5.

168. Biton V, Montouris GD, Ritter F, et al. A randomized, placebo-controlled study of topiramate in primary generalized tonic-clonic seizures. Topiramate YTC Study Group. *Neurology* 1999;52:1330–1337.

169. Faught E, French J, Harden C. Postmarketing Antiepileptic Drug Survey Group (PADS). Adverse effects of TPM: results from a large post-marketing survey. *Epilepsia* 1997;38[Suppl 8]:97(abst).

170. Faught E, Kuzniecky R, Gilliam F. Cognitive effects of TPM. *Neurology* 1997;48:336a(abst).

171. Martin R, Kuzniecky R, Ho S, et al. Cognitive effects of topiramate, gabapentin, and lamotrigine in healthy young adults. *Neurology* 1999;52:321–327.

172. Shorvon SD. Safety of topiramate: adverse events and relationships to dosing. *Epilepsia* 1996;37[Suppl 2]: S18–S22.

173. Tassanari CA, Michelucci R, Chauvel P, et al. Double-blind, placebo-controlled trial of topiramate (600 mg daily) for the treatment of refractory partial epilepsy. *Epilepsia* 1996;37:763–768.

174. Abou-Khalil B, Fakhoury T. Neuropsychiatric profile of high-dose topiramate. *Epilepsia* 1997;38[Suppl 8]:207(abst).

175. Betts T, Smith K, Khan G. Severe psychiatric reactions to topiramate. *Epilepsia* 1997;38[Suppl 3]:64(abst).

176. Dohmeier C, Kay A, Greathouse N. Neuropsychiatric complications of topiramate therapy. *Epilepsia* 1998;39[Suppl 6]:189(abst).

177. Marcotte D. Topiramate in the treatment of mood disorders. 151st annual meeting of the American Psychiatric Association. Toronto, Canada, 1998:115(abst).

178. Calabrese JR, Shelton MD III, Keck PE Jr, et al. Pilot study of topiramate in acute severe treatment-refractory mania. *Proc 151st Ann Meet Am Psychiatr Assoc* 1998:121–122.

179. Suppes T, Brown ES, McElroy SL, et al. A pilot trial of adjunctive topiramate in the treatment of bipolar disorder: application of the Stanley Foundation Bipolar Network (SFBN) prospective protocol. *Proc 37th Annu Meet Am Coll Neuropsychopharmacol* 1998: 306(abst).

180. Sherman C. Topiramate may curb bingeing in bipolar patients. *Clin Psychiatry News* 1999:4.

181. Reid SA. Surgical technique for implantation of the neurocybernetic prosthesis. *Epilepsia* 1990;31[Suppl 2]:S38–S39.

182. Walker BR, Easton A, Gale K. Regulation of limbic motor seizures by GABA and glutamate transmission in nucleus tractus solitarius. *Epilepsia* 1999;40: 1051–1057.

183. Ben-Menachem E, Hellstrom K, Waldton C, et al. Evaluation of refractory epilepsy treated with vagus nerve stimulation for up to 5 years. *Neurology* 1999; 52:1265–1267.

184. Helmers SL, Al-Jayyousi M, Madsen J. Adjunctive treatment in Lennox-Gastaut syndrome using vagal nerve stimulation. *Epilepsia* 1998;39[Suppl 6]:169 (abst).

185. Parker APJ, Polkey CE. Vagal nerve stimulation in epileptic encephalopathies. *Pediatrics* 1999;103: 778–782.

186. Clark KB, Krahl SE, Smith DC, et al. Post-training unilateral vagal stimulation enhances retention performance in the rat. *Neurobiol Learn Mem* 1995;63: 213–216.

187. Clark KB, Naritoku DK, Smith DC, et al. Enhanced recognition memory following vagus nerve stimulation in human subjects. *Nat Neurosci* 1999;2:94–98.

188. Harden CL, Pulver MC, Nikolov B, et al. Effects of vagus nerve stimulation on mood in adult epilepsy patients. *Neurology* 1999;52[Suppl 2]:238a(abst).

189. Ettinger AB, Nolan E, Vitale S, et al. Changes in mood and quality of life in adult epilepsy patients treated with vagal nerve stimulation. *Epilepsia* 1999;40: 62(abst).

190. Aman MG, Singh NN. *Aberrant behavior checklist.* East Aurora, NY: Slosson Educational Publications, 1994.

13

Aggressive Behavior in Epilepsy

Steven C. Schachter

Department of Neurology, Harvard Medical School, Boston, Massachusetts 02215

Epilepsy is a model for brain–behavior relationships because seizures affect behavior, and behavior affects seizures. One particularly controversial aspect of this relationship is the disputed association of epilepsy and aggressive or violent behavior (1–7). Many books, papers, and reviews have addressed this topic because of its highly charged medical, legal, and sociological implications (8–19). Nonetheless, there remains considerable debate, uncertainty, and contradictory evidence concerning the extent of the association between epilepsy and aggressive or violent behavior.

A comprehensive review of the neurobiology of aggression, violence, and impulsivity is beyond the scope of this chapter (20,21), but it is pertinent to note that electrical stimulation of limbic structures in animals elicits aggressive or attack behaviors (22–28). Rats with an electrically kindled amygdaloid seizure focus (but no spontaneous seizures) are more aggressive than control rats or those with a kindled focus in the caudate nucleus, suggesting that hippocampal or amygdaloid kindling could be associated with violent behavior even without clinical evidence of a seizure disorder (25). Further, ictal discharges in amygdala, hippocampus, and septal regions have been observed with depth electrodes in several epileptic patients with nonictal episodic aggressive behavior (29) as well as others with ictal aggression (30,31).

The behavioral effects of electrical stimulation and the findings of epileptiform discharges in patients with aggressive behavior do not prove that aggression and epilepsy are related, however. As outlined by Herzberg and Fenwick (32), there are three key questions to be answered:

1. Is the association between aggression and epilepsy due to occurrence of the epileptic seizure itself?
2. Is it due to the associated brain damage that may be the cause of seizures?
3. Is it the result of socioeconomic factors or medication?

This chapter first reviews the available data for these three questions and then outlines the measurement of aggressive behavior, discusses treatment approaches, and highlights legal considerations. The treatment of acute violent behavior in the emergency room is well covered elsewhere (33–35) and will not be discussed here.

IS THE ASSOCIATION BETWEEN AGGRESSION AND EPILEPSY DUE TO OCCURRENCE OF THE EPILEPTIC SEIZURE ITSELF?

Using seizures as a marker in time, aggressive and violent behavior may be considered by their temporal relations to seizures.

Preictal Aggression

In some patients, the seizure prodrome (the minutes, hours, or even days leading up to a seizure) consists of predictable changes in psychological functioning and behavior, including the development of irritability, anxiety, and aggression (36,37).

Ictal Aggression

Directed, purposeful, aggressive, or violent behavior during seizures is generally considered rare. Papers in the literature typically either include cases in which seizures were inferred from the history, or others in which seizures were directly observed by trained professionals or recorded with sophisticated monitoring techniques.

Hindler (38) reported the case of a 19-year-old nanny with a history of febrile convulsions up to the age of 7 years and a positive family history for focal epilepsy in a younger sister. The patient had a more recent history of 5- to 10-minute episodes of strange sensations resulting in a feeling of emptiness and a sensation of her mind becoming separated from her body, followed by intense feelings of hate and aggression directed at the baby in her care. The episodes were triggered by the baby laughing and were only experienced while the nanny and the baby were alone. During one such episode, she swung the baby by the legs and the baby's head hit a cabinet and perhaps the floor, sustaining a fatal brain injury.

After she was incarcerated, her doctor observed her to have a "generalized epileptiform convulsion." An electroencephalogram (EEG) showed epileptiform abnormalities, and she was treated with anticonvulsant therapy with no further abnormal experiences. Hindler concluded that the patient committed murder during an epileptic attack and that she had an unusual form of reflex epilepsy.

One hundred thirty-two prisoners with epilepsy (including 11 who were convicted of murder, attempted murder, rape, attempted rape, and armed violence) were asked if they had ever committed an offense in association with a seizure (39). None of the prisoners admitted to a history of ictal violence, although three reported being arrested for disorderly conduct immediately after a seizure and one had a seizure while a robbery was already in progress.

Directed, purposeful ictal aggression during observed seizures has only been rarely reported (1,40–42). At the Montreal Neurological Institute, Gloor (43) witnessed few, if any, cases of spontaneous or electrically induced ictal aggression. Similarly, Rodin (42) witnessed several hundred spontaneous psychomotor seizures; only one seizure was accompanied by directed aggression, which Rodin concluded was goal directed and an expression of vengeance, rather than related directly to the seizure.

Rodin (42) further reported 57 patients whose bemegride-induced "psychomotor automatisms" were photographed while they were seated in a chair undergoing EEG testing. None of the patients became aggressive during seizures, although two patients were observed to suddenly lunge forward and "show a rather ferocious facial expression." In one case, an unsuccessful attempt by the attending physician to keep the patient seated made the patient clench his fist, adopt a boxer-type stance, and appear imminently violent. The threatening behavior immediately ended once the patient was physically released, suggesting to Rodin a "defensive reaction due to being restrained rather than active trouble-seeking." He postulated that "the patient, if he were to be restrained during his confusional state, might react in a defensive manner that could be misinterpreted as a goal-directed assault." Because the EEG results were not provided, it is possible that this may have been a case of postictal resistive violence (see later).

Ramani and Gumnit (41) recorded focal seizures in 15 epileptic patients with significant histories of episodic aggressive behaviors. No patients showed ictal violent or aggressive behavior.

Delgado-Escueta et al. (1) reviewed the cases of 5,400 patients with epilepsy who underwent inpatient evaluation. They then further studied 19 patients who were believed to have ictal aggression, including three previously reported patients (30,44). Based on a review of 33 seizures, the authors concluded that only one patient committed an aggressive act during a seizure that could have harmed another person (the patient attempted to scratch her psychologist's face). None of the other observed aggressive behaviors threatened the well-being of others, although some behaviors appeared hostile, such as assuming a karate posture and making striking motions, shouting, or spitting; or destroying inanimate objects such as curtains, chairs, and beds.

Other anecdotal reports of aggressive ictal automatisms have documented behaviors such as flailing or chopping movements of the arms, spitting, biting, or physical assaults on nearby objects (31,44,45), which were generally stereotyped and nondirected.

Nonconvulsive status epilepticus may present with psychiatric symptomatology, including psychotic features (46). A report nearly 40 years ago suggested that absence status epilepticus may be associated with hostility, aggression, agitation, and impulsive behavior (47).

Postictal Aggression

Several studies utilizing video EEG monitoring showed that violent behavior may result from attempts at physical restraint during the postictal period, so-called resistive violence (1,45). For example, one patient "exhibited angry facial expressions during ictal episodes and confused, nondirected, aggressive behavior postictally while attempting to free himself of the soft restraints" (41).

Violent behavior may occur during a postictal psychosis, which typically begins within several days of a cluster of complex partial or secondarily generalized seizures and includes hallucinations, paranoia, and delusions (35, 46,48–50). The fear that accompanies the delusions or paranoia may lead to violent behavior, which may be self-directed (51,52).

Kanemoto et al. (52) evaluated aggression in 30 patients with postictal psychosis and 30 patients matched for gender, age, and age of seizure onset with postictal confusion, but no postictal psychosis. All seizures were partial onset, and they were directly observed and documented by trained professionals. A postic-

tal psychosis was diagnosed on the basis of hallucinations, delusions, thought disorder, and affective changes that were clinically demarcated from seizures and the immediate postictal state. Violence was defined as well-directed, well-organized attacks against human beings because of irrational behavior that resulted in a severe injury or a life-threatening situation, such as strangulation. Resistive violence as described earlier was analyzed separately.

In their study, violent attacks occurred in association with 13 (23%) of 57 episodes of postictal psychosis, compared to one of 134 episodes of postictal confusion ($p < 0.001$). In eight postictal psychotic episodes, the violent behavior occurred within 24 hours of the onset of postictal psychosis. Another four patients in the postictal group attempted suicide during their postictal psychosis, compared to none of the controls ($p < 0.005$). On the other hand, four control patients displayed resistive violence during the postictal state compared to none of the patients with postictal psychosis.

Interictal Aggression

Blumer (53,54) described an interictal dysphoric disorder characterized by marked irritability, with troublesome loss of control and often associated with intermittent depressive or euphoric moods, anergia, insomnia, anxiety, and fears. Interictal aggression has generally been studied in selected groups of patients and prisoners with epilepsy. The results in these skewed populations suggest that impulsive, assaultive interictal behavior is seen in up to 56% of patients with temporal lobe epilepsy (TLE) (55–61).

Of 100 children with TLE followed for a mean of 10 years, 36 had outbursts of unspecified "catastrophic rage" (62). Rage outbursts were associated with a history of head injury or cerebral infection, seizure onset under the age of 1 year, and a "disordered" home (defined as gross poverty, deceased mother before the proband was 10 years old, aggressive father, or psychosis or chronic neurosis in one or both parents). There was no relationship between seizure frequency and rage outbursts.

Not all studies find a high incidence of interictal aggression. Rodin (42) reviewed the charts of 700 patients with epilepsy seen at a tertiary referral center over a 5-year period and found that 34 (4.8%) had exhibited "destructive-assaultive" behavior. These aggression-prone patients tended to be young men of lower-than-average intelligence, with a history of behavioral difficulties dating back to school age, who had unspecified signs of diffuse organic disease. There was no association between seizure type or the location of onset and the likelihood of aggressive behavior. Hermann et al. (63) later confirmed these findings.

Ramani and Gumnit (41) studied 19 epileptic patients with significant histories of episodic aggressive behaviors for an average of 6.3 weeks as inpatients with video telemetry. Two patients exhibited repeated aggressive behavior. There was no apparent temporal relationship between the aggression and ictal EEG patterns in one patient, who ripped loose a kitchen sink. Upon admission, 13 patients were irritable and socialized poorly, but this behavior was said to improve in the "supportive ward milieu."

Mendez et al. (64) reviewed the records of 44 epileptic patients attending a university-affiliated neurology clinic who were referred for psychiatric evaluation because of violent interictal behavior (defined as the forceful infliction of injury or harm on persons or property). Most of the violent acts consisted of verbal or minor physical aggression. Compared to nonviolent age- and sex-matched epileptic patients, the violent patients did not differ on seizure variables such as type and frequency of seizures, auras, EEG findings, age of seizure onset, or antiepileptic drug (AED) treatment. The authors concluded that interictal violence in their sample was not associated with epileptiform activity or other seizure variables.

Herzberg and Fenwick (32) retrospectively reviewed the charts of patients admitted to the epilepsy unit of the Maudsley Hospital over a 10-year period with a discharge diagnosis of TLE. Aggressive behavior was associated with male sex, early age of seizure onset, and a history of chronic behavioral difficulties. No relationship was found with specific EEG or computed tomgographic scan findings or a history of psychosis.

Kanemoto et al. (52) studied the incidence of interictal violence in 33 patients with localization-related epilepsy and acute interictal psychosis. Violent attacks occurred in association with three of 62 interictal psychotic episodes, which was significantly less than the incidence of violent attacks that occurred in other patients during postictal psychoses ($p < 0.01$).

Among adolescent and adult prisoners, the prevalence of EEG abnormalities and epilepsy has been reported to be as high as 65% and 18%, respectively (16,39,65–68). Because the prevalence of epilepsy in prisons may be similar to the prevalence of epilepsy in the underprivileged, lower socioeconomic communities from which prisoners typically originate (69), these studies do not necessarily prove that epilepsy is more frequent among prisoners.

Several studies of prisoners attempted to correlate epilepsy with violence. Lewis et al. (65) retrospectively reviewed records of incarcerated adolescent boys and found that the number of "psychomotor symptoms" correlated with degree of violence (as measured by a scale derived by the authors). In contrast, two other studies found that prisoners with epilepsy were not convicted of more serious or more violent crimes than age- and race-matched nonepileptic prisoners (39,66,68).

IS AGGRESSION DUE TO THE ASSOCIATED BRAIN DAMAGE THAT MAY BE THE CAUSE OF SEIZURES OR THE RESULT OF SOCIOECONOMIC FACTORS OR MEDICATION?

Several studies showed a high prevalence of head injury in violent patients with epilepsy, suggesting that brain damage is the more proximate cause of poor impulse control and violent behavior, rather than seizures (65,70,71). Among 18 incarcerated adolescent boys with definite or probable epilepsy, 16 (89%) had histories of severe brain trauma and/or perinatal difficulties (65). In another study, head trauma was the probable cause of seizures in 45% of adult prisoners with epilepsy using rigorous diagnostic criteria (39).

Another cause of violent behavior in patients with epilepsy is psychosis (72,73). Interictal psychosis and other psychopathology are increased in patients with epilepsy (74), and psychosis in nonepileptic patients is associated with violent behavior, especially in conjunction with delusions (75–77). In an unselected Swedish birth cohort followed up to the age of 30 years, men with schizophrenia and major affective disorders were four times more likely than men with no mental disorder to commit a violent offense; among women with major mental disorders there was a 27-fold increase (72).

Among 18 incarcerated adolescent boys with definite or probable epilepsy, paranoid ideation and hallucinations were common and contributed to violent acts (65). In another series, violent epileptic patients were significantly more likely to meet the diagnostic criteria for a schizophrenic disorder compared to nonviolent age- and sex-matched epileptic patients ($p < 0.001$) (64). Although not reaching statistical significance, violent patients also were twice as likely to be diagnosed with depression or bipolar disease and an adjustment disorder. One patient impulsively killed someone with an automobile in association with paranoid ideation; a court-ordered neuropsychiatric evaluation concluded that the violence resulted from a paranoid schizophrenic state.

Cognitive and Behavioral Disorders

Mild-to-severe cognitive deficits, especially in the domains of attention, memory, and motor speed, are associated with epilepsy in many patients (78) and may contribute to violent behavior. In a Swedish study, intellectually handicapped men were five times more likely than men with no handicap to commit a violent offense; among intellectually handi-

capped women there was a 25-fold increase (72). Several studies showed a high incidence of mental retardation and chronic behavioral disorders in violent patients with epilepsy (32). Mendez et al. (64) found that violent epileptic patients were significantly more likely to be mentally retarded compared to nonviolent age- and sex-matched epileptic patients ($p < 0.01$).

Neuroendocrinologic Dysfunction

Measurable hormonal changes accompany seizures (79), epileptiform discharges (80, 81), and AED therapy (82–86). Whether these hormonal changes are surrogate markers for neuronal dysfunction or related to specific behaviors is not known.

Prolactin and cortisol are of particular interest. Low prolactin levels have been linked to psychosis (87,88), and an increase in the rate of metabolism of a radioactive dopa tracer has been demonstrated in the neostriatum of patients with limbic seizures and psychosis (89). Leiderman et al. (90) studied the correlations of neuroendocrine function with psychopathology, seizure variables, and neuropsychological function in 16 male patients with limbic epilepsy and found a correlation between low prolactin concentrations and thinking disturbance on the Brief Psychiatric Rating Scale.

Cortisol concentrations may increase following seizures (91,92), and high serum cortisol concentrations are associated with fear-based defensive aggression in rhesus monkeys (93). The relationships between postictal resistive violence, postictal fear, and postictal cortisol concentrations remain to be explored.

Episodic Dyscontrol

Episodic dyscontrol (*Diagnostic and Statistical Manual of Mental Disorders, Fourth Edition* [DSM-IV] classification 312.34, Intermittent Explosive Disorder) is characterized by episodic violent behavior in patients who do not otherwise have an aggressive personality disorder. The patient's temper escalates over minutes and greatly out of proportion to the nature of the provocation, which is trivial, if any (51). The episodes generally occur in the presence of other people who are emotionally important to the patient and last for 20 to 30 minutes. Patients are unable to terminate the episode once it is in progress. Afterward, patients are remorseful, regretful, or embarrassed, and they understand that their temper was excessive under the circumstances. The relationship of episodic dyscontrol to epilepsy is unclear (94,95) and the etiology is unknown, although epileptiform discharges in limbic structures may play a role (51).

Socioeconomic Factors

Antisocial, violent behavior often is associated with a childhood history of impulsive behavior. Other contributing factors are living in a crowded environment, disrupted and unstable home environments, accessibility of guns, decline of cultural constraints, and violent role models, especially parents who incorporate physical punishment in their child-rearing practices (57,70,76,96).

Iatrogenic Causes

Aggressive or violent behavior may be due to corticosteroids, digitalis, L-dopa, isoniazid, anticholinergic drugs, antihistamines, antabuse, propranolol, indomethacin, bromocriptine, and sedatives (33). In patients with epilepsy, AEDs may cause aggressive behavior, particularly as a consequence of a psychosis associated with complete seizure control (forced normalization) (97) or due to sedation and disinhibition. Thus, before initiating additional pharmacotherapy, reducing the dose of a sedating AED may be reasonable, particularly if seizures are well controlled.

Another unusual cause of iatrogenic aggression due to AEDs is acute intermittent porphyria, which results from inherited abnormalities of the enzyme porphobilinogen deaminase (98–100). Acute attacks can be triggered by many AEDs and last for a day to weeks. Prominent symptoms include abdominal pain, constipation, tachycardia, and seizures. Patients often are delirious and psychotic, and they may exhibit aggressive or violent behavior.

Miscellaneous

Violent behavior may occur during a delirium, which usually is characterized by inattention, agitation, hallucinations, delusions, and restlessness. Delirium may be due to drug (substance) and alcohol abuse or withdrawal in patients with or without a history of psychosis (75,101). Amphetamines, diet pills, cocaine, phencyclidine, opioids, and lysergic acid diethylamide (LSD) are particularly likely to cause aggression. Other medical conditions to consider are hypoxemia, hypoglycemia, and thyrotoxicosis.

INSTRUMENTS FOR MEASURING AGGRESSIVE BEHAVIOR

There is no widely used instrument for measuring aggressive behavior in patients with epilepsy, in part because of the problems inherent in assessing aggression in this population (102,103). Even so, the Resentment-Aggression scale on the Minnesota Multiphasic Personality Inventory (MMPI) and the Aggression scale of the Bear-Fedio Inventory have been utilized for research purposes in epilepsy patients, as have several other tools (57,63,65,104).

Many scales and inventories have been developed, validated, and used in studies of aggressive behavior in nonepileptic populations, such as head-injured and demented patients. The Behavior Rating Scale for Dementia was designed to measure behaviors, including irritability and aggression, in patients with dementia (105). The Neurobehavioral Functioning Inventory addresses somatic, cognitive, behavioral, communication, and social problems and has been used in head-injured patients (106,107).

Other available instruments include the Buss-Durkee Hostility Inventory, which is completed by self-report, and includes subscales for indirect assault, irritability, verbal assault, and direct assault (108); the Subtraction Aggression Paradigm, a computerized test designed to provoke aggressive behavior (109); the Barratt Impulsiveness Scale (110); the Agitated Behavior Scale (111); and several others (112–118).

TREATMENT CONSIDERATIONS

Aggressive behavior probably is underreported to physicians for a variety of reasons, including embarrassment, the desire to keep such behavior personal, and a lack of appreciation that it may be treatable. Most neurologists, in turn, do not take sufficiently detailed histories of aggressive behavior. Thus, the assessment of aggressive behavior must begin with heightened awareness by physicians, who should inform patients and families in a reassuring manner that aggressive behavior can occur in association with epilepsy for a number of reasons, some of which are reversible. The physician should ask patients and their families specific and directed questions to determine whether the behavior in question is disruptive, destructive, or dangerous and, therefore, necessary to further evaluate and address. Aggressive behavior can be viewed along a spectrum; the point at which it requires evaluation and possible treatment will depend on the individual circumstances and cultural setting.

In general, the appropriate treatment of aggressive or violent behavior in a patient with epilepsy depends on the cause. Ictal aggression due to isolated seizures or nonconvulsive status epilepticus responds to AED therapy. Postictal resistive violence is avoided by limiting physical restraint during the postictal period when possible (44,119). Aggression or violence during a postictal psychosis is prevented by eliminating clusters of seizures and treated acutely with benzodiazepines and dopamine blockers, particularly haloperidol (11,46). Psychiatric hospitalization is recom- mended if the patient is at risk of impulsive, potentially self-injurious behavior.

Interictal aggression is somewhat more complicated to treat because it does not necessarily improve with complete seizure control (9,120). Controlled studies are unavailable, but AEDs and psychoactive drugs have been used empirically.

Antiepileptic Drugs

AEDs have been used to treat aggressive and violent behavior in nonepileptic patients. Carbamazepine (CBZ) has been shown effective for episodic dyscontrol (121,122) as well as for violent behavior in patients with psychiatric disorders and no evidence of EEG abnormalities (123). An open trial of CBZ 400 to 800 mg per day for 8 weeks in ten nonepileptic patients with agitation and anger outbursts following closed head injuries reduced irritability and disinhibition, and resulted in improvement on the Agitated Behavior Scale in eight patients (80%) (111). A placebo-controlled, double-blind, randomized trial of CBZ for treatment of agitation and aggression in 51 nursing home residents with dementia showed statistically significant efficacy for CBZ (mean serum level 5.3 µg/mL) compared to placebo (124). CBZ also may be beneficial for agitation in patients with Alzheimer's disease whose behavior fails to improve with neuroleptics (125).

Other AEDs may be beneficial. Valproate shows possible efficacy in the treatment of agitation, impulsive aggression, and episodic dyscontrol (51,126). There have been several reports of a beneficial effect of gabapentin and lorazepam for agitation in nonepileptic patients, including patients with Alzheimer's disease (127–129).

Psychoactive Drugs

Clozapine, an atypical antipsychotic agent that does not cause extrapyramidal side effects, reduces aggressive and violent behavior associated with a psychosis, including self-mutilating behavior (130,131). However, dose-related seizures occur in 3% to 5% of treated patients (35). Other atypical neuroleptic agents with lower propensity for reducing seizure threshold may be considered as alternative choices. Antidepressants may be useful for the interictal dysphoric disorder described by Blumer (53).

Psychosurgery

From the 1950s through the 1970s, amygdalectomies were recommended by some proponents for treatment of aggressive behavior, including use in patients with epilepsy (102,132). No controlled studies were performed, behavioral outcomes were not quantified, and selection criteria are not yet understood (11,51,103).

LEGAL CONSIDERATIONS

From 1889 through 1981, epilepsy was used as a defense against charges of murder, homicide, manslaughter, or disorderly conduct in 15 appellate cases (1). From 1977 through 1981, epileptic automatisms were used as part of a "diminished legal responsibility" or "insanity" defense against 12 charges of violent crimes, including five murder cases in 1979 (1). In one well-publicized case, a New York City policeman pleaded "mental illness" to a charge of murder (133). A psychiatrist testifying for the defendant stated that the police officer shot and killed a 15-year-old boy, apparently without being provoked, either during a seizure or because of a "psychosis associated with epilepsy." The defendant had no prior history of epilepsy, and neurologists testified he did not have epilepsy. The jury found him not guilty, and he was committed to a state hospital. Other psychiatrists and neurologists concluded he did not have epilepsy. He subsequently was released upon order from the court because there was no documented proof that he had mental illness and posed a danger to others.

Physicians may be called on to render an opinion whether a particular patient committed an aggressive or violent act in conjunction with a seizure. In 1981, a panel of epileptologists suggested five relevant criteria to determine whether a violent crime resulted from an epileptic seizure (1):

1. The diagnosis should be established by at least one neurologist with special competence in epilepsy.
2. The presence of epileptic automatisms should be documented by the history and by closed-circuit television and EEG monitoring.
3. The presence of aggression during epileptic automatisms should be verified in a videotape-recorded seizure in which ictal epileptiform patterns also are recorded on the EEG.
4. The aggressive or violent act should be characteristic of the patient's habitual seizures.
5. A clinical judgment should be made by the neurologist, attesting to the possibility that the alleged crime was part of a seizure.

In 1989, Hindler (38) suggested the following less stringent criteria for determining that a crime was committed during a seizure:

1. An unequivocal past history of epileptic attacks,
2. The crime is out of character with the accused person's previous personality,
3. The crime is motiveless and unpremeditated,
4. EEG studies are compatible,
5. An altered state of consciousness during the event, and
6. Total or partial amnesia for the crime.

CONCLUSIONS

There are multiple determinants to violent and aggressive behavior, and new techniques, such as neuroimaging studies, are expanding our understanding of the neurobiology of these behaviors (134,135). However, the practical limitations of studying epilepsy and violence and the methodologic problems reported in the literature have hampered our understanding of the causal relationships between seizures and aggression, even though, as observed by Devinsky and Bear (56), "it would be difficult to cite, either from case reports or a literature review, another medical or neurologic illness in which aggressive behavior is described so regularly." Nonetheless, the available evidence suggests that seizures and the brain pathology that underlies seizures may give rise to aggression in some patients with postictal confusion who are restrained, patients with postictal psychosis, and some patients during the interictal period.

Studies of ictal aggression have been limited by a number of factors. Patients are observed in unnatural environments, such as hospital rooms, and seize under circumstances that may be unusual for them, for example, in bed or in a locked room (32). Observers are generally trained professionals who are taught not to apply restraint during or after seizures. These factors probably influence the incidence and nature of seizure-related behavior (44).

Recording seizures in patients with very violent behavior is technically difficult and ethically problematic. Therefore, it is unlikely that a case of ictal or postictal violence that involves a series of organized purposeful behaviors, if it exists, could ever be electrographically confirmed. Although the current evidence argues against the possibility of goal-directed ictal aggression, absence of proof is not necessarily proof of absence.

Studies of ictal aggression generally are performed in tertiary referral centers with patients who are referred for evaluation of particularly severe or unusual seizures. Such patients tend to have significant cognitive and behavioral disorders and psychosocial difficulties. The highly selected nature of this population may bias the likelihood of documenting aggressive behavior. Similarly, studies of interictal aggression generally rely on specific cohorts, such as incarcerated prisoners or subjects at detention centers or group homes, rather than a random sampling of patients with epilepsy in the community, and the reliability of medical information and data acquisition varies substantially between studies.

Many previous studies have lacked adequate control groups. Numerous confounding and interrelated variables must be considered in future studies of epilepsy and aggression (Table 13.1), including seizure type, specific auras, ictal automatisms, postictal behavior, whether the patient is already engaged in a threatening situation when the seizure begins, seizure medications, and fluctuations in serum concentrations. Other important variables are a history of violence prior to the onset of seizures, history of drug or alcohol abuse, intelligence level, brain injury/pathology, comorbid cognitive and psychiatric disorders, neuroendocrine function, and psychosocial variables, such as coping mechanisms, socioeconomic status, and family structure.

In addition to adequate controls, studies must be sufficiently powered; otherwise, negative findings are inconclusive. Further, researchers must develop a practical taxonomy of aggressive behavior (Intermittent Explosive Disorder is the only DSM-IV diagnosis that recognizes aggressive behavior), precise terminology (20), and tools for measuring aggressive and violent behavior in patients with

TABLE 13.1. *Variables that should be controlled in studies of epilepsy and aggression*

Seizure-related variables
  Seizure type(s) and age of onset
  Etiology of seizures/epilepsy syndrome/
    electroencephalographic findings
  Nature of auras and ictal automatisms
  Postictal behavior/psychosis
  Temporal relationship between aggression and
    seizures
  Activity that patient was engaged in at start of
    seizure
  Seizure medications taken; evidence of
    neurotoxicity
Other medical variables
  Drug or alcohol abuse
  Head injury/brain pathology
  Intelligence quotient
  Concomitant cognitive and psychiatric disorders
  Neuroendocrinologic function
Psychosocial variables
  Socioeconomic status
  History of violence prior to onset of seizures
  Family background/structure
  Coping skills

epilepsy that are easy to complete and validated for this patient population.

Well-controlled studies of aggression and epilepsy will better characterize the etiologic factors that give rise to socially disruptive behavior and help establish more effective treatments. In addition, such studies will reduce the stigma of epilepsy, which is based in part on the misconception that violence and epilepsy are inextricably linked (11).

REFERENCES

1. Delgado-Escueta AV, Mattson RH, King L, et al. Special report. The nature of aggression during epileptic seizures. *N Engl J Med* 1981;305:711–716.
2. Gunn J. Can violence be a manifestation of epilepsy? [Letter]. *Neurology* 1981;31:1204–1205.
3. Pincus JH. Temporal lobe epilepsy and violence [Letter]. *Neurology* 1982;32:574–575.
4. Pincus JH. Can violence be a manifestation of epilepsy? *Neurology* 1980;30:304–307.
5. Jaffe R. Can violence be a manifestation of epilepsy? [Letter]. *Neurology* 1980;30:1337.
6. Stone AA. Violence and temporal lobe epilepsy [Letter]. *Am J Psychiatry* 1984;141:1641–1642.
7. Parker N. Murderers: a personal series. *Med J Aust* 1979;1:36–39.
8. Nassi AJ, Abramowitz SI. From phrenology to psychosurgery and back again: biological studies of criminality. *Am J Orthopsychiatry* 1976;46:591–607.
9. Taylor DC. Aggression and epilepsy. *J Psychosom Res* 1969;13:229–236.
10. Beresford HR. Legal implications of epilepsy. *Epilepsia* 1988;29[Suppl 2]:S114–S121.
11. Fenwick P. Aggression and epilepsy. In: Devinsky O, Theodore WH, ed. *Epilepsy and behavior.* New York: Wiley-Liss, 1991:85–96.
12. Geschwind N. The clinical setting of aggression in temporal lobe epilepsy. In: Fields WH, Sweet WS, eds. *Neural basis of violence and aggression.* St. Louis: Warren H. Green, 1975.
13. Walter RD. Violence and aggression: the state of the art. In: Burch N, Altshuler HL, eds. *Behavior and brain electrical activity.* New York: Plenum Publishing, 1975.
14. Crichton M. *The terminal man.* New York: Alfred A. Knopf, 1972.
15. Lewis JA. Violence and epilepsy. *JAMA* 1975;232:1165–1167.
16. Mark VH, Ervin FR. *Violence and the brain.* New York: Harper & Row, 1970.
17. Knox SJ. Epileptic automatism and violence. *Med Sci Law* 1968;8:96–104.
18. Treiman DM. Epilepsy and violence: medical and legal issues. *Epilepsia* 1986;27[Suppl 2]:S77–S104.
19. Treiman DM. Violence and the epilepsy defense. *Neurol Clin* 1999;17:245–255.
20. Kavoussi R, Armstead P, Coccaro E. The neurobiology of impulsive aggression. *Psychiatr Clin North Am* 1997;20:395–403.
21. Engel J, Caldecott-Hazard S, Bandler R. Neurobiology of behavior: anatomic and physiological implications related to epilepsy. *Epilepsia* 1986;27:S3–S13.
22. Persinger MA. Geomagnetic variables and behavior: LXXXIII. Increased geomagnetic activity and group aggression in chronic limbic epileptic male rats. *Percept Mot Skills* 1997;85:1376–1378.
23. Kaada B. Brain mechanisms related to aggressive behavior. *UCLA Forum Med Sci* 1967;7:95–133.
24. Singer JL, ed. *The control of aggression and violence.* New York City: Academic Press, 1971.
25. Pinel JPJ, Treit D, Rovner LI. Temporal lobe aggression in rats. *Science* 1977;197:1088–1089.
26. Fernandez de Molina A, Hunsperger RW. Organization of the subcortical system governing defence and flight reactions in the cat. *J Physiol* 1962;160:200–213.
27. Robinson BW, Alexander M, Browne G. Dominance reversal resulting fom aggressive responses evoked by brain telestimulation. *Physiol Behav* 1969;4:749–752.
28. Clemente CD, Chase MH. Neurological substrates of aggressive behavior. *Annu Rev Physiol* 1973;35:329–356.
29. Heath RG. Correlation of electrical recordings from cortical and subcortical regions of the brain with abnormal behavior in human subjects. *Confin Neurol* 1958;18:305–315.
30. Saint-Hilaire JM, Gilbert M, Bouvier G. Epilepsy and aggression: two cases with depth electrode studies. In: Robb P, ed. *Epilepsy updated: causes and treatment.* Chicago: Year Book Medical Publishers, 1980:145–176.
31. Weiser HG. Depth-recorded limbic seizures and psychopathology. *Neurosci Biobehav Rev* 1983;7:427–440.
32. Herzberg JL, Fenwick PBC. The aetiology of aggression in temporal-lobe epilepsy. *Br J Psychiatry* 1988;153:50–55.
33. Rabin PL, Koomen J. The violent patient—differential diagnosis and management. *J Tenn Med Assoc* 1982;75:313–317.
34. Reischel UA, Shih RD. Evaluation and management of psychotic patients in the emergency department. *Hosp Physician* 1999;10:26–38.
35. Torta R, Keller R. Behavioral, psychotic, and anxiety disorders in epilepsy: etiology, clinical features, and therapeutic implications. *Epilepsia* 1999;40[Suppl 10]:S2–S20.
36. Fenwick P. Psychiatric disorders in epilepsy. In: Hopkins A, ed. *Epilepsy.* London: Chapman and Hall, 1987:511–553.
37. Blanchet P, Frommer GP. Mood change preceding epileptic seizures. *J Nerv Ment Dis* 1986;174:471–476.
38. Hindler CG. Epilepsy and violence. *Br J Psychiatry* 1989;155:246–249.
39. Whitman S, Coleman TE, Patmon C, et al. Epilepsy in prison: elevated prevalence and no relationship to violence. *Neurology* 1984;34:775–782.
40. King D, Ajmone Marsan C. Clinical features and ictal patterns in epileptic patients with EEG temporal lobe foci. *Ann Neurol* 1977;2:138–147.
41. Ramani V, Gumnit RJ. Intensive monitoring of epileptic patients with a history of episodic aggression. *Arch Neurol* 1981;38:570–571.
42. Rodin EA. Psychomotor epilepsy and aggressive behavior. *Arch Gen Psychiatry* 1973;28:210–213.

43. Gloor P. Discussion. In: Kaada B. Brain mechanisms related to aggressive behavior. *UCLA Forum Med Sci* 1967;7:95–133.

44. Ashford JW, Schulz SC, Walsh GO. Violent automatism in a partial complex seizure. Report of a case. *Arch Neurol* 1980;37:120–122.

45. Treiman DM, Delgado-Escueta V. Aggression during fear and fight in complex partial seizures: a CCTV-EEG analysis. *Epilepsia* 1981;22:243.

46. Lancman M. Psychosis and peri-ictal confusional states. *Neurology* 1999;53[Suppl 2]:S33–S38.

47. Goldensohn E, Gold A. Prolonged behavioral disturbances as ictal phenomena. *Neurology* 1960;10:1–9.

48. Logsdail SJ, Toone BK. Postictal psychoses. *Br J Psychiatry* 1988;152:246–252.

49. Savard G, Andermann F, Olivier A, et al. Postictal psychosis after partial complex seizures: a multiple case study. *Epilepsia* 1991;32:225–231.

50. Levine DN, Finklestein S. Delayed psychosis after right temporoparietal stroke or trauma: relation to epilepsy. *Neurology* 1982;32:267–273.

51. Fenwick P. Episodic dyscontrol. In: Engle J, Pedley TA, eds. *Epilepsy: a comprehensive textbook.* Philadelphia: Lippincott-Raven Publishers, 1997: 2767–2774.

52. Kanemoto K, Kawasaki J, Mori E. Violence and epilepsy: a close relation between violence and postictal psychosis. *Epilepsia* 1999;40:107–109.

53. Blumer D. Antidepressant and double antidepressant treatment for the affective disorder of epilepsy. *J Clin Psychiatry* 1997;58:3–11.

54. Blumer D. Evidence supporting the temporal lobe epilepsy personality syndrome. *Neurology* 1999;53 [Suppl 2]:S9–S12.

55. Moyer KE. *The psychobiology of aggression.* New York: Harper & Row, 1976.

56. Devinsky O, Bear D. Varieties of aggressive behavior in temporal lobe epilepsy. *Am J Psychiatry* 1984;141: 651–656.

57. Mungas D. An empirical analysis of specific syndromes of violent behavior. *J Nerv Ment Dis* 1983; 171:354–361.

58. Currie S, Heathfield KWG, Henson RA, et al. Clinical course and prognosis of temporal lobe epilepsy—a survey of 666 patients. *Brain* 1971;92:173–190.

59. Falconer MA. Reversibility by temporal-lobe resection of the behavioral abnormalities of temporal-lobe epilepsy. *N Engl J Med* 1973;289:451–455.

60. Glaser GH. Limbic epilepsy in childhood. *J Nerv Ment Dis* 1967;144:391–397.

61. Serafetinides EA. Aggressiveness in temporal lobe epilepticsand its relation to cerebral dysfunction and environmental factors. *Epilepsia* 1965;6:33–42.

62. Ounsted C. Aggression and epilepsy rage in children with temporal lobe epilepsy. *J Psychosom Res* 1969; 13:237–242.

63. Hermann BP, Schwartz MS, Whitman S, et al. Aggression and eplepsy: seizure-type comparisons and high-risk variables. *Epilepsia* 1980;22:691–698.

64. Mendez MF, Doss RC, Taylor JL. Interictal violence in epilepsy. Relationship to behavior and seizure variables. *J Nerv Ment Dis* 1993;181:566–569.

65. Lewis DO, Pincus JH, Shanok SS, et al. Psychomotor epilepsy and violence in a group of incarcerated adolescent boys. *Am J Psychiatry* 1982;139:882–887.

66. Gunn JC. The prevalence of epilepsy among prisoners. *Proc R Soc Med* 1969;62:60–63.

67. Williams D. Neural factors related to habitual aggression. *Brain* 1970;92:503–520.

68. Gunn J, Bonn J. Criminality and violence in epileptic prisoners. *Br J Psychiatry* 1971;118:337–343.

69. Treiman DM. Epilepsy and violence: medical and legal issues. *Epilepsia* 1986;27[Suppl 2]:77–104.

70. Elliott FA. Violence. The neurologic contribution: an overview. *Arch Neurol* 1992;49:595–603.

71. Fenwick P. Aggression and epilepsy. In: Trimble MR, Bolwig TG, eds. *Aspects of epilepsy and psychiatry.* Chichester: John Wiley and Sons, 1986:31–60.

72. Hodgins S. Mental disorder, intellectual deficiency, and crime. Evidence from a birth cohort. *Arch Gen Psychiatry* 1992;49:476–483.

73. Mouridsen SE, Tolstrup K. Children who kill: a case study of matricide. *J Child Psychol Psychiatry* 1988; 29:511–515.

74. Trimble MR. *The psychosis of epilepsy.* New York: Raven Press, 1991.

75. Arboleda-Florez J. Mental illness and violence: an epidemiological appraisal of the evidence. *Can J Psychiatry* 1998;43:989–996.

76. Eronen M, Angermeyer MC, Schulze B. The psychiatric epidemiology of violent behaviour. *Soc Psychiatry Psychiatr Epidemiol* 1998;33[Suppl 1]:S13–S23.

77. Taylor PJ. When symptoms of psychosis drive serious violence. *Soc Psychiatry Psychiatr Epidemiol* 1998;33 [Suppl 1]:S47–S54.

78. Perrine K, Kiolbasa T. Cognitive deficits in epilepsy and contribution to psychopathology. *Neurology* 1999; 53[Suppl 2]:S39–S48.

79. Schachter SC. Neuroendocrine aspects of epilepsy. In: Devinsky O, Theodore WH, eds. *Epilepsy and behavior.* New York: Alan R. Liss, 1991:303–333.

80. Hughes JR. The significance of the interictal spike discharge: a review. *J Clin Neurophysiol* 1989;6: 207–226.

81. Molaie M, Cruz A, Culebras A. The effect of epileptiform discharges on neurohormonal release in epileptic patients with complex partial seizures. *Neurology* 1988;38:759–762.

82. Brunet M, Rodamilans M, Martinez-Osaba MJ, et al. Effects of long-term antiepileptic therapy on the catabolism of testosterone. *Pharmacol Toxicol* 1995;76: 371–375.

83. Duncan S, Blacklaw J, Beastall GH, et al. Antiepileptic drug therapy and sexual function in men with epilepsy. *Epilepsia* 1999;40:197–204.

84. Isojarvi JI, Laatikainen TJ, Pakarinen AJ, et al. Polycystic ovaries and hyperandrogenism in women taking valproate for epilepsy. *N Engl J Med* 1993;329: 1383–1388.

85. Isojarvi JI, Repo M, Pakarinen AJ, et al. Carbamazepine, phenytoin, sex hormones, and sexual function in men with epilepsy. *Epilepsia* 1995;36:366–370.

86. Stoffel-Wagner B, Bauer J, Flugel D, et al. Serum sex hormones are altered in patients with chronic temporal lobe epilepsy receiving anticonvulsant medication. *Epilepsia* 1998;39:1164–1173.

87. Kleinman JE, Weinberger DR, Rogol AD, et al. Plasma prolactin concentrations and psychopathology in chronic schizophrenia. *Arch Gen Psychiatry* 1982;39: 655–657.

88. Csernansky JG, Prosser E, Kaplan J, et al. Possible associations among plasma prolactin levels, tardive dysknesia, and paranoia in treated male schizophrenics. *Biol Psychiatry* 1986;21:632–642.

89. Reith J, Benkelfat C, Sherwin A, et al. Elevated dopa decarboxylase activity in living brain of patients with psychosis. *Proc Natl Acad Sci USA* 1994;91:11651–11654.

90. Leiderman DB, Csernansky JG, Moses JA. Neuroendocrinology and limbic epilepsy: relationships to psychopathology, seizure variables, and neuropsychological function. *Epilepsia* 1990;31:270–274.

91. Takeshita H, Kawahara R, Nagabuchi T, et al. Serum prolactin, cortisol and growth hormone concentrations after various epileptic seizures. *Jpn J Psychiatry Neurol* 1986;40:617–623.

92. Abbott RJ, Browning MCK, Davidson DLW. Serum prolactin and cortisol concentrations after grand mal seizures. *J Neurol Neurosurg Psychiatry* 1980;43:163–167.

93. Kalin NH. Primate models to understand human aggression. *J Clin Psychiatry* 1999;60[Suppl 15]:29–32.

94. Bach-y-Rita G, Lion JR, Climent CE, et al. Episodic dyscontrol: a study of 130 violent patients. *Am J Psychiatry* 1971;127:1473–1478.

95. Maletzky BM. The episodic dyscontrol syndrome. *Dis Nerv Syst* 1973;34:178–184.

96. Menuck M, Voineskos G. The etiology of violent behavior. An overview. *Gen Hosp Psychiatry* 1981;3:37–47.

97. Pakalnis A, Drake ME, John K, et al. Forced normalization. Acute psychosis after seizure control in seven patients. *Arch Neurol* 1987;44:289–292.

98. Bylesjo I, Forsgren L, Lithner F, et al. Epidemiology and clinical characteristics of seizures in patients with acute intermittent porphyria. *Epilepsia* 1996;37:230–235.

99. Krauss GL, Simmons OBE, Campbell M. Successful treatment of seizures and porphyria with gabapentin. *Neurology* 1995;45:594–595.

100. Tatum WO, Zachariah SB. Gabapentin treatment of seizures in acute intermittent porphyria. *Neurology* 1995;45:1216–1217.

101. Swanson J, Borum R, Swartz M, et al. Violent behavior preceding hospitalization among persons with severe mental illness. *Law Hum Behav* 1999;23:185–204.

102. Kligman D, Goldberg DA. Temporal lobe epilepsy and aggression. *J Nerv Ment Dis* 1975;160:324–341.

103. Lion JR. Pitfalls in the assessment and measurement of violence: a clinical view. *J Neuropsychiatry Clin Neurosci* 1991;3:S40–S43.

104. Devinsky O, Ronsaville D, Cox C, et al. Interictal aggression in epilepsy: the Buss-Durkee Hostility Inventory. *Epilepsia* 1994;35:585–590.

105. Mack JL, Patterson MB, Tariot PN. Behavior Rating Scale for Dementia: development of test scales and presentation of data for 555 individuals with Alzheimer's disease. *J Geriatr Psychiatry Neurol* 1999;12:211–223.

106. Kreutzer JS, Marwitz JH, Seel R, et al. Validation of a neurobehavioral functioning inventory for adults with traumatic brain injury. *Arch Phys Med Rehabil* 1996;77:116–124.

107. Weinfurt KP, Willke R, Glick HA, et al. Towards a composite scoring solution for the Neurobehavioral Functioning Inventory. *Qual Life Res* 1999;8:17–24.

108. Buss AH, Durkee A. An inventory for assessing different kinds of hostility. *J Consult Psychol* 1957;2:343–349.

109. Pope HG Jr, Kouri EM, Hudson JI. Effects of supraphysiologic doses of testosterone on mood and aggression in normal men: a randomized controlled trial. *Arch Gen Psychiatry* 2000;57:133–140.

110. Seroczynski AD, Bergeman CS, Coccaro EF. Etiology of the impulsivity/aggression relationship: genes or environment? *Psychiatry Res* 1999;86:41–57.

111. Azouvi P, Jokic C, Attal N, et al. Carbamazepine in agitation and aggressive behaviour following severe closed-head injury: results of an open trial. *Brain Inj* 1999;13:797–804.

112. Yudofsky SC, Silver JM, Jackson W, et al. The Overt Aggression Scale for the objective rating of verbal and physical aggression. *Am J Psychiatry* 1986;143:35–39.

113. Silver JM, Yudofsky SC. The Overt Aggression Scale: overview and guiding principles. *J Neuropsychiatry Clin Neurosci* 1991;3:S22–S29.

114. Bjorkly S. Report form for aggressive episodes: preliminary report. *Percept Mot Skills* 1996;83:1139–1152.

115. Bjorkly S. Interrater reliability of the Report Form for Aggressive Episodes in group ratings. *Percept Mot Skills* 1998;87:1405–1406.

116. Arthur HM, Garfinkel PE, Irvine J. Development and testing of a new hostility scale. *Can J Cardiol* 1999;15:539–544.

117. Cook WW, Medley DM. Proposed hostility and pharisaic-virtue scales for the MMPI. *J Appl Psychol* 1954;38:414–418.

118. Pope MK, Smith TW, Rhodewalt F. Cognitive, behavioral, and affective correlates of the Cook and Medley Hostility Scale. *J Pers Assess* 1990;54:501–514.

119. Keats MM, Mukherjee S. Antiaggressive effect of adjunctive clonazepam in schizophrenia associated with seizure disorder. *J Clin Psychiatry* 1988;49:117–118.

120. Bear DM, Fedio P. Quantitative analysis of interictal behavior in temporal lobe epilepsy. *Arch Neurol* 1977;34:454–467.

121. Lewin J, Summers D. Successful treatment of episodic dyscontrol with carbamazepine. *Br J Psychiatry* 1992;161:261–262.

122. Stone JL, McDaniel KD, Hughes JR, et al. Episodic dyscontrol disorder and paroxysmal EEG abnormalities: successful treatment with carbamazepine. *Biol Psychiatry* 1986;21:208–212.

123. Luchins DJ. Carbamazepine for the violent psychiatric patient. *Lancet* 1983;1:766.

124. Tariot PN, Erb R, Podgorski CA, et al. Efficacy and tolerability of carbamazepine for agitation and aggression in dementia. *Am J Psychiatry* 1998;155:54–61.

125. Gleason RP, Schneider LS. Carbamazepine treatment of agitation in Alzheimer's outpatients refractory to neuroleptics. *J Clin Psychiatry* 1990;51:115–118.

126. Davis LL, Ryan W, Adinoff B, et al. Comprehensive review of the psychiatric uses of valproate. *J Clin Psychopharmacol* 2000;20[Suppl 1]:1S–17S.

127. Low RA, Brandes M. Gabapentin for the management of agitation [Letter]. *J Clin Psychopharmacol* 1999;19:482–483.

128. Regan WM, Gordon SM. Gabapentin for behavioral agitation in Alzheimer's disease [Letter]. *J Clin Psychopharmacol* 1997;17:59–60.

129. Modell JG. Further experience and observations with lorazepam in the management of behavioral agitation [Letter]. *J Clin Psychopharmacol* 1986;6:385–387.

130. Volavka J. The effects of clozapine on aggression and substance abuse in schizophrenic patients. *J Clin Psychiatry* 1999;60[Suppl 12]:43–46.

131. Chengappa KN, Ebeling T, Kang JS, et al. Clozapine reduces severe self-mutilation and aggression in psychotic patients with borderline personality disorder. *J Clin Psychiatry* 1999;60:477–484.

132. Kiloh LG, Smith JS. The neural basis of aggression and its treatment by psychosurgery. *Aust N Z J Psychiatry* 1978;12:21–28.

133. Matter of Torsney, 394 NE 2d 799, Court of Appeals, New York, 1979.

134. Raine A, Lencz T, Bihrle S, et al. Reduced prefrontal gray matter volume and reduced autonomic activity in antisocial personality disorder. *Arch Gen Psychiatry* 2000;57:119–127.

135. Woermann FG, van Elst LT, Koepp MJ, et al. Reduction of frontal neocortical grey matter associated with affective aggression in patients with temporal lobe epilepsy: an objective voxel by voxel analysis of automatically segmented MRI. *J Neurol Neurosurg Psychiatry* 2000;68:162–169.

14

Psychiatric Complications of Epilepsy in the Geriatric Patient

Diagnostic and Treatment Considerations

Marlis Frey

Department of Neurology, Rush Presbyterian-Saint Luke's Medical Center, Chicago, Illinois 60612

Trends in demographic data document the significant increase in the number of older adults. People 65 years and older currently represent 13% of the population (1). By the year 2030, this group is expected to increase to 20% of the population. The most striking increase in the elderly is expected to be seen in the year 2010, when the baby boom generation will begin to turn 65. In addition, the older population itself is getting older. The age group 85 years and older comprises the fastest growing segment of the older population.

These statistics are astounding by themselves, but they gain new significance when one considers the epidemiology of seizures in the elderly. Recent studies demonstrated that epilepsy, typically thought of as a disorder or syndrome starting early in life, is the third most common neurologic disorder in the elderly, after stroke and Alzheimer's disease (2). The incidence of epilepsy increases sharply after the age of 50 and by the age of 80 exceeds that of children. The highest incidence has been reported in the oldest age group, those over 75 years of age (139/100,000) (3). This represents a significant increase from the younger group (100/100,000) and the age group up to 50 years (15/100,000). Because the older segment of the population is not only the fastest growing but also the

one with the highest incidence of seizures, the significance of epilepsy is becoming very apparent.

Although seizures in the elderly generally are related to secondary factors, the etiology of the largest group of new onset of seizure disorders remains idiopathic (2). Acute symptomatic seizures, which are seizures secondary to a toxic, metabolic, traumatic, or vascular event, are very frequent in the elderly, with an incidence of 100 per 100,000 after the age of 60 years (4). These seizures often present in the form of status epilepticus or as clusters of seizures. Stroke is the most frequent cause, followed by systemic metabolic disorders, acute brain trauma, central nervous system infection, and toxic insults (2).

The relationship between epilepsy and psychiatric disorders has received increased attention over the last few decades. Most studies and reviews explored mood, anxiety, personality, and psychotic disorders in the general epilepsy population. A review of the literature reveals little information on the psychiatric aspects of the geriatric epileptic patient. Although epidemiologic studies have shown that the second highest incidence of epilepsy occurs in the geriatric population, only recently has this age group received specific attention as to psychiatric manifestations. Although many of the observations made in younger patient groups with epilepsy will apply to geriatric epileptic patients, some may not. For example, as discussed in other chapters of this book, psychopathology is more likely to occur among patients with poorly controlled partial epilepsy. Yet, in 80% to 90% of geriatric patients, seizure disorders beginning after the age of 60 have a very benign course. Thus, do geriatric epileptic patients have a lower incidence of psychopathology related to the epileptic disorder than younger patients? The answer, unfortunately, is yet to be established.

This chapter will review the epidemiology, symptomatology, and assessment of the three major psychiatric disorders: anxiety disorder, depressive disorder, and psychosis, in the elderly in general and in the elderly with epilepsy specifically. Current treatment recommendations for these disorders in the elderly and their specific implications for this patient population will be discussed.

ANXIETY DISORDERS

Epidemiology

In comparison to studies of depressive disorders in the aged, little formal research investigating anxiety disorders in the elderly is available. This is somewhat surprising, given that the prevalence of anxiety disorders in the elderly is greater than that of depressive disorders (5). Anxiety disorders are the most prevalent psychiatric disorder in the elderly. The age-adjusted prevalence rates range from 10% to 20% (6), with even higher rates among those over the age of 75 (7). Incidence data suggest a lower rate of development of new cases of anxiety in the elderly. Larkin and colleagues (8) reported an incidence of 4.4 per 1,000 per year of anxiety disorders in the elderly. Kramer et al. (9) reported a higher incidence of 10.1% in the elderly over the age of 75. These studies show, however, that new onset of anxiety disorders occurs at a much lower rate in the elderly than in the younger population.

Flint (10) reviewed eight community-based survey studies investigating anxiety disorders in persons over 60 years of age. The results of this review suggested that phobias and generalized anxiety disorders are the most prevalent for that age group. However, prevalence rates are very low for obsessive-compulsive disorder (11) and panic disorders (12) in the elderly. Lindesay (12) found agoraphobia to be the only late-onset phobia in the elderly population. The onset of the agoraphobia most often was related to the occurrence of a new medical condition or a traumatic event. Matt et al. (5) analyzed data collected from 1,131 community elderly and found the prevalence of phobias, such as social and simple phobias, was invariably higher in women and that the prevalence of phobias increased with advancing age.

Lindesay (12) reported rates of up to 30% of comorbidity between anxieties and depression in a geriatric community sample. Even higher rates (over 75%) were reported more recently in a study of institutionalized patients (13). Some studies suggested that anxiety arises secondary to depressive episodes (6). In contrast to this suggestion, Coryell (14) argued that anxiety disorders and depressive disorders are two separate and distinct disorders. He based this position on a review of the literature investigating the relationship between anxiety and depressive disorders, from which he concluded that genetic, epidemiologic, and diagnostic evidence supported the lack of dependent comorbidity.

Medical conditions such as endocrine disorders, cardiovascular conditions, and pulmonary conditions may cause symptoms of anxiety in the elderly (15). Additionally, increased sensitivity to pharmacologic agents and frequent use of polypharmacy cannot be underestimated as causative factors in the development of anxiety disorders in this patient population. Primarily, steroids, thyroid preparations, stimulants, anticholinergic medications, and antidepressants may produce anxiety-related physical and psychic symptoms in elderly patients.

Symptomatology of Anxiety in the Elderly

The *Diagnostic and Statistical Manual of Mental Disorders,* Fourth Edition (DSM-IV) (16) sets forth extensive criteria for all mental disorders. Generalized anxiety disorder is defined as "...at least 6 months of persistent and excessive anxiety and worry" (p. 393). It is the intensity, duration, and irrational proportion of the feeling that warrants the diagnosis of anxiety disorder. Individuals may report psychiatric or physiologic symptoms as expressions of anxiety (17). Physiologic symptoms may be either motor signs, such as restlessness and trembling, or autonomic signs, such as sweating and dizziness. Hypervigilance and irritability may be expressions of psychiatric symptoms. Patients may report difficulties with concentration or trouble falling asleep due to anxiety (18). Elderly patients often do not meet all the criteria set forth for a diagnosis of anxiety, but their symptoms still cause functional impairment. This situation is termed subsyndromal anxiety (17).

Assessment of Anxiety

Assessment of anxiety in the elderly can be difficult for two major reasons. First, elderly patients often have an atypical presentation of physical and psychiatric conditions (e.g., a urinary tract infection can present as confusion or a myocardial infarction can present without chest pain). Second, different psychological tools used in the assessment of anxiety are, in general, designed and validated for a younger *(nonepileptic!)* population (19) and may not consider unique social and medical conditions in the elderly. Wording of questions also has been found to be important in the assessment of anxiety in the elderly. Schramke (19) found that, on further questioning, patients who initially reported feeling nervous and anxious actually were not referring to internal feelings of anxiety but rather to physiologic tremors. To help control for some of these confounding effects, a complete assessment of anxiety in the elderly must include a review of medical and psychiatric illness, a review of current drugs that can cause symptoms of anxiety, as well as the patient's current psychosocial situation.

Differential diagnosis of anxiety in the elderly should include primary anxiety disorders, such as generalized anxiety disorder and panic disorder, versus anxiety secondary to medical illness or drugs. Once a diagnosis of primary anxiety disorder has been established, it will be essential to distinguish between the various anxiety disorders (18).

Anxiety and Epilepsy

Limited information can be found when investigating the relationship between anxiety and epilepsy. Betts (20) gave a comprehensive description of the various relationships between anxiety and epilepsy. He argued that anxiety can occur as a reaction to the perceived psychosocial impact of having seizures or as a physical part of the periictal experience. Accordingly, anxiety in the patient with epilepsy can be a reaction to having seizures. This may be true especially for the elderly patient who is newly diagnosed and may feel very frightened and overwhelmed with the diagnosis, especially when other chronic medical conditions already exist. At times, this anxiety may lead to a true phobic response that may prevent the patient from leaving the house.

Anxiety may be part of the periictal experience. A detailed description of the actual seizure will be necessary to determine whether the anxiety is physiologic or psychological in nature. This may be particularly challenging in the geriatric patient who has more than the usual age-related memory problems.

Anxiety in the elderly epileptic patient may be difficult to assess. Keeping in mind that anxiety is the most prevalent psychopathology in the elderly, the challenge for the clinician is to determine whether or not the anxiety is preexisting, part of the ictal event, or a psychological response to the seizures. A thorough seizure history, medical and psychiatric history, as well as drug history, are necessary to arrive at an accurate diagnosis.

Treatment of Anxiety in the Elderly

Prior to initiating any type of treatment, the clinician needs to spend time with the patient and family and discuss the natural course of seizures in the elderly, explaining treatment options and exploring the medical and psychosocial impact of the diagnosis on the patient. Should pharmacologic treatment be indicated, clinicians need to consider the following pharmacokinetic and pharmacodynamic changes caused by the natural aging process: (i) pharmacokinetic changes (what the body does to the drug) in the elderly affect the absorption, distribution, metabolism, and excretion of the drug; and (ii) pharmacodynamic changes (what the drug does to the body) are poorly understood in the elderly (21) and will not be discussed in this chapter. It should be kept in mind at all times, however, that elderly patients are more sensitive to negative psychotropic properties of antiepileptic drugs; therefore, attempts to use the lowest doses possible are of the essence.

The pharmacokinetic changes commonly identified in the elderly can be summarized as follows.

Absorption. Absorption of drugs in the elderly has generally been reported to be similar to that in younger individuals. Exceptions to this include reports of an increase in gastric acidity, which may cause an increase or decrease in absorption with some drugs (22).

Distribution. Distribution is affected by the increase in lipid body mass and the decrease in water associated with age. Therefore, lipophilic drugs in the elderly may have an increased volume of distribution, whereas the volume of distribution for hydrophilic drugs may be decreased. Distribution of a drug is further affected by plasma protein levels. Plasma albumin levels have been reported to be decreased by approximately 20% in healthy elderly patients (22). For drugs that are highly protein bound, this can lead to an increase in the free fraction (unbound) of the drug. This can be of important clinical significance if the drug has a narrow therapeutic index.

Metabolism. There is a decrease in size of the liver as well as a 40% to 49% decrease in hepatic blood flow in aging. Phase I metabolism (such as oxidation, reduction, and hydroxylation) has been reported to decrease with age, whereas drug metabolism by conjugation (phase II metabolism) has been reported to remain stable with age (22).

Excretion. Renal blood flow and glomerular filtration rate decreases with age, leading to a decrease in elimination of drugs and drug metabolites (22). This may lead to an increase in a drug's half-life for compounds depending on renal excretion.

Benzodiazepine

Schneider (18) reviewed data from a private marketing research firm for selected minor tranquilizers from January to December 1995. He found that the majority of anxiolytics prescribed in the elderly were medications without active metabolites, such as lorazepam and oxazepam. The extensively metabolized alprazolam, which is usually the medication of choice for treatment of acute anxiety in younger patients, was relatively seldom prescribed in the elderly. The use of extensively metabolized, long-acting benzodiazepines in the elderly has been associated with an increase in hip fractures (23) and motorist fatalities in older male drivers (24).

The properties of benzodiazepines make them very effective as hypnotics, anxiolytics, anticonvulsants, and muscle relaxants (25). Benzodiazepines are well known to cause sedation in the elderly patient. At toxic levels, which in the elderly may be reached at relatively low doses, benzodiazepines may cause cognitive impairment, confusion, and unsteadiness. One of the major disadvantages of benzodiazepines is that patients may develop physical and psychological tolerance. Benzo-diazepines can have either a short half-life (oxazepam, lorazepam, and alprazolam) or a longer half-life (chlordiazepoxide, diazepam, and clorazepate). Lorazepam and oxazepam are the only benzodiazepines not extensively metabolized by the liver.

Buspirone

Buspirone belongs to a relatively new class of psychotropic medications called aza-pirones. This class of medication has both anxiolytic and antidepressant properties (26). Buspirone is considered an effective alterna-tive to benzodiazepines because of its safety record (27). Buspirone has been shown to be effective for treatment of generalized anxiety disorder, as well as for treatment of depres-sion either in conjunction with a serotonin se-lective reuptake inhibitor (SSRI) or alone (28). Buspirone is not effective against panic attacks (29). Buspirone has been used exten-sively in the treatment of anxiety and depres-sion with anxiety in elderly patients (30). One of the drawbacks of using buspirone is that it may take several weeks before a thera-peutic response is achieved. Cadieux (29) re-ported that patients can be switched safely from benzodiazepines to buspirone without causing benzodiazepine withdrawal symp-toms by following these recommendations: an initial switch of the patient to a long-act-ing benzodiazepine if he or she is not already taking one. Next starting the patient on 5 mg of buspirone t.i.d. and increasing the dose to 30 mg per day. Once this dose is reached, starting the taper of benzodiazepines over the next 60 to 90 days.

β-Adrenergic Receptor Antagonists

These medications are mainly used to treat the physiologic symptoms of anxiety, such as tremors and palpitations. One of the major limitations of using these medications in the elderly is their hypotensive effect.

Antihistamines

Antihistamines have a history of use for treatment of anxiety in elderly patients. They are less effective than benzodiazepines and have anticholinergic effects, such as dry mouth, blurred vision, and cognitive impair-ment (30). For these reasons, they are not an ideal medication for the elderly.

Antidepressant Drugs

Antidepressants have long been used in the treatment for anxiety (31). The drawback with older tricyclics, however, is that, like bus-pirone, they may take several weeks before they become effective. In addition, their side-effect profile is poorly tolerated in the elderly. Monoamine oxidase inhibitors (MAOIs), the classic treatment for phobic anxiety (32), are poorly tolerated in the elderly because of the postural hypotension associated with their use.

SSRIs often have been thought to be too stimulating for patients with anxiety (18,33). Sadavoy and LeClair (33) state that some of the SSRI side effects, such as gastrointestinal upset, anorexia, and insomnia, may be intol-erable for the elderly. However, Lader and An-cill (30) consider SSRIs as the ideal treatment for generalized anxiety disorders, panic disor-ders, and obsessive-compulsive disorders in the elderly. They found that SSRIs in general are very well tolerated in the elderly, and that the feeling of anxiety experienced with their use generally is limited to the initial couple of weeks. The authors were able to decrease the stimulating side effect by starting the patients on half-doses and then slowly titrating the dose upward.

Other Medications

Barbiturates and neuroleptics have been used for treatment of anxiety in the elderly. Given their unfavorable side-effect profile in the elderly, their use should be limited in this patient population.

The use of the anticonvulsant gabapentin for the long-term treatment of anxiety in psychiatric patients has been described (34). Relatively low doses of 200 to 1,800 mg daily were found to have beneficial effects on anxiety-related symptoms, such as generalized anxiety, somatic complaints, panic, and obsessive-compulsive symptoms.

Nonpharmacologic Approaches

In discussing nonpharmacologic approaches for treatment of anxiety in the elderly, Small (31) reported that both "...cognitive-behavioral and psychodynamic group therapy..." (p. 45) have proven beneficial in the elderly depressed and anxious patient population. He goes on to stress the importance of educating elderly patients about the biologic basis of anxiety, as these patients may be more reluctant to acknowledge psychological problems. Cognitive therapy, relaxation training, and teaching problem-solving skills have been reported to be beneficial in the treatment of anxiety disorders in the elderly (35). Often such interventions will take longer than medications for results to become evident, but in the long-term the results may be more beneficial.

Treatment Recommendations for the Geriatric Epileptic Patient with Anxiety

From the earlier review, several conclusions can be drawn for the elderly epileptic patient with anxiety. First, benzodiazepines are not the long-term drug of choice, despite their anticonvulsant efficacy. This class of drugs is used in epilepsy mainly for short-term management of seizure exacerbation; when used continuously, they lose their anticonvulsant efficacy. Therefore, epileptologists in general prefer patients to be treated with another class of drugs. If benzodiazepines need to be used on a short-term basis, oxazepam and lorazepam should be considered, given their short half-lives and absence of active metabolites. Second, buspirone and SSRIs are good choices for elderly epileptic patients because of their favorable side effect profiles. Buspirone has been well tolerated in the geriatric population when started at 5 mg

three times a day, with gradual increases over 7 to 10 days to a total daily dose of 20 to 30 mg. Another advantage is buspirone's minimal interactions with anticonvulsant medications. The pharmacokinetic interaction of some of the SSRIs with antiepileptic and other drugs demands caution in the use of these agents. The use of SSRIs in the elderly will be discussed under treatments for depression.

The most exciting new information in the treatment of anxiety in the elderly epileptic patient pertains to the recent report on gabapentin. New seizure onset in the elderly often takes a rather benign course, and seizures should be easily controlled with an anticonvulsant such as gabapentin. It seems ideal to take advantage of gabapentin's anticonvulsant and anxiolytic properties, as well as its well-tolerated side-effect profile for the elderly epileptic patient with anxiety. In our experience, elderly patients with adequate serum creatinine clearance benefit from daily total doses of up to 1,800 mg taken in three divided doses for seizure control. An initial starting dose of 100 mg three times a day with a gradual increase usually is well tolerated. This daily dose was shown to be beneficial in the treatment of anxiety-related disorders in an adult population and, therefore, would be expected to be therapeutic in the geriatric population. Patients with impaired creatinine clearance may have a therapeutic response at a dose of 900 mg per day.

DEPRESSION

Epidemiology

Estimates of the prevalence of depression in the elderly vary greatly according to setting and type of depression (36). In community-dwelling elderly, the prevalence of major depression is approximately 1%, whereas rates for nursing home patients have been reported to range from 9% to 38%. Depressive symptoms have been reported in approximately 8% to 15% of community elderly and approximately 30% in long-term settings. For both major depression and depressive symptoms in the elderly, there is higher prevalence in women as well as in the "old" old population.

Blazer (37) reported that the majority of elderly do not fit the criteria for depression set forth in the DSM but rather have depressive symptoms associated with physical illness or adjustment to life stresses. Elderly patients will present with the same clinical symptoms of depression, except they may have significant weight loss and deny feelings of worthlessness and guilt. Blazer considers depression in the elderly the most treatable of the psychiatric disorders in that age group, even though that group is at highest risk of problems associated with depression, such as suicide.

Several investigators explored in detail the relationship between epilepsy and depression (38–42). The results suggested a comorbid prevalence between 30% to 50% for interictal depression in epileptic patients. Patients with epilepsy also have been reported to have a suicide rate five times higher than in the general public (43). The risk factors for interictal depression in epilepsy are reviewed in detail in Chapter 5 on affective disorders in epilepsy. In brief, these risk factors include iatrogenic, psychosocial, genetic, and neurobiologic changes related to seizure disorder, per se. The iatrogenic risk factors are of utmost importance in geriatric patients, given their greater vulnerability for adverse events. The negative effects of some anticonvulsant medications on mood have been well established, predominantly as they pertain to drugs such as phenobarbital, primidone, tiagabine, topiramate, and felbamate, which are well known to cause depression. Such side effects need to be explained to patients prior to starting these medications, and patients need to be closely monitored for occurrence of side effects. This is discussed below in greater detail.

It is not clear whether the same psychosocial and neurobiologic risk factors identified in younger patient populations are operant and have the same impact (or greater) in elderly patients. To give a couple of examples, Betts (20) demonstrated the occurrence of endogenous symptoms of depression after patients were informed that they suffer from epilepsy. Hermann and Wyler (44) suggested a relationship between a perceived loss of external locus of control and depression in epilepsy. Given the impact that a diagnosis of epilepsy has on the causation of anxiety in the elderly (20), we would not be surprised if this type of psychosocial risk had a greater impact in the generation of depression in geriatric than in younger patients with epilepsy.

The location of the seizure focus in the left hemisphere is among the neurobiologic risk factors that may have special relevance in the geriatric patient (40,41,45). Victoroff et al. (46) found that patients with a left-sided seizure focus and a left-sided temporal lobe hypometabolism were more likely to have a history of major depressive episodes. Other studies confirmed this association (47). This has led to speculation that, rather than being a reactive event or a familial or genetic phenomenon, interictal depressive disorder somehow is related to repeated seizures arising particularly from the left hemisphere (47). By the same token, patients who suffer a stroke in left frontal structures have been found to be at an increased risk of developing depression (48). Given that stroke accounts for approximately 30% of epilepsy in the elderly (2,4,49), it would be expected for patients with a left frontal stroke and a related seizure disorder to have a significantly higher prevalence of depression. This question is yet to be examined.

Symptomatology

The recognition of depressive disorders in the geriatric patient with epilepsy may not be an easy task. The atypical presentation of symptoms of depression in the elderly patient is compounded by the *not infrequent* atypical presentation of depressive disorders in the patient with epilepsy (see Chapter 5 on affective disorders in epilepsy). Elderly patients often will not admit to symptoms of depression;

rather, they complain of somatic problems such as chronic pain or difficulties with memory and concentration (50). In rare instances, depression can present as a cognitive impairment in the form of a pseudodementia (39).

Few studies have investigated the specific depressive symptoms in the epilepsy population. Mendez et al. (39) compared the clinical characteristics of 20 epilepsy inpatients to 20 depressed nonepileptic patients. The two groups both had psychomotor retardation and neurovegetative signs. Whereas the nonepileptic group reported more neurotic traits, the epilepsy group reported more psychotic traits, such as paranoia, irritability, delusional thinking, and persecutory auditory hallucinations.

Depressive disorders in epilepsy can be classified according to their temporal relation with the seizure occurrence into periictal, ictal, and interictal events. In evaluating periictal depressive events, investigators have described a decline in mood during the hours or days prior to the seizure, with an improvement in mood following the seizures (51,52). Sudden mood changes, anhedonia, guilt, and suicidal ideation may be expressions of simple partial seizures (52) and, therefore, are part of the ictal experience. Kanner and Pollac (53) reported symptoms of postictal depression in 48 of 100 patients, with a median duration of 24 hours in most symptoms. Postictal depressive symptoms have been reported to cause patients to commit suicide (20).

Interictal depression is the most common psychiatric complication of epilepsy (47). It may present as a major depressive or bipolar disorder. As stated earlier, depression in epilepsy more often than not has an atypical presentation. In 1923, Kraepelin (54) recognized this form of depression among patients with epilepsy. More recently, Blumer (41) coined the term "interictal dysphoric disorder" in referring to this type of depression. Characteristically, interictal dysphoric disorder includes expressions of anxiety, uncontrolled irritability, and somatic symptoms, and brief euphoric moods occur intermittently within a chronic dysthymic state.

Assessment

The initial assessment of any geriatric patient with depression should include a thorough history and physical assessment, a medication assessment, and laboratory testing. Both prescribed and over-the-counter medication use should be assessed. Laboratory testing should include vitamin B_{12} levels, folic acid levels, and thyroid panel (55). A clinical interview will further assist in establishing whether the patient meets specific criteria set forth in DSM-IV (16). Clinicians need to keep in mind that the assessment of depression in elderly patients with epilepsy varies to some degree from that of elderly patients without epilepsy. Whereas depressed elderly patients without epilepsy may often meet DSM criteria, patients with epilepsy often will not because of their atypical presentation. Therefore, for elderly patients with epilepsy, a thorough clinical history may be the best available assessment instrument at this time (56). In addition, elderly patients with either long-standing seizures or new-onset seizures need to be assessed for prior history of depression or current psychological reaction to the new diagnosis, reaction to anticonvulsant medication used for treatment of the seizures, as well as a thorough examination of a possible underlying medical condition.

Treatment

Pharmacotherapy

In the 1992 consensus report on diagnosis and treatment of depression in late life, pharmacotherapy was advocated as the treatment of choice for elderly patients (36). One of the key obstacles to pharmacotherapy, however, was stated as patient noncompliance. The report stated that up to 70% of patients took only 50% to 75% of the prescribed dose of a medication. Therefore, the importance of compliance for successful treatment of depression needs to be thoroughly discussed with patients at the onset of antidepressant therapy.

Before initiating antidepressant therapy in the elderly epileptic patient, several issues must be considered. Elderly patients often are more resistant to treatment than patients in younger age groups (55). Elderly patients often are taking a number of prescription and over-the-counter medications; possible drug interactions are a well-founded concern in this population. This is an especially important concern with SSRIs, because they can cause substantial inhibition of cytochrome P-450, which can lead to toxic serum concentrations of other drugs metabolized via that pathway. Finally, an elderly patient's economic status should always be considered prior to choosing a medication to ensure its cost will not jeopardize patient compliance.

Tricyclic Antidepressants

Tricyclic antidepressants have long been the first choice of treatment for patients with depression. The secondary amines nortriptyline and desipramine have been shown to cause fewer side effects than the tertiary amines in elderly patients (56). Tertiary amines are more anticholinergic and antihistaminic than desipramine and nortriptyline. However, even these medications can cause increased heart rate and orthostatic hypotension (55). Of particular importance to elderly epileptic patients is that the use of tricyclic antidepressants has been associated with an increase in seizure frequency. Dailey and Naritoku (57) argued, however, that tricyclic antidepressants in low doses have anticonvulsant properties and only at high serum concentrations will such medications actually cause seizures. Regardless, tricyclic antidepressants should not be the first choice of treatment for the elderly epileptic patient with depression.

Monoamine Oxidase Inhibitors

Because of their impact on tyramine-rich foods that may result in hypertensive events, MAOIs usually are only considered for treatment-resistant depression (23). MAOIs also should not be considered for elderly patients in general because they can cause orthostatic hypotension.

Selective Serotonin Reuptake Inhibitors

The SSRIs are a newer class of antidepressants with a more favorable side-effect profile than either tricyclics or MAOIs. Nausea and insomnia are the most common side effects of these medications. The one concern with using this medication in the elderly population has been the associated weight loss (58). As previously discussed, possible drug interactions need to be evaluated prior to starting patients on SSRIs. These interactions are more likely to occur with fluoxetine, paroxetine, and fluvoxamine and to a lesser degree with sertraline and citalopram (52).

New Agents

Little information exists about the use of the three newest available antidepressants in the elderly: venlafaxine, nefazodone, and mirtazepine. In one review of the use of these agents in the elderly, Nelson (55) cited reports that stressed the efficacy of venlafaxine, especially at higher doses. However, these higher doses were associated with increase in blood pressure. Nefazodone has been reported to be very sedating in the elderly, as well as cause an increase in blood pressure. Mirtazepine has been associated with a potential to cause weight gain, which may be considered a beneficial side effect in anorectic elderly.

Use in Geriatric Epileptic Patients

The general recommendation has been to start geriatric patients on an SSRI. Fluoxetine, paroxetine, sertraline, and citalopram can all be given as a once-a-day dose. Fluoxetine, which has an active metabolite with a half-life of 5 to 7 days, is less than ideal in the geriatric population. Paroxetine and sertraline have been recommended as the agents of choice in the geriatric population because of their low side-effect profile and their increased safety in overdose. Paroxetine is recommended for more agitated depression. For paroxetine, a starting dose of 10 mg per day for 1 week, with increments up to a total dose of 40 mg per day is recommended in the elderly. Sertraline should be started at 25 mg per day for 1 week, with increments up to a total dose of 200 mg per day. Reynolds et al. (59) state that a time period of 4 to 5 weeks should be allowed in the elderly when using SSRIs to determine reliable discrimination between remittance and nonremittance. They further recommend not decreasing the maintenance therapy from the initial therapeutic dose. Venlafaxine might be more appropriate in anergic patients and can be dosed once a day in the extended release form.

Whenever starting an elderly epileptic patient on antidepressant medication, possible medication interactions with anticonvulsant and other medications need to be considered. Keeping in mind that many newer antidepressants have not been extensively studied in the elderly, these medications should be started slowly at low doses and slowly titrated up in small increments to avoid or minimize side effects.

Nonpharmacologic Treatment

The increase of success in treating elderly depressed patients with a combination of pharmacologic agents and appropriate psychotherapy has been advocated by several authors (41,44). Reynolds et al. (59) reported a decrease in recurrence of depressive symptoms in patients receiving adjunct interpersonal psychotherapy following a year of maintenance therapy. Cognitive and behavioral therapy have been advocated as the therapies of choice (37).

PSYCHOSIS

Epidemiology

Psychotic disorders of the elderly have not been studied as extensively as psychotic disorders of younger patients. Paranoid states

are the more frequent expression of psychosis in the elderly. Paranoia may occur in the context of a "delirium" caused by toxic or metabolic states; not infrequently it is common in Alzheimer's dementia. In addition, paranoid states can occur in the aftermath of a stroke or trauma. On the other hand, psychotic disorders in the elderly can present as an expression of a schizophreniform disorder. Schizophrenia currently is considered an episodic disorder with intermittent symptoms that at times require hospitalization and at other times are well controlled (60). In general, schizophrenia is thought of as a biologic disorder due to a pathologic event occurring in the brain early in life. Some investigators stipulated that the brain areas involved include the prefrontal region (61) or the left temporal-limbic system (62). Eastham et al. (21) reported that approximately 60% of patients with schizophrenia are expected to remain stable over their lifetime. Of the remaining 40%, half will improve, but the remainder will worsen. Epidemiologic data on schizophrenia in late life are limited. Previous studies reported an onset of symptoms after the age of 45 years in approximately 15% of all schizophrenia patients. More recently, schizophrenia with onset after the age of 45 years (late-onset schizophrenia) has been reported as more common than previously thought (63), with a higher prevalence in women. Another condition associated with onset after the age of 55 is paraphrenia, which is characterized by paranoid symptoms. A sensory loss, mainly deafness, often is associated with this disorder, which in turn makes patients unresponsive to pharmacotherapy.

The comorbidity of psychosis and epilepsy was first described to be more than coincidental by Slater and Beard (64). Results from an uncontrolled descriptive study that took place from 1957 to 1959, found that patients with epilepsy and schizophrenia differed from patients with pure schizophrenia by having less catatonia and more affective responsiveness. In addition, the authors reported an average of 14 years between onset of epilepsy and onset of psychotic symptoms. The long-term outcome of patients diagnosed with both epilepsy and schizophrenia was more favorable than the outcome of patients with schizophrenia alone. More recently, Moore (47) reviewed data from ten studies that investigated the relationship between epilepsy and psychosis. Except for one study, the prevalence data for psychosis in epileptic patients ranged from 3.09% to 15.0%.

Symptomatology

Psychotic symptoms in patients with epilepsy have been classified according to their onset in relation to seizures as either ictal, postictal, or interictal (65). Often, ictal psychosis presents with psychotic symptoms in some cases of nonconvulsive status epilepticus (absence and complex partial status). Electroencephalographic abnormalities aid identification of the epileptic nature of this presentation but may be absent in some patients with simple partial status (66). Clinicians need to be especially alert to geriatric patients presenting in any acute confusional state with psychotic features, because new-onset seizures in this age group often present in status epilepticus (2).

Postictal psychotic symptoms have been recognized for many decades (64,67). Kanner et al. (68) reported that patients with partial epilepsy have a 6.7% annual incidence of postictal psychosis when they undergo a prolonged video electroencephalographic monitoring study. The actual prevalence and incidence in the general population of epileptic patients are yet to be established. Such patients usually have a history of seizures dating back more than 10 years. The psychotic episodes usually occur 12 to 72 hours after the last seizures and have a mean duration of 70 hours (68). Patients normally are treated with small doses of neuroleptics, such as haloperidol, for 2 to 3 days until their sensorium clears.

Slater and Beard (64) characterized the onset of interictal psychosis in their patients as insidious, acute, or episodic. They stated that patients who developed interictal psychosis

through episodic psychotic events had ever shorter intervals between such events until they finally became continuous. The presentation of psychotic symptoms was similar for patients with schizophrenia and epilepsy and those with schizophrenia alone, with the exception of preserved warm affect in patients with epilepsy.

Patients with 11 to 15 years' duration of temporal lobe epilepsy have been identified to be at higher risk of developing interictal psychosis (69). Umbricht et al. (70) compared clinical, neuropsychological, and seizure-related variables between patients with epilepsy and no history of psychotic episodes and patients with epilepsy and either chronic or postictal psychosis. They found the two psychotic groups differed from the nonpsychotic group by the "...preponderance of bitemporal seizure foci, a relative absence of histories of febrile convulsions, and the presence of histories of clusters of seizures" (p. 227). The authors also found a greater number of women in the chronic psychosis group as well as lower verbal and full-scale IQ and earlier onset of seizures than in the postictal psychosis group. Investigating the relationship between psychosis, neuropathology, and epilepsy, Bruton et al. (71) compared brains of epileptic patients with psychosis to those with epilepsy without psychosis. The found three features distinguishing the two groups. Compared to epileptic patients without psychosis, patients with psychosis had "...enlarged ventricles, periventricular gliosis, and excess of acquired focal brain damage..." (p. 39). Such findings of structural abnormalities arising during fetal development were shown recently in patients with schizophrenia without epilepsy (72).

Assessment

In the geriatric epileptic patient, psychosis may be due to several factors. First, a new-onset epileptic patient in this age group has a significantly higher chance of presenting in nonconvulsive status epilepticus, with signs and symptoms presenting as an acute onset confusional episode. Second, a patient with late-onset schizophrenia or paraphrenia may not come to medical attention until the development of a new-onset–independent seizure disorder. Third, a long-term epileptic patient may start developing postictal or interictal psychosis in old age.

Ictal and postictal psychoses need to be considered in the differential diagnosis of acute-onset psychosis in the geriatric patient with epilepsy (47). In geriatric patients with new onset of seizures and psychosis, the differential diagnosis should include a slowly growing temporal lobe mass, limbic encephalitis, lupus erythematosus, and alcoholic hallucinosis or paranoia.

Treatment

Optimally, treating seizures in an attempt to improve patients lives and to prevent seizure-associated psychiatric symptoms is a treatment priority. In the elderly patient, the choice of appropriate anticonvulsant medication is essential given the previously discussed pharmacokinetic and pharmacodynamic changes. (For a comprehensive review on management of epilepsy in the elderly, see Kanner and Frey [73]). When the use of psychotropic medications is considered in patients with epilepsy, the effect of such medication on anticonvulsants, as well as on the seizures themselves, needs to be considered.

Neuroleptic Medications

Neuroleptic medications are divided into either typical or atypical. Typical neuroleptics are divided further into either low- or high-potency drugs. This distinction is made on the drug's potency to block D_2 receptors. Low-potency neuroleptics, such as chlorpromazine and thioridazine, have a lower risk of extrapyramidal symptoms (EPS) but have a high degree of sedation, adrenergic-blocking, and anticholinergic activity compared to high-potency drugs such as haloperidol (21). Haloperidol is less sedating and has lower adrenergic-blocking and anticholinergic prop-

erties than low-potency neuroleptics. However, it has a higher risk of EPS, with akathisia and tardive dyskinesia being most common in the elderly. Both groups of typical neuroleptics have been reported to be effective in the elderly. The side effects of sedation, hypotension, central anticholinergic effects, and electrocardiographic changes make low-potency neuroleptics less ideal for patients at risk of sedation and cardiac problems. High-potency neuroleptics, such as haloperidol, are not ideal for patients at risk of developing parkinsonism.

Atypical Antipsychotics

The newer atypical antipsychotic medications, such as clozapine, sertindole, olanzapine, quetiapine, ziprasidone, and risperidone, are characterized by causing less EPS than typical neuroleptics (21). Although all neuroleptics have the potential to cause seizures by lowering the seizure threshold, clozapine should be avoided in patients with epilepsy because it is the most likely of all the neuroleptics to cause seizures. The only other atypical neuroleptic that has been studied in middle-aged and frail elderly is risperidone. Eastham et al. (21) reported on their findings with risperidone in three different patient populations. In one trial, they studied inpatients in a tertiary-care county hospital with diagnosis of schizophrenia, organic delusional disorder, or bipolar disorder. Patients responded well to low doses of risperidone (range 0.5 to 8 mg per day). Side effects generally could be decreased by lowering the dose. In two other studies, one an open-label trial with schizophrenia patients in an outpatient clinic and the second with frail nursing home patients with severe agitation or psychosis, small doses of risperidone seemed effective and well tolerated (21).

Treatment Recommendations for the Elderly Epileptic Patient with Psychotic Features

From the overview, the following recommendations can be made. First, it is essential to rule out any underlying medical condition that could cause psychotic symptoms in this age group. Treatment of such a cause ultimately will resolve the symptoms. Second, haloperidol should be the drug of choice for the acute treatment of psychosis in the elderly patient with seizures. Doses of 0.5 mg p.o. once or twice a day should be used initially and slowly titrated up until symptoms subside. Third, risperidone should be considered for long-term treatment. Starting doses of 0.25 mg per day are indicated in the elderly. Finally, it is important to assure elderly patients and their families that psychotic episodes have a biologic basis and are not psychological. This is especially important in view of the increased sensitivity to mental disorders in the elderly.

CONCLUSION

There is limited information available in the scientific literature pertaining to psychiatric disorders in the elderly epileptic patient. Epidemiologic data for this patient population are sparse. Geriatric psychopharmacology is just beginning to investigate its implications for elderly patients, and few controlled studies are available. The impact of psychopharmacology on the elderly epileptic patient has not yet been investigated. In the context of the "graying" of the population, continued research is required to ensure the best possible treatments for elderly patients in general and elderly epileptic patients with psychiatric symptoms in particular.

REFERENCES

1. American Association of Retired Persons. *A profile of older Americans: 1999.* Washington, DC: AARP Fulfillment, 1999.
2. Hauser WA. Epidemiology of seizures and epilepsy in the elderly. In: Rowan AJ, Ramsay RE, eds. *Seizures and epilepsy in elderly.* Boston: Butterworth-Heinemann, 1997:7–18.
3. Hauser WA, Annegers JF, Kurland LT. The incidence of epilepsy in Rochester, Minnesota, 1935–1984. *Epilepsia* 1993;34:453.
4. Annegers JF, Hauser WA, Lee JRJ, et al. Acute symptomatic seizures in Rochester, Minnesota, 1935–1984. *Epilepsia* 1995;36:327.
5. Matt GE, Dean A, Wang B, et al. Identifying clinical syndromes in a community sample of elderly persons. *Psychol Assess* 1992;4:174–184.
6. Blazer D, George LK, Hughes D. The epidemiology of anxiety disorder: an age comparison. In: Salzman C, Lebowitz B, eds. *Anxiety in the elderly: treatment and research.* New York: Springer, 1991:17–30.
7. Raj BA, Corvea MH, Dagon EM. The clinical characteristics of panic disorders in the elderly: a retrospective study. *J Clin Psychiatry* 1993;54:150–155.
8. Larkin BA, Copeland JRM, Dewey ME, et al. The natural history of neurotic disorder in an elderly urban population: findings from the Liverpool longitudinal study of continuing health in the community. *Br J Psychiatry* 1992;160:681–686.
9. Kramer M, German PS, Anthony JC, et al. Geriatric psychiatry consultations in a university hospital. *Int Psychogeriatr* 1985;2:161–168.
10. Flint AJ. Epidemiology and comorbidity of anxiety disorders in the elderly. *Am J Psychiatry* 1994;151:640–649.
11. Salzman C. Conclusion. In: Salzman C, Lebowitz B, eds. *Anxiety in the elderly: treatment and research.* New York: Springer, 1991:305–312.
12. Lindesay J. Phobic disorders in the elderly. *Br J Psychiatry* 1991;159:531–541.
13. Casten RJ, Parmelee PA, Kleban MH, et al. The relationships between anxiety, depression, and pain in a geriatric institutionalized sample. *Pain* 1995;6:271–276.
14. Coryell W. Anxiety secondary to depression. *Psychiatr Clin North Am* 1990;13:685–698.
15. Sheikh JI, Salzman C. Anxiety in the elderly: course and treatment. *Psychiatr Clin North Am* 1995;18:871–883.
16. American Psychiatric Association. *Diagnostic and statistical manual of mental disorders*, 4th ed. Washington, DC: American Psychiatric Press, 1994.
17. Mach JR Jr, Maleta G. Anxiolytic and sedative/hypnotic use in the elderly. *Strategies Geriatr* 1995;2:1–5.
18. Schneider LS. Overview of generalized anxiety disorder in the elderly. *J Clin Psychiatry* 1996;57[Suppl 7]:34–45.
19. Schramke CJ. Anxiety disorders. In: Nussbaum PD, ed. *Handbook of neuropsychology and aging.* New York: Plenum Press, 1997:80–97.
20. Betts TA. Depression, anxiety and epilepsy. In: Reynolds EH, Trimble MR, eds. *Epilepsy and psychiatry.* London: Churchill Livingstone, 1981:60–71.
21. Eastham JH, Lacro JP, Lohr JB, et al. Treatment of psychosis in late life. In: Nelson JC, ed. *Geriatric psychopharmacology.* New York: Marcel Dekker, 1998:301–326.
22. Bernus I, Dickinson RG, Hooper WD, et al. Anticonvulsant therapy in aged patients: clinical pharmacokinetic considerations. *Drugs Aging* 1997;10:278–289.
23. Ray WA, Griffin MR, Downey W. Benzodiazepines of long and short elimination half-life and the risk of fractures. *JAMA* 1989;262:3303–3307.
24. Johansson K, Bryding G. Traffic dangerous drugs are often found in fatally injured older male drivers [Letter]. *J Am Geriatr Soc* 1997;45:1029–1031.
25. Zimmer B, Grossberg G. Geriatric psychopharmacology: an update and review. In: Nussbaum PD, ed. *Handbook of neuropsychology and aging.* New York: Plenum Press, 1997:483–507.

26. Baughman OL. The safety record of buspirone in generalized anxiety disorder. In: *Buspirone: seven-year update* [Monograph]. Memphis, TN: Physicians Postgraduate Press, 1994:37–43.

27. Schweizer E, Rickels K. New and emerging clinical uses for buspirone. In: *Buspirone: seven-year update (monograph).* Memphis, TN: Physicians Postgraduate Press, 1994:46–54.

28. Sussman N. The uses of buspirone in psychiatry. In: *Buspirone: seven-year update (monograph).* Memphis, TN: Physicians Postgraduate Press, 1994:3–19.

29. Cadieux RJ. Azapirones: an alternative to benzodiazepines for anxiety. *Am Fam Physician* 1996;53: 2349–2353.

30. Lader M, Ancill R. The treatment of generalized anxiety disorder, panic disorder, and obsessive-compulsive disorder in the elderly. In: Nelson JC, ed. *Geriatric psychopharmacology.* New York: Marcel Dekker, 1998: 367–380.

31. Small GW. Recognizing and treating anxiety in the elderly. *J Clin Psychiatry* 1997;58:41–47.

32. Burke WJ, Folks DG, McNeilly D. Effective use of anxiolytics in older adults. *Clin Geriatr Med* 1998;14: 47–63.

33. Sadavoy J, LeClair JK. Treatment of anxiety disorders in late life. *Can J Psychiatry* 1997;42:28S–34S.

34. Chouinard G, Beauclair L, Belanger M-C. Gabapentin: long-term antianxiety and hypnotic effects in psychiatric patients with comorbid anxiety-related disorders [Letter]. *Can J Psychiatry* 1998;43:305.

35. Gelder M. Psychological treatment for anxiety disorder: adjustment disorder with anxious mood, generalized anxiety disorders, panic disorder, agoraphobia, and avoidant personality disorder. In: Coryell W, Winokur G, eds. *The clinical management of anxiety disorders.* New York: Oxford University Press, 1991:10–27.

36. Schneider LS, Reynolds CF, Lebowitz DB, et al., eds. *Diagnosis and treatment of depression in late life: proceedings of the NIH consensus development conference.* Washington, DC: American Psychiatric Press, 1994.

37. Blazer D. Current concepts: depression in the elderly. *N Engl J Med* 1989;320:164–166.

38. Lewis A. Melancholia: a historical review. *J Ment Sci* 1934;80:1–42.

39. Mendez MF, Cummings JL, Benson DF. Depression in epilepsy: significance and phenomenology. *Arch Neurol* 1986;43:766–770.

40. Robertson M. The organic contribution to depressive illness in patients with epilepsy. *J Epilepsy* 1989;2: 189–230.

41. Blumer D. Epilepsy and disorders of mood. In: Smith D, Treiman D, Trimble MR, eds. *Neurobehavioral problems in epilepsy.* New York: Raven Press, 1991: 185–195.

42. Devinsky O, Bear DM. Varieties of depression in epilepsy. *Neuropsychiatry Neuropsychol Behav Neurol* 1991;4:49–61.

43. Barraclough B. Suicide and epilepsy. In: Reynolds EH, Trimble MR, eds. *Epilepsy and psychiatry.* Edinburgh: Churchill Livingstone, 1981:72–76.

44. Hermann BP, Wyler AR. Depression, locus of control, and the effects of epilepsy surgery. *Epilepsia* 1989;30: 332–338.

45. Indaco A, Carrieri PB, Nappi C, et al. Interictal depression in epilepsy. *Epilepsy Res* 1992;12:45–50.

46. Victoroff JI, Benson DF, Grafton ST, et al. Depression in complex partial seizures: electroencephalography and cerebral metabolic correlates. *Arch Neurol* 1994;51: 155–163.

47. Moore DP. *Partial seizures and interictal disorders: the neuropsychiatric elements.* Boston: Butterworth-Heinemann, 1997.

48. Starkstein SE, Robinson RG. Depression in cerebral vascular disease. In: Starksten SE, Robinson RG, eds. *Depression in neurologic disease.* Baltimore: The Johns Hopkins University Press, 1993:28–49.

49. Hasegawa H, Kanner AM. Seizure control following chronic pharmacotherapy in epileptic disorders beginning after 40 years of age. *Clin Neuropharmacol* 1995; 18:13–22.

50. Jenike MA. *Handbook of geriatric psychopharmacology.* Littleton, MA: PSG Publishing, 1985.

51. Perrine K, Congett S. Neurobehavioral problems in epilepsy. *Neurol Clin North Am* 1994;12:129–152.

52. Kanner AM, Nieto JCR. Depressive disorders in epilepsy. *Am Acad Neurol* 1999;53[Suppl 2]:S26–S32.

53. Kanner AM, Pallac S. Depression in epilepsy: a common but often unrecognized comorbid malady. *Epilepsy and Behavior* 2000;1:37–51.

54. Kraepelin E. *Clinical psychiatry.* New York: Delmar, Scholars Facsimilies and Reprints, 1981. Diefendorf AR, translator.

55. Nelson CJ. Treatment of major depression in the elderly. In: Nelson CJ, ed. *Geriatric psychopharmacology.* New York: Marcel Dekker, 1998:61–97.

56. Salzman C. A primer on geriatric psychopharmacology. *Am J Psychiatry* 1982;139:67–76.

57. Dailey JW, Naritoku DK. Antidepressants and seizures: clinical anecdotes overshadow neuroscience. *Biochem Pharmacol* 1996;52:1323–1329.

58. Brymer C, Winogard CH. Fluoxetine in elderly patients: is there cause for concern? *J Am Geriatr Soc* 1992;40: 902–905.

59. Reynolds CF III, Alexopoulos G, Katz I, et al. Treatment of geriatric mood disorders. In: Rush JA, ed. *Mood and anxiety disorders.* Philadelphia: Current Science, 1998:122–144.

60. Goldstein G. Psychotic disorders in late life. In: Nussbaum PD, ed. *Handbook of neuropsychology and aging.* New York: Plenum Press, 1997:98–110.

61. Goldberg TE, Weinberger DR. Probing prefrontal function in schizophrenia with neuropsychological paradignms. *Schizophr Bull* 1988;14:179–183.

62. Gruzelier JH. Hemispheric imbalance syndromes of schizophrenia, premorbid personality, and neurodevelopmental influences. In: Steinhauer SR, Gruzelier J, Zubin J, eds. *Handbook of schizophrenia.* London: Elsevier, 1991:599–650.

63. Jeste DV. Late-life schizophrenia: editor's introduction. *Schizophr Bull* 1993;19:687–689.

64. Slater E, Beard AW. The schizophrenia-like psychoses of epilepsy, V: discussion and conclusions. *J Neuropsychiatry Clin Neurosci* 1995;7:37–378. Reprinted from *Br J Psychiatry* 1963;109:143–150.

65. Sachdev P. Schizophrenia-like psychosis and epilepsy: the status of the association. *Am J Psychiatry* 1998;155: 325–336.

66. Devinsky O, Kelly K, Porter RJ, et al. Clinical and electroencephalographic features of simple partial seizures. *Neurology* 1988;43:1347–1352.

67. Penfield W, Jasper H. *Epilepsy and the functional anatomy of the human brain.* Boston: Little, Brown, 1954.
68. Kanner AM, Stagno S, Kotagal P, et al. Postictal psychiatric events during prolonged video-electroencephalographic monitoring studies. *Arch Neurol* 1996;53:258.
69. Trimble MR. *The psychoses of epilepsy.* New York: Raven, 1991.
70. Umbricht D, Degreef G, Barr, WB, et al. Postictal and chronic psychoses in patients with temporal lobe epilepsy. *Am J Psychiatry* 1995;152:224.
71. Bruton CJ, Stevens JR, Frith CD. Epilepsy, psychoses, and schizophrenia: clinical and neuropathologic correlations. *Neurology* 1994;44:34–42.
72. Trimble MR, Schmitz B. The psychoses of epilepsy: a neurobiological perspective. In: McConnell H, Snyder P, eds. *Psychiatric comorbidity in epilepsy.* Washington, DC: American Psychiatric Press, 1998: 169–186.
73. Kanner AM, Frey M. The management of epileptic seizures in the elderly patient. *Clin Geriatr* 1998;6: 12:542–548.229

15

Psychiatric Issues in Epilepsy Surgery

Dietrich P. Blumer and *Keith Davies

*Departments of Psychiatry and *Neurosurgery, University of Tennessee, Memphis, Tennessee 38105*

Although epilepsy surgical techniques were developed more than 50 years ago, treatment of epilepsy has undergone a change in the last 20 years with the expansion of the number of epilepsy surgery programs throughout North America and, to a lesser degree, in other parts of the world (1). Epilepsy surgery has had a major impact on the treatment of epilepsy conditions such as mesial temporal sclerosis (MTS), in which antiepileptic drugs are expected to yield a seizure-free rate in only 25% of patients (2). Conversely, a unilateral anterior temporal lobectomy can be expected to render 60% to 80% of these patients seizure-free (3). Identification of candidates for surgical treatment among patients with various forms of drug-resistant seizure disorders has become routine in most major epilepsy centers.

Surgically, the problem of treating epilepsy may be approached in three different ways that are not mutually exclusive:

1. Resection of a "focus" or epileptogenic area, if one can be identified. This may require electroencephalographic monitoring with intracranial electrodes in the absence of good agreement of data from noninvasive monitoring, with structural abnormalities demonstrated on imaging studies. Stimulation mapping may be necessary if the onset is believed to be in areas of eloquent cortex. A basic principle of resection is that, although the epileptogenic area is removed, the integrity of functioning, eloquent cortex (e.g., language, memory, sensorimotor) should be preserved.
2. Prevention of propagation of a discharge, either interhemispheric as with corpus callosum section, or locally with multiple subpial transection.
3. Chronic stimulation of the left vagus nerve, which is a novel modality introduced recently and which has been shown to have antiepileptic effects.

Anterior temporal lobectomy is the most frequently performed procedure in most, if not all, centers. It yields the best seizure control in patients with MTS. The seizure-free rate falls to about 40% to 50% in patients with temporal onset without MTS (4). In selective amygdalohippocampectomy, resection of the mesial temporal structures is undertaken in the presence of imaging-demonstrated MTS or when the ictal onset is shown to be mesial temporal with intracranial monitoring (5). The results are similar to those for anterior temporal lobectomy. Partial seizures are much less frequently of extratemporal origin, and their surgical treatment yields a seizure remission rate that depends on the demonstration of a structural abnormality, being 60% to 70% in the presence of a lesion but 30% to 50% in the absence of a lesion (3). Unilateral frontal lobectomy is the most frequently performed type of extratemporal resection. The psychiatric changes among patients who undergo frontal lobectomy have not been well studied, but they appear to be similar to those of patients treated with temporal resection, a not surprising finding if one considers the intimate connection of the temporal and frontal limbic systems.

For patients with infantile hemiplegia and widespread hemisphere damage, complete hemispherectomy yielded excellent results for seizure control, and there was remarkable improvement of patients' behavior (6). However, enthusiasm for the procedure waned when late complications of hemosiderosis became apparent (7). Modification of the procedure either by obliteration of the resection cavity (8) or functional disconnection with preservation of frontal and occipital lobes (9) has resulted in a decline in the late complication rate and renewed enthusiasm in appropriate candidates. The most recent modification is periinsular hemispherotomy, whereby the entire hemisphere is disconnected without the need to remove any brain substance (10).

Corpus callosotomy has been used for the treatment of generalized epilepsy or partial epilepsy with secondary generalization when the onset cannot be localized. It is particularly effective for the drop seizures of Lennox-Gastaut syndrome. Freedom from seizures is achieved infrequently (11). Apart from a postoperative syndrome of mutism and lethargy, no specific neuropsychiatric complications are reported. Anterior partial callosotomy does not usually have significant cognitive consequences, but complete callosotomy often produces a hemisphere disconnection syndrome resulting in disabling symptoms of intermanual conflict (12). The failure of interhemispheric transfer can be demonstrated in the conventionally organized patient (left hemisphere dominant for language) by failure of the patient to be able to name an object placed in the left hand (which now has access only to the mute right hemisphere). Similarly, objects placed in the left visual field cannot be named, although the left hand (connected to the same hemisphere) can retrieve the same object.

Local disconnection of epileptogenic cortex can be achieved by the technique of multiple subpial transection developed by Morrell et al. (13). The theoretical basis of this technique is that horizontal intragriseal fibers are transected, thereby preventing local synchronization of epileptogenic activity. Because columnar organization is maintained, eloquent cortex is amenable to the technique without loss of function.

Finally, vagus nerve stimulation, which entails the subcutaneous implantation of a battery-driven pulse generator in the left upper chest connected to electrodes applied to the left vagus nerve, is a novel treatment for intractable epilepsy. It reduces seizure frequency and severity, but it is unlikely to render patients seizure-free (14). Application of a magnet at the onset of a seizure will terminate the seizure in many instances. Vagus nerve stimulation may be associated with the same psychiatric complications that follow significant reduction in seizures by antiepileptic medications or intracranial surgery.

Patients who are candidates for intracranial surgery for intractable epilepsy are routinely administered a battery of neuropsychological tests, and the evaluation contributes information on localization of dysfunction. The evaluation of memory and language (especially naming) is of particular importance. Temporal resection almost invariably includes the hippocampal formation, an area that mediates acquisition of memory. It is imperative that consideration be given to potential risk to memory. The risk for memory seems to be significant almost entirely for surgery on the left, language-dominant side (15). In addition, the risk (for both memory and naming) is greater for late-onset (postadolescent) temporal lobe epilepsy, which is less likely to be associated with hippocampal sclerosis, than for early-onset (childhood) temporal lobe epilepsy, where hippocampal sclerosis is a frequent finding. The functional integrity of nonsclerotic hippocampus is essential for maintaining function, whereas the already damaged, nonfunctioning sclerotic hippocampus may be resected with impunity. The intracarotid amobarbital (Wada) test is an invaluable technique for determining the laterality of language function, as well as the relative functional adequacy of the hippocampi.

Surgical treatment of epilepsy can greatly improve the lives of many patients with drug-resistant epilepsy, but it often is associated with psychiatric complications. Despite the high frequency and significant impact of psychiatric disorders in this type of patients, the role of psychiatrists in presurgical evaluations has been limited to a few epilepsy centers. At a majority of surgical programs, psychiatric profiles, if performed at all, are derived from the completion of self-rating scales and computerized personality inventories (i.e., Minnesota Multiphasic Personality Inventory) as part of the neuropsychological evaluation.

Temporal lobectomy is by far the most common surgical treatment carried out for intractable epilepsy, and the literature on the psychiatric aspects of epilepsy surgery deals almost exclusively with the outcome of temporal lobectomy. For an understanding of the topic, it is necessary to first review phenomenology, pathogenesis, and treatment of the psychiatric disorders that are specifically associated with temporal lobe epilepsy and then to consider the findings of lobectomy in the animal experiment.

PHENOMENOLOGY, PATHOGENESIS, AND TREATMENT OF PSYCHIATRIC DISORDERS ASSOCIATED WITH TEMPORAL LOBE EPILEPSY

Prior to about 1950, psychiatrists were very familiar with the psychiatric disorders specific for epilepsy. In fact, chapters in premodern textbooks of psychiatry tended to focus as much on epilepsy as on schizophrenia or manic-depressive disease (16,17). The psychiatric knowledge of that time was based largely on the observations of institutionalized patients with chronic epilepsy who, in a majority of cases, had shown the neuropathologic finding of MTS (18), the same finding that is common among patients treated surgically since 1951 (19) for temporal lobe epilepsy in the absence of visible structural

lesions. The modern focus on epilepsy as a neurologic disorder has been associated with remarkable progress in understanding seizures and their treatment, but also with conspicuous neglect of the psychiatric aspects of epilepsy and uncertainty about their identity.

In the modern era, the study of patients with mesial temporal lobe epilepsy treated by unilateral anterior temporal lobectomy has been an important factor in prompting renewed interest in the psychiatric aspects of epilepsy. When Bailey and Gibbs (19) introduced the surgical treatment of epilepsy by resection of an anterior temporal interictal focus, they explicitly hoped to improve the psychosocial plight of their patients. Because chronic epilepsy of temporal origin tends to be associated with the development of psychiatric disorders (20–22), the psychiatric study of patients who undergo surgical treatment that can eliminate the seizure disorder is of exceptional psychiatric interest.

The premodern longitudinal study of institutionalized patients with epilepsy had led to the recognition of an intermittent and pleomorphic dysphoric disorder as the most common psychiatric disorder associated with epilepsy. Kraepelin (16) observed that dysphoric symptoms occurred commonly at the time of seizures, during the prodromal and postictal phases, but more prominently independent of seizures, as an interictal disorder. Interictal psychotic episodes were viewed as distinct from schizophrenic psychoses, and Kraepelin considered such episodes as expansion of the dysphoric disorder. The existence of the interictal dysphoric disorder, overlooked by modern cross-sectional analyses of the psychiatric changes among patients with epilepsy, was reconfirmed recently (23). The interictal dysphoric disorder occurs at various intervals, it tends to last a few hours to a couple of days, and the presence of at least three symptoms coincides with significant disability. It consists of eight affective-somatoform symptoms: irritability, depressive moods, anergia, insomnia, pains, anxiety, phobic fears, and euphoric moods. The disorder tends to respond promptly to the addition of modest doses of antidepressant-type medication and meets the four criteria for validity in psychiatric disorders outlined by Robins and Guze (24): clinical phenomenology, genetics (etiology), course, and treatment response. A classification of the major interictal psychiatric disorders is listed in Table 15.1.

Interictal dysphoric disorders tend to develop 2 years or longer following onset of epilepsy (21), whereas interictal psychoses develop on the average 14 years after the first seizure (25), at a time when seizures have decreased or ceased (26). Engel (27) and Stevens (28) postulated that the psychiatric disorders of epilepsy may result from the inhibitory activity that develops in reaction to the excessive excitatory activity of the chronic seizure disorder. Mechanisms to suppress seizure activity and to terminate seizures obviously exist, but their action presently can be assessed only indirectly. The emergence of psychiatric changes with predominant inhibition, at the time when seizure activity has subsided, is well known as the phenomenon termed "forced normalization" by Landolt (29). Landolt's initial observation of forced normalization concerned a patient whose epileptiform electroencephalogram normalized each time he was dysphoric; later observations have focused chiefly on the absence of seizures that tends to be associated with interictal psychoses (alternating psychoses) (30,31). The following findings suggest that the presence of predominant or enhanced inhibitory mechanisms, operating in homeostasis with the excitatory activity, may produce the psychiatric disturbances of the interictal and periictal phases of temporal lobe epilepsy:

1. The development of interictal dysphoric and psychotic disorders is delayed following onset of the epilepsy (21,25), as inhibitory mechanisms become increasingly established. This finding is in accordance with the particular linkage of the psychiatric disorders of epilepsy with its most prominent chronic form, mesial temporal lobe epilepsy.
2. Upon decrease and particularly upon full control of seizures, dysphoric symptoms and psychoses tend to be exacerbated or to emerge *de novo* (forced normalization or alternating psychosis) (29,31).

TABLE 15.1. *Classification of the interictal psychiatric disorder*

Dysphoric disorder	Psychosis

Eight affective-somatoform symptoms
   Depressive moods
   Anergia
   Irritability
   Pain
   Insomnia
   Fears
   Anxiety
   Euphoric moods
	Marked dysphoric disorder with
	   Hallucinations
	   Paranoia
	   Delusions

The interictal dysphoric disorder is defined by the presence of at least three of the eight affective-somatoform symptoms, each to a troublesome degree, in a patient with epilepsy. The symptoms tend to be intermittent (duration of hours to a few days) and occur at a frequency of every few days to every few months.

The interictal psychoses are characterized by a preexisting and concomitant severe dysphoric disorder. The psychotic symptoms need to be present in a more than fleeting pattern. Psychotic episodes can be differentiated from chronic psychoses by their briefer duration (few days to a few weeks vs. months) and may be better termed dysphoric disorders with psychotic features.

Data from Kraepelin E. *Psychiatrie,* 8th ed. Leipzig: Barth, 1923; and Blumer D. Dysphoric disorders and paroxysmal affects: recognition and treatment of epilepsy-related psychiatric disorders. *Harvard Rev Psychiatry* 2000;8:8–17, with permission.

3. There is a delayed phasing-out of the psychiatric changes after surgical elimination of the epileptogenic zone, presumably with only gradual fading of inhibitory mechanisms (32).

4. Psychiatric changes emerge also at times when acute exacerbation of the seizure activity engages an enhanced inhibitory response; thus, dysphoric symptoms commonly occur periictally, in the prodromal and particularly in the postictal phases (16). Dysphoric symptoms also may intensify with the increased seizure activity of the premenstrual phase (33), and a rare type of psychosis termed "paraictal" (34) may occur upon increased seizure frequency.

If exacerbation of seizure activity prompts acute enhancement of inhibitory activity resulting in dysphoric or psychotic disturbance (as in the last described conditions), improved antiepileptic medication is of primary importance. In all other circumstances, when chronic suppression of seizure activity predominates, the pharmacologic treatment has to be directed against the inhibitory mechanisms (26,32,35–38).

The proconvulsant antidepressant drugs at modest doses appear to serve as effective antagonists to excessive inhibition and are indispensable for successful treatment of the interictal dysphoric and psychotic disorders. Gastaut et al. (21) pointed out that, as measured by response to pentylenetetrazol (Metrazol), patients with temporal lobe epilepsy (in contrast to those with primary generalized epilepsy) show a higher interictal seizure threshold than do persons without epilepsy. The bias against the use of antidepressants for the psychiatric disorders of epilepsy, on the grounds that they may lower the seizure threshold (39), is erroneous on both empirical and theoretical grounds. Modest amounts of antidepressant medication do not increase seizure frequency in patients with chronic epilepsy whose dysphoric disorder indicates the presence of marked inhibition. Most antidepressants tend to lower the seizure threshold more than other psychotropic drugs, and their proconvulsant effect may serve to mitigate the psychotoxic effects of excessive inhibition.

The following recommendations for the pharmacotherapy of the psychiatric disorders of epilepsy are based on one of the author's (D.B.) experience at the Epi-Care Center in Memphis over the last 13 years. During that period, the author (D.B.) evaluated and treated every patient with psychiatric complications from a population of over 10,000 patients with epilepsy. (Alternative approaches are discussed in Chapter 5.) The treatment results of a consecutive series of patients with severe dysphoric disorders (37) and of a consecutive series of patients with interictal psychosis (26) have been reported; in both series, the patients had been previously judged intractable. An earlier report of a series of patients with epilepsy treated for their psychiatric complications preceded the author's (D.B.) experience at the Epi-Care Center (35).

Imipramine 100 mg (up to 150 mg) is added at bedtime to the antiepileptic medication, making sure that the common insomnia (consisting of difficulty initiating and maintaining sleep) is corrected. Amitriptyline, doxepin, trimipramine, or nortriptyline may have to be substituted for that purpose. If the patient does not respond well, a selective serotonin reuptake inhibitor (SSRI) is added to the tricyclic, which then usually is kept at 100 mg. Paroxetine 20 mg once or twice daily has been the preferred SSRI, but sometimes a different SSRI may be more effective. One also may proceed in the reverse order by starting with the SSRI and then adding a tricyclic drug, if necessary. When the dysphoric disorder is severe, risperidone about 2 mg once or twice daily may have to be added to the double antidepressant medication. Response to this treatment can be seen not only in the symptoms commonly associated with depressive mood (anergia, insomnia, pains), but also in all the symptoms of the dysphoric disorder, including irritability and anxiety. Response can be expected as soon as the therapeutic dose is reached, allowing a rapid escalation of the dose as necessary. The mechanism of action of the antidepressant drugs for the dysphoric disorder appears to be different from that for traditional depressive disorders: they are effective rapidly, they are effective at lower doses, and they have a broad-spectrum effect for the entire range of the symptomatology.

If interictal dysphoric disorder is associated with suicidality or with psychotic features, it is advisable to start treatment with double antidepressant medication and to add a small dose of a neuroleptic, if necessary. Interictal psychosis can be viewed as dysphoric disorder with predominantly psychotic features (16) and should be treated in identical fashion, not simply with neuroleptics (26).

Interictal dysphoric disorder, recognized by premodern psychiatrists as presenting in a characteristic intermittent and pleomorphic pattern in hospitalized patients with chronic epilepsy, can be recognized nowadays by obtaining a longitudinal history from patient and next of kin in a semistructured manner (Appendix 15.1). The customary modern cross-sectional psychological assessment of patients with epilepsy (usually carried out with methods validated for use in patients who did not have epilepsy) is insensitive to the task. Some patients may have a baseline of depressive mood and anergia that was not reported in the premodern literature and may result from modern antiepileptic medication. However, all the dysphoric symptoms tend to be subject to marked episodic fluctuations, presumably related—as are the seizures—to the intermittent ebb and flow of excitatory and inhibitory influences in the brain. The dysphoric disorder usually can be distinguished from depressive, bipolar, and anxiety disorders without difficulty, even when, in the absence of seizures, it presents as subictal dysphoric disorder (33,40,41). Patients who have brain lesions without an epileptiform component (e.g., frontal lobe lesions) differ by the absence of the intermittent and pleomorphic symptoms characteristic of epilepsy-related psychiatric disorders.

TEMPORAL LOBE SYNDROME AFTER BILATERAL TEMPORAL LOBECTOMY AND IN THE PRESENCE OF A MESIAL TEMPORAL EPILEPTOGENIC FOCUS

Klüver and Bucy (42) first described the remarkable behavioral changes that take place in animals after bilateral temporal lobectomy: placidity, inability to stay focused (hypermetamorphic impulse to action), and hypersexuality. Based on a series of his own studies, Gastaut (43) noted that patients with chronic mesial temporal lobe epilepsy tend to show changes opposite to those seen in Klüver-Bucy syndrome. He pointed out that this finding was not surprising, considering that, because of the effect of the irritative lesion, patients with temporal lobe epilepsy interictally present a state of increased (excitatory and inhibitory) activity of the temporal-limbic system as opposed to the state of globally decreased activity following the ablation experiment (Table 15.2).

The most prominent symptoms of the heightened emotional intensity among patients with chronic mesial temporal lobe epilepsy are the pleomorphic and intermittent changes of interictal dysphoric disorder: intensified moods, angry affect, anxiety, and fears. These global intermittent changes tend to be associated with more subtle habitual changes consisting of a general deepening or intensification of emotionality and a serious, highly ethical, and spiritual demeanor that contrasts starkly with the intermittent and usually regretted outbursts of angry temper, as noted by many observers since premodern times (16,21,41,44–47). Another distinct, although often subtle, personality change has been frequently noted: as opposed to the very brief attention span seen in the Klüver-Bucy syndrome, patients with epilepsy have been noted to be particularly detailed, persistent, and orderly in speech and behavior (16,17, 22). These traits have been referred to by several different names, including "viscosity," "stickiness," and "ixothymia," and in premodern times were often viewed as the leading as-

TABLE 15.2. *Comparison of behaviors after bilateral temporal lobectomy (Klüver-Bucy syndrome) and in the presence of a mesial temporal epileptogenic focus*

Modifications of animal behavior after bilateral ablation of rhinencephalon (principally basal)	Human behavior difficulties in the intervals between psychomotor fits according to case histories, observations, and psychometric examinations of 100 patients
Modifications of general activity	
Augmentation: Animals move about in their cages without cease; are interested in everything and touch everything, as anything attracts transitory attention ("hypervigilance" of attention).	Diminution: Subjects are slow in their movements, gestures, facial expressions, elocution, ideation, voluntary deliberation, and in the association or recollection of ideas. Psychometric tests reveal this slowness, which is accompanied by exactitude in case of normal intelligence.
Modifications of social behavior	
Amelioration: Animals become placid, caressing, lose their combative faculties, and present defensive or aggressive reactions with difficulty.	Aggravation: Subjects become impulsive, aggressive, and inclined to angry and sometimes violent reactions.
Modifications of sexual behavior	
Augmentation: Animals try unceasingly to have sexual relations with any other kind of animal regardless of age, sex, or species.	Diminution: Many subjects become progressively impotent, indifferent, or both.
Modifications of alimentary behavior	
Qualitative but not quantitative modification: Animals put everything to their mouths to smell or taste; they ingest unhabitual aliments.	No modification, neither quantitative nor qualitative.

Adapted from Gastaut H. Interpretation of the symptoms of psychomotor epilepsy in relation to physiological data on rhinencephalic function. *Epilepsia* 1954;3:84–88.

pects of the "epileptic personality." A third pattern among patients with temporal lobe epilepsy that is opposite to what is seen in Klüver-Bucy syndrome is a global hyposexuality, including decreased libidinous and genital arousal. Gastaut and Collomb (48) first described these findings among patients with temporal lobe epilepsy, and their findings have since been frequently confirmed (49,50).

As the result of a fully successful surgical treatment for chronic mesial temporal lobe epilepsy with psychiatric changes, one would expect a reversal of excessive emotionality, viscosity, and hyposexuality, i.e., changes in the direction of the Klüver-Bucy syndrome.

Apart from the three major behavioral effects of removing both temporal lobes listed by Gastaut, the Klüver-Bucy syndrome also includes behavior indicating lack of recognition of objects (psychic blindness), as well as strong oral tendencies in examining objects by licking, biting, chewing, and touching with lips. The oral tendencies have no consistent correlates in humans with temporal lobe epilepsy or after unilateral temporal lobectomy for epilepsy. The "psychic blindness" (not listed by Gastaut, Table 15.2), on the other hand, corresponds clearly to the severe memory deficit that becomes apparent after unilateral lobectomy if the contralateral hippocampal zone is damaged.

REPORTS OF PSYCHIATRIC OUTCOME OF TEMPORAL LOBECTOMY FOR EPILEPSY

Whereas some series of patients who underwent temporal lobectomy either excluded patients with psychiatric complications or ignored the latter, others included a large number of patients who had been cared for in psychiatric institutions (51). Falconer's Guys-Maudsley series of lobectomies included 45% who "had experience of life in institutions" (52), and the Danish series of Jensen and Vaernet (53) consisted entirely of patients who had been "socially incapacitated." The psychiatric history of the patients often was reported insufficiently, and a major problem was the lack of satisfactory diagnostic criteria defining the psychiatric disorders associated with epilepsy. However, the report of psychosis or of suicide can be considered an unequivocal statement.

In Falconer's initial series (51), 11 of 27 patients treated by unilateral temporal lobectomy became depressed postoperatively (with five requiring electroconvulsive therapy). Taylor and Marsh (54) reported that nine patients from Falconer's larger series of 193 patients had committed suicide (six within 4 years, and two within 7 years after the operation); six more patients died in unclear circumstances (54). In a series of 100 of Falconer's patients, Taylor (55) reported seven with *de novo* postoperative psychosis. The report, from the Danish series of 74 patients with temporal lobectomy, of six patients with *de novo* postoperative psychosis and of six suicide attempts during the first postoperative month is striking (56,57). Trimble (58) reviewed all data available from temporal lobectomy series and calculated that postoperative *de novo* psychoses developed in 3.8% to 35.7% (mean 7.6%) of patients and concluded that, in at least some cases, a causal relation by way of forced normalization was suggested.

On the positive side, the heightened tendency to react with anger or violence (usually termed "aggression") may be improved after surgery (59,60), and the preoperative hyposexuality tends to be normalized postoperatively (or rarely reversed to a less welcome prolonged hypersexual phase) if the seizures are completely eliminated (49,60). Both the latter improvements were noted in the Johns Hopkins series of 50 patients reevaluated a mean of 17 years (range 2 to 30 years) after unilateral temporal lobectomy (50). Before surgery, fewer than one-fourth of the patients could be considered socially incapacitated, and only ten patients had been in psychiatric hospitals for brief stays before

surgery. Four patients had *de novo* psychoses with onset a mean 11.6 months (range 6 weeks to 24 months) after left temporal lobectomy; long-term follow-up indicated that these patients were not seizure-free after surgery. A high prevalence of postoperative depressive symptoms was assessed inadequately at the time. One patient committed suicide 4 years after surgery, and a second patient may have died by suicide 10 years after the operation; both patients had continued to have seizures.

Depression, assessed in a global fashion, has been reported to be the most common psychiatric complication following epilepsy surgery. In our more recent experience, depressive episodes after surgery for epilepsy tend to be intermittent and pleomorphic. They should be viewed as postoperative dysphoric disorders with prominent depressive mood (32).

A 20- to 30-year follow-up study by Stevens (61) of 14 patients who had undergone unilateral temporal lobectomy reported an abstract of every case. Of the six patients with poor psychiatric outcome after temporal lobectomy, five developed psychoses (two had been psychiatrically intact prior to surgery) and one became depressive and irritable. Only one of the six patients had become seizure-free. Both patients whose psychiatric status was greatly improved after temporal lobectomy had been rendered seizure-free. The other six patients from the series were rated as mentally normal both before and after surgery, and all but one were rendered seizure-free by the temporal lobectomy. Complete relief from seizures appears to be of significant importance for good psychiatric outcome.

A recent report of the early psychiatric outcome of unilateral temporal lobectomy indicated a high incidence of early postoperative psychiatric disturbances (62). Sixty patients were interviewed before surgery, at 6 weeks, and again at 3 months after the operation. Preoperatively, just over half the patients had displayed significant psychopathology or personality or psychosocial difficulties. At 6 weeks after surgery, half of those without preoperative psychopathology had developed symptoms of anxiety or depression, and 45% of all patients were noted to have increased emotional lability. By 3 months after surgery, emotional lability and anxiety symptoms had diminished, whereas depressive states tended to persist. The authors stated that it had become their practice to warn patients prior to surgery that changes in their mental state may occur in the weeks after the operation.

Although surgery for partial epilepsy can achieve splendid results, better psychiatric outcomes must be aimed for. Psychiatric complications must be determined by finer measures than the presence or absence of postoperative psychosis or suicide, and the evaluation of patients must focus on the psychiatric changes specific for chronic epilepsy. Our Epi-Care Center follow-up study of 50 patients operated on for partial epilepsy reflects a significant improvement in the approach to the psychiatric complications of epilepsy (32). First, the approach was based on the diagnostic concept of the interictal dysphoric disorder consisting of eight key symptoms, with or without psychotic features, allowing an assessment of the quality of life resulting from the seizure disorder and its postoperative modification. Second, it proceeded with pharmacotherapeutic intervention for the psychiatric complications from the time of the preoperative evaluation through the follow-up period. The patients were seen both preoperatively and postoperatively by the same team. The Seizure Questionnaire used in the study is found in Appendix 15.1, together with an illustrative case.

Fifty consecutive patients treated surgically for focal epilepsy (44 temporal and six frontal) were evaluated by established neuropsychiatric methods (Seizure Questionnaire, semistructured interview, and Neurobehavioral Inventory, see Appendix 15.1) before surgery and over a mean period of 2 years after surgery. The patients with interictal dysphoric disorders, with or without psychotic episodes, were treated with tricyclic antidepressant medication alone or combined with

an SSRI and, if necessary, risperidone. The small number of patients who underwent unilateral frontal lobectomies showed similar psychiatric changes as the main group with unilateral temporal lobectomies. We focus here on the findings in the main group of temporal lobectomies.

An exceptional psychiatric morbidity was associated with the months after temporal lobectomy. Before surgery, 25 (57%) of the 44 patients with temporal lobe epilepsy had dysphoric disorders. After surgery, 17 (39%) of the 44 patients experienced either *de novo* psychiatric complications (six psychotic episodes, six dysphoric disorders, and two depressive episodes) or exacerbation of preoperative dysphoric disorders (three patients). Among the 19 patients who had been psychiatrically intact prior to surgery, eight (42%) developed postoperative dysphoric disorders (two with psychotic features) that were significantly related to recurrence of seizures. All psychiatric complications occurred in the first 2 months after surgery, except for the six patients intact before surgery who had a recurrence of seizures and became for the first time dysphoric between 5 and 8 months after the operation. Thus, a similar proportion of the two groups (preoperatively intact vs. dysphoric) experienced postoperative complications. The extent of the postoperative psychiatric complications probably was influenced by the fact that several patients had failed to continue their preoperative psychotropic medication after surgery. A significant predictor of ultimate excellent psychiatric outcome was complete absence of seizures after surgery. All postoperative psychiatric complications remitted on treatment with psychotropic medication in the compliant patients.

ANALYSIS OF PSYCHIATRIC CHANGES ASSOCIATED WITH TEMPORAL LOBECTOMY FOR EPILEPSY

A slight majority of the patients with mesial temporal lobe epilepsy who become candidates for surgical treatment experience troublesome dysphoric and sometimes also psychotic symptoms, presumably as a result of the development of chronic inhibition in reaction to the presence of the epileptogenic zone. If the operation achieves the optimal effect of eliminating the epileptogenic zone *in toto* with lasting freedom from seizures, the dysphoric disorder will disappear gradually 6 to 18 months after surgery, presumably as the inhibitory mechanisms gradually fade. If the surgical effect is suboptimal, patients tend to continue to have seizures, although usually at a much reduced rate. Concomitantly, the psychiatric disorder tends to persist and may be exacerbated, or the seizure disorder may become latent while a "subictal" psychiatric disorder persists. Treatment with psychotropic medications is of crucial importance for many patients with suboptimal surgical effect.

It appears from the literature that patients with epilepsy and marked psychiatric complications may have a higher risk of a stormy psychiatric outcome after surgery (51–57). However, patients who were psychiatrically intact before surgery are likewise at significant risk of postoperative *de novo* dysphoric or psychotic disorders (32,62). The presence of a dysphoric disorder or an interictal psychosis is not a contraindication for epilepsy surgery. The overall outcome is optimal if the epileptogenic zone is abolished, but persistent or *de novo* psychiatric complications are well treated by psychopharmacologic intervention. Clearly, the high risk of postoperative psychiatric complications calls for both a warning to the patients before surgery and ready intervention with psychotropic medication postoperatively. We observed occasional dysphoric or psychotic episodes while patients are still hospitalized after surgery. Therefore, psychotropic medication of preoperatively dysphoric patients should be resumed the day after the operation, and the patients need to be reminded of the importance of continuing the psychotropic together with the antiepileptic medication until they are free from seizures and psychiatric symptoms 6 to 18 months after the operation.

Postictal psychoses obviously are eliminated if the operation renders the patient seizure-free. Most patients with interictal psychosis reported in the literature have generally remained psychotic after temporal lobectomy, even though they may be free from clinical seizures (63,64). This result suggests that seizure activity sustaining the psychosis may not be confined to a well-definable epileptogenic zone. However, there are exceptions. One of our patients with malignant interictal psychosis became completely seizure-free following wide resection of a left frontal epileptogenic zone, and her hallucinatory state with self-mutilation and suicide attempts first diminished then cleared up completely 16 months after the operation (26).

It may be presumed that the postoperative lessening of excitatory activity with enhanced predominance of inhibition favors both the worsening and the *de novo* emergence of dysphoric disorders and psychotic episodes. Presumably, the inhibitory mechanisms will fade only gradually after optimal removal of the epileptogenic zone, resulting in a delayed recovery from psychiatric disorders. With suboptimal surgical results, on the other hand, as there is a recurrence of seizures after surgery, renewed seizure-suppressing activity again may favor psychiatric complications. Beyond the proximate postoperative phase, presumably upon the development of more predominant inhibition as the seizure disorder persists, a psychiatric disorder may become more severe, requiring more vigorous psychotropic treatment. Stevens (61) suggested that postoperative worsening of the psychiatric status may result from anomalous synaptic regeneration following temporal lobectomy, but her findings confirm that persistence of the seizure disorder appears to be the decisive factor for poor psychiatric outcome of epilepsy surgery.

The changes, after an operation has eliminated the epileptogenic zone, are clearly in the direction of the Klüver-Bucy syndrome: heightened emotionality with dysphoric symptomatology is diminished and sexual arousal is increased, occasionally to the extreme of a hypersexuality that will subside upon recurrence of seizures or spontaneously about 2 years after surgery, a time span identical to the duration of the hypersexuality of the Klüver-Bucy syndrome. Reversal of viscosity has not been documented by clinical observations and may require the use of psychometric testing as carried out for patients with mesial temporal lobe epilepsy by Gastaut (20).

The team at an epilepsy center that surgically treats for epilepsy includes a neuropsychologist. Neuropsychologists have developed fine skills for assessing the cognitive functions of patients with epilepsy and, in particular, the memory functions of those considered for surgical treatment. A modern comprehensive epilepsy center also must include a psychiatrist who is able to recognize and treat the specific psychiatric changes associated with chronic epilepsy.

REFERENCES

1. Penfield W, Baldwin M. Temporal lobe seizures and the technic of subtotal temporal lobectomy. *Ann Surg* 1952;136:625–634.
2. Glaser GH. Natural history of temporal lobe-limbic epilepsy. In: Engel J Jr, ed. *Surgical treatment of the epilepsies.* New York: Raven Press, 1987:13–30.
3. Engel J Jr, Van Ness P, Rasmussen TB, et al. Outcome with respect to epileptic seizures. In: Engel J Jr, ed. *Surgical treatment of the epilepsies,* 2nd ed. New York: Raven Press, 1993:609–621.
4. Davies KG, Hermann BP, Dohan FC Jr, et al. Relationship of hippocampal sclerosis to duration and age of onset of epilepsy, and childhood febrile seizures in temporal lobectomy patients. *Epilepsy Res* 1996;24:119–126.
5. Wieser HG. Selective amygdalohippocampectomy. In: Wyler AR, Hermann BP, eds. *The surgical management of epilepsy.* Boston: Butterworth-Heinemann, 1994: 155–170.
6. Krynauw RA. Infantile hemiplegia treated by removing one cerebral hemisphere. *J Neurol Neurosurg Psychiatry* 1950;13:243–267.
7. Wilson PJ. Cerebral hemispherectomy for infantile hemiplegia: a report of 50 cases. *Brain* 1970;93: 147–180.
8. Adams CBT. Hemispherectomy—a modification. *J Neurol Neurosurg Psychiatry* 1983;46:617–619.
9. Rasmussen T. Hemispherectomy for seizures revisited. *Can J Neurol Sci* 1983;10:71–78.
10. Villemure JG, Mascott CR. Peri-insular hemispherotomy: surgical principles and anatomy. *Neurosurgery* 1995;37:975–981.
11. Wyler AR. Corpus callosotomy. In: Wyler AR, Her-
mann BP, eds. *The surgical management of epilepsy.* Boston: Butterworth-Heinemann, 1994:139–145.
12. Reeves AG, Risse G. Neurological effects of callosotomy. In: Reeves AG, Roberts DW, eds. *Epilepsy and the corpus callosum 2.* New York: Plenum Press, 1995: 241–251.
13. Morrell F, Whisler WW, Bleck T. Multiple subpial transections: a new approach to the surgical treatment of focal epilepsy. *J Neurosurg* 1989;70:231–239.
14. Schachter SC, Saper CB. Vagus nerve stimulation. *Epilepsia* 1998;39:677–686.
15. Hermann BP, Seidenberg M, Haltimer A, et al. Relationship of age at onset, chronological age, and adequacy of preoperative performance to verbal memory change after anterior temporal lobectomy. *Epilepsia* 1995;36:137–145.
16. Kraepelin E. *Psychiatrie,* 8th ed. Leipzig: Barth, 1923.
17. Bleuler E. *Lehrbuch der Psychiatrie,* 8th ed. Berlin: Springer, 1949.
18. Gastaut H. État actuel des connaissances sur l'anatomie pathologique des épilepsies. *Act Neurol Psychiatr Belg* 1956;56:5–20.
19. Bailey P, Gibbs FA. The surgical treatment of psychomotor epilepsy. *JAMA* 1951;145:365–370.
20. Gastaut H, Roger J, Lesèvere N. Différenciation psychologique des épileptiques en fonction des formes électrocliniques de leur maladie. *Rev Psychol Appl* 1953;3:237–249.
21. Gastaut H, Morin G, Lesèvre N. Étude du comportement des épileptiques psychomoteurs dans l'intervalle de leurs crises: les troubles de l'activité globale et de la sociabilité. *Ann Med Psychol (Paris)* 1955;113:1–27.
22. Blumer D. Temporal lobe epilepsy and its psychiatric significance. In: Benson DF, Blumer D, eds. *Psychiatric aspects of neurologic disease.* New York: Grune & Stratton, 1975:171–197.
23. Blumer D, Montouris G, Hermann B. Psychiatric morbidity in seizure patients on a neurodiagnostic monitoring unit. *J Neuropsychiatry Clin Neurosci* 1995;7: 44–56.
24. Robins E, Guze SB. Establishment of diagnostic validity in psychiatric illness: its application to schizophrenia. *Am J Psychiatry* 1970;126:983–987.
25. Slater E. Beard AW. The schizophrenia-like psychoses of epilepsy. *Br J Psychiatry* 1963;109:95–150.
26. Blumer D, Wakhlu S, Montouris G, et al. Treatment of the interictal psychoses. *J Clin Psychiatry* 2000;61: 110–122.
27. Engel J. *Seizures and epilepsy.* Philadelphia: FA Davis Co., 1989.
28. Stevens JR. Interictal clinical manifestations of complex partial seizures. In: Penry JK, Daly DD, eds. *Advances in neurology,* Volume 11. *Complex partial seizures and their treatment.* New York: Raven Press, 1975:85–112.
29. Landolt H. Serial electroencephalographic investigations during psychotic episodes in epileptic patients and during schizophrenic attacks. In: de Haas L, ed. *Lectures on epilepsy.* Amsterdam: Elsevier, 1958: 93–133.
30. Landolt H. Über Verstimmungen, Dämmerzustände und schizophrene Zustandsbilder bei Epilepsie: Ergebnisse klinischer und elektroenzephalographischer Untersuchungen. *Schweiz Arch Neurol Psychiatrie* 1955;76: 313–321.

31. Landolt H. Die Dämmer und Verstimmungszustände bei Epilepsie und ihre Elektroenzephalographie. *Deutsche Zeitschr Nervenheilk* 1963;185:411–430.

32. Blumer D, Wakhlu S, Davies K, et al. Psychiatric outcome of temporal lobectomy for epilepsy: incidence and treatment of psychiatric complications. *Epilepsia* 1998;39:478–486.

33. Blumer D, Herzog AG, Himmelhoch J, et al. To what extent do premenstrual and interictal dysphoric disorder overlap? Significance for therapy. *J Affect Disord* 1998; 48:215–225.

34. Schmitz B, Wolf P. Psychoses in epilepsy. In: Devinsky O, Theodore WH, eds. *Epilepsy and behavior.* New York: Wiley-Liss, 1991:97–128.

35. Blumer D, Zielinski J. Pharmacologic treatment of psychiatric disorders associated with epilepsy. *J Epilepsy* 1988;1:135–150.

36. Blumer D. Postictal depression: significance for the treatment of the neurobehavioral disorder of epilepsy. *J Epilepsy* 1992;5:214–219.

37. Blumer D. Antidepressant and double antidepressant treatment for the affective disorder of epilepsy. *J Clin Psychiatry* 1997;58:3–11.

38. Blumer D. Diagnosis and treatment of psychiatric problems associated with epilepsy. In: Smith DB, ed. *Epilepsy: current approaches to diagnosis and treatment.* New York: Raven Press, 1990:193–209.

39. McConnell HW, Duncan D. Treatment of psychiatric comorbidity in epilepsy. In: McConnell HW, Snyder PJ, eds. *Psychiatric comorbidity in epilepsy: basic mechanisms, diagnosis and treatment.* Washington, DC: American Psychiatric Press, 1998:245–361.

40. Blumer D, Heilbronn M, Himmelhoch J. Indications for carbamazepine in mental illness: atypical psychiatric disorder or temporal lobe syndrome? *Compr Psychiatry* 1988;29:108–122.

41. Blumer D. Dypshoric disorders and paroxysmal affects: recognition and treatment of epilepsy-related psychiatric disorders. *Harvard Rev Psychiatry* 2000;8:8–17.

42. Klüver H, Bucy PC. Preliminary analysis of functions of the temporal lobes in monkeys. *Arch Neurol Psychiatry* 1939;42:979–1000.

43. Gastaut H. Interpretation of the symptoms of psychomotor epilepsy in relation to physiological data on rhinencephalic function. *Epilepsia* 1954;3:84–88.

44. Freud S. Dostoevsky and parricide. In: Strachey J, ed. *The standard edition of the complete works of Sigmund Freud,* Volume 21. London: Hogarth, 1961: 177–196.

45. Szondi L. *Schicksalanalytische Therapie: ein Lehrbuch der passiven und activen analytischen Psychotherapie.* Bern: Huber, 1963.

46. Geschwind N. The clinical setting of aggression in temporal lobe epilepsy. In: Fields WS, Sweet WH, eds. *Neural bases of violence and aggression.* St. Louis: Green, 1975:273–281.

47. Blumer D. Epilepsy and violence. In: Madden DJ, Lion JR, eds. *Rage, hate, assault and other forms of violence.* New York: Spectrum, 1976:207–221.

48. Gastaut H, Collomb H. Étude du comportement sexuel chez les épileptiques psychomoteurs. *Ann Med Psychol (Paris)* 1954;112:657–696.

49. Blumer D, Walker AE. Sexual behavior in temporal lobe epilepsy. *Arch Neurol* 1967;16:37–43.

50. Walker AE, Blumer D. Behavioral effects of temporal lobectomy. In: Blumer D, ed. *Psychiatric aspects of epilepsy.* Washington, DC: American Psychiatric Association Press, 1984:295–323.

51. Hill D, Pond DW, Mitchell W, et al. Personality changes following temporal lobectomy for epilepsy. *J Ment Sci* 1957;103:18–27.

52. Taylor DC. Psychiatric and social issues in measuring the input and output of epilepsy surgery. In: Engel J Jr, ed. *Surgical treatment of the epilepsies.* New York: Raven Press, 1987:485–503.

53. Jensen I, Vaernet K. Temporal lobe epilepsy: follow-up investigation of 74 temporal lobe resected patients. *Acta Neurochirurg* 1977;37:173–200.

54. Taylor DC, Marsh SM. Implications of long-term follow-up studies in epilepsy. In: Penry JK, ed. *Epilepsy: 8th international symposium.* New York: Raven Press, 1977:27–34.

55. Taylor DC. Mental state and temporal lobe epilepsy. *Epilepsia* 1972;13:727–765.

56. Jensen I, Larsen JK. Mental aspects of temporal lobe epilepsy. *J Neurol Neurosurg Psychiatry* 1979;42: 256–265.

57. Jensen I, Larsen JK. Psychoses in drug resistant temporal lobe epilepsy. *J Neurol Neurosurg Psychiatry* 1979; 42:948–954.

58. Trimble MR. Behaviour changes following temporal lobectomy, with special reference to psychosis [Editorial]. *J Neurol Neurosurg Psychiatry* 1992;55:89–91.

59. James IP. Temporal lobectomy for psychomotor epilepsy. *J Ment Sci* 1960;106:543–558.

60. Walker AE, Blumer D. Long-term effects of temporal lobe lesions in sexual behavior and aggressivity. In: Fields WS, Sweet WH, eds. *Neural basis of violence and aggression.* St. Louis: Green, 1975:392–400.

61. Stevens J. Psychiatric consequences of temporal lobectomy for intractable seizures: a 20–30-year follow-up of 14 cases. *Psychol Med* 1990;20:529–545.

62. Ring HA, Moriarity J, Trimble MR. A prospective study of the early postsurgical psychiatric associations of epilepsy surgery. *J Neurol Neurosurg Psychiatry* 1998; 64:601–604.

63. Serafetinides EA, Falconer MA. The effects of temporal lobectomy in epileptic patients with psychoses. *J Ment Sci* 1962;108:584–593.

64. Reutens DC, Savard G, Andermann F, et al. Results of surgical treatment in temporal lobe epilepsy with chronic psychosis. *Brain* 1977;120:1929–1936.

65. Blumer D. Personality in epilepsy. *Semin Neurol* 1991; 11:155–166.

66. Blumer D. Personality disorders in epilepsy. In: Ratey JJ, ed. *Neuropsychiatry of personality disorders.* Boston: Blackwell Science, 1995:230–263.

67. Blumer D. Evidence supporting the temporal lobe epilepsy personality syndrome. *Neurology* 1999;53[5 Suppl 2]:S9–S12.

APPENDIX 15.1

Case with Severe Interictal Dysphoric Disorder and Optimal Outcome of Right Temporal Lobectomy

At age 24 years, this male patient was evaluated for seizures that began at age 17 and had become intractable. His father had been alcoholic and abusive toward the mother; she left her husband when the patient was 5 years old and she remarried 2 years later. The mother suffered from migraines as well as depressive episodes, and an aunt had epilepsy. The patient obtained only a tenth-grade education but had average intelligence. At one time he had the ambition to become a preacher, but merely did some manual labor until 1 year prior to evaluation. At age 17, he entered a marriage without enthusiasm, had two children, then divorced at age 23. Complex partial seizures had begun to occur daily with about monthly secondary generalization, despite trials with various antiepileptic drugs.

Within 1 year of seizure onset, he developed an interictal dysphoric disorder that became critical at age 22. He had sudden and severe depressive moods that occurred about 2 days per week. During the 2 years prior to surgery, he made four serious suicide attempts, each requiring intensive care and then psychiatric hospitalization. He never received antidepressant medication, was treated by counseling only, and the family was resigned to finding him dead one day. Frequent outbursts of anger remained, usually but not always verbal, and contrasted with his more predominant good-natured behavior. Hypersomnia and frequent anxieties also were present.

Upon evaluation for surgery at age 24, double antidepressant treatment (desipramine 100 mg and paroxetine 20 mg daily) was initiated and led to prompt remission of the dysphoric disorder. A right temporal resection performed 3 months later revealed the presence of end folium sclerosis and abolished further seizures. Dysphoric symptoms persisted 2 months after surgery, but they subsided once he resumed regular intake of the antidepressant medication together with phenytoin. His

sexual arousal increased from monthly to daily about 1 month after surgery, and he pursued female companionship with new enthusiasm. "Everything is in tune now," was the comment of his brother. About 6 months after surgery, he chose to discontinue all his medications and remained in remission from both the epilepsy and the dysphoric disorder.

Comment: The patient was fortunate to survive when his psychiatrists had failed to prescribe antidepressant medication, perhaps because of the brevity of his depressive moods or for fear of causing more seizures. The postoperative delay in recovery from the dysphoric disorder after optimal surgical result was relatively short (few months), perhaps as a result of the relatively brief duration of his epilepsy (7 years). Successful surgery not only abolished the dysphoric disorder but also resulted in a marked increase of his sexual arousal. The patient's temporal lobe syndrome of epilepsy was normalized, in the direction of the Klüver-Bucy syndrome.

Optimal outcome with, in effect, total removal of the epileptogenic zone, as in this patient, is achieved in a minority of patients. In a majority of patients, the surgeon cannot remove the epileptogenic zone *in toto,* and the antiepileptic medication must be continued indefinitely. The patient at risk of a dysphoric or psychotic disorder will then also need to continue psychotropic medication. With modern psychopharmacologic treatment, the poor psychiatric outcomes of unilateral temporal lobectomy for epilepsy reported in the past can be avoided as long as the patients are compliant with therapy.

The Seizure Questionnaire

The *Seizure Questionnaire* was developed at the Epi-Care Center over a number of years to its present form to assess systematically the seizures and the broad psychiatric variables of patients with seizures. It has become indispensable in our practice for the comprehensive and expedient evaluation of patients with seizures, including those with nonepileptic seizures, and it allows for accurate research data. The questionnaire is submitted to the patient and next of kin competent to answer the questions (rarely, because of illiteracy of the informants, it must be completed by the interviewer). The answers are reviewed for completeness and accuracy by the interviewer, who thus obtains a complete set of data by semistructured interview of patient and next of kin together or separately if more straightforward responses need to be facilitated.

The *Seizure Questionnaire* begins with questions about the seizures, including the prodromal and postictal phases (questions 1–11). The second section deals with significant past and present life events (12–21). The third section addresses the physical and emotional health before and after onset of the seizures and includes questions about the history of past abuse, the effects of the epilepsy on emotional life, and the influence of the menstrual cycle on seizures and on moods (22 and 23). Then follow the important specific questions about the eight key symptoms of the interictal dysphoric disorder (24–32) and their course in time (question 29 addresses not a key symptom but the general lability of moods); the number of any key symptom that is troublesome by itself is circled. Two questions address psychotic symptomatology (33 and 34). This main section ends with questions about confusional episodes apart from seizures, personality traits, history of addiction, and religious orientation (35–39). Finally, there is a list of important illnesses in the family history to be reported by the patient and next of kin (40). On the last page, the interviewer will establish a relatively detailed family tree of the patient for documentation of illnesses as well as of social achievements (occupations) and difficulties in the family.

The *Neurobehavioral Inventory* is used as an adjunct to the *Seizure Questionnaire*. This inventory consists of 100 true/false questions presented in two different formats for patient and next of kin. It is used only if the patient has at least average intelligence and is not of crucial importance if the *Seizure Questionnaire* is completed properly. The inventory is geared for patients with epileptic seizures, serves to detect data perhaps not fully revealed in the questionnaire, helps clarify differences in the responses of patient and next of kin, and reveals more refined aspects of the patient's personality. The *Neurobehavioral Inventory* has been published elsewhere together with discussion of its validity (65–67).

QUESTIONNARE FOR SEIZURE PATIENTS

NAME OF PATIENT _____ DATE _____

DATE OF BIRTH _____ AGE _____ SEX _____

RACE _____

OCCUPATION(S) _____ EDUCATION _____

MARITAL STATUS _____

ADDRESS (IN FULL) _____

TELEPHONE NUMBER _____

HANDEDNESS _____

ASSISTED BY _____ RELATIONSHIP _____ AGE _____

EDUCATION _____

TELEPHONE _____

EMERGENCY CONTACT NAME AND NUMBER _____

_____

_____

Please answer the following questions as precisely as possible. If you do not understand a question, place a question mark (?) beside it. You may use the back of the pages or additional sheets if there is not enough space for your answers.

Some of the questions can best be answered by a close relative or friend. Please get the appropriate assistance to complete the questionnaire.

1. At what age did your seizures begin?

   Minor (small) seizures   Major (generalized) seizures

2. Have your seizures become worse over time? If yes, in what way?

3. What may have caused the seizures (birth injury, febrile convulsions, head injuries, etc.)?

4. List your present and previous medications

   Present   In the Past

5. How often do your minor and major seizures occur? (Please circle: per day, week or month)

   Minor seizures
   The most I have _____
   The least _____
   The average _____

   Major seizures
   The most I have _____
   The least _____
   The average _____

6. What, if anything, may bring about a seizure?

7. Describe any changes occurring regularly *for hours or days before the seizures:*

   How long does this last before the seizure takes place?

8. What do you remember about your seizures? (Include a detailed description of any aura or warning you may have.)

   Is this always the same?

   How long does this last?

9. What do others observe at the time of a seizure?

   Do others tell you that the seizures vary or do they say they are always the same?

   How long do observers of your seizures tell you they last?

10. Describe what happens after the seizure is over:

    How long does it take?

11. List other medical problems you may have:

12. Your years of education:

13. What type of work did you wish to pursue?

14. Your work experience:

    When did you work last?

15. Your present living situation:

16. Your marital history:

17. Has sex been important in your life?

18. What effect has epilepsy had on your sex life?

    Since about when?

19. Do you have many close friends?

20. What effect has epilepsy had on your social life?

21. Briefly list your hobbies and other things you enjoy doing:

22. How was your physical and emotional health *before onset of epilepsy*? (List any counseling, psychiatric treatment, medication, or hospital stay.)

    Have you ever been in an abusive situation? If so, please describe:

23. Describe the effects of epilepsy on your emotional life:

    List any counseling, psychiatric treatment, medication, or hospital stay:

For Female Patients:

How does your menstrual cycle affect your seizures?

How does your menstrual cycle affect your moods?

24. Do you have frequent depressive moods?

    Since about when?

    Are they present all the time or off and on?

    How long do they last (hours, days, or weeks)?

    How often do they occur?

25. Do you often lack energy?

    Since about when?

    Do you lack energy all the time or episodically?

    If episodically, indicate how often and how long this lasts (hours, days, weeks)?

26. Do you have trouble with your sleep?

    Since about when?

    How often and what kind of trouble?

27. Do you have many aches and pains? (Please describe pain and location.)

    Since about when?

    How often and for how long?

247

28. Do you have sudden moods of happiness?

    Since about when?

    How often and for how long?

29. Do your moods often change out of the blue?

    Since about when?

    How frequently do your moods change unpredictably (by hours, days, or weeks)?

30. Are you often very irritable?

    Do you have outbursts of temper?

    Since about when?

    How often do you become very irritable?

31. Do you have frequent worries (anxieties)?

    Since about when?

    How often do you feel very worried?

32. Do you have fears of certain situations?

    Since about when?

    What fears do you have (being in crowds, being alone, or other)?

33. Do you often mistrust others?

    Do you imagine things?

    Since about when?

34. Do you sometimes hear or see things that are not there?

    Since about when? Please describe:

35. Do you have periods of confusion or loss of memory, even without a seizure?

    Since about when?

36. Do you tend to be very good-natured and conscientious?

    Since about when?

37. Do you tend to be very orderly, strong on details, persistent in your actions? (Please circle which one[s] apply to you.)

Since about when?

38. Have you ever suffered from a drug or alcohol addiction?

About when?

39. What are your religious (spiritual) beliefs and practices?

Since about when?

Please list your pattern of religious practices or spiritual experiences:

40. List family members who have suffered from:
Epilepsy
Migraine
Stuttering
Neurologic disorder
Psychiatric disorder
Alcoholism
Drug addiction

To be completed by Examiner:

Family Tree (with occupations and exceptional traits of first-degree relatives; include any second-degree relative with significant illness)

Examiner: _____

Date: _____

16

Anticonvulsants and Psychiatric Disorders

Ahmad Beydoun and Erasmo A. Passaro

Department of Neurology, University of Michigan Health System, Ann Arbor, Michigan 48109

Anticonvulsants have had a significant impact on the treatment of psychiatric illnesses, especially in their role as mood stabilizers and for treatment of anxiety disorders. Although lithium remains a first-line treatment for bipolar disorders, it is effective only in a proportion of patients (1–3) and is of limited benefit in specific subgroups, including patients with rapid cycling (1,4), dysphoric mania, or when associated with alcohol or substance abuse (5). In addition, lithium appears to lose its efficacy over time in some patients, possibly because of the development of tolerance (6,7). Although neuroleptics were shown to have efficacy in affective disorders, alternative treatment with safe drugs has been sought, with anticonvulsants leading the pack. Following the success of valproate and carbamazepine for treatment of psychiatric conditions, recent studies have evaluated the safety and efficacy of some of the newer anticonvulsants introduced to the market. This chapter reviews experience with antiepileptic drugs in the treatment of psychiatric conditions. The reader is referred to Chapter 12 for a review of the psychotropic property considerations of anticonvulsants in the treatment of epilepsy.

VALPROATE

History

Valproic acid was first synthesized in the United States in 1882 and was used as an organic solvent (8). In 1963, Meunier discov-ered its antiepileptic potential serendipitously when he learned that nonepileptic compounds that were dissolved in valproic acid developed anticonvulsant activity (9). Valproate is a simple branched-chain carboxylic acid that is structurally distinct from other antiepileptic and psychotropic drugs. Valproate has been available in Europe as an anticonvulsant since the late 1960s and initially was approved by the United States Food and Drug Administration (FDA) for generalized tonic-clonic seizures in 1978 (10).

Valproate's efficacy in affective disorders was first recognized in 1966. The French investigator Lambert demonstrated that valpromide, the primary amide of valproic acid, was effective in affective disorders in hospitalized psychiatric patients with "melancholia" (11). This early study was an open-label study in patients with descriptive diagnoses, as diagnostic research criteria for affective illnesses such as unipolar depression and bipolar illness were not yet developed. As a result, some patients with personality disorders or psychotic disorders may have been included. In addition, some of these patients were treated with other psychotropic medications, such as antidepressants and neuroleptics. Later in 1980, Emrich et al. (11a) found that valproate also was useful in bipolar illness.

Acute Mania

Recent open-label and controlled clinical trials evaluated the efficacy of valproate for treatment of acute mania. A total of seven controlled clinical trials demonstrated the superiority of valproate over placebo and its equivalent efficacy to lithium and haloperidol for the short-term treatment of mania. Pope et al. (12) conducted a placebo-controlled, double-blind, randomized clinical trial of valproate in 36 patients who failed to respond to or were intolerant of lithium. The 17 patients randomized to valproate had a 53% median improvement compared to a 5% median improvement for placebo-treated patients. More recently, Bowden et al. (13) completed a large randomized, double-blind, parallel-group study of 179 acutely manic patients who met diagnostic research criteria for mania. Half of their patients previously were unresponsive to lithium. They randomly assigned patients to valproate, lithium, or placebo for 21 days after a 3-day washout period. Treatment with valproate and lithium led to an improvement in 48% and 49% of patients, respectively. These results were significantly better than the 25% improvement seen in placebo-treated patients. In that study, the efficacy of valproate appeared to be independent of prior response to lithium. In their review of previously published studies of valproate in acute mania, Keck and McElroy (14) found that 71 (53%) of 134 patients who received valproate had a moderate or marked reduction in acute manic symptoms. In these studies, the antimanic response to valproate occurred within several days to 2 weeks of achieving a serum valproate concentration greater than 50 mg/L. Typically, valproate is started at a dose of 20 mg per kg per day in divided doses (15), with serum levels between 45 and 125 mg/L usually associated with good efficacy and tolerability (16). The possibility of oral or intravenous loading with valproate is useful for achieving rapid stabilization in acutely manic patients. Valproate is the only drug other than lithium approved by the FDA for treatment of bipolar disorders.

Rapid-Cycling Bipolar Illness

In a double-blind, placebo-controlled clinical trial, valproate was found to be equally effective for patients with rapid- or nonrapid-cycling bipolar illness (13). This finding is of clinical relevance, because many patients with rapid cycling fail to respond to lithium therapy (1,4). Calabrese et al. (17) reported similar findings in an open-label prospective study of valproate in 101 patients with rapid-cycling bipolar I and II disorder followed for an average of 17 months. They reported that valproate was effective for both the symptomatic treatment of acute mania and as a prophylactic agent in this rapid-cycling group. Other open-label trials suggest that this drug may be effective for prophylactic treatment of depression in this group of patients (18,19).

Acute Mania with Depressive Symptoms (Mixed Mania)

Similar to patients with rapid cycling, those with mixed mania are less responsive to treatment with lithium (20). In a study of 179 patients, valproate was found to be equally effective for treatment of manic patients with and without depressive symptoms (20).

Major Depression

Controlled studies of valproate in acute unipolar or bipolar depression have not been performed. Although valproate is highly effective in the treatment of acute mania, several open-label studies indicate that valproate has a marginal effect in major depression.

In a review of four open-label trials, McElroy et al. (21) found that treatment with valproate resulted in a significant antidepressant response in only 30% of 195 patients. More recently, Davis et al. (22) found a 66% response rate by week 8 in an open-label, intent-to-treat analysis of valproate in major depression. Because up to 25% to 50% of patients receiving placebo in controlled trials may have a therapeutic antidepressant response (23), valproate's efficacy in the treatment of acute depression remains unresolved. Double-blind, placebo-controlled clinical trials are necessary to clarify this issue.

Prophylactic Treatment of Bipolar Disorder

The efficacy of valproate for maintenance treatment of patients with bipolar disorder was demonstrated in two controlled clinical trials. In a comparative study of 83 patients with bipolar disorder, patients were randomly assigned to treatment with lithium or valpromide, the primary amide form of valproate, which is available in Europe, and were followed up for 2 years (24). There was no significant difference in recurrence rates between the two groups. A more recent unpublished randomized double-blind study of bipolar patients treated for 1 year with valproate, lithium, or placebo demonstrated that valproate was slightly more effective than lithium (25).

Several open-label trials also demonstrated the efficacy of valproate for prophylactic treatment of bipolar illness (18,21,26). The valproate dosage and plasma levels are similar for acute and for maintenance treatment.

Use of combination therapy has become commonplace in the treatment of refractory bipolar disorders. In a recent placebo-controlled clinical trial, patients treated with a combination of lithium and valproate were significantly less likely to suffer a relapse than patients who received lithium and placebo (27). The combination of valproate and carbamazepine might be effective (28,29); however, serum level monitoring is needed because of the drug–drug interactions that are likely to occur when this combination is used.

Secondary Mania

Secondary mania is defined as mania due to an acquired etiology, such as cerebral infarction or traumatic brain injury. Lithium usually is ineffective in secondary mania. One report showed valproate efficacy in a small group of patients with organic brain syndromes (30). However, this issue is unresolved, because a controlled clinical trial addressing this question has not been performed.

Anxiety Disorders

Valproate may be useful for treatment of panic disorders. In a study of 12 patients with panic disorder, treatment with valproate led to a reduction in the intensity and duration of the panic attacks (31). In a 6-week, open-label trial of 12 patients with panic disorder, 75% of patients were purported to have marked improvement in their symptoms, and efficacy was sustained for up to 6 months (32). In a prospective study of 16 patients with panic disorder challenged with lactate infusion to induce panic attacks, treatment with valproate was found to be highly effective (33).

Valproate was shown to have efficacy in reducing the symptoms associated with benzodiazepine withdrawal (34). In addition, it was reported to be useful for treatment of agitation in patients with dementia (35).

Mechanisms of Action

Like other anticonvulsants such as phenytoin, carbamazepine, and lamotrigine, valproate blocks the voltage-gated sodium channel during sustained rapid repetitive neuronal firing (36). Valproate also modulates γ-aminobutyric acid (GABA) activity through multiple mechanisms. For example, chronic valproate treatment results in an increase in whole-brain GABA levels in animals (37) and increased cerebrospinal fluid GABA levels in both volunteers and epileptic patients (38). It also is a weak inhibitor of GABA transaminase, the enzyme responsible for GABA catabolism, and it increases the activity of the GABA-synthesizing enzyme glutamic acid decarboxylase. However, many of these animal studies used valproate doses that are several fold higher than what is clinically used in humans.

Valproate also appears to affect basal ganglia circuits, which are important in cortical hyperexcitability and seizure spread. For example, valproate increases the excitability threshold for caudate-thalamocortical systems (39), possibly by increasing GABA levels in the substantia nigra pars reticulata

(SNr) (40). The SNr, which is GABA-ergic, provides a powerful gating mechanism for generalization of seizures (41).

Frontal-subcortical circuits may be important in behavioral disturbances (42). These circuits consist of parallel segregated loops for motor control, cognition, and behavior. The cognitive/behavioral loop consists of striatal projections from the caudate to the globus pallidus (GP) and the SNr. The SNr and the GP, which comprise the basal ganglia outflow pathway, provide inhibitory GABA-ergic output to the ventral anterior thalamus, which then projects to the dorsolateral prefrontal cortex and the orbitofrontal cortex. Lesions at different levels within this circuit may produce mood disorders such as depression or mania (43). In this regard, valproate may exert its therapeutic effect in mania by enhancing GABA-ergic outflow in the SNr, thereby influencing the activity of thalamocortical projections.

It has been hypothesized that lithium exerts its therapeutic antimanic effect by inhibiting the turnover of the second messenger phosphoinositide (PI). When an agonist binds to a PI-linked receptor, a series of events occur that result in G-protein activation and subsequent activation of the enzyme phospholipase C. This enzyme cleaves phosphatidylinositol 4,5-biphosphate (PIP_2) into inositol triphosphate (IP_3) and diacylglycerol. IP_3 causes calcium release from the endoplasmic reticulum, and diacylglycerol activates protein kinase C, which then activates other proteins via phosphorylation. Both IP_3 and diacylglycerol are cleaved by inositol monophosphatases to free inositol, which then is available to regenerate PIP_2 for the next cycle. Chronic lithium inhibits the enzyme inositol monophosphatase, thereby preventing the regeneration of PIP_2 and disrupting the PI cycle (44). Valproate also appears to have a similar effect on PI turnover (45). In addition, both lithium and valproate reduce protein kinase C α and ε isozyme activity (46,47), and both reduce myristolated alanine-rich C kinase substrate (MARCKS) protein, which is linked to G-protein signal transduction and is involved in cellular processes associated with cytoskeletal restructuring and signaling (48).

CARBAMAZEPINE

Suggestion of the potential usefulness of carbamazepine in the treatment of acute mania was first reported in 1971 (49). Subsequently, carbamazepine became the first anticonvulsant used for treatment of bipolar disorders.

Acute Mania

The efficacy of carbamazepine in the treatment of acute mania was documented in a number of randomized clinical trials. In a comparative, monotherapy trial, 60 patients with acute mania were randomized to carbamazepine (up to 550 mg per day) or chlorpromazine (up to 275 mg per day) (50). There was no significant difference between the two groups over the 3- to 5-week trial duration, with moderate-to-marked improvement seen in 70% and 60% of carbamazepine- and chlorpromazine-treated patients, respectively (50). Other comparative trials versus neuroleptics for treatment of mania reported comparable efficacy but better tolerability with carbamazepine (51–53). Carbamazepine was compared to lithium therapy in randomized, double-blind, clinical trials. These trials showed that both drugs had comparable efficacy and tolerability (54–57), except in one trial where the efficacy of lithium was reported to be significantly better (58). In that 4-week trial, in which a total of 14 patients were evaluated in each group, the median carbamazepine and lithium doses at week 4 were 1,400 mg (1,200 to 1,600 mg) and 2,100 mg (900 to 3,900 mg), respectively. This resulted in a median carbamazepine serum level of 8.8 mg/L and lithium level of 0.87 mEq/L. Although there was a statistical trend for the Mean Brief Psychiatric Scale score and Manic State Rating Scale favoring lithium-treated patients, it did not reach statistical significance. The Clinician Global Impression of Change significantly favored lithium-treated patients because of a more consistent response across patients (58).

Although the combination of lithium and carbamazepine is used frequently in clinical practice for treatment of refractory bipolar patients (59,60), the efficacy of this treatment modality was never established in a placebo-controlled clinical trial. In a retrospective study of 16 rapid-cycling patients given lithium alone or in combination with carbamazepine, improvement was noted earlier in the group receiving combination therapy (61). A number of other open-label studies support the use of this combination (62–65). Carbamazepine also can be added successfully to neuroleptics, but its combination with clozapine is relatively contraindicated because of the potential for hematologic side effects (66) and drug–drug interactions (67).

Controlled clinical trials demonstrated the efficacy of carbamazepine as a prophylactic agent, with efficacy reported in up to 72% of patients. Larger uncontrolled clinical trials using carbamazepine as monotherapy or adjunctive therapy reported a 64% response rate.

Although the rate of tolerance to carbamazepine has not been studied adequately, some data suggest that patients with rapid cycling are more likely to develop tolerance with long-term treatment with carbamazepine (68).

Depression

Limited data suggest that carbamazepine may be effective for treatment of unipolar or bipolar depression (69,70).

Anxiety

Carbamazepine was not found to be effective in the treatment of panic disorders (71). It had moderate benefit in reducing the distress associated with the discontinuation of benzodiazepines (72).

Mechanisms of Action

It is well established that one of the mechanisms of action of carbamazepine responsible for its anticonvulsant effects is via modulation of the sodium channels during high-frequency repetitive firing (73). Al-

though this effect is not believed to play a role in its mood stabilizing properties (6), carbamazepine has a number of other actions that affect a number of neurotransmitters (6). For example, it was found to decrease glutamate release and GABA turnover and to act as an adenosine receptor antagonist (6). The mechanisms responsible for its effect on mood have not yet been elucidated (74).

GABAPENTIN

Bipolar Disorders

The first suggestion of the potential role of gabapentin in mood disorders was derived from the results of clinical trials in patients with epilepsy. In those trials, patients treated with gabapentin had improvement in mood and quality of life, often unrelated to changes in seizure frequency (75). Its efficacy in bipolar disorders has so far only been reported in open-label studies, in which gabapentin was predominantly used as adjunctive therapy for patients with a partial or inadequate response to their treatment regimen. In a retrospective series of 73 patients with refractory bipolar or schizoaffective disorders, the addition of gabapentin at daily doses of 200 to 3,500 mg led to a positive response in 67 patients (76). In another series of nine refractory patients, the addition of gabapentin titrated up to 4,800 mg daily led to significant improvement in manic or hypomanic symptoms in eight patients (77). In an open-label study of 12 patients with treatment-resistant bipolar spectrum disorders, the addition of gabapentin at a median daily dose of 2,400 mg resulted in a marked response in one patient and a moderate response in seven (78). Other uncontrolled studies reported its efficacy for treatment of mania in patients with bipolar disorders (79–82).

Because of its favorable pharmacokinetic profile and lack of drug–drug interaction, gabapentin can be added to other drugs in patients with refractory bipolar disorders without affecting the serum level or metabolism of those drugs.

Depression

In an open-label, 6-week study of 15 patients with bipolar depression, adjunctive treatment with gabapentin at a mean daily dose of 1,050 mg (range 300 to 2,400 mg) led to a significant but modest reduction in the Hamilton Depression Rating Scale (83). Eight patients (53%) responded to treatment (three with a marked response and five with a partial response), and the drug was well tolerated overall (83). This preliminary report needs confirmation in a larger randomized clinical trial.

Anxiety

Gabapentin exhibited anxiolytic effects in a number of animal models of anxiety (84). In an open-label series of 18 patients with a variety of anxiety-related symptoms, the addition of gabapentin at daily dosages of 200 to 1,800 mg led to significant improvement in symptoms (85). In another small series of four patients with panic disorder and generalized anxiety, the use of gabapentin as monotherapy or adjunctive therapy at daily doses of 400 to 1,200 mg led to a marked reduction in symptoms in all four patients (86). Gabapentin also has been anecdotally reported to be useful in the treatment of behavioral agitation associated with dementia (87).

Gabapentin is the first anticonvulsant evaluated in a randomized, placebo-controlled, clinical trial for treatment of social phobia (88). In this 14-week trial, 60 patients with Liebowitz Social Anxiety Scale scores higher than 50 were randomized to treatment with gabapentin (900 to 3,600 mg per day) or placebo. The response rate at the end of the trial was significantly better for gabapentin-treated patients compared to placebo. Higher severity of phobic avoidance at baseline predicted a better response to gabapentin (88).

Mechanisms of Action

The mechanisms of action of gabapentin in psychiatric disorders have not been elucidated. This drug was found to bind to specific and novel receptors in the central nervous system (89). These receptors have been purified and identified as the $\alpha_2\delta$ subunit of a voltage-dependent L-type calcium channel (90). Data from nuclear magnetic resonance spectroscopy showed that, in the presence of gabapentin, the central nervous system level of GABA is increased in a dose-dependent manner and amounted to a 40% increase at a dose of 3,600 mg per day (91). This increase in GABA levels may play a role in its anxiolytic properties. In addition, there is some suggestion that gabapentin modulates the serotonergic system. In one study, there was an increase in the cerebrospinal fluid level of 5-hydroxyindoleacetic acid, the metabolite of serotonin, following gabapentin administration (92). In addition, gabapentin administered to healthy volunteers resulted in an increase in the whole-blood serotonin level (93).

LAMOTRIGINE

Bipolar Disorders

Similar to gabapentin, patients treated with lamotrigine in the epilepsy trials related improvement in their mood and quality of life (94). In an open-label trial, 16 patients with bipolar disorders were treated with lamotrigine as alternative monotherapy or as add-on therapy. At treatment initiation, nine patients were depressed, six were in a mixed state, and one was manic. Eight patients (50%) had a positive response to lamotrigine used at a mean dose of 141 mg per day (range 50 to 250 mg per day) for a mean duration of 5 weeks (95). In a study of seven patients with rapid-cycling bipolar disorders, six of whom were newly diagnosed patients, treatment with lamotrigine at 100 to 500 mg per day resulted in a good response in four of the six newly diagnosed patients within 3 weeks. In the last patient, lamotrigine was added to valproate and resulted in a control of the depressive episodes (96). A number of other open-label studies had concordant results and suggested that lamotrigine as monotherapy or adjunctive therapy is useful for management of treatment-resistant bipolar disorders (97–100).

Although lamotrigine can be used as adjunctive therapy, one has to be careful when using this drug concomitantly with valproate. Valproate inhibits the metabolism of lamotrigine and this combination has been associated with a significantly higher frequency of cutaneous rashes. It is therefore important to start at a low dose and to very gradually increase the lamotrigine dose when this combination is used.

Bipolar Depression

Lamotrigine has been shown to have efficacy in the treatment of bipolar depression. In a study of 22 patients with refractory bipolar depression, the addition of lamotrigine led to improvement, defined as a 50% or better reduction in the Hamilton Depression Rating Scale score in 16 patients (72%) by the end of week 4. By week 6, 14 patients (63%) were reported to be in remission (101).

A recent double-blind, randomized, placebo-controlled clinical trial confirmed the efficacy of lamotrigine for treatment of bipolar depression (102). In that study, 195 patients with bipolar I disorder who experienced a major depressive episode were randomized to 7 weeks of treatment with lamotrigine as monotherapy at daily doses of 50 mg or 200 mg or to placebo. The trial indicated that lamotrigine had a significant and dose-related antidepressant efficacy in bipolar I depression, and that clinical improvement is evident by the third week of treatment. On the Clinician Global Impression Scale for improvement, 51%, 41%, and 26% of patients in the 200 mg per day, 50 mg per day, and placebo groups, respectively, rated their improvement as very much or much improved (102).

Anxiety

There currently are little data on the efficacy of lamotrigine for treatment of anxiety disorders.

Mechanisms of Action

The mechanism of action of lamotrigine in psychiatric disorders has not yet been fully elucidated. Its modulation of sodium-dependent voltage channels, resulting in a decrease in the release of excitatory neurotransmitters (103), could play a role in its mood-stabilization properties.

TOPIRAMATE

Early studies suggest that topiramate may be useful for treatment of affective disorders. In an open-label study, adjunctive therapy with topiramate titrated to 400 mg per day in 44 consecutive patients with refractory mood disorders led to moderate or marked improvement in 52% of patients (104). However, five patients were rated as worse following the addition of topiramate, predominantly because of adverse events consisting of anxiety, confusion, and hallucinations (104). In an open-label study of ten patients with acute mania, treatment with topiramate at daily dosages up to 1,600 mg resulted in a decrease in average mania score (105).

Topiramate has multiple mechanisms of action, including the modulation of voltage-dependent sodium channels, enhancement of GABA activity, inhibition of kainate at the AMPA receptor, and inhibition of carbonic anhydrase (106).

CONCLUSIONS

Carbamazepine and valproate are well established for treatment of some psychiatric disorders. Accumulating data suggest efficacy of newer antiepileptic agents, including gabapentin, lamotrigine, and topiramate. The safety and favorable pharmacokinetic profile of the newer anticonvulsants make them attractive drugs to be considered for treatment of psychiatric conditions. The efficacy of these newer agents to treat psychiatric conditions needs to be established in placebo-controlled, randomized, clinical trials.

REFERENCES

1. Dunner DL, Fieve RR. Clinical factors in lithium carbonate prophylaxis failure. *Arch Gen Psychiatry* 1974; 30:229–233.
2. Grof P. Long-term treatment of bipolar depression. *Psychiatr J Univ Ottawa* 1989;14:390–332.
3. Vestergaard P. Treatment and prevention of mania: a Scandinavian perspective. *Neuropsychopharmacology* 1992;7:249–260.
4. Post RM, Uhde TW, Ballenger JC, et al. Prophylactic efficacy of carbamazepine in manic-depressive illness. *Am J Psychiatry* 1983;140:1602–1604.
5. Post RM. Non-lithium treatment for bipolar disorder. *J Clin Psychiatry* 1990;51[Suppl]:9–16.
6. Post RM, Weiss SR, Chung DM. Mechanisms of action of anticonvulsants in affective disorders: comparisons with lithium. *J Clin Psychopharmacol* 1992;12 [Suppl 1]:23S–35S.
7. Maj M, Pirozzi R, Kemali D. Long-term outcome of lithium prophylaxis in patients initially classified as complete responders. *Psychopharmacology* 1989;98: 535–538.
8. Bowden CL, McElroy SL. History of the development of valproate for treatment of bipolar disorder. *J Clin Psychiatry* 1995;56[Suppl 3]:3–5.
9. Penry JK, Dean JC. The scope and use of valproate in epilepsy. *J Clin Psychiatry* 1989;40:17S–22S.
10. Levy RH, Mattson RH, Meldrum BS, eds. *Antiepileptic drugs,* 4th ed. New York: Raven Press, 1995.
11. Lambert PA, Cavaz G, Borselli S, et al. Action neuropsychotrope d'un nouvel anti-épileptique: le Depamide. *Ann Med Psychol (Paris)* 1966;1:707–710.
11a. Emrich HM, von Zerssen D, Kissling W, et al. Effect of sodium valproate on mania. The GABA-hypothesis of affective disorders. *Arch Psychiatr Nervenkr* 1980; 229:1–16.
12. Pope HG Jr, McElroy SL, Keck PE, et al. Valproate in the treatment of acute mania: A placebo controlled study. *Arch Gen Psychiatry* 1991;48:62–68.
13. Bowden CL, Brugger AM, Swann AC, et al. Efficacy of divalproex vs lithium and placebo in the treatment of mania. *JAMA* 1994;271:918–924.
14. Keck PE Jr, McElroy SL. Antiepileptic drugs. In: Schatzberg AF, Nemeroff CB, eds. *Textbook of psychopharmacology,* 2nd ed. Washington, DC: APA Press, 1998:431–454.
15. Keck PE, McElroy SL, Tugrul KC, et al. Valproate oral loading in the treatment of acute mania. *J Clin Psychiatry* 1993;54:305–308.
16. Bowden CL, Janicak PG, Orsulak P, et al. Relation of serum valproate concentrations to response in mania. *Am J Psychiatry* 1996;153:765–770.
17. Calabrese JR, Woyshville MJ, Kimmel SE, et al. Predictors of valproate response in bipolar rapid cycling. *J Clin Psychopharmacol* 1993;13:280–283.
18. Calabrese JR, Delucchi GA. Spectrum of efficacy of valproate in 55 patients with rapid cycling bipolar disorder. *Am J Psychiatry* 1990;147:431–434.
19. Calabrese JR, Markovitz PJ, Kimmel SE, et al. Spectrum of efficacy of valproate in 78 rapid-cycling bipolar patients. *J Clin Psychopharmacol* 1992;12:53S–56S.
20. Swann AC, Bowden CL, Morris D, et al. Depression during mania: treatment response to lithium or divalproex. *Arch Gen Psychiatry* 1997;54:37–42.
21. McElroy SL, Keck PE Jr, Pope HG Jr, et al. Valproate in bipolar disorder: literature review and treatment guidelines. *J Clin Psychopharmacol* 1992;12: 42S–52S.
22. Davis LL, Kabel D, Patel D, et al. Valproate as an antidepressant in major depressive disorder. *Psychopharmacol Bull* 1996:32:647–652.
23. Depression Guideline Panel. Depression in primary care: volume 2. Treatment of major depression. Clinical practice guideline, number 5. Rockville, MD: US Department of Public Health, Public Health Service, Agency for Health Care Policy and Research, 1993, AHCPR publication no. 93-0551.
24. Lambert PA, Venaud G. Comparative study of valpromide versus lithium as prophylactic treatment in affective disorders. *Nervure* 1994;17:1–19.
25. Bowden CL. Treatment of bipolar disorder. In: Schatzberg AF, Nemeroff CB, eds. *Textbook of psychopharmacology,* 2nd ed. Washington, DC: APA Press, 1998:431–454.
26. Emrich HM, Wolf R. Valproate treatment of mania. *Prog Neuropsychopharmacol Biol Psychiatry* 1992; 16:691–701.
27. Solomon DA, Ryan CE, Keitner GI, et al. A pilot study of lithium carbonate plus divalproex sodium for the continuation and maintenance treatment of patients with bipolar I disorder. *J Clin Psychiatry* 1997;58: 95–99.
28. Schaff M, Fawcett J, Zajecka J. Divalproex sodium in the treatment of refractory affective disorders. *J Clin Psychiatry* 1993;54:380–384.
29. Tohen M, Castillo J, Pope HG Jr, et al. Concomitant use of valproate and carbamazepine in bipolar and schizoaffective disorders. *J Clin Psychopharmacol* 1994;14:67–70.
30. Kahn D, Stevenson E, Douglas CJ: Effect of sodium valproate in three patients with organic brain syndromes. *Am J Psychiatry* 1988;145:1010–1011.
31. Lum M, Fontaine R, Elie R, et al. Probable interaction of sodium divalproex with benzodiazepines. *Prog Neuropsychopharmacol Biol Psychiatry* 1991;15: 269–273.
32. Woodman CL, Noyes R Jr. Panic disorder: treatment with valproate. *J Clin Psychiatry* 1994;55:134–136.
33. Keck PE Jr, Taylor VE, Tugrul KC, et al. Valproate treatment of panic disorder in lactate-induced panic attacks. *Biol Psychiatry* 1993;33:542–546.
34. Roy-Byrne PP, Ward NG, Donnelly PJ. Valproate in anxiety and withdrawal syndromes. *J Clin Psychiatry* 1989;50[Suppl]:44–48.
35. Mellow AM, Solano-Lopez C, Davis S. Sodium valproate in the treatment of behavioral disturbances in dementia. *J Geriatr Psychiatry Neurol* 1993;6: 205–209.
36. McClean MJ, Macdonald RL. Sodium valproate, but not ethosuximide, produces use and voltage dependent limitation of high frequency repetitive firing of action potentials of mouse central neurons in culture. *J Pharmacol Exp Ther* 1986;238:727–732.
37. Nau H, Loscher W. Valproic acid: brain and plasma levels of the drug and its metabolites, anticonvulsant effects and GABA metabolism in the mouse. *J Pharmacol Exp Ther* 1982;220:654–659.
38. Loscher W, Siemens H. Valproic acid increases GABA in CSF of epileptic children. *Lancet* 1984;2:225.

39. Mutani R, Fariello RG. L'azione dell'acido n-dipropi-lacetico (DPA) sulle "caudate spindles" corticali. *Boll Soc Ital Biol Sper* 1969;45:1416–1417.

40. Iadarola MJ, Gale K. Dissociation between drug-induced increase in nerve terminal and non-nerve terminal pools of GABA in vivo. *Eur J Pharmacol* 1979;59: 125–129.

41. Gale K. Subcortical structures and pathways involved in convulsive seizure generation. *J Clin Neurophysiol* 1992;9:264–277.

42. Cummings JL. Frontal-subcortical circuits and human behavior. *Arch Neurol* 1993;50:873–880.

43. Berthier ML. Poststroke bipolar affective disorder: clinical subtypes, concurrent movement disorders and anatomical correlates. *J Neuropsychiatry Clin Neurosci* 1996;8:160–167.

44. Berridge MJ. Neural and developmental actions of lithium: a unifying hypothesis. *Cell* 1989;59:411–419.

45. Dixon JF, Hokin LE. The antibipolar drug valproate mimics lithium in stimulating glutamate release and inositol 1,4,5-triphosphate accumulation in brain cortex slices but not accumulation of inositol monophosphates and biphosphates. *Proc Natl Acad Sci USA* 1997;94:4757–4760.

46. Nishizuka Y. Intracellular signaling by hydrolysis of phospholipids and activation of protein kinase C. *Science* 1992;258:607–614.

47. Chen G, Manji HK, Hawver DB, et al. Chronic valproate selectively decreases protein kinase C alpha and epsilon in vitro. *J Neurochem* 1994;63:2361–2364.

48. Lenox RH, McNamara RK, Watterson JM, et al. Myristolated alanine-rich C kinase substrate (MARCKS): a molecular target for the therapeutic action of mood stabilizers in the brain? *J Clin Psychiatry* 1996; 57[Suppl 3]:23–31.

49. Takezaki H, Hanaoka M. The use of carbamazepine (Tegretol) in the control of manic-depressive psychosis and other manic-depressive states. *Seishin Igaku* 1971; 13:173–183.

50. Okuma T, Inanaga K, Otsuki S, et al. Comparison of the antimanic efficacy of carbamazepine and chlorpromazine: a double-blind controlled study. *Psychopharmacology* 1979;66:211–217.

51. Müller AA, Stoll KD. Carbamazepine and oxcarbazepine in the treatment of manic syndromes: studies in Germany. In: Emrich HM, Okuma T, Müller AA, eds. *Anticonvulsants in affective disorders.* Princeton, NJ: Excerpta Medica, 1984:139–147.

52. Grossi E, Sacchetti E, Vita A, et al. Carbamazepine vs. chlorpromazine in mania: a double-blind trial. In: Emrich HMk, Okuma T, Müller AA, eds. *Anticonvulsants in affective disorders.* New York: Elsevier Science Publishers, 1984:177–187.

53. Brown D, Lilverton T, Cookson J. Carbamazepine vs. haloperidol in acute mania. In: Program and abstracts of the 41st Annual Meeting of the Society for Biological Psychiatry, May 7–11, 1986, Washington, DC, Abstract 229.

54. Placidi GF, Lenzi A, Lazzerine F, et al. The comparative efficacy and safety of carbamazepine versus lithium—a randomized, double-blind 3-year trial in 83 patients. *J Clin Psychiatry* 1986;47:490–494.

55. Lenzi A, Lazzarini F, Grossi E, et al. Use of carbamazepine in acute psychosis: a controlled study. *J Int Med Res* 1986;14:78–84.

56. Lusznat RM, Murphy DP, Nunn CM. Carbamazepine vs. lithium in the treatment and prophylaxis of mania. *Br J Psychiatry* 1988;153:198–204.

57. Small JG, Milstein V, Klapper MH, et al. Carbamazepine compared with lithium in the treatment of mania. *Biol Psychiatry* 1989;25:137A.

58. Lerer B, Moore N, Meyendorff E, et al. Carbamazepine versus lithium in mania: a double-blind study. *J Clin Psychiatry* 1987;48:89–93.

59. Keisling R. Carbamazepine and lithium carbonate in the treatment of refractory affective disorders. *Arch Gen Psychiatry* 1983;40:223.

60. Lovett L, Watkins SE, Shaw DM. The use of alternative drug therapy in nine patients with recurrent affective disorder resistant to conventional prophylaxis. *Biol Psychiatry* 1986;21:1344–1347.

61. DiCostanzo E, Schifano F. Lithium alone or in combination with carbamazepine for the treatment of rapid-cycling bipolar affective disorder. *Acta Psychiatr Scand* 1991;83:456–459.

62. Kramlinger K, Post R. Adding lithium carbonate to carbamazepine: antimanic efficacy in treatment-resistant mania. *Acta Psychiatr Scand* 1989;79:378–385.

63. Small JG, Klapper MH, Marhenke JD, et al. Lithium combination with carbamazepine or haloperidol in the treatment of mania. *Psychopharmacol Bull* 1995;31: 265–272.

64. Kishimoto A. The treatment of affective disorder with carbamazepine: prophylactic synergism of lithium and carbamazepine combination. *Prog Neuropsychopharmacol Biol Psychiatry* 1992;16:483–493.

65. Shukla S, Cook BL, Miller MG. Lithium-carbamazepine versus lithium-neuroleptic prophylaxis in bipolar illness. *J Affect Disord* 1985;9:219–222.

66. Junghan U, Albers M, Woggon B. Increased risk of hematological side-effects in psychiatric patients treated with clozapine and carbamazepine? [Letter]. *Pharmacopsychiatry* 1993;26:262.

67. Tiihonen J, Vartiainen H, Hakola P. Carbamazepine-induced changes in plasma levels of neuroleptics. *Pharmacopsychiatry* 1995;28:26–28.

68. Post RM. Sensitization and oscillation following repeated stimulation: relationship to affective illness and its treatment with lithium and carbamazepine. *Psychopharmacol Bull* 1980;16:50–52.

69. Post RM, Rubinow DR, Uhde TW, et al. Dopaminergic effects of carbamazepine. Relationship to clinical response in affective illness. *Arch Gen Psychiatry* 1986; 43:392–396.

70. Cullen M, Mitchell P, Brodaty H, et al. Carbamazepine for treatment-resistant melancholia. *J Clin Psychiatry* 1991;52:472–476.

71. Uhde TW, Stein MB, Post RM. Lack of efficacy of carbamazepine in the treatment of panic disorder. *Am J Psychiatry* 1988;145:1104–1109.

72. Reis R, Roy-Byrne P, Ward NG, et al. Carbamazepine treatment for benzodiazepine withdrawal. *Am J Psychiatry* 1989;146:536–537.

73. Macdonald RL. Antiepileptic drug actions. *Epilepsia* 1989;30[Suppl 1]:S19–S28.

74. Post RM, Uhde TW, Roy-Byrne PP, et al. Antidepressant effects of carbamazepine. *Am J Psychiatry* 1986; 143:29–34.

75. Dimond KR, Pande AC, Lamoreaux L, et al. Effect of gabapentin (Neurontin) on mood and well-being in pa-

tients with epilepsy. *Prog Neuropsychopharmacol Biol Psychiatry* 1996;20:407–417.

76. Ryback RS, Brodsky L. Gabapentin in bipolar disorder [Letter]. *J Neuropsychiatry* 1997;9:301.

77. McElroy SL, Soutullo CA, Keck PE Jr, et al. A pilot trial of adjunctive gabapentin in the treatment of bipolar disorder. *Ann Clin Psychiatry* 1997;9:99–103.

78. Knoll J, Stegman K, Suppes T. Clinical experience using gabapentin adjunctively in patients with a history of mania or hypomania. *J Affect Disord* 1998;49: 229–233.

79. Stanton SP, Keck PE Jr, McElroy SL. Treatment of acute mania with gabapentin. *Am J Psychiatry* 1997; 154:287.

80. Schaffer CB, Schaffer LC. Gabapentin in the treatment of bipolar disorder. *Am J Psychiatry* 1997;154:291–292.

81. Bennett J, Goldman WT, Suppes T. Gabapentin for treatment of bipolar and schizoaffective disorders [Letter]. *J Clin Psychopharmacol* 1997;17:141–142.

82. Soutullo CA, Casuto LS, Keck PE Jr. Gabapentin in the treatment of adolescent mania: a case report. *J Child Adolesc Psychopharmacol* 1998;8:81–85.

83. Young LT, Robb JC, Patelis-Siotis I, et al. Acute treatment of bipolar depression with gabapentin. *Biol Psychiatry* 1997;42:851–853.

84. Watson WP, Robinson E, Little HJ. The novel anticonvulsant, gabapentin, protects against both convulsant and anxiogenic aspects of the ethanol withdrawal syndrome. *Neuropharmacology* 1997;36:1369–1375.

85. Beauclair L, Sultan S, Balanger MC, et al. Antianxiety and hypnotic effects of gabapentin in psychotic patients with comorbid anxiety related disorders. Proceedings of the 35th Annual Meeting of the American College of Neuropharmacology, December 9–13, 1996, San Juan, Puerto Rico.

86. Pollack MH, Matthews J, Scott EL. Gabapentin for refractory anxiety. *Am J Psychiatry* 1998;155:992–993.

87. Regan WM, Gordon SM. Gabapentin for behavioral agitation in Alzheimer's disease. *J Clin Psychopharmacol* 1997;17:59–60.

88. Pande AC, Davidson JR, Jefferson JW, et al. Treatment of social phobia with gabapentin: a placebo-controlled study. *J Clin Psychopharmacol* 1999;19:341–348.

89. Hill D, Suman-Chauhan N, Woodruff GN. Localisation of [^{3}H]-gabapentin to a novel site in rat brain; autoradiographic studies. *Eur J Pharmacol Mol Pharmacol* 1993;244:303–309.

90. Gee MS, Brown FP, Offord J, et al. The novel anticonvulsant drug gabapentin (Neurontin) binds to the alpha-(2)-delta subunit of a calcium channel. *J Biol Chem* 1996;271:5768–5776.

91. Petroff OA, Rothman DL, Behar KL, et al. The effect of gabapentin on brain gamma-aminobutyric acid on patients with epilepsy. *Ann Neurol* 1996;39:95–99.

92. Ben-Menachem E, Persson LI, Hedner T. Selected CSF biochemistry and gabapentin concentrations in the CSF and plasma in patients with partial seizures after a single oral dose of gabapentin. *Epilepsy Res* 1992;11:45–49.

93. Rao ML, Clarenbach P, Vahlensieck M, et al. Gabapentin augments whole blood serotonin in healthy young men. *J Neural Transm* 1988;73: 129–134.

94. Smith D, Baker G, Davies G, et al. Outcomes of add-on treatment with lamotrigine in partial epilepsy. *Epilepsia* 1993;34:312–322.

95. Sporn J, Sachs G. Anticonvulsants in treatment resistant manic-depressive illness. *J Clin Psychopharmacol* 1997;17:185–189.

96. Kusumaker V, Yatham LN. An open study of lamotrigine in refractory bipolar depression. *Psychiatry Res* 1997;72:145–148.

97. Walden J, Berger M, van Calker D, et al. Addition of lamotrigine to valproate may enhance efficacy in the treatment of bipolar Affective Disorder. *Pharmacopsychiatry* 1996;29:193–195.

98. Fatemi SH, Rapport DJ, Calabrese JR, et al. Lamotrigine in rapid-cycling bipolar disorder. *J Clin Psychiatry* 1997;58:522–527.

99. Fogelson DL, Sternbach H. Lamotrigine treatment of refractory bipolar disorder. *J Clin Psychiatry* 1997;58: 271–273.

100. Mauri MC, Laini V, Somaschini E, et al. Lamotrigine: an alternative drug in the prophylaxis of bipolar disorder. *Eur Neuropsychopharmacol* 1997;6:S161(abst).

101. Kusumaker V, Yatham LN. Lamotrigine treatment of rapid cycling bipolar disorder. *Am J Psychiatry* 1997;154:1171–1172.

102. Calabrese JR, Bowden CL, Sachs GS, et al. A double-blind placebo-controlled study of lamotrigine monotherapy in outpatients with bipolar I depression. Lamictal 602 Study Group. *J Clin Psychiatry* 1999;60: 79–88.

103. Messenheimer JA. Lamotrigine. *Epilepsia* 1995;36 [Suppl 2]:S87–S94.

104. Marcotte DB. Use of the new antiepileptic drug topiramate as a mood stabilizer. In: Syllabus and proceedings summary of the annual meeting of the American Psychiatric Association, May 1998, Toronto, Ontario, Canada, Abstract 115.

105. Calabrese JR, Shelton MD, Keck PE, et al. Emerging trends in the management of psychiatric illness. In: Syllabus and proceedings summary of the annual meeting of the American Psychiatric Association, May 1998, Toronto, Ontario, Canada, Abstract NR202.

106. Shank RP, Gardocki JF, Vaught JL, et al. Topiramate: preclinical evaluation of structurally novel anticonvulsant. *Epilepsia* 1994;35:450–460.

17

Frontal Lobe Dysfunction in Epilepsy

Oscar Doval, *Moises Gaviria, and †Andres M. Kanner

*Departments of Neuropsychiatry and *Psychiatry, University of Illinois,
Chicago, Illinois 60612; and †Department of Neurological Sciences,
Rush Presbyterian-Saint Luke's Medical Center,
Chicago, Illinois 60612*

Frontal lobe dysfunction (FLD) is a frequent contributor to the neurobehavioral complications of epilepsy, occurring in up to 50% of cases in some series (1–3). FLD is reflected in the cognitive disturbances and depressive disorders identified in these patients. It occurs in the presence of extrafrontal seizure foci (4,5), including partial seizure disorders of temporal, parietal, or occipital origin, as well as generalized epilepsy (3). FLD in epileptic patients may result from the seizure disorder, per se, from the brain insult that caused the epilepsy, or from both (4–7). In this chapter, we discuss the relationship between FLD and some of the common psychiatric complications of epilepsy.

NEUROANATOMIC ASPECTS OF THE FRONTAL LOBE

The frontal lobes constitute more than one-third of the brain. The cortex of the frontal lobes is divided into four areas: (i) the motor cortex; (ii) the premotor cortex; (iii) the prefrontal area (Brodmann's areas 9 to 12, the anterior part of Brodmann's area 8, and Brodmann's areas 45 and 47), the largest and most anterior section of the frontal lobe; and (iv) the limbic component (Brodmann's areas 24, 25, and 32). Area IV is located in the basal medial region and includes the an-

terior and subgenual portions of the cingulate gyrus, the posterior sector of the orbitofrontal surface, and the gyrus rectus. The prefrontal area and limbic component form the prefrontal cortex (8–11); its major circuits include the dorsolateral, orbitofrontal, and anterior cingulate circuits. Prefrontal cortex and these circuits are involved in complex cognitive functions, in the regulation of emotional states and behavioral control (8,12,13), and are responsible for many of the behavioral syndromes seen in neuropsychiatry. In fact, "the prefrontal syndrome" is probably a more accurate descriptor of the "frontal lobe syndrome" (8,10,14).

The frontal lobes are richly interconnected to numerous subcortical structures and extrafrontal cortical regions. They have intracortical projections to and from the temporal, parietal, and occipital lobes (9,15). In addition, the aforementioned prefrontal circuits follow a general frontal-subcortical looped pathway that projects from the frontal lobes to striatal components, which then connect to the globus pallidus and substantia nigra. The latter structures connect to specific thalamic nuclei, sending afferents back to the frontal lobe to complete the loop (8). This extensive connectivity provides an explanation for FLD in cases of extrafrontal lesions (Fig. 17.1).

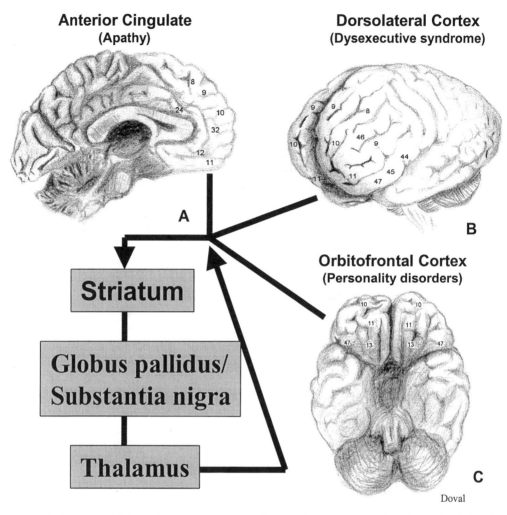

FIG. 17.1. Medial **(A)**, lateral **(B)**, and ventral **(C)** views of the cortex showing the prefrontal regions and a general outline of prefrontal-subcortical circuits.

PREFRONTAL CIRCUITS: FUNCTIONAL AND PSYCHOPATHOLOGIC IMPLICATIONS

Dorsolateral Circuit

The dorsolateral circuit is responsible for carrying out executive functions, which include planning, using past experiences, starting, maintaining, monitoring, shifting, and inhibiting behavioral responses. Hence, "executive dysfunction" is the hallmark of damage to the dorsolateral prefrontal cortex (8,9) and presents as poor organizational strategies (i.e., difficulty in developing hypotheses or goals and in executing plans), motor programming abnormalities (i.e., altered motor sequences), and difficulties in memory search and setup (i.e., poor recall of recent and remote information). It results in concrete interpretation of abstract concepts, such as proverbs and impaired cognitive flexibility. Likewise, completion of any task is not "fluent," as patients have difficulty generating ideas and focusing for a protracted period of time on one task. This results in frequent interruptions, perseveration, and difficulty in reaching completion of given activities (8,10,12,13,16–18). Finally, dysfunction of the dorsolateral circuit results in impairment of working memory (i.e., capacity to briefly store novel information and appropriately retrieve to resolve a given task).

Some authors found that patients with frontal lobe epilepsy have poorer performance on testing of executive functions than patients with epilepsy of extrafrontal origin, i.e., temporal lobe epilepsy (TLE) (6). However, others have related the magnitude of the executive dysfunction to the severity of the seizure disorder, per se, rather than to the specific location of the epileptic focus (i.e., very high frequency [more than 100 over a lifetime] of generalized tonic-clonic seizures, history of convulsive status epilepticus) (7,19).

Orbitofrontal Circuit

The orbitofrontal circuits mediate empathic and socially appropriated behavior. The "orbitofrontal syndrome" is known for impressive personality changes, which consist of increased irritability, disinhibited and impulsive behavior, tactlessness, inappropriate outspokenness, and emotional lability. Other prominent characteristics include poor judgment and insight, decreased concern for the consequences of behavior, loss of empathy, irresponsibility and laziness, and environmental dependency (i.e., imitation behavior and utilization behavior—tendency to touch and use objects around without clear purpose) (8–10, 12,13,16,20–22). The emotional changes are classically referred to as *moria* and *witzelsucht*. Moria is the term given to euphoric and erotic behavior, and witzelsucht refers to inappropriate jokes and factitious behavior. These personality features may be considered an expression of the "frontal lobe personality" (8).

Patients with frontal lobe epilepsy have been reported to exhibit characteristic irritability, poor frustration tolerance, and impulsivity. In addition, interictal aggression, sociopathic behavior, sexual deviancy, disinhibition, and hyperphagia have been described (23). However, these personality traits are not an exclusive manifestation of frontal lobe epilepsy, as similar features have been described in patients with TLE and generalized seizure disorders. These personality changes may be an expression of the FLD associated with different types of epilepsy, but we cannot exclude the role played by the other limbic structures, i.e., amygdala, thalamic nuclei, etc.

Anterior Cingulate Circuit

Motivation is the key function of the anterior cingulate circuit. Bilateral lesions of cingulate gyrus and mesial frontal cortex can lead to profound apathy, abulia (lack of initiative) resulting in paucity of movements and gestures, lack of spontaneous speech, monosyllabic responses, indifference to circumstances, and reduced creative thought. Such passivity may lead the patient to eat and drink only when fed. Patients also may exhibit urinary and fecal incontinence. Some cases may develop akinetic mutism (8,10,15,24,25). Unilateral lesions produce less dramatic apathetic syndromes but may include a transient akinetic mutism (25).

Akinetic mutism and catatonic-like syndromes have been reported occasionally in epileptic patients during nonconvulsive status epilepticus of frontal lobe origin and during the postictal period following a cluster of secondarily generalized tonic-clonic seizures (23,26,27). Catatonic-like symptoms also have been described as an unusual manifestation of TLE and primary generalized epilepsies (28,29).

LATERALITY AND NEUROBEHAVIORAL DISTURBANCES

A vast literature attempted to relate specific psychiatric syndromes with laterality of a frontal lobe lesion. Patients with right frontal lesions, for example, have been reported to display disinhibition, irritability, hypersexuality, and manic-like syndromes (13,30–32), whereas left frontal lesions have been associated with reduced responsiveness, apathy, and depressive syndromes (8,13). The impact of laterality of a frontal seizure focus on the psychiatric profile of patients with epilepsy has yet to be described; therefore, these changes in personality may not apply to patients with frontal lobe epilepsy who do not have a concurrent structural lesion.

FRONTAL LOBE DYSFUNCTION IN EPILEPSY

Cognitive Deficits

Altered executive functions occur in epileptic patients, even in those with extrafrontal epileptogenic foci (4,33–37). Some studies correlated these disturbances with frontal hypometabolism detected by functional neuroimaging procedures (38,39). Giordani (3) illustrated the cognitive deficits found in patients with epilepsy as an expression of FLD:

> Among epileptic patients . . . executive functions appear particularly important in the prediction of social functioning. They are the slowest to improve following apparent recovery from neurologic disorders. Hence, patients achieving good control of their seizure disorder may still require several months to reestablish efficient attention and problem-solving ability. Some patients with seizure disorders and significant difficulties in abstraction and mental flexibility may appear to function quite appropriately during a clinical interview and may demonstrate no apparent evidence of impaired overall intellectual capacity, language, sensory or motor functioning. These same individuals, however, if observed during daily adaptive tasks, may exercise poor judgment or planing, or may show an inability to efficiently benefit from feedback from their environment. In such cases, their families or coworkers may incorrectly assume that lack of motivation or emotional disturbance, alone, accounts for the failures of these individuals.

The Wisconsin Card Sorting Test (WCST) has been the neuropsychological instrument used most frequently to assess executive functions in epileptic patients. This test requires that the patient sort a deck of cards, according to a "flexible" set of rules that must be inferred from the examiner's instructions (8,12). The successful completion of such a task demonstrates reasoning. There are extensive normative data validating this instrument as a sensitive measure of frontal lobe/executive functions (4,8). Recently, neuroimaging studies performed with single photon emission computed tomography (SPECT) and positron emission tomography (PET) have supported the use of WCST, although some authors have voiced concerns (4).

Early in 1976, McDaniel and McDaniel (40) found that intellectually spared epileptic patients presented impairment in WCST and Token Test as an expression of difficulties in sustaining and focusing attention. Hermann et al. (4,33–37) demonstrated impairment in WCST performance in patients with TLE. These findings are suggestive of FLD. They also found a significant relationship between the degree of associated FLD (as assessed by WCST) and dysphoric mood (34). The same paradigm was applied to patients with TLE, before and after undergoing temporal lobe resection. A significant improvement in WCST performance was observed postsurgically, which seems to substantiate the notion that the epileptogenic cortex adversely affects extratemporal regions (33,35).

Other authors using WCST in TLE found similar results (41–46). In addition, some studies using the Stroop Test, Verbal Fluency Tests, and other tests sensitive to executive functions revealed impairment in these capacities in epileptic patients with different seizure types (41,47–50). These findings correlate with frontal lobe hypometabolism or asymmetry detected by functional neuroimaging techniques (38,39).

The specific effects of antiepileptic drugs (AEDs) on executive functions are not well studied. In general, research in both epileptic and healthy subjects has proven that AEDs may affect overall cognitive performance (7). Older drugs such as phenobarbital, phenytoin, and primidone tend to produce greater impairment of cognitive abilities, including executive functions, as well as personality changes, such as disinhibition, impulsiveness, and irritability (51). Drugs such as carbamazepine, valproic, acid and the new generation of AEDs appear to have less cognitive side effects. However, neuropsychological studies in patients treated with new drugs such as lamotrigine have revealed impairment on executive tests (5).

Neuropsychiatric Syndromes

Depression

Depression has been reported as a common complication of epilepsy regardless of the localization of the seizure focus or the clinical characteristics (52). However, some studies argued that rates of depression in TLE are higher than in other type of seizure disorders (4). Others suggested a relationship between depression and left-sided epileptic foci (4, 52–56). Whether this is specific to the temporal lobe per se or related to left hemispheric lesions remains unclear (52).

As suggested by the studies using WCST in patients with TLE and depression, TLE may compromise frontal lobe functions (4,33–36, 41,43,45,57). Furthermore, intraoperative electrocorticography and invasive electroencephalographic investigations of patients with TLE and depression demonstrated interictal epileptiform activity in the frontal lobes (4,57–59). Also, functional brain imaging techniques performed on individuals with TLE demonstrate decreased interictal hypometabolism that extends beyond the epileptogenic area into the thalamus and the frontal lobes (39,52,60–67). It has been suspected that this frontal hypometabolism may contribute to interictal (cognitive and behavioral) symptoms (4,52,65,68). On the other hand, frontal lobe hypometabolism may be seen in patients with primary or secondary depression of any origin (8,13,31,69–75).

The depressive symptoms associated with FLD may simply be due to the close proximity and interconnection from temporal lobe structures to the medial frontal region, with subsequent involvement of the anterior cingulate circuit. On the other hand, the occurrence of depression is not specific to dysfunction of mesial frontal structures. Lesions affecting other frontal lobe areas and the dorsolateral and orbitofrontal cortices, and even extrafrontal domains, such as the caudate nucleus and parietal lobes, hypothalamus, pituitary, and other cerebral regions, can be associated with the presence of depression and anxiety. It is possible that the rich connectivity of the frontal lobe may explain its involvement in depressive disorders, even with extrafrontal lesions (9,31,76–79).

Alternatively, a possible relationship between epilepsy, depression, and FLD may be postulated in neurochemical terms, given that the inferior frontal cortex is the main target of the mesolimbic dopaminergic neurons and the main source of input to midbrain serotoninergic neurons of the dorsal raphe nucleus. Deficits in serotoninergic transmission have been implicated in both primary and secondary depression (52,72,74,80–83).

Mania

Many studies reported a manic-like syndrome in patients with diverse brain lesions that compromise the right frontal lobe and/or the right hemisphere (10,13,30,84–90). As in depression, mania is a frontal lobe circuit-related, but not circuit-specific, syndrome. It may be viewed as a consequence of lesions or injuries affecting the orbitofrontal cortex, caudate nucleus, and perithalamic areas, as well as the temporobasal regions, which include the amygdala and temporal stem (10,90,91). Subcortical lesions involving the caudate nucleus and thalamus tend to generate bipolar pictures, whereas lesions affecting cortical areas tend to produce a manic syndrome void of depressive cycles (92).

Manic and hypomanic episodes are not commonly associated with epilepsy. Interestingly, as in frontal lobe, manic symptoms in epileptic patients appear to be related to right-sided foci or lesions (52,93). Likewise, bipolar syndrome is infrequently found in association with epilepsy, and the focus or lesion is rather vague (94). It has been suggested that the antimanic effect of various AEDs, such as carbamazepine and valproic acid, can possibly explain the relative infrequency of mania and hypomania in patients with epilepsy (52,93).

Psychosis

Psychosis is a rare finding among patients with neocortical extratemporal epilepsy (95–97). Some studies reported a higher rate of psychosis with focal seizures that involve the mesial temporal structures (5,95), especially those involving the left hemisphere. On the other hand, an increased risk of developing psychosis has been reported in epileptic patients after temporal lobe resection, especially in those undergoing a resection that involves the right temporal lobe (95,98). Thus, the relationship between the lateralization of seizure focus and psychosis needs further clarification.

Some studies performed with SPECT of the brain in patients with TLE and psychosis have revealed decreased interictal perfusion in the temporal lobe ipsilateral to the epileptogenic focus (99–102). Mellers et al. (103) compared 12 patients with schizophrenia-like psychosis of epilepsy (SLPE) to 16 patients with epilepsy without psychosis and 11 patients with schizophrenia without epilepsy. They measured brain perfusion changes with SPECT during a verbal fluency task—sensitive to FLD—as an activation paradigm. Normal subjects showed an increase in regional cerebral blood flow within the left prefrontal and anterior cingulate cortices and an increase or a decrease in the left superior temporal cortex. Patients with SLPE differed from both groups by exhibiting diminished blood flow in the left superior temporal gyrus during performance of the imposed task. The nonepileptic schizophrenic group showed a greater increase in blood flow in the anterior cingulate. These findings appear to support an association between left temporal lobe abnormality and SLPE rather than FLD, as observed in schizophrenic patients. The different patterns of activation observed in people with primary

schizophrenia and SLPE may suggest that different pathophysiologic mechanisms play a role in these two groups. In this regard, Petty and Pearlson (104) hypothesized that schizophrenia is a disorder of the heteromodal association cortex and that disruptions in this system lead to the major syndromes in schizophrenia. The major structures of the heteromodal association cortex are the dorsolateral prefrontal cortex, the parietal lobe, including the inferior parietal lobe and the supramarginal gyri, and the superior temporal gyrus. These three important systems are richly connected to the basal ganglia and interlinked with each other. This hypothesis suggests that damage to the superior temporal gyrus and medial temporal structures are responsible for psychosis associated with TLE. The predominance of hallucinations and delusions seen in psychosis linked to epilepsy appear to be secondary to temporal lobe impairment. On the other hand, flat affect, apathy, and cognitive deficits, which are more characteristic of schizophrenia in nonepileptic patients, seem to be a manifestation of FLD (37,103,105). These clinical findings are not present in SLPE, which further supports the above suggestions.

Many pathologic conditions that produce alterations of the prefrontal cortex and/or related subcortical circuits may generate a psychotic syndrome (77,89,105–107). In addition, individuals presenting with psychosis either as a primary disease (i.e., schizophrenia) or associated with brain impairment (i.e., frontotemporal dementia, Huntington's disease, vascular dementia, etc.) tend to demonstrate frontal hypofunctionalism on neuropsychological testing and different brain mapping methods, such as electroencephalographic, functional magnetic resonance imaging, PET, and SPECT (77,89,105–113). Furthermore, studies using functional imaging revealed hypermetabolism in limbic-temporal lobe structures of patients with psychosis, which has been associated with a greater delusional activity and is believed to be a compensatory dopamine receptor up-regulation due to frontal lobe hypofunction (114). Beyond certain phenomenologic analogies and the fact that FLD underlies schizophrenia and other types of psychosis, to date there is no clear evidence linking FLD to psychotic episodes of TLE patients.

Personality Disorders

Understanding of the relationship between epilepsy and personality disorders, as well as any other psychopathologic manifestations, requires a broadly based perspective that takes into account all the relevant biologic, psychosocial, and pharmacologic factors (57). Traditionally, patients with an interictal "epileptic personality," commonly known as "Geschwind's syndrome," have been described as sticky, suspicious, argumentative, aggressive, touchy, pedantic, egocentric, circumstantial, philosophic, hypergraphic, moralistic, and religious (103,115). These features have predominantly been attributed to TLE and have been hypothesized to be due to a hyperconnective limbic-sensorial syndrome, which confers excessive affective significance to sensorial stimuli (116). The specificity of Geschwind's syndrome for TLE, and even its existence, is still being debated. Some authors consider it a nonspecific manifestation of temporal lobe dysfunction (5,23,103,115). Although there is evidence of orbitofrontal dysfunction in TLE, at least from a phenomenologic point of view, no apparent analogies between "epileptic personality" and "frontal lobe personality" appear to exist (57). However, studies have reported Geschwind's syndrome characteristics in patients with frontal lobe epilepsy; conversely, patients with TLE and primary generalized epilepsy have been reported to have frontal lobe personality features (23,103). Therefore, the concept of personality disorders in epilepsy seems to be more complex than simply specifying the type of seizures or regional location of the epileptogenic focus.

Obsessive-Compulsive Disorder

Obsessive-compulsive disorder and perhaps associated entities, such as pathologic gambling, kleptomania, risk-seeking behavior, body dysmorphic disorder, as well as other primary or secondary obsessive syndromes, have been strongly associated with dysfunction in the orbitofrontal cortex and/or its connections to the thalamus and caudate nucleus (10,117). PET and SPECT studies have shown increased activity in the right frontal, mediofrontal, anterior cingulate, and/or orbitofrontal cortices (118–122). However, data from structural imaging and neuropsychological studies are inconsistent (117). In epileptic patients, obsessive-compulsive symptoms are associated infrequently with the ictal and interictal behavior of epileptic patients (123,124). Occasionally, these symptoms have been reported linked to frontal lobe epilepsy, including epileptic forced thinking, described as a psychic aura characterized by "parasitic" or intrusive thoughts resulting from epileptiform activity (125,126). Also, obsessive-compulsive behavior has occasionally been described in TLE (127). This may be expected because, as previously mentioned, FLD has been demonstrated in patients with TLE and depression.

CONCLUSIONS

FLD has been documented as one of the contributors to the behavioral complications of epilepsy. Experimental data derived from neuropsychological and neuroimaging studies support this assertion for depression and cognitive disturbances, regardless of the clinical and electrical type of seizures. The contribution of FLD to other neuropsychiatric complications of epilepsy, such as psychosis, obsessive-compulsive disorder, personality disorder, and bipolar disorder, remains unclear. Because the frontal lobes play a fundamental role in directing, coordinating, integrating, and modulating behavioral responses and their impairment may frankly compromise social function, special attention must be paid to the research of pathogenic mechanisms and neurobehavioral consequences of their dysfunction among epileptic patients, as well as the development of future therapeutic strategies.

REFERENCES

1. Dikmen S, Matthews C. Effect of major motor seizure frequency upon cognitive-intellectual functions in adults. *Epilepsia* 1977;18:21–29.
2. Dodrill CB. Correlates of generalized tonic-clonic seizures with intellectual, neuropsychological, emotional, and social function in patients with epilepsy. *Epilepsy* 1986;27:399–411.
3. Giordani BJ. Intellectual and cognitive disturbances in epileptic patients. In: Sackellares JC, Berent S, eds. *Psychological disturbances in epilepsy*. Newton, MA: Butterworth-Heinemann, 1996:45–97.
4. Seidenberg M, Hermann BP, Noe A. Depression in temporal lobe epilepsy: a possible role for associated frontal lobe dysfunction? In: Sackellares JC, Berent S, eds. *Psychological disturbances in epilepsy*. Newton, MA: Butterworth-Heinemann, 1996:143–157.
5. Trimble MR, Schmitz B. The psychoses of epilepsy. In: McConnel HW, Snyder PJ, eds. *Psychiatric comorbidity in epilepsy*. Washington, DC: American Psychiatric Press, 1998:169–185.
6. Helmstaedter C, Kemper B, Elger CE. Neuropsychological aspects of frontal lobe epilepsy. *Neuropsychologia* 1996;34:399–406.
7. Perrine K, Kiolbasa T. Cognitive deficits in epilepsy and contributions to psychopathology. *Neurology* 1999;53[Suppl 2]:S39–S48.
8. Bartok JA, Gaviria M. Frontal lobe syndrome. In: Jobe TH, Gaviria M, Kovilparambil A, eds. *Clinical neuropsychiatry*. Boston: Blackwell Science, 1997:236–246.
9. Cummings JL. Frontal-subcortical circuits and human behavior. *Arch Neurol* 1993;50:873–880.
10. Chow TW, Cummings JL. Frontal subcortical circuits. In: Miller BL, Cummings JL, eds. *The human frontal lobes, functions and disorders*. New York: Guilford Press, 1998:3–26.
11. Messulam MM, ed. *Principles of behavioral neurology*. Philadelphia: FA Davis Co., 1985.
12. Milner B. Aspects of the human frontal lobe function. In: Jasper HH, Riggio S, Goldman-Rakic PS, eds. *Epilepsy and the functional anatomy of the frontal lobe*. New York: Raven Press, 1995:67–84.
13. Joseph R. The frontal lobes. In: Joseph R, ed. *Neuropsychiatry, neuropsychology, and clinical neuroscience*, 2nd ed. Baltimore: Williams & Wilkins, 1996:393–440.
14. Alexander GE, DeLong MR, Strick PL. Parallel organization of functionally segregated circuits linking basal ganglia and cortex. *Annu Rev Neurosci* 1986;9:357–381.
15. Damasio AR, Anderson SW. The frontal lobes. In: Heilman KF, Valenstein E, eds. *Clinical neuropsychology*, 3rd ed. New York: Oxford University Press, 1993:409–460.
16. Luria A. *Higher cortical functions in man*. New York: Basis Books, 1980.
17. Cummings JL. *Clinical neuropsychiatry*. New York: Grune & Stratton, 1985.
18. Jones-Gotman M, Milner B. Design fluency: the invention of non-sense drawings after focal cortical lesions. *Neuropsychologia* 1977;15:653–674.
19. Upton D, Thompson PJ. Age at onset and neuropsychological function in frontal lobe epilepsy. *Epilepsia* 1997;38:1103–1113.
20. Eslinger P Jr, Warner GC, Grattan LM, et al. "Frontal lobe" utilization behavior associated with paramedian thalamic infarction. *Neurology* 1991;41:450–452.
21. Logue V, Durward M, Pratt RT, et al. The quality of survival after anterior cerebral aneurysm. *Br J Psychiatry* 1968;114:137–160.
22. Lhermitte F, Pillon B, Serdaru M. Human autonomy and the frontal lobes. I: imitation and utilization behavior, a neuropsychological study of 75 patients. *Ann Neurol* 1986;19:326–334.
23. Devinsky O, Najjar S. Evidence against the evidence of a temporal lobe epilepsy personality syndrome. *Neurology* 1999;53[Suppl 2]:S13–S25.
24. Fesenmeier JT, Warner GC, Grattan LM, et al. Akinetic mutism caused by bilateral anterior cerebral tuberculous obliterative arteritis. *Neurology* 1990;40:1005–1008.
25. Damasio H, Damasio AR, eds. *Lesion analysis in neuropsychology*. New York: Oxford University Press, 1989.
26. Aylett SE, Cross JH, Taylor DC, et al. Epileptic akinetic mutism: following temporal lobectomy for Rasmussen's syndrome. *Eur Child Adolesc Psychiatry* 1996;5:222–225.
27. Lim J, Yagnik P, Schraeder P, et al. Ictal catatonia as a manifestation of nonconvulsive status epilepticus. *J Neurol Neurosurg Psychiatry* 1986;49:833–836.
28. Kirubakaran V, Sen S, Wilkinson CB. Catatonic stupor: unusual manifestation of temporal lobe epilepsy. *Psychiatr J Univ Ottawa* 1987;12:244–246.
29. Shah P, Kaplan SL. Catatonic symptoms in a child with epilepsy. *Am J Psychiatry* 1980;137:738–739.
30. Joseph R. Confabulation and delusional denial: frontal lobe and lateralized influences. *J Clin Psychol* 1986;42:845–860.
31. Joseph R. The right cerebral hemisphere: emotion, music, visual-spatial skills, body image, dreams, and awareness. *J Clin Psychol* 1988;44:630–673.
32. Lishman WA. Brain damage in relation to psychiatry disability after head injury. *Br J Psychiatry* 1968;114:373–410.
33. Hermann BP, Wyler AR, Richey ET. Wisconsin card sorting test performance in patients with complex partial seizures of temporal-lobe origin. *J Clin Exp Neuropsychol* 1988;10:467–476.
34. Hermann BP, Seidenberg M, Haltiner A, et al. Mood state in unilateral temporal lobe epilepsy. *Biol Psychiatry* 1991;30:1205–1218.
35. Hermann B, Seidenberg M. Executive system dysfunction in temporal lobe epilepsy: effects of nociferous cortex versus hippocampal pathology. *J Clin Exp Neuropsychol* 1995;17:809–819.
36. Hermann BP, Seidenberg M, Schoenfeld J, et al. Neuropsychological characteristics of the syndrome of mesial temporal lobe epilepsy. *Arch Neurol* 1997;54:369–376.
37. Gold JM, Hermann BP, Randolph C, et al. Schizophrenia and temporal lobe epilepsy. A neuropsychological analysis. *Arch Gen Psychiatry* 1994;53:265–272.
38. Swartz BE, Simpkind F, Halgren E, et al. Visual working memory in primary generalized epilepsy: an 18FDG-PET study. *Neurology* 1996;47:1203–1212.
39. Jokeit H, Seitz RJ, Markowitsch HJ, et al. Prefrontal asymmetric interictal glucosa hypometabolism and

cognitive impairment in patients with temporal lobe epilepsy. *Brain* 1997;12:2283–2294.

40. McDaniel JW, McDaniel ML. Visual and auditory cognitive processing affected by epilepsy. *Behav Neuropsychiatry* 1976;8:78–82.

41. Corcoran R, Upton D. A role for the hippocampus in card sorting test. *Cortex* 1993;29:293–304.

42. Strauss E, Hunter M, Wada J. Wisconsin Card Sorting Performance: effects of age of onset of damage and laterality of dysfunction. *J Clin Exp Neuropsychol* 1993;15:896–902.

43. Horner MD, Flashman LA, Freides D, et al. Temporal lobe epilepsy and performance on the Wisconsin Card Sorting Test. *J Clin Exp Neuropsychol* 1996;18:310–113.

44. Giovagnoli AR, Avanzini G. Forgetting rate and interference effects on a verbal memory distractor task in patients with temporal lobe epilepsy. *J Clin Exp Neuropsychol* 1996;18:259–264.

45. Hempel A, Risse GL, Mercer K, et al. Neuropsychological evidence of frontal lobe dysfunction in patients with temporal lobe epilepsy. *Epilepsia* 1996;37[Suppl 5]:119.

46. Upton D, Corcoran R. The role of the right temporal lobe in card sorting: a case study. *Cortex* 1995;31:405–409.

47. Howell RA, Saling MM, Bradley DC, et al. Interictal language fluency in temporal lobe epilepsy. *Cortex* 1994;30:469–478.

48. Martin RC, Loring DW, Meador KJ, et al. The effects of lateralized temporal lobe dysfunction on formal and semantic word fluency. *Neuropsychologia* 1990;28:823–829.

49. Williams J, Griebel ML, Dykman RA. Neuropsychological patterns in pediatric epilepsy. *Seizure* 1998;7:223–228.

50. Prevey ML, Delaney RC, Cramer JA, et al. Complex partial and secondarily generalized seizure patients: cognitive functioning prior to treatment with antiepileptic medication. *Epilepsy Res* 1998;30:1–9.

51. Ketter TA, Post RM, Theodore WH. Positive and negative psychiatric effects of antiepileptic drugs in patients with seizure disorders. *Neurology* 1999;53[Suppl 2]:S53–S67.

52. Blumer D, Altshuler LL. Affective disorders. In: Engel J, Pedley TA, eds. *Epilepsy: a comprehensive textbook,* Volume II. Philadelphia: Lippincott-Raven Publishers, 1998:2083–2099.

53. Altshuler LL, Devinsky O, Post RM, et al. Depression, anxiety, and temporal lobe epilepsy. *Arch Neurol* 1990;47:284–288.

54. Mendez MF. Disorders of mood and affect in epilepsy. In: Sackellares JC, Berent S, eds. *Psychological disturbances in epilepsy*. Newton, MA: Butterworth-Heinemann, 1996:125–141.

55. Robertson MM, Trimble MR, Townsend HRA. Phenomenology of depression in epilepsy. *Epilepsia* 1987;28:364–368.

56. Victoronoff JI, Benson F, Grafton ST, et al. Depression in complex partial seizures. Electroencephalography and cerebral metabolic correlates. *Arch Neurol* 1994;51:155–163.

57. Hermann BP, Wyler AR, Richey ET. Epilepsy, frontal lobes, and personality. *Biol Psychiatry* 1987;22:1055–1057.

58. Abou-Khalil BW, Siegel GJ, Sackellares C, et al. Positron emission tomography studies of cerebral glucose metabolism in chronic partial epilepsy. *Ann Neurol* 1987;22:480–486.

59. Lieb JP, Dashieff RM, Engel J Jr. Role of frontal lobes in propagation of ictal discharges originating in mesiotemporal regions. *Epilepsia* 1989;30:664.

60. Engel J Jr, Kuhl DE, Phelps ME, et al. Interictal cerebral glucose metabolism in partial epilepsy and its relation to EEG changes. *Ann Neurol* 1982;12:510–517.

61. Engel P Jr, Taylor DC. Neurobiology of behavioral disorders. In: Engel J, Pedley TA, eds. *Epilepsy: a comprehensive textbook,* Volume II. Philadelphia: Lippincott-Raven Publishers, 1998:2045–2052.

62. Engel J Jr, ed. *Surgical treatment of the epilepsies.* New York: Raven Press, 1987:75–100.

63. Theodore WH, Newmark ME, Sato S, et al. Fluorodeoxyglucose positron emission tomography in refractory complex partial seizures. *Ann Neurol* 1983;14:429–437.

64. Theodore WH, Katz D, Kufta C, et al. Pathology of temporal lobe foci: correlation with CT, MRI, and PET. *Neurology* 1990;40:797–803.

65. Theodore WH, Fishbein D, Dubinsky R. Patterns of cerebral glucose metabolism in partial epilepsy and its relation to EEG changes. *Neurology* 1988;38:1201–1206.

66. Henry TR, Mazziotta JC, Engel J Jr. Interictal metabolic anatomy of mesial temporal lobe epilepsy. *Arch Neurol* 1993;50:582–589.

67. Menzel C, Grunwald F, Klemm E, et al. Inhibitory effect of mesial temporal partial seizures onto frontal neocortical structures. *Acta Neurol Belg* 1998;98:327–331.

68. Bromfield EB, Altshuler L, Leiderman DB, et al. Cerebral metabolism and depression in patients with complex partial seizures. *Arch Neurol* 1992;49:617–623.

69. Baxter LR, Schawrtz JM, Phelps ME, et al. Cerebral metabolic rates for glucose in mood disorders: studies with positron emission tomography and fluorodeoxyglucose F18. *Arch Gen Psychiatry* 1985;42:441–447.

70. Baxter LR, Schawrtz JM, Phelps ME, et al. Reduction of the prefrontal cortex glucose metabolism common to three types of depression. *Arch Gen Psychiatry* 1989;46:243–250.

71. Starkstein SE, Robinson RG. Depression and frontal lobe disorders. In: Miller BL, Cummings JL, eds. *The human frontal lobes, functions and disorders.* New York: Guilford Press, 1998:3–26;537–546.

72. Maybert HS, Starkstein SE, Sadzor B, et al. Selective hypometabolism in the inferior frontal lobe in depressed patients with Parkinson's disease. *Ann Neurol* 1990;28:57–64.

73. Robinson RG, Benson DF. Depression in aphasic patients: frequency, severity, and clinical pathological correlations. *Brain Lang* 1981;14:282–291.

74. Robinson RG, Kubos KL, Starr LB, et al. Mood disorders in stroke patients. *Brain* 1984;107:81–93.

75. Sinyour D, Jacques P, Kaloupek DG, et al. Post-stroke depression and lesion location. *Brain* 1986;109:537–546.

76. Irle E, Pepper M, Wowra B, et al. Mood changes after surgery for tumors of the cerebral cortex. *Arch Neurol* 1994;51:164–174.

77. Folstein SE, ed. *Huntington's disease: a disorder of families.* Baltimore: John Hopkins University Press, 1989.

78. Robinson RG, Starkstein SE. Current research in affective disorders following stroke. *J Neuropsychiatry Clin Neurosci* 1990;2:1–14.

79. Starkstein SE, Cohen BS, Fedoroff P, et al. Relationship between anxiety disorders and depressive disorders in patients with cerebrovascular injury. *Arch Gen Psychiatry* 1990;47:246–251.

80. Eisen MS. Serotonin: a common neurobiologic substrate in anxiety and depression. *J Clin Psychopharmacol* 1990;10[Suppl]:26S–30S.

81. Mayeux R, Stern Y, Williams JBW, et al. Clinical and biochemical features of depression in Parkinson's disease. *Am J Psychiatry* 1986;143:756–759.

82. Lipsey JR, Robinson RG, Pearlson GD, et al. Mood change following bilateral hemisphere brain injury. *Br J Psychiatry* 1983;143:266–273.

83. Jorge RE, Robinson RG, Arndt SV, et al. Comparison between acute and delayed-onset depression following traumatic brain injury. *J Neuropsychiatry Clin Neurosci* 1993;5:43–49.

84. Bogousslavsky J, Ferrazzini M, Regli F, et al. Manic delirium and frontal lobe-like syndrome with paramedian infarction of the right thalamus. *J Neurol Neurosurg Psychiatry* 1988;51:116–119.

85. Clark AF, Davison K. Mania following head injury. *Br J Psychiatry* 1987;150:841–844.

86. Devinsky O, Morrel MJ, Vogt BA. Contributions of the anterior cortex to behavior. *Brain* 1995;118:279–306.

87. Cummings JL, Mendez FM. Secondary mania with focal cerebrovascular lesions. *Am J Psychiatry* 1984;41:1084–1087.

88. Forrest DV. Bipolar illness after right hemispherectomy. *Arch Gen Psychiatry* 1982;39:817–819.

89. Miller BL, Benson DF, Cummings JL, et al. Late-life parafrenia: an organic delusional syndrome. *J Clin Psychiatry* 1986;47:204–207.

90. Starkstein SE, Pearlson GE, Boston J, et al. Mania after brain injury. *Arch Neurol* 1987;44:1069–1073.

91. Lykestos C, Stoline AM, Longstreet P, et al. Mania in temporal lobe epilepsy. *Neuropsychiatry Neuropsychol Behav Neurol* 1993;6:19–25.

92. Starkstein SE, Fedoroff P, Berthier ML, et al. Manic-depressive and pure manic states after brain lesions. *Biol Psychiatry* 1991;29:149–158.

93. Robertson M. Mood disorders associated with epilepsy. In: McConnel HW, Snyder PJ, eds. *Psychiatric comorbidity in epilepsy.* Washington, DC: American Psychiatric Press, 1998:133–167.

94. Atre-Vaidya N. Epilepsy. In: Jobe TH, Gaviria M, Kovilparambil A, eds. *Clinical neuropsychiatry.* Boston: Blackwell Science, 1997:207–221.

95. Trimble MR, Schmitz B. The psychoses of epilepsy/schizophrenia. In: Engel J, Pedley TA, eds. *Epilepsy: a comprehensive textbook,* Volume II. Philadelphia: Lippincott-Raven Publishers, 1998:2071–2081.

96. Onuma T. Limbic lobe epilepsy with paranoid symptoms: analysis of clinical features and psychological test. *Fol Psychiatr Neurol Jpn* 1983;37:253–258.

97. Sengoku A, Yagi, Seino M, et al. Risk of occurrence of psychoses in relation to the types of epilepsies and epileptic seizures. *Fol Psychiatr Neurol Jpn* 1983;37:221–226.

98. Engel J Jr. The Hans Berger Lecture: functional explorations of the human brain and their therapeutic implications. *Electroencephalogr Clin Neurophysiol* 1990;76:296–316.

99. Jibiki I, Maeda T, Kubota T, et al. 123I-IMP SPECT brain imaging in epileptic psychosis: a study of two cases of temporal lobe epilepsy with schizophrenia-like syndrome. *Neuropsychobiology* 1993;28:207–211.

100. Marshall EJ, Syed GMS, Fenwick PBC. A pilot study of schizophrenia-like psychosis in epilepsy using single-photon emission computerised tomography. *Br J Psychiatry* 1993;163:32–36.

101. McPherson SE, Cummings JL. The neuropsychology of the frontal lobes. In: Ron MA, David AS, eds. *Disorders of brain and mind.* Cambridge: Cambridge University Press, 1998:11–34.

102. Ring HA. Other psychiatric illnesses. In: Engel J, Pedley TA, eds. *Epilepsy: a comprehensive textbook,* Volume II. Philadelphia: Lippincott-Raven Publishers, 1998:2171–2177.

103. Mellers JDC, Adachi N, Takei N, et al. SPET study of verbal fluency in schizophrenia and epilepsy. *Br J Psychiatry* 1998;173:69–74.

104. Petty RG, Pearlson CD. Temporal lobe laterality and involvement of heteromodal association cortex in schizophrenia. *Neuropsychopharmacology* 1993;29(abst).

105. Fenwick P. Psychiatric disorders and epilepsy. In: Hopkins A, Shorvon S, Cascino G, eds. *Epilepsy,* 2nd ed. Cambridge: Chapman & Hall Medical, 1995:453–502.

106. Hyde TM, Ziegler JC, Weinberger DR. Psychiatric disturbances in metachromatic leukodystrophy. Insights into the neurobiology of psychosis. *Arch Neurol* 1992;49:401–406.

107. Sultzer DL, Mahler ME, Maldenkern MA, et al. The relationship between psychiatric symptoms and regional cortical metabolism in Alzheimer's disease. *J Neuropsychiatry Clin Neurosci* 1995;7:476–484.

108. Cummings JL, Goselfeld LF, Houlihan JP, et al. Neuropsychiatric disturbances associated with idiopathic calcification of the basal ganglia. *Biol Psychiatry* 1983;18:591–601.

109. Akbarian S, Vinuela A, Kim JJ, et al. Distorted distribution of nicotinamide-adenine dinucleotide phosphate-diaphorase neurons in temporal lobe of schizophrenics implies anomalous cortical development. *Arch Gen Psychiatry* 1993;50:178–187.

110. Van der Does AW, Van der Bosch RJ. What determines Wisconsin Card Sorting Test performance in schizophrenia? *Clin Psychol Rev* 1992;12:567–583.

111. Perry W, Swerdlow NR, McDowell JE, et al. Schizophrenia and frontal lobe functioning. In: Miller BL, Cummings JL, eds. *The human frontal lobes, functions and disorders.* New York: Guilford Press, 1998:509–521.

112. Braff DL, Heaton R, Kuck J, et al. The generalized pattern of neuropsychological deficits in outpatients with chronic schizophrenia with heterogeneous Wisconsin Card Sorting Test results. *Arch Gen Psychiatry* 1991;48:891–898.

113. Wilson FA, Scalaidhe SP, Goldman-Rakic PS. Dissociation of object and spatial processing domains in primate prefrontal cortex. *Science* 1993;260:1955–1958.

114. Andreasen NC, Arndt S, Swayze V, et al. Thalamic abnormalities in schizophrenia visualized through magnetic resonance imaging averaging. *Science* 1994;266: 294–298.
115. Reith J, Benkelfat C, Sherwing A, et al. Elevated dopa decarboxylase activity in living brain of patients with psychosis. *Proc Natl Acad Sci USA* 1994;91: 11651–11654.
116. Benson DF, Hermann BP. Personality disorders. In: Engel J, Pedley TA, eds. *Epilepsy: a comprehensive textbook,* Volume II. Philadelphia: Lippincott-Raven Publishers, 1998:2065–2070.
117. Bear DM. Temporal lobe epilepsy: a syndrome of sensory-limbic hyperconnection. *Cortex* 1979;15:357–384.
118. Rubin RT, Ananth J, Villanueva-Meyer J, et al. Regional [133]xenon cerebral flow and ^{99m}Tc-HM-PAO uptake in patients with obsessive-compulsive disorder before and during treatment. *Biol Psychiatry* 1995;38:429–437.
119. Harris GJ, Hoehn-Saric R, Lewis RW, et al. Mapping of SPECT regional cerebral perfusion abnormalities in obsessive-compulsive disorder. *Hum Brain Map* 1994; 1:237–248.
120. Rubin RT, Harris GJ. Obsessive-compulsive disorder and the frontal lobes. In: Miller BL, Cummings JL, eds. *The human frontal lobes, functions and disorders.* New York: Guilford Press, 1998:522–536.
121. Benkelfat C, Nordahl TE, Semple WE, et al. Local cerebral glucose metabolic rates in obsessive-compulsive disorder. *Arch Gen Psychiatry* 1990;47:840–848.
122. Perani D, Colombo C, Bressi S, et al. [18F]FDG PET study in obsessive-compulsive disorder: a clinical/metabolic correlation study after treatment. *Br J Psychiatry* 1995;166:244–250.
123. Kettl PA, Marks IM. Neurological factors in obsessive compulsive disorder: two cases reports and a review on the literature. *Br J Psychiatry* 1986;149:315–319.
124. Baxter LR, Phelps ME, Mazziotta JC, et al. Local cerebral glucose metabolic rates in obsessive-compulsive disorder: a comparison with rates in unipolar depression and in normal controls. *Arch Gen Psychiatry* 1987;44:211–218.
125. Mendez M, Cherrier MM, Perryman KM. Epileptic forced thinking from left frontal lesions. *Neurology* 1996;47:79–83.
126. Levin B, Duchowny M. Childhood obsessive-compulsive disorder and cingulate epilepsy. *Biol Psychiatry* 1991;30:1049–1055.
127. Schmitz EB, Moriarty J, Costa DC, et al. Psychiatric profiles and patterns of cerebral blood flow in focal epilepsy: interactions between depression, obsessionality, and perfusion related to the laterality of the epilepsy. *Neurol Neurosurg Psychiatry* 1997;62: 458–463.

18

Models of Psychopathology in Epilepsy

Lessons Learned from Animal Studies

Thomas J. Hoeppner and Michael C. Smith

Department of Neurological Sciences, Rush Medical College, Chicago, Illinois 60612

Many patients with epilepsy show cognitive, memory, or affective abnormalities even when they are not having seizures. These abnormalities occur more frequently than would be expected by chance (1–4). Several factors may contribute to the association between epilepsy and behavioral abnormalities. One condition may be the etiology of the other, or they both may have a common source.

The three possible relationships are that (i) the epilepsy leads to the psychopathology, (ii) the psychopathology leads to the epilepsy, or (iii) another process is responsible for both.

The first possibility is that the presence of epilepsy might lead to the development of behavioral abnormalities. For instance, the behavioral abnormality might be due to (i) a reaction to the social stigma of having epilepsy (5); (ii) the presence of any chronic, intractable disease (4); (iii) a consequence of epileptic activity itself; or (iv) the treatment of epilepsy (medical or surgical).

The second possibility is that the presence of certain behavioral abnormalities might increase the likelihood of developing epilepsy. For instance, hyperactivity, impulsive behavior, and other socially maladaptive behaviors might increase the likelihood of head trauma or drug and alcohol addiction, with a concomitant increase in posttraumatic epilepsy or other forms of epilepsy. In addition, the treatment of psychiatric disease, by modulation of neuronal circuits, may alter the excitability of

critical neuronal circuits and increase the likelihood of developing epilepsy.

The third possibility is that the presence of epilepsy and of a behavioral abnormality may be due to a common pathophysiologic process. For instance, an insult to the brain that caused the epilepsy also may cause a behavioral abnormality, or there may be a common genetic predisposition for both epilepsy and certain behavioral abnormalities due to abnormal production of a type of γ-aminobutyric acid (GABA) receptor or other neurotransmission factor.

This chapter addresses the thesis that experimental animal studies provide novel information about psychopathology in epilepsy.

BACKGROUND TO THE USE OF ANIMAL MODELS IN STUDYING NORMAL FUNCTION, EPILEPSY, AND PSYCHOPATHOLOGY

Animal studies have provided an extensive understanding of anatomic, physiologic, pharmacologic, and behavioral processes and, in particular, the fundamental mechanisms of normal neuronal excitability and the neuronal elements of emotional behavior. It is upon this substrate that pathologic alterations and therapeutic interventions occur. The basic mechanisms involved in membrane potential and action potential generation and synaptic transmission form the foundation of neuronal physiology. Disturbance of these cellular mechanisms within particular anatomic circuits results in the diverse panoply of neurologic and psychiatric diseases (6,7). Systematic exploration and controlled manipulation of these basic physiologic and anatomic mechanisms can only be accomplished in animals. We will outline the normal physiologic elements and identify their contribution to understanding the nature of epilepsy and behavioral disturbances and their treatment. We then will examine the application of specific animal models of epilepsy and psychopathology.

Our animal models occasionally may appear to be very poor representations of human disease, and the promises offered by the animal models often may exceed their yield (8), but in several instances they have provided a basis for new therapies, an understanding of the mechanism of action of established therapies, an understanding of disease etiologies, or a description of diseases that have not yet been appreciated in humans.

PHYSIOLOGIC PROCESSES OF NEURONAL EXCITABILITY

Action Potential Mechanisms

The distinct function of voltage-gated sodium and potassium channels in a semipermeable membrane described in the squid giant axon provides our understanding of the ionic and molecular basis of action potential generation (9). These macromolecular complexes have been well characterized and are the therapeutic targets for some of the most widely used anticonvulsants, including phenytoin, carbamazepine, valproate, and lamotrigine. These antiseizure agents block sustained repetitive firing of isolated neurons, leaving low-frequency action potentials relatively unaffected (10). Such an action provides symptomatic treatment of seizures, which involve high-frequency discharges while leaving the lower-frequency discharges involved in normal behaviors relatively unaffected. In contrast, the puffer fish poison tetrodotoxin blocks the voltage-gated sodium channel. This prevents the increase in sodium permeability associated with the rising phase of the action potential, altering both normal and pathologic neuronal firing (11). Differentiating the action of an agent on repetitive firing from the action of a direct sodium channel blocker permits the development of less toxic anticonvulsants. Some of the anticonvulsants directed at action potential mechanisms have proven very effective in treating refractory pain (carbamazepine, phenytoin).

Synaptic Transmission

Presynaptic Mechanisms

Synaptic transmission depends on neurotransmitter synthesis, packaging in vesicles, calcium-regulated docking and release at presynaptic release sites, diffusion across the synaptic cleft, and subsequent binding at a postsynaptic receptor. Each of these processes provides a target site for disease and a target site for therapy.

Postsynaptic Mechanisms

The macromolecular postsynaptic receptors are neurotransmitter specific, but the receptors for a given neurotransmitter show remarkable diversity in affinity for the neurotransmitter and other ligands (12,13).

Each neurotransmitter has a family of receptors to which it will bind. The family is composed of various combinations of discrete subunits. The combination of subunits results in neurotransmitter specificity but diversity in affinity for the neurotransmitter and for other ligands. The postsynaptic receptor may have an associated ionophore or a metabotropic effect via a second messenger.

Neurotransmitter receptors commonly show developmental changes in their expression. The developmental changes in particular neurotransmitter systems may underlie the high incidence of seizures in early life (14).

Neurotransmitter receptor subtypes also show distinct cellular and regional distributions. The diversity, regulation of number, and cellular and regional locations of a given neurotransmitter receptor subtype determine its role in neuronal excitability.

Reuptake and/or degradation of neurotransmitters are dependent on specific reuptake pumps, autoreceptors, and enzymes.

This discussion of neurotransmission applies particularly to the small molecule "traditional" neurotransmitters and neuropeptides. The participation of gas neurotransmitters in these processes expands the set of regulatory mechanisms that may be involved in neuronal excitability and in emotional behavior.

Pharmacologic Treatment of Epilepsy and Psychiatric Disorders Directed Extensively at Synaptic Mechanisms Based on *In Vitro* Animal Models

Antiepileptic Drugs Affecting Synaptic Transmission

Many anticonvulsants are characterized according to the synaptic mechanism to which they are directed (15,16).

Utilizing animal models, many currently available anticonvulsants have been demonstrated to have a mechanism of action that enhances neurotransmission that utilizes GABA, the primary inhibitory neurotransmitter in the central nervous system. These include phenobarbital, diazepam, vigabatrin, and tiagabine. Blocking neurotransmission that utilizes glutamate, the primary excitatory neurotransmitter in the central nervous system, appears to be an important function of felbamate, remacemide, and topiramate (15).

Based on this experience, one can design an anticonvulsant based on its ability to enhance GABA neurotransmission or to block glutamate neurotransmission. Although this approach does not guarantee a useful antiepileptogenic drug for clinical purposes, it provides a rational approach to the development of antiepileptic drugs (AEDs). It is generally predictable that agents that act on such ubiquitous neurotransmitter systems as GABA and glutamate will alter the occurrence of seizures, but they also are likely to influence other behaviors (including emotional expression) that utilize these neurotransmitter systems. Thus, barbiturates, which enhance GABA neurotransmission, also are potent sedatives. It seems likely that the use of ligands that are more selective in their action, such as those that act at a specific subtype of a neurotransmitter receptor that has a restricted distribution, generally will have reduced side effects. Ketter et al. (17) proposed that better psychiatric outcomes in patients with epilepsy may be obtained by the judicious use of AEDs that have mechanisms of action that are "sedating" or "activating." Thus, they would utilize the psychotropic action of AEDs for positive benefit. They suggest that the sedating (primarily GABA agonists) AEDs, such as barbiturates, benzodiazepines, valproate, gabapentin, tiagabine, and vigabatrin, might be beneficial in patients with activated baselines involving insomnia, agitation, anxiety, racing thoughts, and weight loss, whereas activating (primarily glutamate antagonists) AEDs, such as felbamate and lamotrigine, might be helpful in patients with sedated baselines involving hypersomnia, fatigue, apathy, depression, sluggish cognition, and weight gain. Of further relevance to psychiatry is the observation that barbiturates may alter the metabolism of tricyclic antidepressants, resulting in the loss of the antidepressant effect (18).

Ethosuximide reduces the low-threshold calcium current (through T-type channels) in thalamic neurons, which seems to be important in the control of absence seizures (19,20).

The low neurotoxicity of ethosuximide may be attributable in part to a more selective mechanism and anatomic distribution of its site of action in the nervous system compared to most other AEDs.

Antipsychotic Drugs Affecting Synaptic Transmission

Many drugs used in the treatment of psychiatric conditions are defined on the basis of the neurotransmitter action they alter in animal models (21).

Neuroleptics generally antagonize dopa-mine-mediated neurotransmission, particularly at D2 receptors, and this is believed to be important to their efficacy (22). D2 receptors are particularly dense in the basal ganglia and in mesocortical and mesolimbic structures. The dopamine hypothesis of schizophrenia is based on the observation that the potency of antipsychotic drugs directly correlates with their affinity for the dopamine receptor (23). In this view, schizophrenia is attributable to an aberration in dopamine neurotransmission. Combined studies using patients with schizophrenia and animal models suggest that a balance between transmission at D1 and D2 receptors and a balance between transmission at D2 and glutamate receptors may be important in the pathophysiology of schizophrenia (23,24).

Antidepressants generally increase the availability of monoamines by blocking their reuptake or inhibiting their metabolism (21,25).

Tricyclic antidepressants inhibit norepinephrine and serotonin reuptake into nerve endings. They reduce the synthesis and release of norepinephrine and decrease the firing of neurons in the locus coeruleus of the rat. They tend to increase the likelihood of seizures.

Monoamine oxidase inhibitors prevent the enzymatic deamination of norepinephrine, serotonin, and dopamine to varying extents. They also interfere with the metabolism of barbiturates and many other drugs that might alter seizure control (26).

Selective serotonin reuptake inhibitors act at presynaptic autoreceptors of serotonin-releasing neurons and are effective in the treatment of depression (25). Some, but not all, selective serotonin reuptake inhibitors can lower the seizure threshold (27).

In the past, anxiety often was treated with barbiturates, but now it more commonly is treated with benzodiazepines (21). The efficacy of benzodiazepines in relief of anxiety has been demonstrated in a conflict punishment model in animals (28). Both benzodiazepines and barbiturates enhance GABA neurotransmission at the postsynaptic macromolecular complex. There are specific bind-ing sites for benzodiazepines associated with GABA receptors and a separate binding site for barbiturates on the GABA macromolecular complex (13).

Note that both benzodiazepines and barbiturates are potent anticonvulsants in both animal models and patients with epilepsy.

That some AEDs and antipsychotic drugs act on the same neurotransmitter systems and that some of the manifestations of the diseases are induced by these treatments (see later) in animal models provide clear bases for interaction between the treatment of one condition and induction of the other.

ANIMAL MODELS: GENERAL CONSIDERATIONS

Animal models of human behavior and disease serve many different purposes. They may be used to provide insight and understanding of normal function or a disease process. Use of animal models for testing the safety and efficacy of therapeutic approaches is standard practice. Animal models minimize or eliminate placebo effects, allow the rapid screening of large numbers of compounds in a short period of time, and minimize cost. The models may give insight to the mechanisms involved in pathophysiology (producing epilepsy or behavioral abnormalities). Note that the models that have been developed reflect a collective understanding of the disease and the attempt to control some of the abnormal features. This frequently leads to animal models of a symptom and consequently to symptomatic therapies. Such approaches may not influence the underlying etiologic processes. Thus, sodium channel blockers are effective in preventing seizures induced by maximal electroshock (MES) and provide symptomatic therapy in epilepsy. Epilepsy is a chronic disease in which recurrent seizures occur. A seizure is defined as a stereotyped, involuntary paroxysmal alteration of behavior (based on an abnormal synchrony of neuronal discharge). Epilepsy is a chronic disease and may be manifest in a variety of syndromes, but many of the animal models are acute seizure models. This may be beneficial for certain therapeutic purposes but will tend to mask or ignore interictal features. Chronic models may be necessary to study the process of epileptogenesis, the interictal state, and the long-term consequences of repeated seizures (29,30).

Epilepsy Models

There are more than 50 different animal models of epilepsy (31–34). The models utilize chemical/pharmacologic convulsants (alumina cream, cobalt, tungstic acid, iron, pentylenetetrazol [PTZ], penicillin, picrotoxin, strychnine, potassium, ouabain, kainate, pilocarpine), electrical stimulation (MES, kindling), sensory stimulation (audiogenic, photogenic seizures), genetic models (genetically epilepsy prone rat, tottering mouse, Papio papio, Genetic Absence Epilepsy Rats from Strasbourg [GAERS]), and physical trauma.

Selective models will be discussed for their impact on our understanding of epilepsy, their role in therapeutics, or their relationship to psychological processes. These are among the most widely utilized. The models of epilepsy share a common marker for the occurrence of seizures: the electrical manifestations of neuronal hyperexcitability and hypersynchrony, i.e., the paroxysmal depolarization shift at the cellular level, epileptic spikes, and/or electrographic seizures in the electroencephalogram (32), and some of them show behavioral seizures. There is no single marker for psychopathology that is as readily available and accepted as is electrical activity for a seizure. Animal models of psychopathology rely primarily on behavioral measures of function. Animal models of epilepsy reflect the major categories of seizures: generalized seizures (absence, myoclonic, and tonic-clonic) and partial seizures (simple, complex, and partial seizures with secondary generalization). The availability of electrographic discharges as a marker for epileptic activity enables the use of *in vitro* preparations for the study of seizures. The use of tissue slices or dissociated neurons derived from several different brain regions in diverse species has contributed enormously to

our understanding of the mechanisms of action of anticonvulsants and of convulsants (10,19,20,32). Although there are several *in vitro* animal models, this discussion will focus on *in vivo* models to facilitate consideration of focal neuroanatomic features and behavioral manifestations.

Models of Generalized Tonic-Clonic Seizures

The MES model involves electrical activation of generalized seizures in normal animals (35). Stimulation through the intact skull (electrodes may be placed at various sites, but most commonly they are applied to the corneas) results in a high frequency generalized epileptic discharge. In the rat and mouse, MES produces tonic bilateral limb flexion and extension followed by clonus. In 1937, Merritt and Putnam (36,37) successfully applied a variant of this model in the search for a nonsedating structural relative of phenobarbital with anticonvulsant properties. Their demonstration of the suppression of electroshock-induced convulsions in cats by diphenylhydantoin (phenytoin) was a landmark in the application of experimental animal techniques to clinical neuroscience questions. It resulted from a systematic screening of compounds in an animal model of epilepsy. Within 1 year of the discovery of its efficacy in suppressing electroshock-induced seizures in animals, phenytoin was introduced on a large scale to humans for the symptomatic treatment of epilepsy (38). The studies of Merritt and Putnam firmly established the validity of an animal model of epilepsy as a test for drug efficacy with important clinical significance. They combined behavioral (nonsedating), pharmacologic (structural analogue of phenobarbital), and therapeutic (anticonvulsant) criteria simultaneously. The discovery of phenytoin was aimed at minimizing an undesirable behavioral effect of phenobarbital (sedation). A comparable approach aimed at reducing the psychiatric manifestations associated with epilepsy might be profitable.

The MES model is recognized as a good predictor of efficacy against generalized tonic-clonic seizures. Drugs that are effective in blocking tonic hindlimb extension in this model generally are effective against partial and generalized tonic-clonic seizures in humans (39). The seizures produced by MES involve widespread, bilateral neural structures, but the tonic hindleg extension appears to be dependent on activation of brainstem structures (40). MES is an acute seizure model. Although it has been widely used for testing potential AEDs, it is not promoted as a model to study behavioral alterations or other interictal effects to any extent. Note, however, that electroconvulsive shock is widely utilized as the treatment of choice for severe clinical depression (41).

Models of Generalized Absence Seizures

Systemic administration of PTZ provides an animal model of absence seizures. The model mimics the bilaterally synchronous spike-and-wave discharge characteristic of absence seizures. There is an associated arrest of behavior. At high doses, this may be followed by myoclonic jerks and may proceed to generalized tonic-clonic seizures. PTZ-induced seizures are blocked by ethosuximide and valproate. PTZ blocks GABA-mediated inhibitory postsynaptic transmission (42). PTZ-induced seizures have been shown to be a good predictor of efficacy against absence seizures (39). High-dose systemic penicillin (another GABA inhibitor) also provides an animal model of absence seizures. Drugs that are effective against PTZ seizures, such as ethosuximide and trimethadione, are not very effective against MES seizures. Some drugs that are effective against MES-induced seizures, such as carbamazepine and phenytoin, are not very effective against PTZ-induced seizures and may actually worsen them (39,43). This double dissociation suggests different mechanisms for the seizure models and different mechanisms of action for the anticonvulsants. As indicated earlier, ethosuximide preferentially blocks the low-threshold calcium current in thalamic neurons and is very effective against the PTZ animal model

and human absence seizures (19). *In vitro* animal models of absence seizures suggest critical involvement of thalamocortical circuitry, with a low-threshold calcium current of neurons in the thalamic reticular nucleus providing a pacemaker function for the typical spike-and-wave discharges (44–46).

The GAERS are an inbred strain that display many of the characteristics of human absence epilepsy (47,48). The occurrence of spontaneous spike-and-wave discharges and behavioral arrest in the GAERS offers the opportunity to evaluate interictal behavioral alteration in a chronic model of a human epilepsy in which there is generally considered to be little or no cognitive or emotional disturbance.

Models of Simple Partial Seizures

Focal application of aluminum hydroxide to the cortex results in a delayed appearance of epileptic spikes and electrographic and behavioral seizures (49,50). The behavioral and electrical characteristics of the seizures reflect the site of application of the alumina. Intracortical alumina provides a chronic model of epilepsy that manifests spontaneous recurring seizures and is considered by some the best validated model of epilepsy with regard to the behavioral and electrographic manifestations of seizures, the temporal and spatial distribution of the seizures, and the response to anticonvulsants that parallels the response of patients with focal epilepsy (32). Decreases in GABA concentrations have been observed around the focus in the alumina model (51). This model would allow for examination of interictal behavioral concomitants of recurrent seizures, but it appears that its use has been limited because of the variability of seizure occurrence (a feature in common with human epilepsy) and the cost of the primate model. The model is not as readily developed in rodents *(personal observation)*.

Recurrent focal partial seizures also are modeled by intracortical application of the metals cobalt, tungsten, zinc, and iron (32). These models are effective in rodents and could be applied to the investigation of inter-ictal behavioral alterations. In contrast to the other models, the use of iron as an epilepto-genic agent mimics the availability of a natu-rally occurring blood component (from hemo-globin) associated with head trauma (52).

Electrical kindling can produce a model of simple partial seizures, but it will be dis-cussed later as a model of complex partial seizures. The difference reflects the site of stimulus application. Stimulation in the motor cortex produces a model of simple partial seizures, whereas stimulation in the amygdala or hippocampus produces a model of complex partial seizures.

Models of Complex Partial Seizures

Kainate

Systemically administered kainic acid pro-duces epileptic seizures originating in the hip-pocampus. The kainic acid binds to glutamate receptors and produces relatively selective death of neurons in the hippocampus (53). This model is particularly useful to evaluate excitotoxic processes, the consequences of hippocampal cell loss, and the resultant neu-ronal circuitry reorganization. In some re-gards, this parallels the pathologic changes of hippocampal sclerosis seen in patients with the syndrome of mesial temporal lobe epilepsy (54). However, it is not well suited to the examination of interictal effects of epilep-tic activity itself due to its subacute duration.

Kindling

In the kindling model of epilepsy, a brief, focal electrical stimulus is applied at an inten-sity that is initially subthreshold for behav-ioral seizures, but elicits an electrical afterdis-charge (55,56). On subsequent days, the same stimulus results in a progressively longer and more widespread afterdischarge and a focal behavioral seizure. After several days of stim-ulation, partial seizures with secondary gen-eralization can be triggered by the previously subthreshold stimuli. After an animal has

reached the point where stimulation produces a secondarily generalized seizure, the animal is said to be kindled. At this point, a general-ized seizure can be produced by a previously subthreshold stimulus, even after a period of several months without stimulation. Kindling models some of the chronic aspects of epilepsy in that kindled animals display an en-during change of excitability after an initial series of seizures (57). After several stimu-lated generalized seizures are produced, spon-taneous seizures may be seen (58,59). Kin-dling occurs most readily in the amygdala, but several other forebrain sites are effective. The initial seizure observed on amygdala kindling involves mild motor automatisms. On subse-quent stimulations, there is a gradual progres-sion to more intense seizures involving facial and forelimb clonus, rearing, and, eventually, loss of equilibrium (60).

Both GABA-ergic and glutamatergic neu-rotransmission may be involved in the kin-dling process (61). GABA neurotransmission is impaired in the region of the kindled epileptic focus (62), and N-methyl-D-aspar-tate (NMDA) receptor antagonists retard the development of kindling (63). The possibility that the neurotransmitter changes are a conse-quence of epileptic activity rather than a cause cannot be excluded (26). The early de-velopment of kindled seizures appears to de-pend on the activation of NMDA-type gluta-mate receptors, but NMDA blockers have much less effect on already kindled seizures (64,65). This suggests a separation between the development of seizures (epileptogenesis) and the chronic condition of epilepsy, with different therapeutic options for each.

Kindling is considered by some the pre-ferred model of complex partial epilepsy, not solely a seizure model (30,32,66). Drug sensi-tivity of kindled seizures in animals parallels that of complex partial seizures in humans (67). Ethosuximide is not effective in block-ing kindled seizures, whereas phenytoin, car-bamazepine, and phenobarbital are effective at nontoxic doses.

Of all the animal models, kindling has been the most widely utilized to examine the relationship between epilepsy and behavioral abnormalities (68–70). These studies show alterations of emotional behavior induced by kindling. The anatomic distribution of the sites most sensitive to kindling corresponds to sites that have been most consistently involved in emotional behavior (compare references 55 and 71). In the cat, amygdala kindling produces an enduring alteration in defensive responses to capture and predatory behavior (68). In the rat, amygdala kindling produces long-term impairment in conditioned emotional response learning (69). Fear conditioning is impaired by amygdala kindling in the rat, and this impairment may be reduced by antiepileptic treatment with valproate during the kindling process (see below, and references 100–102).

Neuronal Elements of Emotional Behavior

Extensive studies of Rolls (71) in rodents and primates utilizing a combination of single unit recording, electrical stimulation, and selective ablation show the physiologic, anatomic, and pharmacologic elements that are the normal underpinning of emotional behavior. Rolls (71, p. 41) defines emotions as states elicited by rewards and punishers. In this view, emotional behavior is dependent on the interplay between rewards and punishment, classical and operant conditioning, and the strength of primary drives.

Several neural structures involved in feeding, drinking, sexual behavior, and temperature regulation have been identified. These behaviors have been dissected to differentiate signals that provide reward value from satiety signals in the control of consummatory behavior. Thus, in the control of feeding behavior, studies of sham feeding in which ingested food is diverted from the stomach by a gastric cannula show that monkeys will continue to eat for an extended period of time if food does not accumulate in the stomach and intestine. The taste, smell, and eating of food provide the reward for food-motivated behaviors (71). The satiety signals are provided by gastric distention (72). Food or fluid introduced directly into the stomach, bypassing the mouth and thus avoiding taste and smell, has little or no reward value for work. Furthermore, the reward value of the food is modulated by the hunger and satiety signals so that the smell and taste of food are rewarding when hunger signals are present and satiety signals are not (71, p. 11). The ability of peripheral signals to modify feeding behavior differentially implies the presence of central control systems that are separate, but able to interact, as satiety signals can alter the reward value of taste and smell signals. Central control of these behaviors is demonstrated by the lateral and ventromedial hypothalamus. Bilateral lesions of the ventromedial hypothalamus lead to hyperphagia and obesity (73,74). This appears to be due to an influence of the ventromedial hypothalamus on insulin secretion mediated by the vagal input to the pancreas. Bilateral lesions of the lateral hypothalamus lead to reduction in feeding and body weight (75). Some of the neurons recorded from the lateral hypothalamus of the monkey fire in response to the taste of certain food substances in the mouth and/or at the sight of food (76). The response of these neurons to the taste or sight of food was present when the animals were hungry and was eliminated when the animals were satiated (71, p. 21).

Olds (77,78) had shown earlier that rats will work for electrical stimulation of certain brain regions, mimicking the effect of natural rewards. Neurons responsive to food reward also are located in the amygdala and orbital frontal cortex. The regions in which neurons are activated by food reward in monkeys overlap with the sites at which animals will self-stimulate in order to receive electrical stimulation. Furthermore, both the electrical self-stimulation and the neuronal activity in response to food presentation were diminished in animals that had been fed to satiety (79).

Experiments on visual, gustatory, and olfactory pathways involved in feeding behavior show a convergence of these pathways on the amygdala and orbital frontal cortex and from there to the hypothalamus. These studies suggest that the amygdala is involved in establishing the reward value of a stimulus based on association of the stimulus with a primary reinforcer, such as food (71, p. 48); thus, its role depends on learning. The orbital frontal cortex appears to be more involved in the rapid readjustment of behavioral responses when the reinforcement value is repeatedly changing, as in discrimination reversal tasks (71, p. 49). Rolls (71, p. 49) notes that the ability to flexibly alter responses based on their changing reinforcement associations is important in motivated behavior, such as feeding, and in emotional behavior, and these are disturbed in animals with orbital frontal lesions.

Orbital frontal cortex lesions in monkeys alter food preferences, impair extinction, impair reversal learning, and produce changes in emotional behavior. Based on a combination of ablation, single unit recording, and electrical stimulation studies in primates, Rolls (71, p. 75) shows that the neural processing of emotion depends on neurons in the amygdala and the orbital frontal cortex. Neurons in these areas are responsive to stimuli in multiple modalities, compute the reward value of positive and negative reinforcers, and are involved in the learned associations between primary (unconditioned stimuli: taste, pleasant touch, pain) and secondary (conditioned stimuli: previously neutral stimuli, which can alter the probability of an arbitrary instrumental response or action) reinforcers. In contrast, neurons in the primary sensory areas and secondary sensory areas, which are sensitive to the physical properties of stimuli, are not responsive to the reward value of stimuli (71).

Subsequent to the monkey studies, Rolls et al. (80) showed using functional magnetic resonance imaging that pleasant tactile stimuli activated the orbital frontal cortex in humans but neutral tactile stimuli did not. Somatosensory cortex was activated by both neutral and pleasant stimuli. The identification of discrete brain sites that are modulated by reward and satiety suggests that these sites may be selectively disturbed to produce behavioral disturbances and that these sites may provide the target for specific therapies. Rolls (71) makes the point that

although the amygdala in rats is well developed, the orbital frontal cortex is not, so that subhuman primates may be the preferred model for orbital frontal function in humans.

Animal Models of Depression

We will focus on animal models of depression, because depression is the most consistently observed psychopathology in patients with epilepsy (81,82) (for review, see reference 26).

Reserpine-Induced Sedation (Pharmacologic Model)

Administration of the sympathetic antagonist reserpine produces sedation and impairs performance in the passive avoidance test. Reserpine depletes the brain of serotonin and norepinephrine. Clinically useful antidepressants antagonize or reverse the sedative effect of reserpine, and this has served as a sensitive screen of putative antidepressants. The animal model mimics the clinical model of reserpine-induced sedation and depression. Reserpine-induced depression is a significant risk in patients being treated for hypertension.

Forced Swimming (Behavioral Model)

An animal (usually a rat) is forced to swim in a tank of water with no possibility of escape. After initial unsuccessful attempts to escape, the rat stops trying to escape (freezes), except for the effort to stay afloat. Effective antidepressants reduce the time of freezing and the model serves as a screen for new antidepressants. The model is referred to as behavioral despair.

Learned Helplessness (Behavioral Model)

If a rat is exposed to repetitive aversive stimuli (usually foot shock) that it can control by an operant behavior (e.g., jumping or pressing a lever), it will quickly learn to press the lever to escape shock. In the learned helplessness model, an animal initially is exposed to repetitive aversive stimuli that it cannot control. When it subsequently is put in a situation in which it can control the occurrence of the aversive stimulus, it fails to make the appropriate response (83). A comparable phenomenon can be demonstrated in humans (84). The model is sensitive to a large number of antidepressants, but it is not used as a routine screening tool for new antidepressants because it is time consuming (26).

Because epileptic seizures generally are unpredictable and may be aversive, epilepsy itself may be considered a condition that leads to learned helplessness in some patients. Manifestations of this may include noncompliance in medical treatment, such as AED therapy, and noncompliance in those behavioral modifications that may reduce the incidence of seizures, such as avoiding alcohol, getting adequate sleep, and managing stress. Effective medical and behavioral therapies may have to overcome the previously learned helplessness. Thus, AEDs with an antidepressant effect may have a direct anticonvulsant action and promote better medical and behavioral compliance.

Olfactory Bulbectomy (Surgical Ablation Model)

Surgical removal of the olfactory bulbs (in rodents) results in impaired acquisition of a passive avoidance. This provides a sensitive screening procedure for antidepressant drugs (26, pp. 827–828). The olfactory bulbs project to the amygdala (uncus) and dorsomedial nucleus of the thalamus, and then to the orbital frontal cortex (85, p. 180). As noted earlier, Rolls (71) found neurons in the amygdala and orbital frontal cortex that were sensitive to the reward value of stimuli. Such neurons are likely to be perturbed in this model of clinical depression. There are strong behavioral, anatomic, and pharmacologic parallels between the olfactory bulbectomized rat and the depressed patient (86,87).

Klüver-Bucy Syndrome (Surgical Ablation Model)

Bilateral ablation of the anterior temporal lobe in monkeys produces a striking syndrome that includes a lack of emotional responsiveness, tameness, excessive manipulation of objects, and eating of objects that normally would not be eaten (88). Weizkrantz (89) showed that most of these effects could be attributed to ablation of the amygdala. Bilateral amygdalectomy in monkeys impairs conditioning to both positive and negative reinforcers (produces a deficit in learning to associate neutral stimuli with a primary reinforcer, reward, or punisher) (71, pp. 90, 91, 99). After Klüver and Bucy described the syndrome in monkeys, the same syndrome was described in humans (92,93). This is one of the interesting situations in which the development of the animal model appears to have preceded the full recognition of the syndrome in humans.

Rolls (71, p. 99) suggests that the symptoms of Klüver-Bucy syndrome, including the emotional changes, are due to a deficit in learning stimulus-reinforcement associations and the deficit is due to bilateral damage to the amygdala.

Bilateral amygdala lesions in rodents impair behavior based on the association between neutral stimuli and positive or negative reinforcers but do not impair the behavior to primary reinforcers (94,95). This applies to sexual responses, drug-seeking behavior, and feeding behavior. Thus, the primary consummatory responses to these stimuli are intact, but the conditioned behaviors are impaired. It appears that the conditioned behaviors linked to these reinforcers are dependent on the amygdala, whereas the primary reinforcing value is dependent on the hypothalamus and surrounding structures (71, p. 100).

The most common form of epilepsy involves a focus in anterior temporal lobe structures, including the hippocampus, amygdala, and surrounding cortex, target sites of the olfactory bulb. Therefore, one might expect some elements of the behavioral alterations seen in animals with an olfactory bulbectomy or Klüver-Bucy syndrome to be manifest by patients with anterior temporal lobe epileptic foci, especially if there is bilateral involvement.

The most common form of surgery for epilepsy involves resection of the anterior temporal lobe structures. This could exacerbate some of the underlying behavioral disturbances by bringing out elements of an olfactory bulbectomy or Klüver-Bucy syndrome. Thus, the surgical treatment of epilepsy may be a double-edged sword, curing the epilepsy and inducing psychopathology. It would be difficult to overlook the Klüver-Bucy syndrome if it were being routinely produced in the many patients who had epilepsy surgery involving the anterior temporal lobe. Therefore, the syndrome might require extensive bilateral damage, as initially suggested (88), or the behavioral disturbances may be more subtle than the full syndrome.

Fear Conditioning (Behavioral Model)

This animal model of fear is based on a classical conditioning paradigm. In a typical example of this model, on each trial a 20-second conditioning stimulus (CS) (e.g., sound) is terminated by onset of an aversive unconditioned stimulus (e.g., foot shock that lasts 0.5 second). Behavioral immobility (freezing) during the 20-second sound CS is the conditioned response. On the first trial, when the sound comes on the animal moves around freely. Within a few trials, the animal freezes when the sound comes on and remains still for most of its duration. The conditioned response—freezing—is used as a measure of fear. The manifestations of the inferred fear state in this animal model closely parallel the clinical criteria of generalized anxiety (96). There is increased heart rate and stroke volume, dry mouth/decreased salivation, stomach ulcers/upset stomach, altered respiration, scanning and vigilance, increased urination and defecation, grooming/fidgeting, as well as freezing/apprehension.

Phillips and LeDoux (95) showed that bilateral lesions of the amygdala (but not of the hippocampus or neocortex) attenuate fear conditioning to sound stimuli in rats. Fear conditioning is dependent on activation of NMDA-type glutamate receptors in the amygdala (96,97). The many manifestations of fear conditioning appear to be dependent on outputs from different portions of the amygdaloid complex to specific targets. Thus, the freezing response, autonomic changes, and cortical arousal components of conditioned fear could be selectively impaired by lesions of the central gray of the midbrain, lateral hypothalamus, and basal nucleus of Meynert, respectively (71, p. 102; 96). Epileptic foci in the structures involved in fear conditioning might impair the normal development of fear and thereby lead to inappropriate behavior in those situations that commonly would evoke fear.

CONJUNCTION OF ANIMAL MODELS OF EPILEPSY AND PSYCHOPATHOLOGY

As indicated earlier ("Models of Complex Partial Seizures"), kindling has been used most widely to study the relationship between epilepsy and psychopathology in animals (68–70,98–102). It provides a chronic model of epilepsy that is particularly potent in those limbic structures that appear to be most involved in emotional behavior.

In an extensive series of studies of cats, Adamec (68,98) showed that amygdala kindling produces an enduring alteration in several species' characteristic emotional behaviors. Cat defensive responses (withdrawal from threat, hissing, and affective attack) satisfy several of the criteria for an animal model of anxiety. These responses generally are enhanced in amygdala-kindled cats and are attenuated by benzodiazepines (68). A study in rats by McIntyre and Molino (69) indicated that amygdala kindling impairs emotional behavior as measured by the conditioned emotional response. However, that study involved prior ablation of the amygdala on the side contralateral to the kindling site, leaving it undetermined whether unilateral amygdala kindling could produce a bilateral functional amygdala deficit (70,99). Because unilateral kindling of the amygdala results in bilateral epileptic discharge in homotopic regions as kindling progresses, it seems likely that the structures receiving the most severe epileptic bombardment may, over time, alter their responsiveness, resulting in a bilateral functional lesion of the amygdala. We utilized the model of conditioned fear in conjunction with the kindling model to determine the impact of epileptic activity in the amygdala on fear conditioning. A preliminary report of these studies has been published (100) and a full presentation is in preparation (101).

Because amygdala kindling produces permanent changes in the excitability of the amygdala and fear conditioning is dependent on the amygdala, we hypothesized that unilateral amygdala kindling would interfere with subsequent fear conditioning.

Rats received amygdala kindling once a day for 15 days or until they had three secondarily generalized seizures (stage 5 in the classification of Racine [60]), whichever came first. To allow any acute effects of seizures to dissipate, the evaluation of fear conditioning commenced 10 to 14 days after kindling was completed. On each trial, a 20-second sound stimulus (the CS) was terminated with a 0.5-second foot shock (unconditioned stimulus). There were two conditioning trials each day for 2 days. The duration of freezing (immobility) during the 20-second CS was the measure of fear conditioning. On the third through the seventh day, the CS was presented without shock and the duration of freezing during CS presentation was measured. Amygdala-kindled rats showed markedly reduced fear conditioning compared to control animals that had electrodes implanted in the amygdala but were not kindled. These findings indicate that epileptic activity associated with kindling of the amygdala provides a functional lesion of the amygdala that lasts for at least 2 weeks after the last seizure, well beyond the immediate postictal period. Because both the kindled rats and the unstimulated control rats had electrodes implanted, the deficit is most likely attributed to the electrographic activation of the kindled animals and the associated neurochemical changes.

Further evidence to support the role of epileptic activity in producing the behavioral deficit in fear conditioning is provided by a parallel study of rats that received valproate throughout the kindling process and then were tested on fear conditioning 10 to 14 days later. The valproate was discontinued immediately after the kindling concluded, so that it would not be in the system when fear conditioning was tested (102). Valproate markedly inhibited amygdala kindling. When animals were tested on fear conditioning, they demonstrated relatively normal fear conditioning; thus, prophylactic treatment with the AED valproate blocked kindling and protected the animals against the behavioral impairment.

These studies indicate that unilateral amygdala kindling resulted in impaired fear conditioning. It appears that a unilateral epileptogenic focus in the amygdala may produce behavioral deficits indicative of bilateral amygdala dysfunction long after the occurrence of seizures and that the deficit is associated with the prior spread of epileptic activity from one amygdala to the other.

Animal studies such as these suggest that social stigma, structural lesions, specific genetic predisposition, or genetic comorbidity are not necessary elements in the development of behavioral abnormalities in epilepsy.

SUMMARY

The large number of animal models of epilepsy and of psychopathology indicate the many different neuronal mechanisms that may contribute to the symptoms of these common disease families.

The impact of epileptic activity on cognitive and affective behaviors will depend on the overlap between the localization and distribution of the epileptic activity and the anatomic and physiologic substrate of the particular behavior under consideration.

Animal models give several insights to the relationship between epilepsy and psychopathology. The animal models of epilepsy strongly reflect the anatomic site of origin (thalamic, neocortical, or limbic) resulting in generalized or partial seizures (simple and complex), respectively. This is consistent with the varieties of human epilepsy and provides a basis for selective therapies. The animal models of some psychopathologies show a striking convergence in the preferential involvement of limbic structures (amygdala, hippocampus, orbital frontal cortex). The anatomic overlap of the models of complex partial seizures and models of psychopathology (especially depression) points directly to limbic structures, particularly the amygdala, as a critical site in the comorbidity of the two conditions.

It is clear that the treatment of one condition can lead to the manifestations of the other condition. This is particularly noticeable in that GABA agonists effective in preventing seizures may have a sedating effect. This can be avoided by the use of alternative AEDs.

Study of experimental animal models of epilepsy and of psychopathology reveals examples of each of the three possible relationships between these conditions. Epilepsy may lead to psychopathology, psychopathology may lead to epilepsy, or another process may produce both. Of particular significance for practitioners in this area is the observation that treatment of one condition may induce, or promote, the appearance of the other.

Just as Merritt and Putnam designed their search for an AED that was nonsedating more than 60 years ago, we can design our search for new AEDs that produce minimal psychotropic impairment themselves and that protect against the behavioral impairment produced by epileptic activity. In addition to the usual acute seizure models, such an approach will require the combined use of chronic models of epilepsy and animal models of behavioral impairment.

The enormous power that animal models have provided in understanding the basic mechanisms of neuronal excitability and in building a testing ground for new treatments is being applied increasingly to these most intricate aspects of behavior.

REFERENCES

1. Waxman S, Geschwind N. The interictal behavior syndrome of temporal lobe epilepsy. *Arch Gen Psychiatry* 1975;32:1580–1586.
2. Bear DM, Fedio P. Quantitative analysis of interictal behavior in temporal lobe epilepsy. *Arch Neurol* 1977; 34:454–467.
3. Smith DB, Craft BR, Collins J. Behavioral characteristics of epilepsy patients compared with normal controls. *Epilepsia* 1986;27:760–768.,
4. Schiffer RB, Babigian H. Behavioral disorders in multiple sclerosis, temporal lobe epilepsy and amyotrophic lateral sclerosis. *Arch Neurol* 1984;41:1067–1069.
5. Blumer D, Benson F. Psychiatric manifestations of epilepsy. In: Benson DF, Blumer D. *Psychiatric aspects of neurologic disease,* Volume II. New York: Grune & Stratton, 1982:25–48.
6. Albert ML. Critique of the neurobiologic paradigm. In: Eisendorfer C, Cohen D, Kleinman A, et al., eds. *Models for clinical psychopathology.* New York: Spectrum, 1981:133–137.
7. Kandel ER. Biology and the future of psychoanalysis: a new intellectual framework for psychiatry revisited. *Am J Psychiatry* 1999;156:505–524.
8. Kornetsky C. Animal models: promises and problems. In: Hanin I, Usdin E, eds. *Animal models in psychiatry and neurology.* Oxford: Pergamon Press, 1977:1–7.
9. Hodgkin AL, Huxley AF. A quantitative description of membrane current and its application to conduction and excitation in nerve. *J Physiol (Lond)* 1952;117: 500–544.
10. Macdonald RL, Kelly KM. Antiepileptic drug mechanisms of action. *Epilepsia* 1993;34[Suppl 5]:S1–S8.
11. Ritchie JM. Tetrodotoxin and saxitoxin and the sodium channels of excitable tissues. *Trends Pharmacol Sci* 1980;1:275–279.
12. Hollman M, Heinemann S. Cloned glutamate receptors. *Annu Rev Neurosci* 1994;17:31–108.
13. Macdonald RL, Olsen RW. GABAa receptor channels. *Annu Rev Neurosci* 1994;17:569–602.
14. Kubova H, Moshe SL. Experimental models of epilepsy in young animals. *J Child Neurol* 1994;9 [Suppl 1]:S3–S11.
15. Meldrum BS. Update on the mechanisms of action of antiepileptic drugs. *Epilepsia* 1996;37[Suppl 6]: S4–S11.
16. Meldrum BS, Chapman AG. Basic mechanisms of Gabatril (tiagabine) and future potential developments. *Epilepsia* 1999;40[Suppl 9]:S2–S6.
17. Ketter TA, Post RM, Theodore WH. Positive and negative effects of antiepileptic drugs in patients with seizure disorders. *Neurology* 1999;53[Suppl 2]:S53–S67.
18. Garey KW, Amsden GW, Johns CA. Possible interaction between imipramine and butalbital. *Pharmacotherapy* 1997;17:1041–1042.
19. Coulter DA, Huguenard JR, Prince DA. Characterization of ethosuximide reduction of low-threshold calcium current in thalamic neurons. *Ann Neurol* 1989; 25:582–593.
20. Coulter DA, Huguenard JR, Prince DA. Differential effects of petit mal anticonvulsants and convulsants on thalamic neurons: calcium current reduction. *Br J Pharmacol* 1990;100:800–806.
21. Baldessarini RJ. Drugs and the treatment of psychiatric disorders. In: Hardman JG, Limbard LE, eds. *Goodman & Gilman's the pharmacological basis of therapeutics,* 9th ed. New York: McGraw-Hill, 1996:399–459.
22. Carlsson A. Early psychopharmacology and the rise of modern brain research. *J Psychopharmacol* 1990;4: 120–126.

23. Lidow MS, Williams GV, Goldman-Rakic P. The cerebral cortex: a case for a common site for antipsychotics. *Trends Pharmacol Sci* 1998;19:136–140.

24. Olney JW, Farber NB. Glutamate receptor dysfunction and schizophrenia. *Arch Gen Psychiatry* 1995;52:998–1007.

25. Baldessarini RJ. Current status of antidepressants: clinical pharmacology and therapy. *J Clin Psychiatry* 1989;50:117–126.

26. Feldman RS, Meyer JS, Quenzer LF. *Principles of neuropsychopharmacology.* Sunderland, MA: Sinauer, 1997:438–439.

27. Kanner AM, Kozak AM, Frey M. The use of sertraline in patients with epilepsy: is it safe? *Epilepsy and Behavior* 2000;1:100–105.

28. Eison ES. Use of animal models: toward anxioselective drugs. *Psychopathology* 1984;17[Suppl 1]:37–44.

29. Cavalheiro EA, Santos NF, Priel MR. The pilocarpine model of epilepsy in mice. *Epilepsia* 1996;37:1015–1019.

30. Engel J Jr. Critical evaluation of animal models for localization-related epilepsies. *Ital J Neurol Sci* 1995;16:9–16.

31. Purpura DP, Penry JK, Tower DB, et al., eds. *Experimental models of epilepsy.* New York: Raven Press, 1972:433–458.

32. Fisher RM. Animal models of the epilepsies. *Brain Res Rev* 1989;14:245–278.

33. Turski W, Cavalheiro EA, Bortolotto ZA, et al. Seizures produced by pilocarpine in mice: a behavioral electroencephalographic and morphological analysis. *Brain Res* 1984;321:237–253.

34. Turski W, Cavalheiro EA, Schwarcz M, et al. Limbic seizures produced by pilocarpine in rats: behavioral electroencephalographic and neuropathologic study. *Behav Brain Res* 1983;9:315–335.

35. Swinyard EW. Electrically induced convulsions. In: Purpura DP, Penry JK, Tower DB, et al., eds. *Experimental models of epilepsy.* New York: Raven Press, 1972:433–458.

36. Merritt HH, Putnam TJ. A new series of anticonvulsant drugs tested by experiments on animals. *Trans Am Neurol Assoc* 1937;63:123–128.

37. Merritt HH, Putnam TJ. A new series of anticonvulsant drugs tested by experiments on animals. *Arch Neurol Psychiatry* 1938;39:1003–1015.

38. Merritt HH, Putnam TJ. Sodium diphenyl hydantoinate in treatment of convulsive disorders. *JAMA* 1938;111:1068–1073.

39. MacNamara JO. Drugs effective in the therapy of the epilepsies. In: Hardman JG, Limbard LE, eds. *Goodman & Gilman's the pharmacological basis of therapeutics,* 9th ed. New York: McGraw-Hill, 1996:461–486.

40. Browning RA. Role of the brain-stem reticular formation in tonic-clonic seizures: lesion and pharmacological studies. *Fed Proc* 1985;44:2425–2431.

41. Bailine SH, Rifkin A, Kayne E, et al. Comparison of bifrontal and bitemporal ECT for major depression. *Am J Psychiatry* 2000;157:121–123.

42. Macdonald RL, Barker JL. Pentylenetetrazol and penicillin are selective antagonists of GABA-mediated post-synaptic inhibition in cultured mammalian neurones. *Nature* 1977;267:720–721.

43. Coulter DA, Huguenard JR, Prince DA. Specific petit mal anticonvulsants reduce calcium currents in thalamic neurons. *Neurosci Lett* 1989;98:74–78.

44. Coulter DA, Lee CJ. Thalamocortical rhythm generation in vitro: extra- and intracellular recordings in mouse thalamocortical slices perfused with low Mg^{2+} medium. *Brain Res* 1993;631:137–142.

45. Zhang YF, Gibbs JW III, Coulter DA. Anticonvulsant drug effects on spontaneous thalamocortical rhythms in vitro: ethosuximide, trimethadione, and dimethadione. *Epilepsy Res* 1996;23:15–36.

46. Coulter DA. Antiepileptic drug cellular mechanisms of action: where does lamotrigine fit in? *J Child Neurol* 1997;12[Suppl]:S2–S9.

47. Talley EM, Solorzano G, Depaulis A, et al. Low-voltage-activated calcium channel subunit expression in a genetic model of absence epilepsy in the rat. *Mol Brain Res* 2000;75:159–165.

48. Danober L, Deransart C, Depaulis A, et al. Pathophysiological mechanisms of genetic absence epilepsy in the rat. *Prog Neurobiol* 1998;55:27–57.

49. Kopeloff LM, Chusid JG, Kopeloff N. Epilepsy in *macacca mulatta* after cortical or intracerebral alumina. *Arch Neurol Psychiatry* 1955;74:523–526.

50. Ward AA. Topical convulsant metals. In: Purpura DP, Penry JK, Tower DB, et al., eds. *Experimental models of epilepsy.* New York: Raven Press, 1972:13–35.

51. Lloyd KG, Bossi L, Morselli PL, et al. Alteration of GABA-mediated synaptic transmission in human epilepsy. *Adv Neurol* 1986;44:1033–1044.

52. Willmore LJ. Recurrent seizure induced by cortical iron injection, a model of post-traumatic epilepsy. *Ann Neurol* 1978;4:329–333.

53. Olney JW, Rhee V, Ho OL. Kainic acid: a powerful neurotoxic analog of glutamate. *Brain Res* 1974;77:501–512.

54. Franck JE, Roberts DL. Combined kainate and ischemia produces "mesial temporal sclerosis." *Neurosci Lett* 1990;118:159–163.

55. Goddard GV, McIntyre DC, Leech CK. A permanent change in brain function resulting from daily electrical stimulation. *Exp Neurol* 1969;25:295–330.

56. Racine R. Modification of seizure activity by electrical stimulation: I. After discharge threshold. *Electroencephalogr Clin Neurophysiol* 1972;32:281–294.

57. Teskey GC, Racine RJ. Increased spontaneous unit discharges following electrical kindling in the rat. *Brain Res* 1993;624:11–18.

58. Wada JA, Sato M. Recurrent spontaneous epileptic seizure state induced by localized electrical stimulation. *Neurology* 1973;23:447.

59. Pinel JP, Rovner LI. Experimental epileptogenesis: kindling-induced epilepsy in rats. *Exp Neurol* 1978;58:190–202.

60. Racine RJ. Modification of seizure activity by electrical stimulation: II. Motor seizure. *Electroencephalogr Clin Neurophysiol* 1972;32:281–294.

61. Bradford HF. Glutamate, GABA and epilepsy. *Prog Neurobiol* 1995;47:477–511.

62. Burnham WM. The GABA hypothesis of kindling: recent assay studies. *Neurosci Biobehav Rev* 1989;13:281–288.

63. Dingledine R, McBain CJ, McNamara JO. Excitatory amino acid receptors in epilepsy. *Trends Pharmacol Sci* 1990;11:334–338.

64. Gilbert ME, Mack CM. The NMDA antagonist, MK-801, suppresses long-term potentiation, kindling, and kindling-induced potentiation in the perforant path of the unanesthetized rat. *Brain Res* 1990;519:89–96.
65. Morimoto K, Katayama K, Inoue K, et al. Effects of competitive and noncompetitive NMDA receptor antagonists on kindling and LTP. *Pharmacol Biochem Behav* 1991;40:893–899.
66. McNamara JO. Kindling: an animal model of complex partial epilepsy. *Ann Neurol* 1984;16[Suppl]:S72–S76.
67. Albright PS, Burnham WM. Development of a new pharmacological seizure model: effects of anticonvulsants on cortical- and amygdala-kindled seizures in the rat. *Epilepsia* 1980;21:681–689.
68. Adamec RE. Does kindling model anything clinically relevant? *Biol Psychiatry* 1990;27:249–279.
69. McIntyre DC, Molino A. Amygdala lesions and CER learning: long term effect of kindling. *Physiol Behav* 1972;8:1055–1058.
70. Boast CA, McIntyre DC. Bilateral kindled amygdala foci and inhibitory avoidance behavior in rats: a functional lesion effect. *Physiol Behav* 1977;8:25–28.
71. Rolls ET. *The brain and emotion.* Oxford: Oxford University Press, 1999.
72. Gibbs J, Maddison SP, Rolls ET. The satiety role of the small intestine in sham feeding rhesus monkeys. *J Comp Physiol Psychol* 1981;95:1003–1015.
73. Grossman SP. *A textbook of physiological psychology.* New York: Wiley, 1967.
74. Dube MG, Xu B, Kalra PS, et al. Disruption in neuropeptide Y and leptin signaling in obese ventromedial hypothalamic-lesioned rats. *Brain Res* 1999;816: 38–46.
75. Anand BK, Brobeck JR. Localization of a feeding center in the hypothalamus of the rat. *Proc Soc Exp Biol Med* 1951;77:323–324.
76. Rolls ET, Burton MJ, Mora F. Hypothalamic neuronal responses associate with the sight of food. *Brain Res* 1976;111:53–66.
77. Olds J. The central nervous system and the reinforcement of behavior. *Am Psychol* 1969;24:114–132.
78. Olds J. *Drives and reinforcements: behavioral studies of hypothalamic functions.* New York: Raven Press, 1977.
79. Rolls ET, Burton MJ, Mora F. Neurophysiological analysis of brain stimulation reward in the monkey. *Brain Res* 1980;164:121–135.
80. Rolls ET, Francis S, Bowtell R, et al. Pleasant touch activates the orbitofrontal cortex. *Neuroimage* 1997;5:S17.
81. Lambert MV, Robertson MM. Depression in epilepsy: etiology, phenomenology, and treatment. *Epilepsia* 1999;40[Suppl 10]:S21–S47.
82. Devinsky O, Vasquez B. Behavioral changes associated with epilepsy. *Neurol Clin* 1993;11:127–149.
83. Seligman ME, Beagley G. Learned helplessness in the rat. *J Comp Physiol Psychol* 1975;88:534–541.
84. Klein DC, Seligman ME. Reversal of performance deficits and perceptual deficits in learned helplessness and depression. *J Abnorm Psychol* 1976;85:11–26.
85. Young PA, Young PH. *Basic clinical neuroanatomy.* Baltimore: Williams & Wilkins, 1997:180.
86. Richardson JS. Animal models of depression reflect changing views on the essence and etiology of depressive disorders in humans. *Prog Neuropsychopharmacol Biol Psychiatry* 1991;15:199–204.
87. Jesberger JA, Richardson JS. Brain output dysregulation induced by olfactory bulbectomy: an approximation in the rate of major depressive disorder in humans. *Intern J Neuroscience* 1988;38:241–265.
88. Klüver H, Bucy PC. Preliminary analysis of functions of the temporal lobes in monkeys. *Arch Neurol Psychiatry* 1939;42:979–1000.
89. Weizkrantz L. Behavioral changes associated with ablation of the amygdaloid complex in monkeys. *J Comp Physiol Psychol* 1956;49:381–391.
90. Rolls ET. Functions of the primate hippocampus in spatial processing and memory. In: Olton DS, Kesner RP, eds. *Neurobiology of comparative cognition.* Hillsdale, NJ: Earlbaum, 1990:339–362.
91. Rolls ET. Neurophysiological mechanisms underlying face processing within and beyond the temporal cortical visual areas. *Phil Trans R Soc* 1992;335:11–21.
92. Marlow WB, Mancall EL, Thomas JJ. Complete Kluver-Bucy syndrome in man. *Cortex* 1975;11:53–59.
93. Tonsgard JH, Harwicke N, Levine SC. Kluver-Bucy syndrome in children. *Pediatr Neurol* 1987;3: 162–165.
94. Everitt BJ, Robbins TW. Amygdala-ventral striatal interaction and reward related processes. In: Aggleton JP, ed. *The amygdala.* Chichester: Wiley, 1992: 401–429.
95. Phillips RG, LeDoux JE. Differential contribution of amygdala and hippocampus to cued and contextual fear conditioning. *Behav Neurosci* 1992;106:274–285.
96. Davis M. Anatomic and physiologic substrates of emotion and anxiety in an animal model. *J Clin Neurophysiol* 1998;15:378–387.
97. Miserendino MJ, Sananes CB, Mekia KR, et al. Blocking of acquisition, but not expression of conditioned fear-potentiated startle by NMDA antagonists in the amygdala. *Nature* 1990;345:716–718.
98. Adamec RE. Kindling and species-characteristic behavior. In: Morrell F, ed. *Kindling and synaptic plasticity.* Boston: Birkhauser, 1991:226–238.
99. Lidsky TI, Levine MS, Kreinick CK, et al. Retrograde effects of amygdaloid stimulation on conditioned suppression (CER) in rats. *J Comp Physiol Psychol* 1970;73:135–149.
100. Hoeppner TJ, Smith MC, deToledo-Morrell L, et al. Amygdala kindling and fear conditioning. *Neurosci Abstr* 1996;22:1117.
101. Hoeppner TJ, Smith MC, deToledo-Morrell L, et al. The effects of amygdala kindling on fear conditioning. 2000 (*in preparation*).
102. Hoeppner TJ, Smith MC, Reimschisel TE, et al. The effects of amygdala kindling on fear conditioning in valproate treated rats. *Epilepsia* 1996;37[Suppl 5]:46.

19

The Social Impact of Epilepsy

Keeping Our Patients "In the Closet"

Antonio Gil-Nagel and *Pilar Garcia-Damberre

*Department of Neurology, Hospital Ruber Internacional, Madrid, Spain 28034; and *Department of Psychiatry, Hospital de la Princesa, Madrid, Spain 28006*

Epilepsy is a disorder with biologic and functional consequences that impact on different areas of social adaptation. Seizures and the postictal phase impose restrictions on the performance of different activities, because transient cognitive impairment, loss of motor control, and loss of sensory input are potential risks of accidents and injuries. Social restrictions of seizures are not limited to the actual events; the mere possibility of their occurrence induces patients and their families to limit their social activities, which in turn may foster isolation and interfere with the establishment of long-lasting relations and employment. The cognitive problems associated with the epileptic syndrome, underlying pathology, and antiepileptic drugs decrease skills and the ability to cope with their disease. Anxiety, depression, poor self-esteem, and other psychiatric problems follow both biologic derangement and poor social adaptation. The impact of epilepsy on social functioning has been explored through different types of studies. Studies using quality-of-life questionnaires show poor health-related quality of life in children, adolescents, and adults with epilepsy. Community-based longitudinal studies indicate that poor social adaptation is common among patients with epilepsy. In studies based on patients' reports, specific difficulties in different aspects of their social life usually are encountered. In this chapter, we illustrate with specific examples the different ways in which seizures can impact on daily social activities and the resulting difficulties that clearly interfere with these patients' quality of life.

APPRAISAL OF THE EXTENT OF THE PROBLEM

Several lines of evidence indicate that, as in other chronic disorders, problems related to epilepsy extend beyond the symptoms of the disease itself. In many ways, the impact of epilepsy on social functions differs from that of other chronic disorders. For example, it is not unusual for people who are not familiarized with the disease to misinterpret the various clinical expressions of complex partial seizures as psychological problems. In so doing, patients are conveyed the message that they have control over their ictal behavior. Historically, epilepsy has been subject to various degrees of stigma. Unfortunately, this problem is not relegated to the past. It persists to date in many cultures, including those of industrialized societies, and leads patients to avoid reporting their disease. Data on the social impact of epilepsy have been derived from various instruments completed by patients and/or family members (i.e., quality-of-life questionnaire) in population-based and small cohort studies.

Quality-of-Life Measures

Health-related quality of life in epilepsy refers to physical health as well as mental and social health. Questionnaires usually provide information about social functioning, mostly focusing on work, fear about having a seizure, general social adaptation, and driving (1,2). These studies showed an improvement in health-related quality of life after successful medical and surgical treatment (3,4). Most studies in quality of life in epilepsy have used the Quality of Life in Epilepsy Inventory (QOLIE) (5,6). This scale has been validated in other languages (7,8) and is instrumental in the evaluation of antiepileptic drug trials and the efficacy of epilepsy surgery. Studies with QOLIE have identified risk factors for poor health-related quality of life. Seizure severity and neurotoxicity are among the most important factors among the different age groups, but other variables related to social integration, such as lower socioeconomic status, need for special education classes, and frequent hospitalizations, were found to have a negative correlation with quality of life (9). An in-depth discussion on quality of life in epilepsy can be found in Chapter 21.

Community-Based Longitudinal Studies

In a large prospective comparative study of 245 children with epilepsy followed over 30 years, a diagnosis of epilepsy was associated with a more than two-fold increase of early school abandonment and more than three-fold increase in unemployment, failure to marry, and having children (10). These outcomes were unrelated to neuropsychological function. The results of this study support the general impression of epilepsy caregivers but are contrary to the findings of a previous study that failed to find any differences in education and professional achievement of patients followed for more than 30 years, except when epilepsy was associated with overt central nervous system pathology (11). A study performed in Massachusetts showed that 65% of patients with epilepsy considered themselves negatively affected by their disease, including

patients with fewer than one seizure per year (12). In a survey carried out with members of the Epilepsy Foundation of America, frequent concerns were voiced with respect to health, financial situation, employability, and marriage (13). In addition, some studies found that approximately 50% of children with epilepsy have behavior problems (14,15), suffer from social isolation, and have low self-esteem at higher rates than children with other learning disabilities (16–18). In another study from Finland, approximately 7% of respondents to a questionnaire reported significant dissatisfaction with their life that was associated with lower income and a poor economic status but was independent of the degree of control of their epilepsy (19). This result suggests that the social adjustment of people with epilepsy does not always parallel improvements in seizure control.

Patients' Reports

Fear and shame about their disease are common among people with chronic disorders such as asthma, diabetes, and epilepsy and result in "self perceived stigmatization" (20). In the case of epilepsy, this has resulted in the failure of many patients to disclose their condition to family members, friends, and employers (21). This reluctance to openly disclose their seizure disorder frequently has been based on well-founded concerns. For example, approximately 18% of people with epilepsy who told their employer about their disorder reported subsequent job problems that impaired their careers. For these reasons, vague terms, such as dizzy spells, fainting, amnesia, or attack, often are used by patients and physicians to mask the diagnosis. Physicians in Spain often use other terms, such as "comicial," to refer to epileptic seizures and avoid the word epilepsy. This term is based on the seizures that ancient Greeks had during their congress. In a report of 160 patients from a neurology clinic in Australia, 44% reported their career had been limited, 39% thought their schooling had been reduced, and 58% complained that their social life was restricted because of epilepsy (22). The problems seem to be similar in Europe, where a large analysis of stigma using self-completed questionnaires showed that 51% felt stigmatized, with 18% feeling "highly stigmatized" (23). The latter study was conducted during the last few years and indicates that negative social impact of epilepsy is still a major problem. According to some studies, "enacted stigma," which is the negative impression that individuals in society may feel about epilepsy, may not be as important in social adaptation as "felt stigma," the negative feeling that patients believe their disease causes in other people (13). Even if this is the case, both types of stigma are highly interrelated; the development of self-stigma is, in part, proportional to the negative experiences that people with epilepsy have encountered through their life—that is, in those situations where enacted stigma has been noticed. Trostle (24) suggested that fear of exposure should not be considered legitimate, even when it does not follow specific acts of discrimination.

Much is known about the limitations imposed by seizures on certain activities and social events that carry a risk of physical trauma (i.e., driving) (25). Less information is available on the effect of seizures during other social situations that are not necessarily associated with physical risks, but nevertheless can negatively impact on the life of the patient and others without the occurrence of physical harm. These may take place when seizures occur in any setting, i.e., during personal, professional, and recreational activities. We evaluated the impact of seizures on patients' social and work functions in a retrospective study of 100 consecutive epileptic patients seen at Programa de Epilepsia during 1998. During the first clinic visit, all patients underwent a semistructured interview, during which they were asked to report if they had experienced one or more seizures that caused some type of social or work-related problem in their life or the life of other people. Children and patients with mental retardation were excluded. A total of 14 patients reported having experienced 15 seizures that caused social and professional difficulties (Table 19.1). Nine events were caused by complex partial seizures, three were simple partial, and three generalized tonic-clonic. We investi-

TABLE 19.1. *Patients who had seizures during performance of their profession or while engaged in social events and the consequence in their life*

Profession or social activity	Moment of occurrence	Seizure type and semiology	Consequence
Student	Written examination	CP with prolonged amnesia	Failed the examination
Student	Written examination	CP with short amnesia	Low score on the examination
Office clerk	Work hours at the office	CP with wandering	Reprimanded
Office clerk	Work hours at the office	CP with wandering	Reprimanded
Bank officer	Carrying bank documentation	CP with wandering	Lost documents
Lawyer	Deposition	SP with aphasia	Worsened performance
Lawyer	Trial	CP with amnesia	Trial ended before he could give his speech
Artist	Television interview	SP with aphasia	Interview was postponed
Physician	Attending a conference	CP with secondary generalization	Talk was interrupted
Audience	Professional Tennis Association match	CP with secondary generalization	Game was interrupted
Squash player	Tournament	CP with amnesia	Lost game
Squash player	Tournament	SP	Lost ball
Fiancée	Being introduced to future father-in-law	Cluster of CP with brief impairment of consciousness	Cancellation of wedding
Pharmacy clerk	Attending clients at pharmacy	GTC	Lost his job
Olive oil auctioneer	Discussing price of oil	CP	Moved to a lower responsibility position

CP, complex partial; GTC, generalized tonic-clonic; SP, simple partial.

gated whether or not the consequences of these seizures could have been avoided if adequate measures had been in place.

Case Presentations

A. Two high school students reported having complex partial seizures during written examinations, and their peers and teachers did not identify their seizures. The consequences (a low score in one case and failure of the examination in the other) could have been avoided if the teachers had been informed about the students' seizure disorder and the students had been allowed to have extra time or to repeat the examination at a different date. Epilepsy centers often provide school talks directed at informing teachers and children about seizures. These talks commonly are given at elementary and middle school levels, but usually are neglected at high school and college levels, where the problem of epilepsy still is relevant.

B. Two office clerks were reprimanded at work by their supervisors. The first clerk was reprimanded for wandering out of the office for a prolonged time period on one occasion and for suddenly walking away from his desk while working with a client. Both situations took place during a complex partial seizure. The second office clerk who worked at a bank lost documentation when he had a seizure in the street on his way to a meeting. In both cases, a medical report from the clinic was useful in clarifying the events and avoiding further disciplinary action against the patients. However, it would have been better if the patients' supervisors had been informed in advance about the workers' seizure disorder, something both had avoided because they perceived this could put their job in jeopardy. One year later, one of these two patients was still working in the same office, but in a different position doing archival work. The office clerk had an early retirement because of his epilepsy.

C. Two lawyers reported having seizures during a trial. In one case, the lawyer performed poorly, but the verdict apparently was not affected by the consequences of the seizure. The second lawyer had a complex partial seizure while delivering his closing statement. He suddenly stopped talking, which the judge interpreted as the conclusion of his remarks. The judge then dictated his verdict before the lawyer was able to complete his presentation in support of the defendant. This case could have had dire consequences had the judge dictated a verdict against his client. Imposing professional restrictions does not seem to be a fair solution, because in these two cases the lawyers were perfectly fitted for their job and performed it successfully. However, designating time for education about epilepsy and other disorders in the workplace, including the courts, may be necessary to help with the integration of people with epilepsy.

D. An artist had a seizure during a recorded television interview. This did not have any consequences, because the interviewer noticed that something was wrong and repeated the recording a few minutes later. Nevertheless, in this scenario, a letter explaining the disease could have been useful if the understanding of the interviewer had not been adequate.

E. Two nonprofessional sports players had seizures during a tournament, each one during a different game. One had a simple partial seizure that had no impact on the final score of the match, but was worrisome enough to stop him from competing because of his concern about having more severe seizures in public. The other sportsman had a complex partial seizure that originated from the temporal lobe of the nondominant hemisphere. This patient also stopped competing and is now a squash trainer. He chose to tell his employer and trainees about his seizure disorder.

F. Two patients with focal epilepsy had secondarily generalized tonic-clonic seizures, one while attending a medical conference and the other while attending a tennis match. In both cases, the events had to be interrupted for a few minutes. Both patients became very concerned of the consequences, expressed shame while relating the event at the clinic, and went through a period of increased social isolation. Fortunately, in both cases, complete seizure control eventually was achieved, which led to increased self-esteem and better social integration.

As other studies have shown, these patients tried to avoid discrimination at work and at school by concealing their disease. These cases show that information about epilepsy among co-workers, clients, teachers, and students may reduce the negative impact of seizures that occur at work and during classes. But the implications of disclosure are complex and cannot always be predicted. Some employers may discriminate against people with epilepsy, and some clients may be lost if patients disclose their disease. Disclosing one's seizure disorder may be easier in certain workplaces, such as a sport center, than in others, such as a law firm. The consequences of seizures in this environment of occultation of disease have a negative impact not only on the patients themselves, but also on other people (such as a defendant during a trial in one case). This is a powerful reason to promote knowledge about epilepsy in society.

SOCIAL INTERVENTION

Coming Out of the Closet

In the last decade, many epilepsy centers and associations have placed great importance on ensuring that patients and their families are well informed about their disease. This marks a large shift in efforts to promote the spread of education about epilepsy. In a survey carried out by the Commission for the Control of Epilepsy and Its Consequences of the International League Against Epilepsy (ILAE) in 1978, education was found to be very scarce (26). Education is best achieved through a combination of brochures, specific programs, support groups, and direct information given in the clinic (27,28). There are several areas that should be systematically included in patient education programs: diagnosis of epilepsy, medication, medical follow-up, lifestyle, informing family and friends, preparation for

school or college, marriage, application for work, and information at the workplace. Severe and frequent seizures, additional neurologic deficits, previous academic failure, comorbidity, and lack of family support are conditions associated with higher social dysfunction. Nevertheless, several large prospective studies showed that the negative effect of epilepsy in social adaptation can occur in all patients, including those with mild forms of epilepsy. Therefore, at least some type of social intervention should be provided early to all patients. A detailed discussion on these issues can be found in Chapter 20.

Providing Information on Epilepsy at the Workplace

It is in the patient's best interest for someone at the workplace to know about his or her disease and the characteristics of the seizures. When seizures occur at work, this person may be of help in explaining the problem to other workers and deciding whether or not to call the paramedics for transport to the emergency room. Choosing the right person to inform may be somewhat tricky. The ideal candidate should be another worker who spends considerable time with the patient, occupies a relevant position, understands the disease, and is capable of confronting the medical and labor implications of a seizure.

Informing Friends

Patients should be able to disclose their seizure disorder to their friends, without fearing that they would frighten and alienate them. This is particularly important among adolescents. In this age group, it is helpful if one or more responsible friends can be educated on what to do in case of a seizure and on when to transfer patients to the emergency room. This education is best accomplished during a visit to the epilepsy clinic.

Information at the School

A diagnosis of epilepsy in a child requires education of teachers and schoolmates. This usually is best accomplished through general talks, given at every school, so that when a child is diagnosed with the disorder, the staff is well prepared to help the child in case of seizures and prevent schoolmates from being unnecessarily frightened if they witness a seizure. However, in most instances this usually is not done in a proactive manner; talks are provided after the child suffers from a seizure in school. We suggest that a separate talk be planned for teachers and students. Teachers should be informed specifically of the type of seizures, medication, side effects, neuropsychological performance, and what to do in case of seizures. For classmates, it is better to provide a general talk about epilepsy, emphasizing the likelihood of having a normal life and not revealing the identity of the sick child.

CONCLUSIONS

The impact of epilepsy on patients extends well beyond the medical consequences of the disease. Epilepsy affects all aspects of life. The effect on social functioning is important and does not necessarily have the same prognosis as the epilepsy itself. Epilepsy centers should be proactive in providing adequate services and counseling to reduce the impact of epilepsy on social function. These services should be available to all patients and not only those with medically refractory seizures.

ACKNOWLEDGMENTS

Supported by Consejería de Servicios Sociales, Comunidad de Madrid, and a grant from Obra Social Caja, Madrid, Spain.

REFERENCES

1. Roper Organization. *Living with epilepsy: report of a Roper poll of patients on quality of life.* New York: Carter-Wallace, 1992.
2. Taylor DC, Falconer MA. Clinical, socio-economic, and psychological changes after temporal lobectomy for epilepsy. *Br J Psychiatry* 1968;114:1247–1261.
3. Vickrey BG, Hays RD, Graber J, et al. A health-related quality of life instrument for patients evaluated for epilepsy surgery. *Med Care* 1992;39:299–319.
4. Vickrey BG, Hays RD, Rausch R, et al. Outcomes in 248 patients who had diagnostic evaluations for epilepsy surgery. *Lancet* 1995;346:1445–1449.
5. Devinsky O, Vickrey B, Hays R, et al. Quality of life in epilepsy: QOLIE-89 instrument development. *Neurology* 1994;44[Suppl 2]:A141.
6. Meador KJ. Research use of the new quality-of-life in epilepsy inventory. *Epilepsia* 1993;34[Suppl 4]:S34–S38.
7. Torres X, Arroyo S, Araya S, et al. The Spanish version of the Quality-of-life in Epilepsy Inventory (QOLIE-31): translation, validity, and reliability. *Epilepsia* 1999; 40:1299–1304.
8. Stavem K, Bjornaes H, Lossius MI. Reliability and validity of a Norwegian version of the quality of life in epilepsy inventory (QOLIE-89). *Epilepsia* 2000;41: 91–97.
9. Devinsky O, Westbrook L, Cramer J, et al. Risk factors for poor health-related quality of life in adolescents with epilepsy. *Epilepsia* 1999;40:1715–1720.
10. Sillanpaa M, Jalava M, Kaleva D, et al. Long-term prognosis of seizures with onset in childhood. *N Engl J Med* 1998;338:1715–1722.
11. Britten N, Wadsworth M, Fenwick P. Sources of stigma following early-life epilepsy: evidence from a national birth cohort study. In: Whitman S, Hermann BP, eds. *Psychopathology in epilepsy.* New York: Oxford University Press, 1986:228–244.
12. Schacter SC, Shafer PO, Murphy W. The personal impact of seizures: correlations with seizure frequency, employment, cost of medical care, and satisfaction with physician care. *J Epilepsy* 1993;6:224–227.
13. Collings JA. Life fulfillment in an epilepsy sample from the United States. *Soc Sci Med* 1995;40:1579–1584.
14. Austin JK, Risinger MW, Beckett LA. Correlates of behavior problems in children with epilepsy. *Epilepsia* 1992;33:1115–1122.
15. Hoare P, Kerley S. Psychosocial adjustment of children with chronic epilepsy and their families. *Dev Med Child Neurol* 1991;33:201–215.
16. Austin JK, Smith MS, Risinger MW, et al. Childhood epilepsy and asthma: comparison of quality of life. *Epilepsia* 1994;35:608–615.
17. Margalit M, Heiman T. Anxiety and self-dissatisfaction in epileptic children. *Int J Soc Psychiatry* 1983;29: 220–224.
18. Matthews WS, Barabas G, Ferrari M. Emotional concomitants of childhood epilepsy. *Epilepsia* 1982;23: 671–681.
19. Sillanpaa M. Social adjustment and functioning of chronically ill and impaired children and adolescents. *Acta Paediatr Scand* 1987;340[Suppl]:1–70.
20. Scambler G, Hopkins A. Being epileptic: coming to terms with stigma. *Soc Health Illness* 1986;8:26–43.
21. Jacoby A. Felt versus enacted stigma: a concept revisited. *Soc Sci Med* 1994;38:269–274.
22. Edwards VE. Social problems confronting a person with epilepsy in modern society. *Proc Aust Assoc Neurol* 1974;11:239–243.
23. Baker GA, Brooks J, Buck D, et al. The stigma of epilepsy: a European perspective. *Epilepsia* 2000;41: 98–104.
24. Trostle JA. Social aspects: stigma, beliefs and measurement. In: Engel J Jr, Pedley TA, eds. *Epilepsy: a comprehensive textbook.* Philadelphia: Lippincott-Raven Publishers, 1997:2183–2189.

25. Hansotia P, Broste SK. The effect of epilepsy or diabetes mellitus on the risk of automobile accidents. *N Engl J Med* 1991;324:22–26.

26. Commission for the Control of Epilepsy and Its Consequences. Plan of nationwide action on epilepsy. Rockville, MD: US Department of Health, Education and Welfare, National Institutes of Health; 1977, Volume I, publication no. 78-276.

27. Austin JK, deBoer HM. Disruptions in social functioning and services facilitating adjustment for the child and adult. In: Engel J Jr, Pedley TA, eds. *Epilepsy: a comprehensive textbook.* Philadelphia: Lippincott-Raven Publishers, 1997:2191–2201.

28. Buck D, Jacoby A, Baker GA, et al. Patients' experiences of and satisfaction with care for their epilepsy. *Epilepsia* 1996;37:841–849.

20

Social Services in Epilepsy

Patricia A. Gibson

Department of Neurology, Wake Forest University, Winston Salem, North Carolina 27157

It has long been recognized that the social, psychological, and behavioral problems that frequently accompany epilepsy can be more handicapping than the actual seizures (1). The comprehensive care of those with epilepsy must include, in addition to medical evaluation and treatment, an assessment of the social needs and concerns of the patient. As Dr. David Taylor, a neuropsychiatrist in Wales, pointed out some time ago, people suffering from epilepsy are in a particular "predicament." How any given predicament is being experienced depends on the history of that person in the world. This history of a person becomes a crucial aspect of diagnosis that is different from the history of the disorder (2). It is the role of the social worker to gather that history and to assure that the whole picture is considered in the treatment and management of epilepsy.

The first national effort to promote comprehensive care of those with epilepsy originated in the 1970s under the direction of Dr. J. Kiffin Penry, then director of the Epilepsy Branch of the National Institutes of Neurological, Communicative Disorders and Stroke. Through the efforts of Dr. Penry and others, National Institutes of Health program project grants were awarded in 1976 to develop three model "Comprehensive Epilepsy Programs," with three additional centers funded a few years later. At its inception, "comprehensive" referred to providing multidisciplinary personnel. Dr. Penry and his colleague, Dr. Fritz Dreifuss, director of one of the first compre-

hensive programs located at the University of Virginia, recognized that the "good physician must know the whole patient" (3). They insisted that a variety of disciplines were needed to assist in the comprehensive care of epilepsy. In these days of managed health care with pressure on physicians to see more and more patients in shorter and shorter periods of time, the assistance of other health professionals is even more important in patient management.

Since the beginnings of these model programs, "comprehensive" has been expanded to include all contemporary diagnostic abilities as well as all available current treatments for epilepsy, including experimental therapies. The infrastructure of these programs also provides an opportunity for research into the basic mechanisms of epilepsy, as well as the social issues, in an effort to develop better treatments for the epilepsies.

HISTORY OF SOCIAL WORK IN MEDICINE

Dr. Richard Cabot first introduced medical social services at Boston's Massachusetts General Hospital in 1905 to contribute to the development of preventive medicine. Dr. Cabot recognized the importance of continuity of care and, therefore, included social workers as home visitors in his clinic. Ida Cannon was hired as the first medical social worker. Social work provided an enlarged understanding of psychosocial conditions that could have an impact on medical conditions (4). Social work is a diverse profession with fluid boundaries. There is much greater understanding of what physicians, nurses, lawyers, and psychologists do than is the case with social workers. According to Gibelman (5), this phenomena results partly from the expansive and expanding boundaries of social work and the difficulty of providing succinct, encapsulated descriptions of a complex and multifaceted profession. At the present time, the field of mental health is the fastest growing area of social work practice. As with other professionals, managed care holds the potential of limiting the role of social workers as well as the quality and quantity of services available to the clients in need of social services.

ROLE OF SOCIAL WORK IN EPILEPSY

In 1997, a task force for the International Professionals in Epilepsy Care conducted a worldwide survey of those providing social services in the field of epilepsy (6). It was found that social workers in the United States have widely varied roles in the treatment of epilepsy. Social workers were found providing patient education and individual, group, and family counseling; coordinating epilepsy monitoring units; monitoring drug studies; administering a variety of programs and services in epilepsy; advocating for patients and their families; and holding educational and research positions. Thus, the role changes from setting to setting. Social workers usually are found in most hospital settings in the United States. They may or may not be specifically assigned to provide services to the epilepsy population. Except in special centers of excellence, most cover many population areas and do not have special expertise in epilepsy. Much of their assistance is directed toward exploring financial assistance or discharge planning for patients.

Although the role of social workers in epilepsy varies greatly, the following are some of the most common areas in which social services are provided.

PATIENT EDUCATION

Patient education is crucial in the treatment of epilepsy. Patients often are ill informed about epilepsy and may harbor a variety of fears and concerns (7,8). Provision of a wide range of information in a systematic format has been shown to benefit patients in a number of ways (9). This education should start at the time of diagnosis, be carried out on an ongoing basis, and involve all members of the treatment team.

Communicating well is not always easy, and it is important to evaluate on a regular basis the patient's understanding of his or her condition and the medical instructions. Effective patient education involves the whole family and any other individuals involved in the care of the patient. Information needs to be given on the level of the patient. For many patients, interacting with their physician can be an intimidating experience, and some patients are hesitant to acknowledge that they do not understand what is being said. The social worker can be very helpful as an intermediary in this communication.

In providing education, written materials are as important as verbal information. Windsor et al. (10) found that people could recall and apply 40% of what they heard and 70% of what they saw. There are a number of sources for educational materials on epilepsy. The Epilepsy Foundation has a listing of materials available through their organization. A number of comprehensive epilepsy centers have designed their own educational materials, such as the Seizureman comic book on first aid for children developed by the social workers at the Wake Forest University Comprehensive Epilepsy Center in North Carolina. Many pharmaceutical companies that market antiepilepsy medications also offer free educational materials on epilepsy. Computer resources are being increasing utilized by persons with epilepsy and their families as a source of information.

PREVENTIVE COUNSELING

Preventive counseling carries patient education a step further and is an important part of the social care of epilepsy. This counseling should begin shortly after diagnosis and involve the patient, family members, and any other individuals involved in the care of the patient. Patients and family members need to ventilate their fears, worries, and concerns. Observing a seizure, especially a tonic-clonic seizure, in a loved one can be one of the most frightening moments a person may have. Dr. David Taylor (11) refers to this event as a "pseudo-death," one that evokes a sense of menace and threatens the onlooker's capacity to cope. Ask a loved one about this experience and observe how deeply etched this moment is in his or her memory. Expressing these concerns is a beginning step in the process of dealing effectively with the psychosocial impact of epilepsy. Listening without interruption to the patient and family's feelings and description of the event is extremely important. In their study of the patient–doctor relationship, Beckman and Frankel (12) found that, in interviews with their doctors, patients were most often redirected after the first expressed concern and after a mean time of only 18 seconds. Additionally, in only one in 52 visits did these redirected patients return to their agenda and complete their offering of concerns. It is important to solicit the patient's concerns and worries and to listen fully to their responses. Studies have shown that doing so actually takes less time than expected and can improve interview efficiency and yield increased data (13). Carl Rogers pointed out a number of years ago that "We think we listen, but very rarely do we listen with real understanding, true empathy. Yet listening of this very special kind, is one of the most potent forces for change that I know."

The social worker early on helps the patient and family deal with irrational fears and crushed ambitions, as well as other worries. During this early stage, groundwork can be laid to help parents realize the important role their attitude toward epilepsy plays in influencing how the child will begin to feel about himself or herself. Parents need to understand how overprotecting can lead to emotional crippling. The disabling potential of epilepsy depends heavily on the manner in which the family adjusts to the disorder and is able to help the child cope with the issues that are a part of epilepsy. Early intervention with counseling by the social worker can help prevent many of the social problems that frequently accompany the diagnosis of epilepsy.

CASE MANAGEMENT

Case management involves the coordination of services from different agencies on behalf of a client. Social workers often are involved as case managers for epileptic patients, especially those patients who have other disabilities and are unable to function independently. Needs are assessed, and follow-up involves planning, locating resources, and monitoring services. A variety of interventions may be required, and the social worker may take on an advocacy role when needed services are not available. An example of case management of a client follows.

J.H. was referred to the social worker by the pediatric neurologist who had recently seen him as a new patient. He was 16 years old and had moved to live with his grandparents a month ago. He had severe and intractable seizures, mental retardation, and cerebral palsy. His mother had left him and his father in his early years. The father eventually remarried, but recently died of a heart attack at age 38. His wife did not want the responsibility of the child, who was not hers. The grandparents were in total shock over these events and lacked any knowledge of resources. The social worker assisted in making application for Medicaid and other services. Arrangements were made for him to be seen by the vocational rehabilitation specialist in an effort to develop future rehabilitation plans. Following this assessment, an application was made to the Special Enrichment Center, where he could learn social and daily living skills, as well as employment skills. It also functions as a sheltered workshop. J.H. entered this program at age 18 and made good progress, although his seizures were still uncontrolled. Unfortunately, 2 years later, the grandfather suddenly died of a heart attack, and the grandmother had difficulty physically managing J.H. because of his sudden falls. The social worker began working with the client and grandmother to help locate an appropriate group home situation and to work with the family in their adjustment to this new living arrangement. A group home was located, and the patient was able to continue attending the Special Enrichment Center. The patient adjusted well to the group home, but after the first year, due to administrative changes in the group home management, the family was informed that the client would have to move to a home with lower functioning clients. The social worker became involved again, this time in an advocacy role, and petitioned the Division of Mental Health to intercede. Eventually the patient was allowed to stay in the more appropriate setting.

INDIVIDUAL COUNSELING

A chronic illness of any type has significant impact on the lives of the people it touches. There are many social and psychological consequences when people do not cope well. For some, epilepsy may be looked upon as a minor inconvenience. They have a few seizures and are prescribed medicine; their seizures come under control and do not interfere with functioning. Others are not so lucky. For this group, epilepsy is a devastating diagnosis and looms large, coloring every aspect of their being. There are various emotional responses to any illness or disorder. Although not everyone with epilepsy needs counseling, on occasion the emotional responses may be maladaptive and require intervention. The major problems that a person with epilepsy faces are functions of a number of factors. The age at onset, severity of the disorder, how the patient/family system copes or responds to the seizures, and the quality of the interactions are among the many systems with which the patient and family must deal (14). When problems begin to interfere with the client's functioning or quality of life, then individual counseling may be needed.

Patients with intractable epilepsy are particularly vulnerable to a number of secondary psychosocial problems, including depression and anxiety (15). In addition, low self-esteem and a feeling of loss of control over their lives are common features of children and adults with epilepsy.

When epilepsy is severe and persistent, it is not surprising that it will be associated with behavioral and cognitive disorder, as social behaviors are every bit as dependent on adequate cerebral functioning as is cognition.

The following case is an example of counseling provided by a social worker.

S.M. is a 35-year-old woman who was referred to the epilepsy social worker by a neurologist following the patient's request for disability status. She had approximately one or two partial seizures a month that occasionally generalized to tonic-clonic seizures. She worked in a factory doing work that involved heavy lifting. She had dropped out of school in the tenth grade to get married. Her husband, who could not read or write, also worked at the factory. They had two young children. When first seen, the patient's hair was cut short in a mannish fashion, and she wore no make-up. Her affect was flattened. In assessing the patient's condition, it was learned that, in addition to uncontrolled seizures, she was having mood swings, irritability, and depression. She did not enjoy her job, but the family badly needed the additional income. She was ashamed of having epilepsy and had very poor self-esteem. Her husband was uncomfortable in social situations, and they never went out to eat or to visit except with close relatives. The first step in the patient's assessment was to evaluate her medicine, primidone, an anticonvulsant well known to have side effects of the symptoms she described. Following discussion with her doctor, it was decided to replace her medicine with carbamazepine and to follow her for individual counseling. After a few seizures associated with withdrawal from primidone, the patient became seizure-free for the first time in a number of years. She responded extremely well to supportive counseling. It was learned that she came from a large family and that, shortly after her birth, her mother had been hospitalized in a state psychiatric institution with what sounded like severe postpartum depression and later died there. Her older sisters reared the patient. When the patient started maturing, her father began making inappropriate advances toward her. She begged an older sister to let her live with her. Unfortunately, the newly wed couple was struggling financially, and her presence caused a lot of tension. The patient admitted marrying to escape her unhappy situation. She had never discussed her childhood pain with anyone, and the relief in the ventilation of pent-up feelings was apparent. Her physical appearance started to change. She came to counseling wearing dresses and make-up and a new hair style. When asked about her dreams, the patient confided that she had always wanted to have an "office" job. She was encouraged to consider getting her general equivalency diploma (GED) through a special program. She talked a friend into going with her and surprised herself by making the top grade in the class. She was encouraged to continue her schooling, and a referral was made to the Division of Vocational Rehabilitation. This agency sponsored her attendance at the local community college, where she received an associate degree in nursing. The patient has been employed for a number of years now at the local health department. Today she is a strong, outspoken advocate for those with epilepsy.

In reviewing the referrals made to the social worker at the Wake Forest University School of Medicine's Comprehensive Epilepsy Center for individual counseling, two key problems stand out in many of the patients: a sense of shame and low self-esteem. It is important for all professionals to remember that communicating a sense of possibility and respect, whether by tone of voice, facial expression, or choice of words, often can make a tremendous difference in working with the patient with epilepsy and his or her family.

GROUP COUNSELING

Group counseling can be a very effective treatment modality for those with epilepsy and their families. It was not until after World War II that group work moved solidly into rehabilitation settings. The big push for group work came from the thousands of soldiers and veterans who needed assistance for physical and emotional problems. In this era of cost cutting and managed care, it is generally recognized that group services are more cost effective than individual interventions (16).

There has been an explosion of self-help groups in recent years. Many epilepsy organizations sponsor groups that offer an opportunity for persons with epilepsy and their families to meet others and to learn more about their disorder, as well as share coping skills and support of one another. These groups also may involve social outings. A number of the comprehensive epilepsy programs conduct more formal groups, in which the focus is on treatment of the individual through a group method. Unlike general self-help groups, the social worker or group leader controls the size and entry into the group. The groups may be specific to age or conditions, such as a teen support group or a group of mothers of babies with infantile spasms. Seizure surgery groups, prior to and following surgery, have been effective. Unfortunately, this is an area that has not been systematically studied. In his study of 107 patients who had undergone temporal lobectomy, Dr. Peter Bladin (17) of Australia stressed the serious need for a preoperative counseling program in an effort to prevent the psychosocial difficulties that often accompany epilepsy surgery.

FAMILY COUNSELING

The impact of having epilepsy can be significant medically, socially, psychologically, and financially (18). Epilepsy upsets the equilibrium of the family system and affects everyone in some way. When epilepsy develops in children, families may feel overwhelmed with the burden of the disorder. Family members of children with epilepsy often are forced into becoming case managers in a fragmented system that is confusing even to the seasoned health care professional. Marital problems, neglect of other siblings, a general breakdown of the family unit, and psychiatric disorders often emerge when early counseling, day care, and respite services are not provided. In a study of parents of children with epilepsy, Eastman et al. (19) found that the majority of parents who were questioned revealed high levels of stress, social isolation, and restrictions in leisure activities. The need for psychosocial intervention was stressed (19). When epilepsy develops in early childhood, much of the adjustment hinges on how the family adjusts to the disorder and then is able to help the young child cope with the ensuing issues and concerns. Certainly the severity of the seizure condition, presence of other handicapping conditions, and the social, emotional, and financial stability of the family are all important variables. How disruptive the family perceives the disorder to be, regardless of whether this perception is accurate, is a key factor in their reaction (18). How the family functions prior to the diagnosis is important in how it copes with this situation. The family's adjustment in turn has a profound impact on how the child reacts. If the parents have a healthy attitude toward epilepsy and encourage normal function, then the child can grow up with epilepsy in its proper place—just one part of what makes up that person.

Although the seizures are the most visible part of the disorder, it is usually the emotional and cognitive effects that devastate a child and his or her family. Epilepsy can affect the growing child's academic career and his or her relationship with family and peers. If not handled properly, it can destroy the child's self-esteem. According to Zeigler (20), the negative impact of epilepsy on a child's self-concept is one of the major long-term complications of childhood epilepsy. It is the family that manages the disorder and sets the stage for adjustment.

When the parent has epilepsy, the child's attitude and adjustment obviously is affected by the parents' attitude and self-acceptance. If there is little or no discussion of the problem, then the child will develop his or her own understanding of the disorder, perhaps feeling somehow to blame. What one can imagine almost always is worse than the reality of the situation. Not only must the child gather information from other sources, which may or may not be reliable, but explanations must be found as to why this is too terrible to discuss. According to Lechtenberg (21), the child is at the greatest disadvantage if he or she is told nothing about the parent's disorder. Parents with epilepsy who are "found out" are compromised in two respects. They are no longer viewed as physically reliable, and they lose their credibility (21). Issues of fear of abandonment, transfer of dependence, and fears

of developing epilepsy are to be explored in family counseling.

There are many emotional issues in the process of care, especially when the course is stormy and the outcome poor. The family unit rests at the core and heart of comprehensive services for the patient with epilepsy. Good care is contingent upon a working partnership between patient and professional that acknowledges both the needs and strengths of families. Family counseling can make a tremendous difference in supporting a healthy adjustment to this disorder.

COMMUNITY EDUCATION

Many social workers provide epilepsy education to the community through one-on-one situations, workshops, seminars, conferences, or symposia. A major thrust of the Comprehensive Epilepsy Center of Wake Forest University of North Carolina has been in the area of patient, family, public, and professional education. In an effort to reach as many people as possible, this center opened the Epilepsy Information Service, a nationwide, toll-free telephone line, in 1979. In an analysis of the first 100,000 calls to this line, approximately 70% of the callers have epilepsy or are close family members, with mothers being the most frequent callers. Four times as many women as men have sought information through this service.

When calls are received, information is recorded about the caller topics, type of seizure, and other demographic information. Approximately 2 weeks later, the caller receives a follow-up questionnaire inquiring about satisfaction with the service, as well as requesting additional demographic information about the caller. This information is entered into a computer.

From the calls received, much has been learned about the impact of epilepsy. Many of the callers with epilepsy were not getting proper medical attention. Some callers had not been properly diagnosed; some were taking the wrong medicines; and others were taking either too little or too much medicine.

Some of the callers were not following medical recommendations because they did not understand the importance of doing so. The Epilepsy Information Service is in a position to help many of the callers through proper education and referral to appropriate agencies.

What do callers want to know? Most often, callers request written materials. The Epilepsy Information Service makes available many brochures and other educational materials. The second most frequent topic is medication. Patients and their family members want to know about their medicines and possible side effects. They are much more sophisticated about medical matters than their parents were and are now able to gather a great deal of medical information from many sources, including the Internet. On occasion, the information gathered may not be accurate. The most common psychosocial concerns voiced by callers over the past 10 years are as follows.

Economic

From an economic standpoint, epilepsy is an expensive disorder to have. It is expensive to see a neurologist who specializes in epilepsy. The tests are expensive. Some patients report paying more than $700 per month for medicine. Much time is spent by social workers exploring resources for financial assistance for many patients with epilepsy. This problem is complicated by the difficulty many patients have obtaining insurance.

Insurance

More and more patients are having difficulty obtaining insurance. Many are unable to afford the premiums when they find a company that will accept them, or they must accept a rider that disallows coverage of their epilepsy. Many businesses are finding it more profitable to hire part-time workers to avoid paying benefits. Those who are under a managed care plan often find themselves unable to be seen by an epilepsy specialist or to have tests that are needed. Their plan may not cover the newer, more expensive medicines for epilepsy.

Driving

Without question, one of the most emotionally charged issues in the management of epilepsy is the area of driving. The social worker often finds himself or herself in the uncomfortable position of bearer of this bad news. There are many restrictions involved with life management of those with epilepsy, and this restriction has broad social and economic repercussions. To walk in with this news for a 40-year-old, long-distance truck driver—a man making an excellent salary who just purchased a nice home, has three children nearing college age, but who has only an ninth-grade education—the news that this seizure means the loss of his livelihood is devastating. For the adolescent, obtaining the driver's license is a rite of passage that denotes the first serious step into adulthood. Accurate information on state driving regulations needs to be relayed without delay to patients and their families and in an empathetic manner.

Employment

According to Lechtenberg (22), one of five adults with epilepsy believes the greatest problem he or she faces is securing and holding a job. We now have federal and often state legislation that prohibits discrimination. These laws make it illegal to inquire on employment applications as to whether or not the person has epilepsy. Although there have been many cases in which patients have been able to legally fight discrimination, there continues to be subtle and not so subtle discrimination against those who have epilepsy. At the same time, there are a small number of patients who are quick to claim discrimination when this is clearly not the case (*personal observation*). Some time ago, Ernst Rodin et al. (23) pointed out that it is not always the seizure frequency that is the problem; rather it is the intellectual level of the patient, his or her motivation, and the absence or presence of personality problems that more often are the problem.

School Problems

A number of children with epilepsy have subtle learning problems. Getting what they need from the school system is not always easy. The best way to help children with learning problems is to obtain a careful psychoeducational evaluation that pinpoints their strengths and weaknesses. Then an appropriate remedial teaching curriculum can be designed to meet their needs. Federal law PL94-142 was passed in 1975, which set forth the right of all handicapped children to receive a free, appropriate education in the least restrictive environment. The law provides funding authority for a variety of education services for children with disabilities, establishes a team approach to determining what services are most appropriate for an individual disabled child, and establishes due process safeguards to protect the educational rights of handicapped children and their parents (24). In July 1998, a law called the Individual with Disabilities Education Act (IDEA) became effective; this law strengthens the original legislation. More information about this can be found at the U.S. Department of Education's Web site *(www.ed.gov)*.

Independent Living

Persons with epilepsy whose seizures are not well controlled and who may have other associated handicaps often have a need for independent living situations. Many of these persons live with their parents, often socially isolated from their peers. As the parents begin to age, this becomes a pressing concern. Many communities are not equipped with appropriate facilities for this population. More advocacy is needed in this area.

Poor Self-Esteem and Social Isolation

There is no question that the onset of a disability brings about changes in persons' perceptions not only of themselves but of their environment. For the individual with seizures, early relationships and life experiences can either give him or her the courage to accept and

to overcome the handicap or instill in him or her a complex of fearful self-consciousness and inferiority and a self-image of a social outcast (25). These changes begin early. In her study of parent's behaviors following new-onset seizures, Joan Austin (26) reported that restriction of activities begins almost immediately and continues long after the seizures are controlled.

Fear of Death During a Seizure

One of the biggest and most immediate concerns of parents and persons with epilepsy, especially the newly diagnosed, is the fear of dying during a tonic-clonic seizure. Mittan (27) found that two-thirds of a group of 333 patients in his study thought they might die with their next seizure. In a survey of 1,000 patients nationwide, Fisher et al. (28) found fear to be the number one concern listed when inquiry was made about the worst thing about having epilepsy. This area of concern needs to be addressed early in the management of epilepsy.

Stigma

Although great strides have been made in public understanding about epilepsy, reports continue to surface to remind us that there continues to be a stigma attached to epilepsy. It has been reported that many people fear rejection in association with their epilepsy. Mittan and Locke (29) found that many people with epilepsy fear rejection, but when asked about actual incidents they had not experienced this very often. Similarly, it has been the author's experience that the actual social slights and rebuffs reported by adults have been low, whereas the fear of such reactions is rampant. Many of our adult patients found that when they confided they had epilepsy to others, most people responded in a supportive manner and often went on to talk of a relative or acquaintance with epilepsy. With children (with or without epilepsy), incidents of rejection or shunning are common. Being made fun of can result in very painful and humiliating experiences for any child. These experiences can leave deep emotional scars that interfere with the child's social and emotional adjustment. How do we help young people deal with the embarrassing experience of having a seizure in public? We can teach them and their parents about seizures, help them understand what is happening, what to do in terms of first aid, and be there for them to express their feelings and fears and embarrassment after it is over. This service is available at some epilepsy centers. But how do we combat the stigma in the public population? Many feel that education is the key to a better understanding. With that in mind, the social work section of the Comprehensive Epilepsy Center of Wake Forest University designed an educational project aimed at intervening with the misconceptions and prejudice associated with epilepsy. This project has been ongoing since 1987 and focuses on teaching students (specifically all fourth graders in Forsyth County, North Carolina) in a positive manner about epilepsy. It has been the author's experience that fourth graders, 8- and 9-year-olds, are the most curious, receptive, and kindest of ages. Research has shown that if you wish to change the world view of children, the most crucial time to attempt this influence is at 8 and 9 years of age (30). At the time of the initial effort, 29 schools were involved, with most schools having four to six classes. The overall goal of this ongoing project is to provide education on epilepsy so that fears and misconceptions about this common disorder can be eliminated or diminished and the necessary understanding and support provided to students with epilepsy. It is believed that appropriate and prompt reactions to seizures in the classroom can prevent or minimize social and emotional problems for children with epilepsy and their peers. The results of this ongoing effort have been rewarding. A book on this project is under way.

SUMMARY

There are many different reactions to the diagnosis of epilepsy and no way to predict the impact of this disorder on a person, family, community, or society. How do we reduce the stresses and hopefully prevent the social and psychological problems that often accompany this disorder? First, we make sure that appropriate education and counseling are available soon after diagnosis. Management of the patient must include social evaluation and follow-up in addition to medical care. Of key importance is knowledge of the resources available. When there are no resources, then we must become advocates and speak out on behalf of these needs and gaps in services.

REFERENCES

1. Livingston S. Psychosocial aspects of epilepsy. *J Clin Child Psychol* 1977;6:6–10.
2. Taylor DC. The components of sickness: disease, illness and predicaments. *Lancet* 1979;ii:1008–1010.
3. Moranti AD. In: Morantz RM, Pomerlleau CS, Fenichel CH, eds. *In her own words: oral histories of women physicians.* Westport, CT: Greenwood Press, 1982:73–98.
4. Gibelman M. *What social workers do.* Washington, DC: NASW Press, 1995:131.
5. Gibelman M. The search for identity: defining social work—past, present, future. *Soc Work* 1999;44:301.
6. Brown R. Personal communication with Robin Brown, Co-Chair, International Epilepsy Professionals in Epilepsy Care, Melbourne, Australia.
7. Mittan RJ. Fear of seizures. In: Whitman S, Hermann BP, eds. *Psychopathology in epilepsy: social dimensions.* New York: Oxford University 1986:90–121.
8. Goldstein J, Seidenberg M, Peterson R. Fear of seizures and behavioral functioning in adults with epilepsy. *J Epilepsy* 1990;3:101–106.
9. Helgeson DC, Mittan R, Tan SY, et al. Sepulveda epilepsy education: the efficacy of a psychoeducational treatment program in treating medical and psychosocial aspects of epilepsy. *Epilepsia* 1990;31:75–82.
10. Windsor R, Green L, Roseman J. Health promotion and maintenance for patients with chronic obstructive pulmonary disease: a review. *J Chronic Dis* 1980;33:5–12.
11. Taylor DC. Psychosocial components of childhood epilepsy. In: Hermann B, Seidenberg M, eds. *Childhood epilepsies: neuropsychological, psychosocial and intervention aspects.* New York: John Wiley and Sons, 1989: 119–140.
12. Beckman HB, Frankel RM. The effect of physician behavior on the collection of data. *Ann Intern Med* 1984; 101:692–696.
13. Marvel MK, Epstein RM, Flowers K, et al. Soliciting the patient's agenda—have we improved? *JAMA* 1999; 281:283–287.
14. Arangio A. A systematic examination of the psychosocial needs of patients with epilepsy: the need for a comprehensive change-approach. In: *Plan for nationwide action on epilepsy,* Volume I, Part 1, Section 1-VI. Washington, DC: Department of Health, Education, and Welfare, 1977:385–396.
15. Arniston P, Droge D, Norton R, et al. The perceived psychosocial consequences of having epilepsy. In: Whitman S, Hermann B, eds. *Psychopathology in epilepsy: social dimensions.* New York: Oxford University Press, 1986:143–161.

16. Toseland R, Siporen M. When to recommend group treatment: a review of the clinical and research literature. *Int J Group Psychother* 1986;36:171–201.

17. Bladin P. Psychosocial difficulties and outcome after temporal lobectomy. *Epilepsia* 1992;33:898–907.

18. Appolone C, Gibson PA, Dreifuss FE. Psychosocial considerations in childhood epilepsy. In: Dreifuss FE, ed. *Pediatric epileptology: classification and management of seizures in the child.* Littleton, MA: PSG Publishing, 1983:277–295.

19. Eastman M, Ritter F, Frost M, et al. Impact of the child with epilepsy on the parent. *Epilepsia* 1998;39:158.

20. Zeigler R. Impairments of control and competence. *Epilepsia* 1981;22:339–346.

21. Lechtenberg R. *Epilepsy and the family.* Cambridge, MA: Harvard University Press, 1999:126–134.

22. Lechtenberg R. *Epilepsy and the family.* Cambridge, MA: Harvard University Press, 1999:43-46.

23. Rodin E, Rennick P, Dennerell RD, et al. Vocational and educational problems of epilepsy patients. *Epilepsia* 1971;13:149–160.

24. Epilepsy Foundation of America. *Epilepsy—legal rights, legal issues.* New York: Demos Publications, 1987.

25. Goldin GJ. Building self esteem in people with epilepsy. *Natl Spokesman* 1984;Jul/Aug:6.

26. Austin JK. Paper presented at the 22nd International Epilepsy Congress, Dublin, Ireland, 1997.

27. Mittan R, Fear of seizures. In: Whitman S, Hermann B, eds. *Psychopathology in epilepsy: social dimensions.* New York: Oxford University Press, 1986:90–121.

28. Fisher R, Vickrey B, Gibson PA, et al. A large community based survey of quality of life and concerns of people with epilepsy: part one. *Epilepsia* 1998;39:223.

29. Mittan R, Locke GE. The other half of epilepsy: psychosocial problems. *Urban Health* 1982;Jan/Feb:38–39.

30. Livesley WJ, Bromley D. *Person perception in childhood and adolescence.* Toronto, Canada: John Wiley and Sons, 1973.

21

Quality of Life in Epilepsy

Janice M. Buelow and *Carol Estwing Ferrans

*Department of Neurology, Rush Presbyterian-Saint Luke's Medical Center; and
College of Nursing, University of Illinois, Chicago, Illinois 60612

Control of seizure episodes is the primary goal of treatment of epilepsy, to enable patients to live normal lives. Although quality of life has always been a major concern, measuring it in epilepsy is a relatively new phenomenon. It has been only in the last decade that measures of the concept have been developed specifically for the person with epilepsy, making it possible to assess treatment outcomes in terms of quality of life. The purpose of this chapter is to address the major issues to consider when measuring quality of life and review instruments for the epilepsy population.

Quality of life is a multidimensional construct that encompasses the whole of life. It is particularly salient for the treatment of epilepsy, because of the far-reaching effects of the disorder. In addition to the physical effects of epilepsy itself, treatment is complicated by the side effects of anticonvulsant medications. There also are psychological sequelae related to the seizures and the fact that the person has very little control over their occurrence. The diagnosis of epilepsy carries a social stigma that potentially impacts all areas of life, as well as perceived stigma that affects the persons' view of themselves. There are social consequences for people who experience seizures and those who witness them (1–3). Measurement of outcomes in terms of quality of life can provide a useful tool to assess the effectiveness of treatment regarding the physical, psychological, and social aspects of life and so provide a more comprehensive and accurate evaluation.

HISTORICAL OVERVIEW OF QUALITY-OF-LIFE MEASUREMENT

The beginnings of western thought about quality of life can be traced to Aristotle. Aristotle (4) considered that the nature of happiness and "the good life" was dependent on virtuous activity of the soul. Good health, wealth, and beauty contributed to happiness, but they were not essential for it. The nature of happiness as more than material well-being also was addressed in the teachings of Jesus in the Beatitudes, in which happiness is described as belonging to those who are merciful, pure in heart, and peacemakers. However, it was not until after World War II that the term "quality of life" entered the American vocabulary (5). It was about this time that measurement of quality of life had its earliest roots in the studies of psychologists and sociologists. The first major studies, based on probability samples of the American population, focused on happiness and satisfaction with life. One of these studies was conducted by Norman Bradburn in 1961, who focused on psychological well-being based on the idea of emotional balance. His work focused on positive and negative affect in four midwestern communities (6). Another early researcher, Hadley Cantril, measured satisfaction with life in America and 13 other countries using his self-anchoring scale, a ten-rung ladder anchored by the respondent's hopes and fears. Cantril's work focused on comparing the satisfaction of residents of different countries, based on aspirations and needs that people identified (7). However, probably the most influential was Angus Campbell, who assessed the quality of American life in terms of a broad spectrum of variables, including satisfaction with life, health, and material well-being. Campbell et al. (8) examined the influence of gender, race, work, and other factors on quality of life in a national sample, targeting the elements that affect people's judgments regarding the quality of their lives.

Within health care, the earliest assessments of quality of life focused either on functional status or social utility. For example, the Karnofsky Performance Status Scale, first published in 1948, frequently has been utilized as a measure of quality of life (9). Using the Karnofsky scale, a patient's ability to perform daily activities is rated on a scale ranging from 100 (able to carry on normal activity and to work) to 0 (dead). Functional status continues to be one of the most commonly used approaches for measuring quality of life.

Social utility focuses on the contributions a person makes to society. Common examples are assessment of quality of life in terms of employment and income. Measures of social utility traditionally have been important regarding the allocation of scarce medical resources. For example, in the early days of hemodialysis before 1972 when access was limited, selection for treatment commonly was made based on quality of life as defined by social utility (10). Early studies of the impact of epilepsy on life also measured employment and income, as well as cognitive impairment (11,12). Social utility has largely been abandoned as a measure of quality of life, although it has not disappeared entirely.

CONCEPT OF QUALITY OF LIFE

A variety of meanings are applied to the term quality of life. Therefore, the term is meaningless without a clarification of the definition. There is no general consensus regarding a single definition of quality of life, nor is there a gold standard for measurement. In most cases, what is meant by quality of life must be construed by examining the instruments used to measure it.

Clarity about what is meant by the term is extremely important, because the way quality of life is defined can affect clinical decisions based on its assessment. For example, one study asked 205 family and internal medicine physicians to decide the appropriate treatment for an elderly man with chronic pulmonary disease, based on their own personal definitions of quality of life. The resulting judgments of quality of life varied so widely that some decided the patient should be treated and others decided that treatment should be withheld (13).

As it is used in health care today, quality of life most commonly is used to mean either health status and functioning in a variety of domains or patient satisfaction with those domains. Gotay et al. (14) argued that both are important to measure in quality of life, because one provides information about actual levels of functioning and the other provides the patients' evaluations of their life. They merged the two components into their definition of the concept (14, p. 376):

> Quality of life is a state of well-being that is a composite of two components: (1) the ability to perform everyday activities that reflect physical, psychological, and social well-being and (2) patient satisfaction with levels of functioning and the control of disease and/or treatment-related symptoms.

These two components provide different information about the patient's quality of life, because evaluations of functional ability can differ from patients' satisfaction with those abilities. Across the health care literature in general, health status and patient satisfaction are only moderately correlated, demonstrating that the two components are related but not redundant. In a study of patients with rheumatoid arthritis, psychological distress was affected more by satisfaction with abilities than by the actual state of those abilities (15). The measurement of both components is particularly important in epilepsy, because individuals adjust and compensate for functional disability with varying degrees of success, resulting in differences in outcomes. Assessment of only one component can result in an incomplete characterization of quality of life.

MULTIDIMENSIONAL NATURE OF QUALITY OF LIFE IN EPILEPSY

One area of general agreement regarding the nature of quality of life is that it is multidimensional (16). Although there are some differences in the characterization of domains, there is general consensus that it is more than health status. A study estimating the relative value to patients of physical, mental, and social health when making treatment decisions found that mental and social health were as important as physical health (17). This suggests that seizure frequency would not be the only factor affecting quality of life. In addition, although it is understood that complete control of seizures is the best method for improving quality of life (1), complete control of seizures is not always possible. Hauser and Hesdorffer (18) estimated that about 30% of those treated for epilepsy are unlikely to gain complete control of seizures.

Spilker (19) summarized the health care literature by describing quality of life in terms of four domains: physical, psychological, social, and economic. Similar domains have been identified across a number of chronic illness groups based on qualitative analysis of patients' perspective (20–22). Studies have identified aspects of life across all four domains that are important in epilepsy. For example, based on their clinical experience and that of others, Dodrill et al. (23) identified family background, emotional adjustment, interpersonal adjustment, vocational adjustment, financial status, adjustment to seizures, medicine and medical management, and overall psychosocial functioning as important aspects of quality of life in epilepsy.

Only a few studies have been conducted to identify what the person with epilepsy feels is important to his or her quality of life. One example was a study that incorporated indepth interviews to identify how epilepsy affected the lives of the respondents (24). The interviews were conducted as part of a larger study directed at measuring social effects of epilepsy. Twenty-one areas were identified as affecting quality of life, such as seizures, employment, relationships and social life, medications, and feelings about self (Table 21.1).

These findings were supported in a later study directed at defining self-management in the person with epilepsy (25). In that study, participants were asked to identify what was necessary for them to feel good about their lives. The aspects of life identified as contributing positively to quality of life were employment, family and friends, independence, and health (Table 21.1). Two subthemes emerged as detractors from a good quality of life: "seizures" and "normal problems." The subtheme "seizures" included anything involving seizures, such as medication, the event itself, and the aftermath of the seizure. "Normal problems" included day-to-day problems that any person could experience, with or without epilepsy.

The relationships among the various domains in epilepsy are complex. Findings from early studies concluded that persons with epilepsy were more likely to have emotional problems related to interpersonal relationships, vocational issues, and financial concerns (23,26–28). In addition, the diagnosis of epilepsy carries with it a social stigma that potentially impacts all areas of life, as well as perceived stigma that affects the persons' view of themselves. A study that looked at enacted stigma versus perceived stigma concluded that perceived stigma is as disabling as stigmatizing actions experienced from other people (29). Seizure control has been associated with successful outcomes in employment and education. For example, one study followed children over a 30-year period and looked at outcome measures such as employment and education (12). They found that seizure freedom and not having to take anticonvulsant medication correlated with a feeling of independence and with successful employment. They also concluded that good communication ability, intelligence, and seizure freedom were predictors of social competence.

TABLE 21.1. *Comparison of patient-identified concerns and quality-of-life domains from two studies*

Areas affecting the lives of people with epilepsy[a]	Quality-of-life domains[b]
Attitudes toward accepting the attacks	Health (necessity to feel good about physical and emotional well-being)
Lethargy/lack of energy	
Sleep disturbance	
Change of outlook on life/self	
Attitude toward the label epilepsy	
Fear of having seizures	
Problems with taking medicine	
Depression or emotional reactions	
Distrust of the medical profession	
Misconception about epilepsy	
Concern about housing	Independence (being able to function as desired without interference with others)
Lack of confidence about traveling	
Lack of confidence about the future	
Adverse reaction on leisure pursuit	
Concern about sexual relationships	Social (need for interaction with others: family, friends, acquaintances)
Concern about platonic relationships	
Adverse reaction on social life	
Difficulty in communicating with the family	
Feeling of increased social isolation	
Fear of stigma in employment	Employment/education (issues surrounding work or school that affect positive feelings about life)
Concern about performance at work	

[a]Adapted from Chaplin JE, Yepez R, Shorvom S, et al. A quantitative approach to measuring the social effects of epilepsy. *Neuroepidemiology* 1990;9:151–158.
[b]Adapted from Buelow J. *Perception of self-management in the person with epilepsy* [Ph.D. diss., University of Illinois at Chicago]. 2000.

WHO SHOULD EVALUATE QUALITY OF LIFE

Evaluation of quality of life requires a value judgment, such as good/bad or high/low. The person rating quality of life uses his or her own internal standards for what the rater considers a desirable or undesirable quality of life (16). There have been a number of studies showing a disparity in the reports of quality of life between physician and patient and between family members and the patient (30,31). A study that examined well-being and epilepsy suggested two models to study psychosocial issues in people with epilepsy (3). The first model indicates a linear relationship between seizure severity and psychosocial problems. It predicted that, by controlling seizures, the person with epilepsy should be able to lead a normal life. The second model suggests that the *perception* of the severity of disease has the greatest impact on psychosocial status.

However, there is general agreement that the most appropriate person to judge quality of life is the patient, rather than an outside observer (16,32). Quality of life commonly is viewed as a judgment of the experience of life, and so it is dependent on the individual's own values, perspective, and expectations. Devinsky (33) supports this idea in his introduction to quality-of-life issues in epilepsy. He stated that the patient is the only one who knows how he or she feels and how he or she is able to function in the world. Although the patient's opinion may hold bias, it is the only one that counts. It is the person with the disorder who must define his or her quality of life.

INSTRUMENTS FOR EPILEPSY POPULATIONS

There are many generic quality-of-life tests, but most are too general to address specific issues that are related to the underlying disorder. Disease-specific quality-of-life assessment tools address the issues of the population to whom they are directed. In the last decade, several measures have emerged that are directed specifically at measuring the quality of life of the person with epilepsy. The following section provides an overview of some of the tests that have been developed.

Epilepsy Surgery Inventory-55

Description of Instrument

The Epilepsy Surgery Inventory-55 (ESI-55) was developed to assess the quality of life in persons with epilepsy who underwent surgery as treatment for seizures and is a health-related quality-of-life (HRQOL) tool. The ESI-55 conceptualizes quality of life as perception of well-being in the domains of life that are affected by epilepsy. The domains include physical, mental, social, and general health status (34). The foundation for the ESI-55 is the RAND 36-Item Health Survey (SF-36). The SF-36 is widely used as a health status measure in medical outcomes studies, surveys, clinical research, and in clinical practice that assesses eight HRQOL domains (32). The domains are limitations in physical activities, limitations in social activities, limitations in usual role activities, vitality, pain, general mental health, and general health perceptions (32,35). The original SF-36 was supplemented with 19 epilepsy-specific items (34). Twelve of the items were specific for epilepsy, looking at cognitive function, role limitations due to memory problems, and epilepsy-specific health-related functioning (34). Seven more generic items were added to the health perceptions, role limitations, and overall quality-of-life scales.

Research Context and Use

The ESI-55 has been used extensively to better quantify the quality-of-life outcome of epilepsy surgery. This measure is important to provide evidence that the outcome of surgery is worth its overall cost. Vickrey et al. (36) evaluated the impact of epilepsy surgery on seizures, medication use, employment, and quality of life. Two hundred-two surgery patients and 46 nonsurgery patients were compared through chart review and self-administered quality-of-life questionnaires. Surgery patients had fewer monthly seizures than the nonsurgery patients, but the two groups were otherwise similar. Following surgery, there was not a significant difference in employment status or prospectively assessed quality of life. This study suggests that the impact of surgery on quality of life and employment needs to be assessed in larger prospective studies (36).

McLachlan et al. (37) evaluated HRQOL and seizure control in temporal lobe epilepsy. Seventy-two patients completed the study: 51 surgical patients and 21 medically treated patients. The prospective study was conducted over 24 months to compare HRQOL in surgically and medically treated patients with intractable temporal lobe epilepsy. The quality-of-life scores (ESI-55) were similar in both groups prior to surgery. At 24 months following surgery, seizure-free patients and those with a 90% reduction in seizures reported a significant improvement in quality of life. These findings suggest that quality of life is improved with significant seizure reduction (37).

Rose et al. (38) used the ESI-55 to evaluate changes between preoperative and postoperative HRQOL in 47 patients who underwent a temporal lobectomy. There were significantly improved scores postoperatively. The greatest improvements were in those patients who had low-to-medium HRQOL scores prior to surgery. Those with high scores prior to surgery continued to have high scores following surgery (38).

Measurement Properties

Reliabity and Validity

Internal consistency reliability coefficients (Cronbach α) exceeded 0.70 in all scales except for social function ($\alpha = 0.68$). Construct validity was established through correlations of the ESI-55 to a mood profile measure and an analysis of the relationship of the ESI-55 scale scores to seizure outcome. It was hypothesized that mood profile would correlate significantly with the emotional well-being scale, and the findings supported this hypothesis. There was a significant negative correlation between the mood profile scores of depression and anger to the ESI-55 well-being scale ($p < 0.0001$). There also was a significant relationship between seizure outcomes and the ESI-55 scores ($p < 0.05$). Seizure-free patients scored better on the ESI-55 than patients who continued to have seizures (34).

Quality of Life in Epilepsy

Description of Instrument

The Quality of Life in Epilepsy (QOLIE) was developed to provide a quality-of-life instrument that addressed the specific concerns of the person with epilepsy and could be used both in the clinical setting to measure treatment outcome and for research. The QOLIE is an HRQOL measure designed to address the patient's perception of the impact of epilepsy and its treatment on his or her life (39). As with the ESI-55, the generic core of the scale is the SF-36. The generic core was expanded in several domains. The areas that supplemented the generic core were issues commonly reported by epileptic patients with moderately controlled epilepsy. Forty-eight epilepsy-specific items were added to provide a more comprehensive overview of epilepsy. These included epilepsy-targeted health perception, social function, working and driving limitations, and cognitive function. Other areas addressed in the QOLIE included health perception, seizure worry, physical function, role limitation, overall quality of life, emotional well-being, energy/fatigue, attention/concentration, memory, language, medication effects, and isolation (39).

There are three versions of the QOLIE available for clinical and research use. The QOLIE-89 or QOLIE-1 is the original 89-item instrument developed primarily for research use. It provides an indepth assessment that takes approximately 25 minutes to complete. The QOLIE-31 (QOLIE-2) is composed of 31 items and takes approximately 15 minutes to complete. It provides a less detailed evaluation

and was developed as an indepth clinical evaluation or for abbreviated research. The QOLIE-10 (QOLIE-3) is a ten-item evaluation that takes only a few minutes to complete. It is meant to provide a quick clinical evaluation of quality of life in the clinical setting (33).

Research Context

The QOLIE was developed to provide a comprehensive assessment and outcomes tool. An example is the use of the QOLIE to evaluate the effectiveness of new antiepileptic drugs (AEDs). Several studies have been conducted that evaluate not only the efficacy of the medication but also the affect of the medication on quality of life (40–42). The QOLIE has been evaluated for use in multiple patient populations. Devinsky et al. (43) conducted a study to establish the risk factors for poor HRQOL in adolescence. The QOLIE was adjusted for an adolescent population (44). One hundred ninety-seven adolescents who had a diagnosis of epilepsy were enrolled. Risk factors for poor quality of life in the adolescent population included older age, severity of epilepsy, neurotoxicity, hospitalizations, fewer extracurricular activities, stigma, and lower socioeconomic status. The QOLIE-89 also has been adapted for use in multiple cultures (45,46).

Reliability and Validity

Perrine (47) reported that internal consistency reliability for 16 of the 17 multiitem scales ranged from 0.73 to 0.88. Test–retest reliability ranged from 0.56 to 0.88, with medication effects being the lowest (47). Construct validity was supported by correlations between the QOLIE and established measures. Correlations between the QOLIE emotional well-being and the Profile of Moods (POMS) tension and depression and anger scale ranged from −0.62 to −0.79 ($p < 0.0001$). The QOLIE energy/fatigue scale with the POMS vigor and fatigue scale correlated at 0.61 and 0.65 ($p < 0.0001$) (47). Leidy et al. (48) had similar findings in a telephone validation of the QOLIE-89 ($p < 0.001$).

Liverpool Assessment Battery

Description of Instrument

The Liverpool Assessment Battery was developed to address several issues in quality-of-life research. The developers acknowledged that the measurement of quality of life must include physical and social functioning, burden of symptoms, and a sense of well-being (49). To adequately address these domains, four scales were developed: the Seizure Severity Scale, Impact of Epilepsy Scale, The Epilepsy Specific Mastery Scale, and the Adverse Drug Events Scale. In addition, two well-established generic measures are included in the battery. The scales can be used in different combinations, depending on the needs of the study. Two instruments assess psychological status in terms of self-esteem (Rosenberg Self-Esteem Scale) and anxiety and depression (Hospital Anxiety and Depression Scale). The Rosenberg Self-Esteem Scale was developed to measure the patient's perception of self-esteem. The Hospital Anxiety and Depression Scale was developed as a screening tool for mood disorders in patients with physical illness. These instruments were independently developed and validated, and they have been used extensively in a variety of studies. The psychometric properties of these well-established instruments have been reported elsewhere and so are not presented here.

The Seizure Severity Scale is composed of two subscales. The percept scale assesses the patient's perception of control over the seizures and seizure predictability. The ictal and postictal subscales measure the effect of events experienced during and immediately after a seizure (49). The Impact of Epilepsy Scale is an eight-item scale that allows the patient to assess how the condition affects all areas of his or her life, including personal relationships, work, self-image, and social relationships. The Adverse Drug Events Scale is a 20-item scale that addresses the effects of AEDs on the patient and his or ability to carry on with life. The Epilepsy Specific Mastery Scale represents the patient's perception of control relative to the epilepsy.

Research Context and Use

In a study to measure quality of life and the clinical course of epilepsy, Jacoby et al. (50) mailed questionnaires to 769 subjects and had a 71% return rate. There was a clear relationship between seizure activity and the subjects' psychological well-being, the subjects' perceptions about the impact of epilepsy, and treatment on their daily lives. This study provides valuable data about the overall effect of epilepsy (46). A similar study was conducted throughout Europe, representing 15 countries and more than 5,000 patients (51).

The instruments have been used in drug trials to provide insight into the impact of AEDs on the patient. Smith et al. (52) used the Seizure Severity Scale and other measures of social and psychological status to study the efficacy of lamotrigine. Wagner et al. (53) used the Seizure Severity, Impact of Epilepsy, and Epilepsy Specific Mastery Scales to measure the effect of both the disorder and the use of AEDs (53).

In 1998, the Liverpool Assessment Battery was adapted to the American population. Modifications were made in the instruments based on the recommendations of focus groups of patients with epilepsy and epilepsy specialists (54).

Reliability and Validity

Data to support the reliability and validity of the Liverpool Assessment Battery instruments have been reported. Cronbach α for these scales range from 0.60 to 0.85 (52,55). Cronbach α for the Seizure Severity Scale percept has been as low as 0.43. This suggests that this portion of the tool should be used with caution (52).

Validity of seizure severity has been assessed in several studies. The ictal scale successfully differentiated 94 patients into seizure type ($p < 0.001$) (52). The Impact of Epilepsy Scale was correlated to other scales in the Liverpool Assessment Battery: the Hospital Anxiety and Depression Scale, Self-Esteem Scale, Affect Balance, and Mastery ($r = 0.45$ to -0.54, $p < 0.001$). The Affect Balance

Scale successfully differentiated patients with epilepsy and matched seizure-free patients (p < 0.003) (48).

Quality of Life Index—Epilepsy Version

Description of Instrument

The Quality of Life Index (QLI) was developed by Ferrans and Powers (56) to measure quality of life in terms of satisfaction with life. Quality of life is defined by Ferrans as "a person's sense of well-being that stems from satisfaction or dissatisfaction with the areas of life that are important to him/her" (57, p. 15). The QLI measures both satisfaction and importance of various aspects of life. Importance ratings are used to weight the satisfaction responses, so that the scores produced reflect the respondents' satisfaction with the aspects of life they value. Items that are rated as more important have a greater impact on scores than those of lesser importance. Scores are calculated for quality of life overall and in four domains: health and functioning, psychological/spiritual, social and economic, and family. The instrument consists of two parts: the first measures satisfaction with 35 aspects of life and the second measures importance of those same aspects. Respondents are asked to rate their satisfaction on a six-point scale ranging from "very satisfied" to "very dissatisfied." Importance is rated on a six-point scale ranging from "very important" to "very unimportant." The instrument takes approximately 10 minutes to complete as a self-administered questionnaire (57–59).

Research Context and Use

A number of versions of the QLI have been developed for use with various disorders and in the general population and have been reported in approximately 100 published studies. A common set of items forms the basis for all versions, and items pertinent to each disorder have been added to create the illness-specific versions. Scores for all versions range from 0 to 30, which facilitates comparisons of findings across different versions. General population data are available for interpretive purposes. The instrument has been used both as a self-administered questionnaire and in an interview format. The QLI-Epilepsy Version was used with 305 persons with epilepsy, ranging in age from 15 to 76 years. The mean overall quality-of-life score for this group was 18.62 (SD = 5.33), which was significantly lower than the general population (59).

Reliability and Validity

Substantial evidence of internal consistency reliability of the QLI has been provided by Cronbach α values ranging from 0.85 to 0.98 across 18 published studies. For the QLI-Epilepsy Version, reliability was supported by Cronbach α values of 0.94 for the total scale, and 0.84, 0.89, 0.80, and 0.63 for the four subscales, when used with 305 persons with epilepsy (59). Evidence of stability reliability has been provided for the common items by test–retest correlations of 0.87 with a 2-week interval and 0.81 with a 1-month interval (59).

Evidence of construct validity for the common items was provided by factor analysis, which revealed four dimensions underlying the QLI and explained 91% of the total variance (54). Construct validity also was supported using the contrasted groups approach. Subjects who had less pain and less depression or were coping better with stress were found to have higher quality-of-life scores, which was consistent with predictions (53). For the QLI-Epilepsy Version, support for validity was provided by a strong correlation (r = 0.81) between the overall QLI score and another instrument measuring satisfaction with life, when used with 305 persons with epilepsy (59).

Summary of Instruments

As seen in the previous discussion, each instrument has strengths that can be translated into use by both the researcher and the clinician (Table 21.2). The ESI-55 was developed

TABLE 21.2. *Comparison of four quality-of-life tools for epilepsy*

Name of tool	ESI-55	QOLIE	QLI	Liverpool Assessment Battery
Conceptualization of quality of life	Perception of well-being in the domains of life that are affected by epilepsy	A measure to address the patient's perception of the impact of epilepsy and its treatment on life	Life satisfaction	Addresses several issues of QOL (physical, social functioning, burden of symptoms, sense of well-being)
Description of tool	A 55-item scale. Items 1–3 rate health and quality of life in general. Questions are either Likert-type or yes/no in format.	An 89-item scale that rates multiple domains. Two shorter versions are available that allow for multiple uses of the scale. Questions are Likert-type and yes/no.	Two 35-item, Likert-type scales. The first 35 items rate satisfaction and the second 35 items rate how important each item is. This allows for a weighted score.	Multiple scales that can be used individually or together for a more comprehensive study
Domains	Health perceptions, energy/ fatigue, overall quality of life, social function, emotional well-being, cognitive function, physical function, pain, role limitations	Health perception, seizure worry, physical functions, role limitations (physical and emotional), pain, overall quality of life, attention/concentration, energy/fatigue, memory, language, working/driving limitation, medication effects, social function, social support, social isolation	Overall quality of life, health and functioning, psychological/spiritual, social and economic, family	Patients' assessment of seizure severity, life fulfillment, impact of epilepsy and its treatment, adverse effects of antiepileptic medications
Uses	Can be used both for research and to assess outcome of surgery	QOLIE-89 is indepth and used primarily for research purposes. QOLIE-31 can be used both for research or in clinical settings. QOLIE-10 is primarily for clinical settings.	QLI has been used primarily for research purposes. It has been used in multiple chronically ill populations and, therefore, provides useful comparison data between groups.	Used primarily for research.

ESI-55, Epilepsy Surgery Inventory-55; QLI, Quality of Life Index; QOLIE, Quality of Life in Epilepsy.

specifically to measure outcomes for epilepsy surgery patients and provides valuable information about the effect of surgery on the person with epilepsy. Therefore, it is primarily a research tool, but the results can be applied to the clinical setting. The QOLIE was developed to measure HRQOL in persons with epilepsy. This is important because it provides a standard on which to measure issues surrounding living with epilepsy. It can be used both in the research setting and for clinical practice. The QOLIE can provide valuable information regarding the impact of anticonvulsant medications. However, because it also is available in a shorter form, it can be used by the clinician as a quick way to measure the effect of the current treatment regimen.

The Liverpool Assessment Scales are unique because each tool addresses a specific topic in quality-of-life issues. The clinician and the researcher have the potential to address specific subjects and answer specific questions related to quality-of-life issues. For example, the Seizure Severity Scale provides insight into both the severity of seizures and the patient's perception of seizure severity. Finally, the QLI is an important tool because, although it measures the perception of quality of life, it also allows the patients to identify the importance of each item in the scale. This gives a weighted quality-of-life score. The QLI has been developed for multiple disease processes and provides a comparison of actual quality of life across diseases. This is one of the few tools that has this capability while still addressing disease-specific issues.

CONCLUSION

Epilepsy as a chronic illness presents multiple complex problems to everyday living. The primary goal of treatment is to control seizures, but treatment also should be targeted to overcome the broad spectrum of physical, psychological, and social effects of the disorder. Assessment of the number of seizures and anticonvulsant levels is only a part of the picture. As Devinsky (33) points out, the patient is the only one who knows how he or she feels

and is the only person who can evaluate treatment outcome. If quality-of-life issues are not addressed, then important factors may be overlooked by the clinician. A decrease in seizure frequency may not guarantee an increase in quality of life. If seizure frequency has been decreased at the expense of greater medication side effects, then quality of life may be negatively affected. Second, other factors may be missed, such as the impact of seizures at work or on social life. These are important issues that should be addressed by the clinician and the patient together, to work to improve quality of life.

There are several mechanisms with which to measure quality of life. This chapter presented some options to quantitatively measure quality of life. Discussion with the patient about quality-of-life issues is a legitimate manner in which to assess the success of treatment. Regardless of how quality of life is assessed, including the concept as part of the overall outcome measure is the important issue.

REFERENCES

1. Jacoby A. Epilepsy and quality of everyday life. *Soc Sci Med* 1992;34:657–666.
2. Scamber G, Hopkins A. Generating a model of epileptic stigma: the role of qualitative analysis. *Soc Sci Med* 1990;30:1187–1194.
3. Collings JA. Psychosocial adjustment of adults with epilepsy. *Patient Educ Counsel* 1990;29:418–426.
4. Aristotle. De Anima. In: McKeon R, ed. *Introduction to Aristotle*. New York: Modern Library, 1947:148–153.
5. Campbell A. *The sense of well-being in America*. New York: McGraw-Hill, 1981.
6. Bradburn N, Caplovitz, D. *Reports on happiness*. Chicago: Aldine, 1965.
7. Cantril H. *The pattern of human concerns*. New Brunswick, NJ: Rutgers University Press, 1965.
8. Campbell A, Converse P, Rodgers W. *The quality of American life*. New York: Russell Sage Foundation, 1976.
9. Karnofsky D, Abelmann W, Craver L. The use of nitrogen mustards in the palliative treatment of carcinoma. *Cancer* 1948;4:634–656.
10. Ferrans CE. Quality of life as a criterion for allocation of life-sustaining treatment. In: Anderson G, Glesnes-Anderson V, eds. *Health care ethics*. Rockville, MD: Aspen, 1987:129–136.
11. Rodin E, Rennick P, Denneril R, et al. Vocational and educational problems of epileptic patients. *Epilepsy* 1972;13:149–160.
12. Sillanpaa M, Helenius H. Social competence of people with epilepsy: a new methodological approach. *Acta Neurol Scand* 1993;87:335–341.

13. Pearlman R, Jonsen A. The use of quality of life considerations in medical decision making. *J Am Geriatr Soc* 1985;33:344–352.

14. Gotay C, Korn E, McCabe M. Quality-of-life assessment in cancer treatment protocols: research issues in protocol development. *J Natl Cancer Inst* 1992;84: 575–579.

15. Blalock S, DeVellis B, DeVellis R, et al. Psychological well-being among people with recently diagnosed rheumatoid arthritis. *Arthritis Rheum* 1992;35: 1267–1272.

16. Osoba D. Lessons learned from measuring health-related quality of life in oncology. *J Clin Oncol* 1994;12: 608–616.

17. Sherbourne CD, Sturm R, Wells KB. What outcomes matter to patients? *J Gen Intern Med* 1999;14:357–363.

18. Hauser WA, Hesdorffer DC. Epilepsy: frequency, causes, and consequences. Landover, MD: Epilepsy Foundation of America, 1990.

19. Spilker B. Introduction. In: Spilker B, ed. *Quality of life and pharmaeconomics in clinical trials,* 2nd ed. Philadelphia: Lippincott-Raven Publishers, 1996:1–10.

20. Ferrans C. Development of a conceptual model of quality of life. *Scholar Inquiry Nurs Pract* 1996;10: 293–304.

21. Ferrell B, Grant M, Padilla G. Experience of pain and perceptions of quality of life: validation of a conceptual model. *Hospice J* 1991;7:9–24.

22. Padilla G, Ferrell B, Grant M, et al. Defining the content domain of quality of life for cancer patients with pain. *Cancer Nurs* 1990;13:108–115.

23. Dodrill C, Beier R, Kasparich M, et al. Psychosocial problems in adults with epilepsy: comparison of findings from four countries. *Epilepsia* 1984;25:176–183.

24. Chaplin JE, Yepez R, Shorvom S, et al. A quantitative approach to measuring the social effects of epilepsy. *Neuroepidemiology* 1990;9:151–158.

25. Buelow J. *Perception of self-management in the person with epilepsy* [Ph.D. diss., University of Illinois at Chicago]. 2000.

26. Dodrill CB, Batzel LW, Queisser HR, et al. An objective method for assessment of psychological and social problems among epileptics. *Epilepsia* 1980;21:123–135.

27. Cofield R, Austin J. Psychosocial adjustment of adults with epilepsy. *Patient Educ Counsel* 1984;6:125–130.

28. Fraser RT, Clemmons DC, Dodrill CB, et al. The difficult-to-employ in epilepsy rehabilitation: problems of response to an intensive intervention. *Epilepsia* 1986; 27:220–224.

29. Ryan R, Kamper K, Emlen AC. The stigma of epilepsy as a self-concept. *Epilepsia* 1980;21:433–444.

30. Hays RD, Sherbourne C, Mazel E. The RAND 36-item health survey 1.0. *Health Econ* 1993;2:212–227.

31. Sprangers MA, Aaronson NK. The role of health care providers and significant others in evaluating the quality of life of patients with chronic disease: a review. *J Clin Epidemiol* 1992;45:743–760.

32. Nayfield S, Ganz P, Moinpour C, et al. Report from a national cancer institute (USA) workshop on quality of life assessment in cancer clinical trials. *Qual Life Res* 1992;1:203–210.

33. Devinsky O. Clinical uses of the quality-of-life in epilepsy inventory. *Epilepsia* 1993;34[Suppl 4]: S39–S44.

34. Vickrey BG. A procedure for developing a quality-of-life measure for epilepsy surgery patients. *Epilepsia* 1993;34[Suppl 4]:S22–S27.

35. Ware JE, Sherbourne CD. A 36-item short-form health survey (SF-36): I. Conceptual framework and item selection. *Med Care* 1992;30:473–483.

36. Vickrey BG, Hays RD, Rausch R, et al. Outcomes in 248 patients who had diagnostic evaluations for epilepsy surgery. *Lancet* 1995;346:1445–1449.

37. McLachlan RS, Rose KJ, Derry PA, et al. Health-related quality of life and seizure control in temporal lobe epilepsy. *Ann Neurol* 1997;41:482–489.

38. Rose KJ, Derry PA, Wiebe S, et al. Determinants of health-related quality of life after temporal lobe epilepsy surgery. *Qual Life Res* 1996;5:395–402.

39. Devinsky O, Veckrey BG, Cramer J, et al. Development of the quality of life in epilepsy inventory. *Epilepsia* 1995;36:1089–1104.

40. Bruni J. Gabapentin as adjunctive therapy for seizures. *Epilepsia* 1999;40[Suppl 6]:S27–S28.

41. Mirza WU, Rak IW, Thadani VM, et al. Six month evaluation of Carbatrol (extended release carbamazepine) in complex partial seizures. *Neurology* 1998;51: 1727–1729.

42. Jones MW. Topiramate—safety and tolerability. *Can J Neurol Sci* 1998;25:s13–s15.

43. Devinsky O, Westbrook L, Cramer J, et al. Risk factors for poor health-related quality of life in adolescents with epilepsy. *Epilepsia* 1999;40:1715–1720.

44. Cramer JA. Quality of life assessment in clinical practice. *Neurology* 1999;53[Suppl 2]:S49–S52.

45. Staven K, Bjornaes H, Lossius MI. Reliability and validity of a Norwegian version of the quality of life in epilepsy inventory (QOLIE-89). *Epilepsia* 2000;41: 91–97.

46. Cramer JA, Perrine K, Devinsky O, et al. Development and cross-cultural translations of a 31-item quality of life in epilepsy inventory. *Epilepsia* 1998;39:81–88.

47. Perrine KR. A new quality-of-life inventory for epilepsy patients: interim results. *Epilepsia* 1993;34[Suppl 4]: S28–S33.

48. Leidy NK, Elixhauser A, Rentz AM, et al. Telephone validation of the quality of life in epilepsy inventory-89 (QOLIE-89). *Epilepsia* 1999;40:97–106.

49. Baker GA. Health-related quality of life issues: optimizing patient outcomes. *Neurology* 1995;45[Suppl 2]: S29–S34.

50. Jacoby A, Baker GA, Steen N, et al. The clinical course of epilepsy and its psychological correlates: findings from a UK community study. *Epilepsia* 1996;37: 148–161.

51. Baker GA, Jacoby A, Buck D, et al. Quality of life of people with epilepsy: a European study. *Epilepsia* 1997; 38:353–362.

52. Smith D, Baker GA, Davies G, et al. Outcomes of add-on treatment with lamotrigine in partial epilepsy. *Epilepsia* 1993;34:312–322.

53. Wagner AK, Keller SD, Kosinski M, et al. Advances in methods for assessing the impact of epilepsy and antiepileptic drug therapy on patients' health-related quality of life. *Qual Life Res* 1995;4:115–134.

54. Rapp S, Shumaker S, Smith T, et al. Adaptation and evaluation of the Liverpool quality of life battery for American epilepsy patients. *Qual Life Res* 1998;7: 353–363.

55. Baker GA, Jacoby A, Smith DF, et al. Development of a

novel scale to assess life fulfillment as part of the further refinement of a quality of life model for epilepsy. *Epilepsia* 1994;35:591–596.

56. Ferrans C, Powers M. Quality of life index: development and psychometric properties. *Adv Nurs Sci* 1985; 8:15–24.

57. Ferrans CE. Development of a quality of life index for patients with cancer. *Oncol Nurs Forum* 1990;17: 15–19.

58. Ferrans C, Powers M. Psychometric assessment of the quality of life index. *Res Nurs Health* 1992;15:29–38.

59. Ferrans CE, Cohen FL. Quality of life: persons with epilepsy and the general population. *Epilepsia* 1993;34 [Suppl 6]:25.

22

Psychosocial Aspects of Pediatric Epilepsy

Joan K. Austin

School of Nursing, Indiana University, Indianapolis, Indiana 46202

A chronic illness in childhood, such as epilepsy, poses special challenges for both the children with the condition and their families. In addition to the normal developmental tasks of childhood, these children are confronted with other psychosocial stressors related to coping with a chronic health condition. Both children and families need to make a successful adaptation to epilepsy to facilitate the optimal development of the child. Furthermore, failure to make a satisfactory adaptation can lead to psychosocial adjustment problems throughout childhood that continue into adulthood. Unfortunately, children with epilepsy are a population at risk for reduced quality of life because of high rates of adjustment problems, especially mental health and academic achievement problems.

In this chapter, rates of mental health and school problems found in children with epilepsy are presented and followed by a description of common psychosocial issues confronting these children and their families. These issues, which can vary both by duration of the seizure condition and by the age of the child, are reviewed next. The most common factors associated with these mental health and school problems are described along with how psychosocial issues might be related to these factors. The chapter concludes with a discussion of the psychosocial care needs of children with seizures and their parents.

PSYCHOSOCIAL PROBLEMS

Mental Health Problems

Rates of mental health problems in children with epilepsy are more than four times higher than for children in the general population [1,2]. It also appears that epilepsy places children at greater risk of mental health problems than do other physical chronic conditions, especially those without neurologic involvement. In one epidemiologic study, the prevalence rate of behavior problems was 6.6% in the general childhood population, 11.6% in children with physical conditions without neurologic involvement, 28.6% in children with idiopathic epilepsy, and 58.3% in children with both seizures and central nervous system damage [2]. Other studies compared the rates of psychological problems in children with epilepsy to rates in children with other chronic conditions. Austin et al. [3] found children with epilepsy to have higher rates of psychological and social problems than a comparison sample of children with asthma. In addition, Hoare [4] found 48% of children with epilepsy to have psychological problems compared to 17% of children with diabetes. McDermott et al. [1] found children with epilepsy to have higher rates of psychiatric problems (31%) than children with cardiac problems (21%) or controls (8.5%).

Academic Achievement Problems

Problems at school are overrepresented in children with epilepsy, whose academic performance has consistently been found to be poorer than what would be expected by their intellectual ability (5). A large epidemiologic study found that children with uncomplicated epilepsy were, on average, about 1 year delayed in overall reading ability and approximately 20% of them demonstrated severe deficits (6). More recent studies also indicate that children with epilepsy make less academic progress in arithmetic, reading, comprehension, and word recognition than would be expected for their age and intelligence level (7,8). In research with children, Austin et al. (9–11) found 32.6% were receiving some form of special education service and 44% repeated at least one grade in school. They also found children with epilepsy to have significantly lower academic achievement scores than children with asthma. Boys with more severe epilepsy were the group most at risk of underachievement (12). When they explored change in academic achievement 4 years later, they found that children with epilepsy continued to perform significantly worse academically, even though half of them had inactive epilepsy (i.e., no seizures and no medication). No changes in academic achievement were found over time, even for those whose seizure conditions had improved (9). There also is empirical evidence that these achievement problems can continue into adulthood. A recent 35-year follow-up study of adults with childhood onset of epilepsy found that their vocational problems were significantly more common than in a control sample (13,14).

These high rates of mental health and academic achievement problems strongly indicate that attention to psychosocial adjustment should be a critical component in the overall management of the child with epilepsy. A first step in addressing these problems is to understand better the psychosocial stressors confronting children with epilepsy and their families.

PSYCHOSOCIAL ISSUES

Psychosocial issues can vary by the duration of the seizure disorder. Some issues occur early in the course of the disorder, and others occur or become more paramount when the child's condition continues over time. Also, because psychosocial issues can vary by the age of the child, it is important to consider these issues within a developmental context. In this section, psychosocial issues by duration (new onset and chronic) and child age are reviewed.

Duration of Seizure Disorder

Issues at Onset

It can be safely assumed that parents desire children who are healthy and otherwise conform to societal ideals. Consequently, when parents are confronted with having a child with any potentially chronic physical condition, they often have a strong negative response. Seeing their child have the first seizure has been reported by parents to be a most frightening and confusing experience. Parents often react to a first seizure with a range of strong emotions including shock, fear, sadness, anger, and guilt (15).

Once parents are informed that their child has a seizure condition, they have many concerns and fears. Ward and Bower (16) found parents of children with newly diagnosed seizures to express fear surrounding the seizures. These fears were related to the nature of the seizures including noise, interruptions in breathing, loss of consciousness, twisting and jerking, and eye movements such as staring. Other commonly mentioned concerns were related to their child having a social handicap and to their child being physically injured.

In a more recent study, Austin et al. (17) found the concerns and fears of parents whose children recently had a first seizure to be focused in two areas: (i) the effect of seizures and their treatment, and (ii) managing their child's epilepsy (17). Parents were most concerned about the cause of the seizure and the future course of the condition. Early concerns focused on the effects of the seizure on their child's brain, mental health, activities, and future vocation. Parents' management concerns were grouped into four areas: (i) seizures, (ii) responses of others, (iii) lifestyle, and (iv) mental health (17). In the area of seizures, they were unsure how to handle their child's future seizures, including when to take them to the hospital and when to call the physician. They also were worried about potentially negative side effects of the antiepilepsy medication on their child. They were concerned about knowing which side effects to report to the physician. Interestingly, even though these children had just had their first seizure, their parents were already concerned about the stigma associated with epilepsy, including how to handle potentially negative responses to their child by others. Parents also were worried about how to tell others about their child's epilepsy in such a way that they would not treat the child differently. When the children were school aged, their parents were especially concerned about their peers teasing them because of the seizures. In the area of lifestyle changes, parents were concerned about keeping their child safe without overprotecting them or interfering with their normal development. Finally, parents were worried about their child developing mental health problems. For example, some parents were aware of the association between epilepsy and mental illness and were worried about how to prevent their child from developing problems.

When children are old enough to understand what is happening, they also find the onset of seizures to be frightening. Austin (18) found school-aged children to have many concerns about seizures, antiepilepsy medication, and responses of others. Children were worried about what caused their seizure, and some attempted to identify possible causes. They had many questions about the nature of seizures, including what causes the jerking and shaking during a seizure. Some were con-

cerned about their prognosis and if their condition would get worse. Some children experienced anxiety associated with the context of the first seizure. For example, those who had their first seizures in bed often were afraid to be alone in bed; likewise, those who had their first seizures at school were fearful of returning to school. Finally, some children were concerned that seizures might hurt them. For example, several children were concerned about dying, and some were concerned about becoming mentally ill or not being able to grow up normally. Treatment-related concerns of children, which focused on the tests (electroencephalogram, blood tests, and imaging), included worry about what the tests were for and what the results were. Children were worried when they saw other severely disabled children in physicians' waiting rooms; children with epilepsy thought that they might become like them because they were seeing the same doctor (18). Children also were concerned about the possibility that their peers would make fun of them or tease them about having seizures.

Issues with a Chronic Condition

As time passes and families realize that their child has a chronic seizure condition, they realize they must deal with the ramifications of living with a chronic seizure condition. There can be a relentlessness to having a chronic condition, such as epilepsy, because it is always there at some level. Even in periods of good seizure control, the possibility of a period of seizure hangs over the families' heads (19). The uncertainty of when the next seizure will occur is a major psychosocial stressor for these children and their families. Although over time parents and children can gain experience in dealing with seizures, they also are confronted with new and continuing issues related to epilepsy. As children age, they are able to comprehend more about the ramifications of living with seizures and become aware of new psychosocial issues that need to be addressed. As the ability of the child who has the seizure condition as well as the ability of siblings to understand increases, parents need to teach them how to cope with the seizure condition.

These families are confronted with incorporating the epilepsy into their daily lives and helping the child make a satisfactory adjustment. Knafl (20) points out that families of children with chronic conditions have many tasks, including making sense of the condition, mastering treatments, creating a normal life for the child, adapting the family's routine to the condition, and negotiating with school and health care professionals. Families of children with epilepsy need to become competent in managing their child's seizure condition and in teaching the child to take over responsibility for their own treatment when they are old enough. Over time, the family is confronted with continuing inconveniences, including regular trips to the doctor and pharmacy, as well as their associated costs.

In addition to the psychosocial issues common to all chronic childhood conditions, epilepsy presents unique challenges for the child and family. First, there continue to be issues related to stigma (21,22). Parents and children have concerns about disclosure of the epilepsy, including who, when, and what to tell persons about the epilepsy so that negative effects can be minimized. Perceptions of stigma being related to epilepsy have been associated with an increase in mental health problems, especially low self-esteem (23). The high rates of mental health problems in children with epilepsy increase the likelihood that families will be confronted with some mental health-related problems over the course of chronic epilepsy. The most common mental health problems are behavior disturbances, poor self-concept, social isolation, and depression (2–4,24,25). Having a child with these mental health problems also leads to more psychosocial stressors for the whole family.

The longer the child has seizures and the more frequent the seizures, the more urgent is the need to have a plan for dealing with possible seizures at school. Each year, parents are faced with informing the child's teacher about their child's seizures and developing a strategy with the teacher for handling seizures at school. Moreover, the high rates of academic achievement problems mean that many children with epilepsy will experience these problems. These problems are a source of stress for both the child and the parents. In addition to dealing with the school system about their child's learning problems and helping the child with homework issues, parents worry about the long-term effect of their child's poor school performance. Will the child be able to handle college work or vocational training? Finally, youth with epilepsy who also have problems with school achievement are even more at risk of mental health problems (26). For example, doing poorly at school can contribute to poor self-esteem.

Psychosocial Issues Related to Child's Age

Infancy and Early Childhood

Infants need a safe, nurturing environment and attachment to a stable adult in order to learn trust (27), which is the major developmental task of infancy. If parents are so burdened by their own inability to cope with the epilepsy that they are unable to respond adequately to the infant's needs, the infant might not learn to trust. In early childhood, children need a family environment where they are able to become increasingly independent. They have daily routines, become socialized, master toilet training and other self-care activities, and learn to communicate with others (28). For optimal psychosocial development, these children need an environment where they can develop autonomy and initiative (29). If parents have a poor response to the epilepsy that involves overprotection or overindulgence, it could deprive the child of experiencing feelings of competence (30). If parents are overly protective and concerned about injury from a seizure, they may overrestrict the child's activities and hinder his or her development of life skills.

Middle Childhood

In middle childhood, developmental tasks include becoming more independent from parents and more attached to peers. Active involvement in a peer group is critically important to the psychosocial development of the child. It also is important for children in middle childhood to experience success in school to facilitate the development of industry. Achievement in school can provide an opportunity for the child to receive recognition from others and to experience a sense of accomplishment. Epilepsy can interfere with the accomplishment of these tasks. Children with epilepsy recognize that they have a condition that most other children do not have. If they associate negative feelings with their seizure condition, it could lead to feeling different, withdrawal from peers, and poor self-esteem. According to Massie (31), children with chronic conditions incorporate the illness into their self-concept. Because negative feelings are associated with their seizure condition, it can lead to negative feelings about themselves.

There is empirical evidence in the literature that children with epilepsy can have problems with completion of some of these developmental tasks. For example, children with epilepsy have been found to be more dependent than children with tonsillectomies (32). Child social development has been associated with parenting behaviors. Social maturity and social skills in children with epilepsy were found to be positively related to parental strictness (33). In their investigation of parenting behaviors in mother–child interactions, Lothman et al. (34) found maternal praise to be related to child competence and child positive affect. Conversely, intrusive and overcontrolling parenting behaviors were related to decreased child autonomy and child confidence.

Adolescence

The primary developmental task of adolescence is to consolidate one's identity (28). Ideally, adolescents should emerge into adulthood with a strong sense of identity, with both positive and negative feelings of self integrated into a coherent whole. Other major tasks include the achievement of independence from parents, establishment of intimate relationships outside the family, and identification of a vocation. Peer group membership plays an important role in the social development of adolescents and in their becoming independent from their family. The presence of a chronic condition such as epilepsy can interfere with the accomplishment of these developmental tasks and lead to a prolonged adolescence period (35). Compared to their healthy peers, adolescents with chronic conditions are more likely to be overprotected, to have less experience with peers, and to have fewer appropriate role models (35). The failure to develop a strong sense of self as competent can lead to problems with poor self-esteem and feelings of being different from others.

When youth with epilepsy are overprotected and sheltered by their parents, it reduces their opportunities to interact with peers. Youth with epilepsy can have problems meeting the developmental accomplishments of adolescence. The occurrence of seizures and the need to take medication can lead to a reduced sense of physical competence. The stigma associated with epilepsy can have a negative impact on how youth perceive themselves, socially and physically. Even youth with newly diagnosed epilepsy have been found to feel different from their peers and to worry about being teased by peers (18). The episodic loss of control caused by seizures can make it more difficult for these adolescents to become independent and to separate from families. The inability to drive a car at an age-appropriate time can be a major problem for adolescents with epilepsy, because it limits opportunities for developing independence and participation in social activities (36). Parental overprotection can deprive the child of experiencing the feelings of competence and subsequently affect later self-esteem (30).

A final area where the presence of epilepsy might affect social functioning is in academics. Success in school facilitates the development of industry. School achievement also provides an opportunity for the youth to receive recognition from others and to derive a sense of accomplishment. Not only do these school problems reduce opportunities for the development of a sense of pride and accomplishment, but they also place these youth at risk for later vocational problems.

FACTORS ASSOCIATED WITH PSYCHOSOCIAL ADJUSTMENT PROBLEMS

Although factors accounting for the mental health and academic achievement problems in children with epilepsy have not been well delineated (5), research has identified some factors associated with higher rates of problems. Before interventions can be designed to prevent or reduce these problems, it is important to identify causal factors. Four broad factors have been identified as being associated with higher rates of child psychosocial adjustment problems: (i) neurologic dysfunction, (ii) high seizure frequency and more antiepileptic drugs, (iii) negative family response, and (iv) negative child response. Evidence for the association of each of these factors with increased problems and how they might interact with psychosocial issues for the child and the family are reviewed.

Neurologic Factors

Children with epilepsy and accompanying deficits in neurologic functioning have long been known to be at increased risk of both mental health and academic achievement problems (37–39). That the rate of problems is higher in children with neurologic conditions than in chronic childhood physical conditions without neurologic involvement (2,40,41) suggests that neurologic deficits might be involved to some degree in the development of both mental health and academic achievement problems. Also, the high rate of behavior problems in children with both epilepsy and mental retardation (59%)

found by Steffenburg et al. (42) further supports that neurologic dysfunction is an important risk factor. Finally, studies showing that children with new-onset seizures have higher than expected rates of psychological problems suggest that an underlying neurologic dysfunction might play a role in the development of behavior problems in children with epilepsy. For example, Dunn et al. (43) found that 24% of children who recently had their first recognized seizure had behavior problem scores in the at-risk range on a standardized scale. In addition, Hoare (4) found 45% of children with new-onset epilepsy had a psychiatric disturbance.

The specific ways that neurologic deficits might cause psychosocial adjustment problems in children with epilepsy have not been specified. One hypothesis is that underlying brain structure and function abnormalities cause neuropsychological functioning deficits, such as poor attention, slow psychomotor speed, memory and learning problems, and poor executive skills (e.g., abstract reasoning) and that these deficits, in turn, lead to mental health and academic achievement problems (44). Another reason these children have more adjustment problems might be because they are experiencing more psychosocial stressors than children without neurologic deficits. These children must cope with seizures and neurologic deficits. Because these children also are experiencing problems in neuropsychological functioning, they probably have fewer available cognitive resources to deal with the demands of having a chronic health condition. For example, if they have limited ability to engage in abstract reasoning, it might be more difficult for them to engage in problem-solving coping. In other words, children with epilepsy who also have deficits in neurologic functioning might experience more psychosocial problems and have more difficulty coping with them. Neurologic dysfunction can lead to serious learning problems, causing additional stress related to doing poorly in school. Finally, having these additional problems could contribute to the child feeling even more different from his or her peers, which can negatively affect the child's self-concept.

Seizures and Antiepileptic Medications

Factors such as seizure characteristics and antiepileptic medication side effects have been identified as being associated with an increase in psychosocial problems in children with epilepsy. Seizure variables that have been found to be related to psychological problems include early age of onset, long duration of epilepsy, high seizure frequency, and multiple seizure types (4,45,46). The most consistent finding has been a link between higher seizure frequency and psychosocial functioning problems. There also is some evidence that antiepileptic medication is associated with psychosocial problems. For example, the barbiturates have been associated with depression, irritability, conduct disorder, and hyperactivity (47). It also appears that polytherapy (treatment with more than one antiepileptic medication) is more likely to be associated with poorer psychological functioning than monotherapy (47,48).

The consistent finding appears to be that the more severe the seizure condition (i.e., the longer the time the child has had seizures, the more seizures he or she has had, and the more types of seizures he or she has experienced), the more likely the child is to have mental health and academic achievement problems. Aicardi (49) proposes that transient cognitive impairment caused by subclinical epileptiform discharges leads to disorganization and suppression of normal brain functioning. Children with more severe seizure conditions would be more likely to have more subclinical epileptiform discharges and, therefore, more mental health and academic achievement problems. Another potential cause of more adjustment problems might be that children who are having more seizures also have more psychosocial stressors because of living with uncontrolled seizures. For example, more frequent seizures could lead to more opportunities for the child to be confronted with the stigma and to be teased by peers. Having a more severe seizure condition could lead to these children having more academic achievement problems and feeling different from their healthy peers.

Negative Parental Response

The family not only is affected by the epilepsy in a child, but the family's response also is hypothesized to affect the child's adjustment to the epilepsy. Poor parent response to the epilepsy is believed to complicate the child's psychosocial adjustment to the epilepsy. Episodic conditions that are unpredictable, such as epilepsy, present unique stressors for the family. Families must cope with this unpredictability, help the child with seizures deal with the experience, and help others associated with the child to cope with the epilepsy (50). Negative parental attitudes toward the epilepsy are proposed to be associated with psychosocial adaptation problems in the child (51). Austin et al. (45) found family stress and fewer family adaptive resources (low extended family social support and lower levels of family mastery) to be positively associated with child mental health problems.

Parent response has been found to be important in child academic achievement. It has been suggested that parental expectations for academic achievement are reduced in children with epilepsy, and these reduced expectations are associated with poorer school performance (52). In addition, Mitchell et al. (53) found that academic achievement was predicted by high parent education, educational materials in the home, and family participation in developmentally stimulating activities. The child's environment is important in helping the child make a satisfactory adjustment to a chronic health condition. When the child is in an environment where the parents are having problems coping with the seizure condition, the child has fewer family resources to help them deal with the condition.

Psychosocial issues can increase for these children because their parents' negative response to their health condition could lead to increased family conflict. For example, if the family overprotects or overrestricts the child's activities, it can lead to conflict about the child's activities. In addition, a negative family response to the epilepsy could lead to the child having a negative attitude toward having epilepsy. Research indicates that negative attitudes toward having epilepsy and lower levels of youth satisfaction with family relationships are associated with depression in adolescents with epilepsy (54).

Negative Child Response

A poor response to the epilepsy on the part of the child has been identified as a potential cause of mental health and academic achievement problems. Poor child response generally includes the child adopting a negative attitude toward having epilepsy and using negative coping strategies, such as becoming irritable, withdrawing from others, and resisting taking medication. The few studies that have been conducted on the relationships between child response and adjustment problems support the relationship. Austin and Huberty (55) found children's negative attitudes toward having epilepsy to be related to behavior problems, symptoms of depression, and poor self-concept. When Austin et al. (56) investigated the relationship between child coping and psychological functioning, positive coping strategies of developing competence, optimism, treatment compliance, and seeking support were associated with fewer behavior problems. In contrast, negative coping strategies of irritability, feeling different, and social withdrawal were related to more behavior problems.

One child characteristic that is thought to influence the child's response is temperament, which refers to the child's behavioral style in activity, mood, and emotional response (57). A more difficult temperament has been linked to mental health problems in normal childhood populations and in children with chronic health conditions, including neurologic conditions (58). In contrast, more positive temperamental characteristics may help the child in dealing with a chronic condition and the

stressors associated with living with epilepsy. Temperament also may play a role in academic achievement problems. Child temperament has been found to be related to cognitive functioning in healthy children (59) and to predict problem-solving ability and mother–child interactions during problem-solving tasks in early childhood (60). Finally, aspects of child temperament, such as task orientation, have been found to influence teacher-student interactions (61).

Children with a more negative response to having epilepsy most likely will have a negative response to the psychosocial stressors associated with having epilepsy. For example, they may have heightened anxiety about dying, or they may be overly concerned about the negative effects of seizures on the brain or the side effects of medication. A child with a negative attitude about having epilepsy could view the additional psychosocial stressors as further reasons for having a negative attitude and for not trying. Also, a child who uses negative coping strategies might have more problems coping with the learning problems associated with epilepsy. Children with a difficult temperament may find the additional challenges of a chronic health condition to be much more disruptive than a child with an easy temperament.

PSYCHOSOCIAL CARE NEEDS

Recently, there has been an increase in emphasis on family satisfaction with care and on how well psychosocial care needs of children with epilepsy and their parents are being met by health care personnel. Two scales (Parent Report of Psychosocial Care, and Child Report of Psychosocial Care) were developed recently by Austin et al. (12) to measure psychosocial care needs of both children with new-onset seizures and their parents. Three areas of care are measured by each of the scales: satisfaction with information received, needs for information or support, and concerns and fears. Other researchers focused more on satisfaction with care and the factors associated with satisfaction.

Parent Psychosocial Care Needs

Parental satisfaction with care has been addressed in several studies. Good communication with health care personnel has consistently been associated with satisfaction with care for children with epilepsy. Suurmeijer (62) studied the communication and relationship between patient or family and the providers of health care. The major outcome variable, patient and family's satisfaction with care, was conceptualized as the match between care provided and needs of the patient and family. He found that one-third of the parents or partners of individuals with epilepsy believed there was inadequate access to, and/or communication with, care providers and were not satisfied with the care given.

Shore et al. (63) administered the Parent Report of Psychosocial Care Scale to 125 parents of children with recent-onset seizures. In general, the level of satisfaction with information received from doctors and nurses was relatively high. Parents were most satisfied with information related to administration of medication and least satisfied with the amount of information they received about handling their child's seizure condition at school. About half of the mothers reported being less than satisfied with the information they received on handling seizures at school. Approximately two-thirds of mothers and about half of the fathers had at least some need for more information in the following areas: seizures, treatment information, possible causes of seizures, handling future seizures, restriction of their child's activities, and how to prevent their child from being injured. Approximately half of the mothers and one-third of the fathers had at least some need for support, including the need for general support and encouragement, help with handling responses of others, discussing fears about their child's future, discussing fears about seizures, discussing mental heath concerns, and help with handling their child's response to the seizures. About two-thirds of mothers and about half of the fathers wanted their child to have an opportunity to discuss their seizure condition with another child who also had seizures. Mothers had more needs for support than did fathers, and these needs did not appear to decrease during the first 6 months after seizure onset.

Parental satisfaction with epilepsy services, including overall quality of amount of information given, attitude of clinic staff, time spent with staff, recommendations for clinic use to other parents, and comfort in contacting clinic staff, was studied by Williams et al. (64). In general, parents found the overall quality of the clinic to be excellent. Their overall rating was most highly associated with the amount of information they received related to diagnosis and treatment of seizure disorders. A large majority (84%) of the parents indicated that the clinic staff had helped them deal more effectively with the epilepsy and increased their understanding of their child's developmental needs. In this study, the number of clinic visits was not associated with satisfaction with care.

Webb et al. (65) made a general assessment of care for children with epilepsy. The first part of their study was an audit on correspondence, prescription of medication, and laboratory use. They also mailed a 13-item questionnaire measuring parental satisfaction with epilepsy care, with specific questions about courtesy, communication, and the process of the clinic visit. Results indicated that parents were satisfied with the clinic visits and the courtesy of staff, but only half were mostly or very satisfied with the explanation of epilepsy, information given, or questions answered. Hanai (66) sent questionnaires about seizures, medication, behavior, school, and future prospects to parents. He found parents to be worried about their child's seizures, school performance, and their child's future. The author highlighted the importance of comprehensive care that would meet the needs of children with epilepsy and their families.

Child Psychosocial Care Needs

Fewer studies have been carried out to identify children's self-reported needs for psychosocial care and satisfaction with care. McNelis et al. (67) and Brown (68) both questioned children. McNelis et al. (67) studied children with first seizures and found that, 6 months after seizure onset, up to 40% were less than satisfied with the information they had received and over half wanted more information in several areas. They found that 38% of children felt that they were not fully informed about how the antiepileptic medication worked. A similar proportion felt that they were not given sufficient opportunity to talk about their fears and worries about their seizure condition and its effect on their life. Over two-thirds of the children wanted information on handling future seizures, preventing injuries during seizures, and the possible causes of their seizures. Brown (68) sent questionnaires to children with seizures. Approximately one-third of them reported that their physicians had not talked to them about their seizures. Moreover, of the group whose physicians had talked to them about their seizures, about half reported that they did not understand what the doctor said. These results suggested that children had other concerns that needed to be addressed. Approximately two-thirds described fatigue from the antiepileptic drug, and half experienced feelings of helplessness, being scared, or being different from others. As a whole, these studies strongly indicate that children have many psychosocial care needs that are not being addressed adequately in the clinical setting.

SUMMARY AND CONCLUSIONS

Children with epilepsy are a vulnerable population. They have high rates of mental health and academic achievement problems that can reduce their quality of life both in childhood and into adulthood. Epilepsy presents unique psychosocial stressors for both the child and the family because of its unpredictability, sometimes frightening display of symptoms, and associated stigma. Children with more severe epilepsy, neuropsychological deficits, or a difficult temperament are at special risk for poor psychosocial outcomes.

It is essential that a regular assessment of the child's mental health and academic functioning be conducted. It also is important that children who are at greater risk of problems be targeted for prevention programs.

Parents of children with epilepsy have additional stressors with which to cope. They need to make a successful adjustment to their child's epilepsy. They must help their child with the condition and help other members of the family make a satisfactory accommodation to the epilepsy. It is important that the parents' response to the epilepsy be systematically assessed in the clinical setting so that negative responses can be immediately identified and addressed. Finally, it is important that the psychosocial care needs of the child and the family be routinely assessed and strategies implemented to provide them with needed information and support.

ACKNOWLEDGMENT

The author acknowledges support from the National Institute for Neurological Disorders and Stroke (NS22416) and the National Institute of Nursing Research (NR04536) in preparation of this chapter.

REFERENCES

1. McDermott S, Mani S, Krishnaswami S. A population-based analysis of specific behavior problems associated with childhood seizures. *J Epilepsy* 1995;8:110–118.
2. Rutter M, Graham P, Yule W. A neuropsychiatric study in childhood. *Clin Dev Med* 1970;35/36.
3. Austin JK, Smith MS, Risinger MW, et al. Childhood epilepsy and asthma: comparison of quality of life. *Epilepsia* 1994;35:608–615.
4. Hoare P. The development of psychiatric disorder among school children with epilepsy. *Dev Med Child Neurol* 1984;26:3–13.
5. Seidenberg M, Berent S. Childhood epilepsy and the role of psychology. *Am Psychol* 1992;47:1130–1133.
6. Yule W. Educational achievement. In: Kerley BM, Meinardi H, Stores G, eds. *Epilepsy and behavior.* Lisse, The Netherlands: Swets and Zeitlinger, 1980: 162–168.
7. Seidenberg M, Beck N, Geisser M, et al. Academic achievement of children with epilepsy. *Epilepsia* 1986; 27:753–759.
8. Seidenberg M, Beck N, Geisser M, et al. Neuropsychological correlates of academic achievement of children with epilepsy. *J Epilepsy* 1988;1:23–29.

9. Austin JK, Huberty TJ, Huster GA, et al. Does academic achievement in children with epilepsy change over time? *Dev Med Child Neurol* 1999;41:473–479.
10. Huberty TJ, Austin JK, Risinger MW, et al. Relationship of selected seizure variables in children with epilepsy to performance on school-administered achievement tests. *J Epilepsy* 1992;5:10–16.
11. Huberty TJ, Austin JK, Risinger MW, et al. Classroom performance and adaptive skills in children with epilepsy. *J School Psychol* 1992;30:331–342.
12. Austin JK, Huberty TJ, Huster GA, et al. Academic achievement in children with epilepsy or asthma. *Dev Med Child Neurol* 1998;40:248–255.
13. Jalava M, Sillanpaa M, Camfield C, et al. Social adjustment and competence 35 years after onset of childhood epilepsy: a prospective controlled study. *Epilepsia* 1997;38:708–715.
14. Sillanpaa M, Jalava M, Kaleva O, et al. Long-term prognosis of seizures with onset in childhood. *N Engl J Med* 1998;338:1715–1722.
15. Voeller KK, Rothenberg MB. Psychosocial aspects of the management of seizures in children. *Pediatrics* 1973;51:1072–1082.
16. Ward F, Bower BD. A study of certain social aspects of epilepsy in childhood. *Dev Med Child Neurol* 1978;20:1–63.
17. Austin JK, Oruche UM, Dunn DW, et al. New-onset childhood seizures: parents' concerns and needs. *Clin Nurs Pract Epilepsy* 1995;2:8–10.
18. Austin JK. Concerns and fears of children with seizures. *Clin Nurs Pract Epilepsy* 1993;1:4–6.
19. Rolland JS. A conceptual model of chronic and life-threatening illness and its impact on families. In: Chilman CS, Nunnally EW, Cox FM, eds. *Chronic illness and disability.* Newbury Park, CA: Sage Publications, 1988:1–68.
20. Knafl KA. Meeting the challenges of chronic illness for children and families. In: Broome ME, Knafl K, Pridham K, et al., eds. *Children and families in health and illness.* Thousand Oaks, CA: Sage Publications, 1998:236–245.
21. Baumann RJ, Wilson JF, Wiese J. Kentuckians' attitudes toward children with epilepsy. *Epilepsia* 1995;36:1003–1008.
22. Gordon N, Sillanpaa M. Epilepsy and prejudice with particular relevance to childhood. *Dev Med Child Neurol* 1997;39:777–781.
23. Westbrook LE, Bauman LJ, Shinnar S. Applying stigma theory to epilepsy: a test of a conceptual model. *J Pediatr Psychol* 1992;17:633–649.
24. Margalit M, Heiman T. Anxiety and self-dissatisfaction in epileptic children. *Int J Soc Psychiatry* 1983;29:220–224.
25. Matthews WS, Barabas G, Ferrari M. Emotional concomitants of childhood epilepsy. *Epilepsia* 1982;23:671–681.
26. Sturniolo MG, Galletti F. Idiopathic epilepsy and school achievement. *Arch Dis Child* 1994;70:424–428.
27. Lipsitt LP. Stress in infancy: toward understanding the origins of coping behavior. In: Garmezy W, Rutter M, eds. *Stress, coping and development in children.* New York: McGraw-Hill, 1983:161–180.
28. Billingham KA. *Developmental psychology for health care professions.* Boulder, CO: Westview Press, 1982.
29. Freiberg KL. *Human development: a life span approach,* 2nd ed. Monterey, CA: Wadsworth Health Sciences Division, 1983.
30. McCollum AT. *The chronically ill child: a guide for parents and professionals.* New Haven, CT: Yale University Press, 1981.
31. Massie RK. The constant shadow: reflections on the life of a chronically ill child. In: Hobbs N, Perrin JM, eds. *Issues in the care of children with chronic illness.* San Francisco: Josey-Bass Publishers, 1985:13–23.
32. Hartlage LC, Green JB, Offutt L. Dependency in epileptic children. *Epilepsia* 1972;13:27–30.
33. Hartlage LC, Green JB. The relation of parental attitudes to academic and social achievement in epileptic children. *Epilepsia* 1972;13:21–26.
34. Lothman DJ, Pianta RC, Clarson SM. Mother-child interaction in children with epilepsy: relations with child competence. *J Epilepsy* 1990;3:157–163.
35. Strax TE. Psychological issues faced by adolescents and young adults with disabilities. *Pediatr Ann* 1991;20:507–511.
36. Dean P, Austin JK. Adolescent psychosocial issues in epilepsy. *Clin Nurs Pract Epilepsy* 1996;3:4–6.
37. Hermann BP. Deficits in neuropsychological functioning and psychopathology in persons with epilepsy: a rejected hypothesis revisited. *Epilepsia* 1981;22:161–167.
38. Hermann BP. Neurological functioning and psychopathology in children with epilepsy. *Epilepsia* 1982;22:703–710.
39. Rutter M. Psychological sequelae of brain damage in children. *Am J Psychiatry* 1981;138:1533–1544.
40. Breslau N. Psychiatric disorder in children with physical disabilities. *J Am Acad Child Psychiatry* 1985;24:87–94.
41. Howe GW, Feinstein C, Reiss D, et al. Adolescent adjustment to chronic physical disorders—I. Comparing neurological and non-neurological conditions. *J Child Psychol Psychiatry* 1993;34:1153–1171.
42. Steffenburg S, Gillberg C, Steffenburg U. Psychiatric disorders in children and adolescents with mental retardation and active epilepsy. *Arch Neurol* 1996;53:904–912.
43. Dunn DW, Austin JK, Huster GA. Behavior problems in children with new-onset epilepsy. *Seizure* 1997;6:283–287.
44. Papero PH, Howe DW, Reiss D. Neuropsychological function and psychosocial deficit in adolescents with chronic neurological impairment. *J Dev Phys Disabil* 1992;4:317–340.
45. Austin JK, Risinger MW, Beckett L. Correlates of behavior problems in children with epilepsy. *Epilepsia* 1992;33:1115–1122.
46. Hermann BP, Whitman S, Dell J. Correlates of behavior problems and social competence in children with epilepsy, aged 6–11. In: Hermann BP, Seidenberg M, eds. *Childhood epilepsies: neurological, psychological and intervention aspects.* New York: John Wiley and Sons, 1989:143–157.
47. Trimble MR, Cull CA. Children of school age: the influence of antiepileptic drugs. *Epilepsia* 1988;29[Suppl 3]:15–19.
48. Trimble MR, Cull CA. Antiepileptic drugs, cognitive function, and behavior in children. *Cleve Clin J Med* 1989;56[Suppl Pt 1]:140–146.
49. Aicardi J. Epilepsy as a non-paroxysmal disorder. *Acta Neuropediatr* 1996;2:249–257.

50. Austin JK. A model of family adaptation to new-onset childhood epilepsy. *J Neurosci Nurs* 1996;28:82–92.

51. Bagley C. Social prejudice and the adjustment of people with epilepsy. *Epilepsia* 1972;13:33–45.

52. Green JB, Hartlage LC. Comparative performance of epileptic and nonepileptic children and adolescents. *Dis Nerv Syst* 1971;32:418–421.

53. Mitchell WG, Chavez JM, Lee H, et al. Academic underachievement in children with epilepsy. *J Child Neurol* 1991;6:65–72.

54. Dunn DW, Austin JK, Huster GA. Symptoms of depression in adolescents with epilepsy. *J Am Acad Child Adolesc Psychiatry* 1999;38:1132–1138.

55. Austin JK, Huberty TJ. Development of the Child Attitude Toward Illness Scale. *J Pediatr Psychol* 1993;18:467–480.

56. Austin JK, Patterson JM, Huberty TJ. Development of the Coping Health Inventory for Children (CHIC). *J Pediatr Nurs* 1991;6:166–174.

57. Bates JE. Concepts and measurement of temperament. In: Kohnstamm GA, Bates JE, Rothbart MK, eds. *Temperament in childhood.* New York: John Wiley and Sons, 1989:3026.

58. Wallander JL, Hubert NC, Varni JW. Child and maternal temperament characteristics, goodness of fit, and adjustment in physically handicapped children. *J Clin Child Psychol* 1988;17:336–344.

59. Plumert JM, Schwebel DC. Social and temperamental influences on children's overestimation of their physical abilities: links to accidental injuries. *J Exp Child Psychol* 1997;67:317–337.

60. Fagot BI, Gauvain M. Mother-child problem solving: continuity through the early childhood years. *Dev Psychol* 1997;33:480–488.

61. Rothbart MK, Jones LB. Temperament: developmental perspectives. In: Gallimore R, Bernheimer LP, MacMillan DL, et al., eds. *Developmental perspectives on children with high-incidence disabilities.* Mahwah, NJ: Lawrence Erlbaum Associates, 1999:33–53.

62. Suurmeijer TPBM. Quality of care and quality of life from the perspective of patients and families. *Int J Adolesc Med Health* 1994;7:281–288.

63. Shore C, Austin J, Musick B, et al. Psychosocial care needs of parents of children with new-onset seizures. *J Neurosci Nurs* 1998;30:169–174.

64. Williams J, Sharp GB, Griebel ML, et al. Outcome findings from a multidisciplinary clinic for children with epilepsy. *Child Health Care* 1995;24:235–244.

65. Webb DW, Coleman AF, Fielder A, et al. An audit of paediatric epilepsy care. *Arch Dis Child* 1998;79:145–148.

66. Hanai T. Quality of life in children with epilepsy. *Epilepsia* 1996;37:28–32.

67. McNelis A, Musick B, Austin J, et al. Psychosocial care needs of children with new-onset seizures. *J Neurosci Nurs* 1998;30:161–165.

68. Brown SW. Quality of life—a view from the playground. *Seizure* 1994;3:11–15.

23

Psychiatric and Psychological Impact of Sexual Problems in Epilepsy

Donna C. Bergen and *Sandra D. Hamberger

*Department of Neurological Sciences, Rush Medical College, Chicago, Illinois 60612;
and *Comprehensive Epilepsy Center, Long Island Jewish Health Systems,
New Hyde Park, New York 11040*

Chronic epilepsy can have a profound effect on sexual function in both men and women. Although many people with well-controlled seizure disorders (who make up the majority of those with epilepsy) experience little alteration in their sexual lives, others find that vital areas of their lives, such as sexual relations, marital life, and child-bearing, can be seriously distorted by epilepsy or its treatment. Clinicians' awareness of these complications and appropriate and timely interventions can prevent them or, at the least, minimize their impact on the sexual lives of these patients.

Whereas a limited literature on sexuality in epilepsy focuses on potential physiologic dysfunction, there is virtually nothing written about the impact of having epilepsy on quality of life related to sexuality issues. In preparing this chapter, the authors surveyed several epilepsy social service institutions and psychiatrists regarding concerns about sexuality expressed by their epileptic patients. We were surprised to find that this topic almost never was discussed. Our own experience and the paucity of information in the medical literature suggest that professionals do not address intimate details of their patients' sexual experiences. Future studies will need to address the impact of epilepsy and its treatment on sexual desire, sexual arousal, and the capacity for satisfactory sexual functioning.

The following case study exemplifies the need to investigate these issues in our epileptic patients. In this example, sexual problems developed when a husband's seizure disorder became a major stressor in a marital relationship. These consequences affected the patient, the partner, and, ultimately, the entire family.

CASE REPORT

The patient was a 45-year-old white man with a history of simple and complex partial seizures since the age of 6 years, who was referred for counseling because of symptoms of depression. These symptoms began following a series of misfortunes that included the death of his mother, the impending loss of his job, and the ending of his 18-year marriage. He had intractable seizures with a frequency of one to two seizures per month. A salient element of his psychosocial history revolved around the potential impact of seizures on his marital relationship. Before getting married, he experienced great timidity toward women and ascribed it to his seizure disorder. He could not conceive achieving a marital relationship and was passive in pursuing relationships to avoid being rejected. The patient met his future wife the night of a New York City blackout; they helped each other find their ways home. There was an immediate attraction, and she initiated the first contact. He informed her of his epilepsy on their first date; however, she assured him that his seizures would not interfere with their "budding relationship."

Her background was notable for a history of childhood emotional and sexual abuse; she had been raped twice. Her parents expressed their disapproval of her relationship with "a man with epilepsy." However, over time, he perceived that he had won them over using his warmth, sense of family values, and decency. This opened the way for their marriage 1 year later. Sue had a high-paying position and earned a higher salary than he. The patient was unwilling to advance to a supervisory position for fear that the anticipated stress could increase his seizure frequency.

During the first 5 years of marriage, he experienced occasional auras during sexual contacts with her. During these times, he would lose his erection and was unable to perform. She would feel rejected and was left with feelings of inadequacy. She expressed a feeling of failure as a sex partner. The patient also confided that if a seizure had occurred at work during the day, he would be fearful of having sexual relations that night and afraid that sexual activity could provoke more seizures. However, if he did engage in intercourse, he would "pray and take deep breaths" to assuage these fears.

In their sixth year of marriage, he had a major seizure during coitus. After that incident, she suffered from anticipatory anxiety that he would experience seizure recurrences during intercourse. In response to her own concerns, she prepared alcoholic drinks prior to intercourse to "relax both of them." However, the patient declined, to avoid mixing alcohol with antiepileptic drugs (AEDs). She drank by herself and expressed a feeling of being alone. After 17 years of marriage, she became involved in an extramarital relation that she did not hide from her husband. The patient refused to see that his marriage was deteriorating and did not confront his wife. Finally, she separated from him and moved out of state with their children "because of his epilepsy; I can't live with it anymore."

The patient felt that his wife had left him out of anger, because he made her feel rejected and sexually inadequate. In this way, he thought, she could act to spite her husband as well as prove to herself that she was desirable and good sexual partner. Recently, the patient secured a better job and started dating other women. Nevertheless, he continues to avoid pursuing women and instead waits for them to initiate contact. His feeling of manhood, already tenuous because of his seizures, appears to have been injured further by the collapse of his marriage.

This case illustrates some of the common problems experienced by patients with epilepsy and the direct impact of these problems on their sexual lives. These include (i) a feeling of inferiority because of having epilepsy that translates into a pervasive fear of rejection and, in turn, a tendency to avoid seeking out relations with women; (ii) a fear of having seizures in the midst of sexual intercourse, which, in turn, leads to avoidance of sexual intercourse, resulting in the partner's feeling of rejection, guilt, and, eventually, a distancing between the sexual partners; and (iii) the inevitability of anticipatory anxiety regarding sexual intercourse. These vicious cycles evolve into an interminable spiraling process of sexual problems that ultimately result in the break of the relationship, as it occurred with this patient.

The fear of rejection and the heightened sensitivity toward being the target of stigmatization by the general population are unfortunate widespread problems that patients with epilepsy must face. This issue is discussed in greater detail in Chapters 19 and 20. Such problems undoubtedly contributed to this patient's feelings of sexual inadequacy and explained his timidity toward women. There is no question that the marital difficulties of this couple went beyond the more common complications of the sexual life of patients with epilepsy. Yet, it is conceivable that a timely inquiry on the part of his treating physician into the problems of his sexual life may have averted the ultimate outcome. For example, a referral for sexual counseling could have helped the couple overcome their anxieties with respect to their sexual relations.

Clearly, this patient's sexual problems were directly related to his seizure disorder. Treatment should have been directed toward these problems as vigorously as was the pharmacotherapy to abolish his seizures, for both had a negative impact on his quality of life. The reluctance of physicians to address these problems is puzzling and merits close scrutiny. Any physician treating patients with epilepsy is well aware of the stigma, fears, and misinformation surrounding sexual issues in epilepsy. For example, until careful, open-minded investigations by Henri Gastaut in

1954, epilepsy was associated both in the public and in the medical mind with hypersexuality and sexual deviancy (1). Such opinions can be found in early writings of diverse cultures: the Ayurveda of India, considered to be the oldest medical text in the world, suggests that epilepsy results from sexual excess (2). In Hippocrates' writings, we find statements suggesting that complete abstinence or excessive intercourse may be the cause of epilepsy (3). Unfortunately, the widespread misconceptions of sexual issues in epilepsy contrast with the limited literature addressing the very common psychological and psychiatric consequences of sexual problems of patients with epilepsy.

As suggested by Kanner and Weisbrot in Chapter 3, clinicians should include in the initial evaluation of patients with epilepsy an evaluation of the psychological impact of seizures on the different aspects of their lives. This includes their marital, social, and sexual lives. We believe that patients would be more forthcoming with this type of information if clinicians were open to hearing about it.

We present below a series of questions clinicians can use to explore these issues.

1. Patients with epilepsy often feel that having seizures has interfered with establishing new relations, for fear of being rejected or stigmatized. Has that happened to you?
2. Has your epilepsy interfered with your ability to make new friends, establish romantic relations with men/women?
3. It is not rare for people with epilepsy to be afraid of having sexual relations for fear that they would cause a seizure. Has that happened to you?
4. Has your epilepsy had an impact on your sexual life?
   There are many situations where misinformation causes patients and/or their partners to avoid sexual activity. For example:
5. Have you had any situation where a partner has avoided sexual intercourse for fear that you may have a seizure?
6. Some people have been told that masturbating can cause seizures. Have you ever

been told that? Have you ever avoided masturbation for fear of having a seizure?

EFFECTS OF EPILEPSY AND SEIZURES ON SEXUAL FUNCTION

Since the seminal studies of Gastaut and Collomb (1), others investigators have left no doubt that *hypo*sexuality is characteristic of many men and women with epilepsy (4–6). Hyposexuality is not a universal problem among all patients with epilepsy, but it is consistently reported in a substantial number of both men and women. It may take the form of reduced libido, erectile dysfunction, or lack of sexual satisfaction. Dyspareunia is not uncommon. Some patients report a lifelong indifference to sexual drives or activities that may even predate the first seizure.

In addition, irregular or dysfunctional menstrual cycles, anovulatory cycles, and polycystic ovaries occur at a higher rate than in the general population (7,8). Reproductive endocrine disorders, such as hypogonadotropic hypogonadism, hyperprolactinemia, and hypergonadotropic hypogonadism, have been found in men with seizures arising from the temporal lobe (9). Some of these problems appear to be iatrogenic. For example, valproate has been associated with an increased incidence of polycystic ovaries (10).

Various reasons for these abnormalities of sexual function have been offered. The psychosocial effects of chronic disease, especially in those patients with active or medically intractable epilepsy, may be important, but they have been difficult to identify or measure. Prejudice and suspicion directed toward those with epilepsy may affect social relationships. Common complications of epilepsy, such as depression, poor self-esteem, and social and physical isolation, may contribute to ineffective sexual partnering and/or sexual dysfunction.

Most investigations, however, have focused on physiologic factors. Suspicion has fallen on the possible role of epileptogenic damage to the limbic system. Some studies found the highest prevalence of hyposexuality in patients with epilepsy arising from the temporal lobe, suggesting limbic injury or dysfunction as the possible cause (9). Supporting the "temporal lobe hypothesis" is the observation of normalization of sexual function in patients made seizure-free by temporal lobectomy (11). In a recent study, Kanner et al. (12) reported a loss of sexual drive in 26% of 100 consecutive patients with intractable partial epilepsy during the postictal period, with a median duration of 39 hours (mean 42 ± 31). Seventy-nine of these patients suffered from temporal lobe epilepsy.

The impact of epilepsy on the hypothalamus and an abnormal pituitary secretory pattern of sexual hormones have been suggested. For example, the role of prolactin has been questioned in the hyposexuality of patients with epilepsy. It is well known that prolactin-secreting pituitary tumors commonly cause loss of libido or impotence (13). Seizures are associated with an increase of prolactin secretion. Some of the first careful observations of the effects of tonic-clonic seizures on serum levels of sex hormones were made in patients who did not have epilepsy but had psychiatric disorders and who were undergoing electroconvulsive therapy. A sharp increase in serum prolactin levels was found after tonic-clonic seizures provoked by such treatments and after spontaneous tonic-clonic and complex partial seizures (14–16). Whether this abnormal prolactin activity is relevant to the hyposexuality reported by many patients with epilepsy is not yet established. In addition, modest but sustained increases in plasma prolactin levels, for example, have been reported in men with complex partial seizures, even when no seizures are observed (17).

Certain AEDs, most notably phenytoin, carbamazepine, primidone, and other barbiturates, have long been known to be associated with reduced libido and impotence (18). The induction of abnormally high levels of sex hormone-binding globulin and consequent low serum levels of free testosterone have been cited as possible mechanisms (19). Although total (bound plus unbound) serum testosterone levels are lower in men taking carbamazepine or phenytoin, free testosterone

levels frequently are found to be reduced in this population (20). Whether abnormal testosterone levels, either in free or total form, play a role in the sexual complaints of patients is not yet established.

Sexual Function in Chronic Epilepsy

The effect of chronic epilepsy on marriage rates is not clear. Although lower marriage rates in those with epilepsy have been claimed by some investigators, others agree with the prospective British study, which found no difference in marriage rates between people with epilepsy and a control group (21,22). Even in those with epilepsy unassociated with other neurologic disease or abnormalities, fertility rates have been found in some studies to be low, or pregnancies to occur late (23). One careful study demonstrated that yearly fertility rates for married people with nonsymptomatic epilepsy dropped only after the epilepsy was diagnosed (24). A population study in Finland, however, found that only patients with coexisting mental retardation or cerebral palsy had fewer children than did a control group (25).

Management of Chronic Sexual Dysfunction Associated with Epilepsy

In men, it is not clear whether some drugs are more associated with sexual dysfunction than others, but sometimes a change from one AED to another relieves the problem. Some success has been claimed using testosterone injections in men (26). The efficacy of sildenafil (Viagra) in this population has not yet been studied carefully, but the drug has been effective for some men with epilepsy (D.B., *personal observation*). Therapeutic interventions in women with epilepsy-related hyposexuality have yet to be reported.

EFFECTS OF SEXUALITY ON SEIZURES AND EPILEPSY

Normal sexual maturation appears to influence the incidence and course of many epilepsies. Juvenile myoclonic epilepsy and juvenile absence epilepsy, for example, usually begin near or following puberty, and girls who already have absence seizures may begin to have tonic-clonic seizures around the time of menarche (27). In other children, seizure frequency may actually decrease at menarche, and benign rolandic epilepsy in both girls and boys uniformly goes into permanent remission at adolescence (28). Whether these age-related changes in epilepsy are related to hormonal changes or to some other feature of cerebral maturation is not known.

The coupling of seizure worsening or *de novo* appearance of generalized tonic-clonic seizures at the start of adolescence, with its discovery of masturbation and development of interest in the opposite sex and sexual fantasies, may be the source of significant guilt at this age. It is conceivable that some adolescents may blame the seizures on their sexual fantasies, masturbation, etc. One needs to recall the ancient medical texts to find such association between epilepsy and sexual activities (3,4). Pediatricians, pediatric neurologists, and epileptologists who treat adolescents must discuss these issues openly.

In uninformed patients (adolescents and adults), the temporal relation of seizure exacerbation with other sexual-related phenomena, such as ovulation and menstruation, may further feed unnecessary preoccupations and guilt feelings. One should remember that sexual drive is enhanced around the time of ovulation. Some women with epilepsy experience seizures exclusively within a short time before and during the first few days of menses (29). Others experience more frequent seizures during that part of the menstrual cycle or near the time of ovulation. The cause of such catamenial epilepsy is unknown, but shifts in hormonal levels or ratios are thought to be responsible (29). This information should be included in the education of every female patient from the start of therapy or children when they are about to start adolescence.

Seizures associated with sexual intercourse probably are feared by patients more often than they actually occur. Patients may associate the loss of control experienced during a seizure with the excitement of sexual activity. Patients generally should be reassured that seizures during coitus are unusual. Nevertheless, rare patients with "reflex epilepsy" triggered by sexual intercourse have been reported (30).

PREGNANCY AND EPILEPSY

Pregnancy has been a source of conflict for many patients with epilepsy, men and women, alike. Much of it results from misinformation, prejudice, and lack of proper counseling by the treating physician. It is clear that one of the most complex and difficult aspects of the care of young women with epilepsy, even with well-controlled disease, is pregnancy, which presents both physical and psychological challenges. Although the management of epilepsy during pregnancy has been made more systematic and less fearsome by the recent appearance of guidelines drafted by the American Academy of Neurology, the International League Against Epilepsy, and the American College of Obstetric and Gynecologic Physicians (31–33), education of our patients and of many treating physicians remains a major task, including those in developed countries. For example, most pregnancies of women with epilepsy who are taking AEDs are successful. Yet, a surprising number of patients still are advised by their physicians not to have children, sometimes in highly directive and absolute terms. Such advice usually stems from misinformation about physical or mental competence, genetic risk, or all three.

There is an approximately two-fold increased risk of fetal malformations (relative to the rate of offspring of healthy mothers) associated with the use of AEDs, especially in the first trimester (34). Although midline facial and palatal clefts, cardiac malformations, and delayed development often are cited, the most commonly demonstrated abnormality is generally described as the fetal AED syndrome, a cluster of relatively minor facial and digital anomalies that are not specific to any single drug (35). A not uncommon phenomenon is overwhelming fear as well as a guilty feeling that their AEDs are causing harm to their babies. Such concerns lead these patients to stop or lower the dose of their medication, which results in worsening seizures. The same guilt feelings lead some women to chose abortion as an option, without having a clear understanding of the relatively small teratogenic risk of AEDs. The magnitude of this problem has yet to be established.

Education of our patients from the start of treatment is the only solution. Patients need to be advised that the effects specific to different drugs have been difficult to demonstrate, with the exception of spina bifida. The incidence of spina bifida is estimated to be about 1% to 2% in fetuses with first-trimester exposure to chronic valproate and about 0.5% to 1% with exposure to carbamazepine (36,37). Folic acid supplementation has been shown to reduce the incidence of spina bifida in the general population and in those with a family history of spinal malformations. It is recommended for all women taking AEDs. Patients must understand that the occurrence of convulsions, especially during the first trimester, can result in harm to the baby (38–41).

The use of new AEDs does not help assuage the anxiety of potential parents with respect to teratogenic risks of these drugs. Almost all of the clinical reports of pregnancy outcomes associated with AED use relate only to drugs in use before 1993. The effects of the newer AEDs (felbamate, gabapentin, lamotrigine, topiramate, tiagabine, vigabatrin, oxcarbazepine, levetiracetam, zonisamide) on human fetal development have not been studied systematically. An ongoing prospective pregnancy registry now under way in the United States should provide useful information about the effects of specific antiepileptics within the next few years (42).

Many women and men worry about the risk of epilepsy in their children. The impact of a seizure disorder on a person's life often is so pervasive and destructive that the presumption of such genetic risks may be a powerful disincentive to child-bearing. Only a small percentage of adult-onset epilepsies are famil-

ial; most are acquired, even though a specific cause may not be discoverable in most patients. Many of the truly familial epilepsy syndromes, which may make up as many as 25% of those presenting in the first two decades of life, are relatively benign disorders that can be easily controlled with medication. Such epilepsies have a high rate of permanent remission in adulthood. Finally, most of the genetically determined epilepsy syndromes either have a low rate of penetrance (incidence of disease in carriers) or are thought to be polygenetic, so that the risk to offspring may be low. Such counseling requires a firm clinical diagnosis of the patient's epilepsy syndrome, which usually can be made accurately on the basis of the age at presentation, family history, type of seizure(s), electroencephalogram, and response to treatment.

Clearly, the fear of pregnancy of many women with epilepsy is best countered by a frank discussion of the facts and by firm reassurance that most pregnancies of women with epilepsy are successful. Women taking AEDs have a two-fold risk of obstetric complications relative to healthy women. These include toxemia, preeclampsia, bleeding in pregnancy, placental abruption, and premature labor (42). Although most studies have not found an increased risk of spontaneous abortion in women with epilepsy, there almost certainly is a higher perinatal mortality rate (42). Whether these increased risks are associated with the epilepsy itself, its treatment, or genetic factors that increase the risk both of epilepsy and pregnancy complications is unknown. As already mentioned, fetal loss has been reported to follow tonic-clonic seizures (41).

After delivery, a decision about breast-feeding often is a source of anxiety. Many AEDs are not delivered to the infant in sufficient amounts to be of concern, and most women breast-feed without problems. Anxieties and fantasies about dropping or injuring the baby during a seizure are almost universal. Counselling the patient during the pregnancy has been associated with a very low risk of seizure-related neonatal injury in the puerperium.

Pamphlets and articles on these complex and emotionally fraught subjects are available from the Epilepsy Foundation of America. These materials often provide a dispassionate, reassuring summary of current knowledge to the uncertain patient and her spouse. In the end, physicians' assurance that more than 90% of pregnancy outcomes are normal may relieve some of the patients' anxieties.

Impact of Pregnancy on Epilepsy

An additional source of apprehension about pregnancy in patients with epilepsy is the effect of pregnancy on the course of epilepsy, and the fact that it is impossible to predict it in an individual case. Group studies generally have shown no change in seizure frequency in most women, worsening in some, and improvement in a few. Careful comparisons with a group of nonpregnant women with a similar severity of illness have not been made.

Most women fear the occurrence of seizures during labor. They may be reassured that this is uncommon, occurring in 1% to 2% of women during delivery or with 24 hours postpartum (42). Women need to be reassured that if a seizure should occur, special treatment generally is not required.

MENOPAUSE

Virtually nothing is known about the effect of menopause on epilepsy or on the ability of women with epilepsy to cope with the physical and psychological complications of menopause. This is not just a theoretical question; it bears close scrutiny because patients with epilepsy, especially those with poorly controlled seizures, have a higher prevalence of depression and anxiety disorder. Whether this comorbidity has a negative impact on menopause of women with epilepsy is yet to be established.

Although the incidence of seizure disorders rises sharply in the elderly of both sexes, there is no evidence linking the increased risk to hormonal changes. No consistent change in the pattern or severity of a preexisting seizure disorder has been reported in women experiencing menopause (43). Although some women reported the first onset of epilepsy at about the time of menopause, this is not a common occurrence and may not exceed that of chance. Surgical sterilization has not been reported to increase the risk of epilepsy or seizures.

The benefits of postmenopausal hormone replacement therapy seem clear: reduction of risk for osteoporosis, coronary artery disease, and even Alzheimer's disease, as well as symptomatic relief of vasomotor and genital symptoms during the climacteric period (44). There is no evidence that hormone replacement increases the risk of seizures in women with epilepsy (45).

EFFECTS ON QUALITY OF LIFE

The impact of sexual issues on the patient's quality of life cannot be understated, as they encompass issues such as self-esteem, basic social interactions, sexual function, and marriage and child-bearing choices.

The most common psychiatric disturbance found in surveys of most patients with epilepsy is depression (46,47). Risk factors include a high frequency of seizures, left temporal seizure focus, and certain AEDs (47). Although the presumed role of the psychosocial consequences of epilepsy in producing depression has been acknowledged, the explicit relationship between hyposexuality and depression in those with epilepsy has never been analyzed. It is not known, for example, whether sexual dysfunction in this population is a risk factor for serious depression, or vice versa. Although the past 15 years has seen a welcome emphasis on exploring the quality of life of patients with epilepsy and addressing problem areas, some standard instruments used specifically to investigate quality of life in patients with epilepsy do not explicitly ask about sexual function (48). Because patients may not spontaneously reveal sexual difficulties to their physicians, the latter should routinely ask questions about sexual well-being, particularly in cases of depression.

CONCLUDING REMARKS

The impact of sexual problems on the life of patients with epilepsy is significant, yet it remains an unexplored area with respect to prevalence, causes, and, to an even lesser extent, treatment approaches. The biggest culprit is physicians' timidity in openly facing these issues with their patients. Were physicians to "destigmatize" sexual issues, patients would feel comfortable discussing their sexual fears and problems.

REFERENCES

1. Gastaut H, Collomb H. Etude de comportement sexuel chez les epileptigues psychomoteurs. *Ann Med Psychol* 1954;20:657–696.
2. Manyam BV. Epilepsy in ancient India. *Epilepsia* 1992; 33:373–475.
3. Temkin O. *The falling sickness. A history of epilepsy from the Greeks to the beginnings of modern neurology,* 2nd ed. Baltimore: Johns Hopkins Press, 1971.
4. Taylor DC. Sexual behaviour and temporal lobe epilepsy. *Arch Neurol* 1969;21:510–516.
5. Toone B, Wheeler M, Nanjee M, et al. Sex hormones, sexual activity and plasma anticonvulsant levels in male patients. *J Neurol Neurosurg Psychiatry* 1983;46:824–826.
6. Morrell MJ, Guldner GT. Self-reported sexual function and sexual arousability in women with epilepsy. *Epilepsia* 1996;37:204–1210.
7. Cummings LN, Giudice L, Morrell MJ. Ovulatory function in epilepsy. *Epilepsia* 1995;36:355–359.
8. Herzog AG, Klein P, Ransil BJ. Three patterns of catamenial epilepsy. *Epilepsia* 1997;38:1082–1088.
9. Herzog A, Seibel MM, Schomer DL, et al. Reproductive endocrine disorders in men with partial seizures of temporal lobe origin. *Arch Neurol* 1986;43:347–350.
10. Isojarvi JIT, Lastikainen TJ, Pakarinen AJ, et al. Polycystic ovaries and hyperandrogenism in women taking valproate for epilepsy. *N Engl J Med* 1993;329:1383–1388.
11. Cogan PH, Antunes JL, Correll JW. Reproductive function in temporal lobe epilepsy: the effect of temporal lobectomy. *Surg Neurol* 1979;12:243–246.
12. Kanner AM, Soto A, Gross-Kanner H. There is more to epilepsy than seizures: a reassessment of the postictal period. *Neurology* 2000;54[Suppl 3]:A352.
13. Yung WKA, Janys T. Primary neurological tumors. In: Goetz CG, Pappert EJ, eds. *Textbook of clinical neurology.* Philadelphia: WB Saunders, 1999:948.
14. Meldrum BS, McWilliam JR. Hormone changes following seizures. In: Dam M, Gram L, Penry JK, eds. *Advances in epileptology:* XIIth Epilepsy International Symposium. New York: Raven Press, 1981:441–448.
15. Collins WCJ, Lanigan O, Callaghan N. Plasma prolactin concentrations following epileptic and pseudoseizures. *J Neurol Neurosurg Psychiatry* 1983;46:505–508.
16. Sperling MR, Pritchard PB III, Engel J Jr, et al. Prolactin in partial epilepsy: an indicator of limbic seizures. *Ann Neurol* 1986;20:716–722.
17. Molaie M, Culebras A, Miller M. Nocturnal plasma prolactin rise in patients with complex partial seizures. *Ann Neurol* 1985;18:719–722.
18. Mattson RH, Cramer JA, Collins JF, et al. Comparison of carbamazepine, phenobarbital, phenytoin, and primidone in partial and secondary generalized tonic-clonic seizures. *N Engl J Med* 1985;313:145–151.
19. Victor A, Lundberg PO, Johansson EDB. Induction of sex hormone binding globulin by phenytoin. *Br Med J* 1977;11:934–935.
20. Duncan S, Blacklaw J, Beastall GH, et al. Antiepileptic drug therapy and sexual function in men with epilepsy. *Epilepsia* 1999;40:197–204.
21. Lechtenberg R. *Epilepsy and the family.* Boston: Harvard University Press, 1984.
22. Britten N, Morgan K, Fenwick PBC, et al. Epilepsy and handicap from birth to age 36. *Dev Med Child Neurol* 1985;28:719–728.
23. Jalava M, Sillanpaa M. Reproductive activity and offspring health of young adults with childhood-onset epilepsy: a controlled study. *Epilepsia* 1997;38:523–540.
24. Schupf N, Ottman R. Reproduction among individuals with idiopathic/cryptogenic epilepsy: risk factors for reduced fertility in marriage. *Epilepsia* 1996;37:833–840.
25. Olafsson E, Hauser WA, Gudmundsson G. Fertility in patients with epilepsy: a population-based study. *Neurology* 1998;51:71–73.
26. Daniels O, Fenwick PBC, Lelliott P, et al. Sex hormone replacement therapy in male epileptics. In: Porter RJ, ed. *Advances in epileptology: XVth Epilepsy International Symposium.* New York: Raven Press, 1984:291–297
27. Pearl PE, Holmes GL. Absence seizures. In: Dodson WE, Pellock JM, eds. *Pediatric epilepsies: Diagnosis and therapy.* New York: Demos Publications, 1993:163.
28. Diamantopoulos N, Crumrine PK. The effect of puberty on the course of epilepsy. *Arch Neurol* 1986;43:873–876.
29. Cramer JA, Mattson RH. Hormones and epilepsy. In: Wyllie E, ed. *The treatment of epilepsy: principles and practice.* Philadelphia: Lea & Febiger, 1998:686–691.
30. Hoenig J, Hamilton CM. Epilepsy and sexual orgasm. *Acta Psychiatr Scand* 1960;35:448–456.
31. Practice parameter. Management issues for women with epilepsy (summary statement). *Neurology* 1998;51:944–946.
32. Commission on genetics, pregnancy, and the child, International League Against Epilepsy. Guidelines for the care of women of childbearing age with epilepsy. *Epilepsia* 1993:34:588–589.
33. Seizure disorders in pregnancy. *Am Coll Obstet Gynecol Physicians Educ Bull* 1996;231:1–13.
34. Yerby MS. Treatment of epilepsy during pregnancy. In: Wyllie E, ed. *The treatment of epilepsy: principles and practice.* Philadelphia: Lea & Febiger, 1993:844–857.
35. Koch S, Losche G, Jager-Roman E. Major and minor birth malformations and antiepileptic drugs. *Neurology* 1992;42[Suppl 5]:83–88.
36. Lindhaut D, Schmidt D. In-utero exposure to valproate and neural tube defects. *Lancet* 1986;II:1392–1393.
37. Rosa FW. Spina bifida in infants of women treated with

carbamazepine during pregnancy. *N Engl J Med* 1991; 324:674–667.

38. Resources for women with epilepsy and health care providers. *Epilepsia* 1998;39[Suppl 8]:S44–S46.

39. Hiilesmaa VK. Pregnancy and birth in women with epilepsy. *Neurology* 1992;42[Suppl 5]:8–11.

40. Annegers JF, Baumgartner KB, Hauser WA. Epilepsy, antiepileptic drugs, and the risk of spontaneous abortion. *Epilepsia* 1988;29:451–458.

41. Nelson KB, Ellenberg JH. Maternal seizure disorder, outcome of pregnancy, and neurologic abnormalities in the children. *Neurology* 1982;32:1247–1254.

42. Bardy A. Epilepsy and pregnancy. A prospective study of 154 pregnancies of epileptic women. Dissertation, University of Helsinki, Helsinki, Finland, 1982.

43. Abbasi F, Krumholz A, Kittner SJ, et al. Effects of

menopause on seizures in women with epilepsy. *Epilepsia* 1999;40:205–210.

44. Hormone replacement therapy. *ACOG Techn Bull* 1992; 166:1–8.

45. El-Sayed YY. Obstetric and gynecologic care of women with epilepsy. *Epilepsia* 1998;39[Suppl]:S17–S25.

46. Hauser A, Kurland L. The epidemiology of epilepsy in Rochester, Minnesota 1935–1967. *Epilepsia* 1975;15: 1–66.

47. Wiegartz P, Seidenberg M, Woodard A, et al. Co-morbid psychiatric disorder in chronic epilepsy: recognition and etiology of depression. *Neurology* 1999;53[Suppl 2]:S3–S8.

48. The Liverpool quality of life questionnaire. In: Trimble MR, Dodson WE, eds. *Epilepsy and quality of life.* New York: Raven Press, 1994:267–279.

24

Psychogenic Pseudoseizures

A General Overview

Marcelo E. Lancman, *Christos C. Lambrakis, and †Michael I. Steinhardt

*Epilepsy Program, Saint Agnes Hospital, White Plains, New York 10605; and
*Northeast Regional Epilepsy Group and †Pediatric Neuroscience Institute,
Hackensack University Medical Center, Hackensack, New Jersey 07601*

An epileptic seizure is defined as a sudden, involuntary, time-limited alteration in behavior, motor activity, autonomic function, consciousness, or sensation, accompanied by an epileptiform electrographic ictal pattern (1). A pseudoseizure is a paroxysmal "nonepileptic event" that derives its name from its clinical similarity to epileptic seizures, in the absence of a concurrent electrographic ictal pattern. Pseudoseizure events may result from organic or psychogenic processes. A wide variety of organic pseudoseizures have been recognized. These include syncope (2), sleep disorders presenting as cataplectic or sleep paralysis episodes of narcolepsy (3), the automatic behavior displayed during episodes of excessive daytime somnolence in obstructive sleep apnea, and parasomnias presenting as sleep walking, rapid eye movement behavior disorder, and night terrors (4). In addition, pseudoseizures may present as breath-holding spells (5), gastrointestinal reflux (6), complicated migraines (7), startled responses (8), and certain types of movement disorders. *Psychogenic* pseudoseizures are the most frequent type of nonepileptic paroxysmal events. The advent of video electroencephalographic (EEG) telemetry has demonstrated that 17% to 30% of patients referred to tertiary epilepsy centers with a diagnosis of intractable epilepsy ultimately are found to experience nonepileptic events (9–17), most of which are of psychogenic origin. Because the management of pseudoseizures is completely different from that of epileptic seizures, establishing the correct diagnosis is of paramount importance.

In this chapter, we review the clinical characteristics of psychogenic pseudoseizures and discuss the different diagnostic strategies available to help clinicians distinguish pseudoseizures from epileptic seizures. The term "pseudoseizure" was advanced by Liske and Forster (9) to describe clinical events that, by their nature, resemble an epileptic seizure but lack the necessary paroxysmal electrophysiologic patterns seen in epileptic seizures (9). Other terms include psychogenic seizures, hysterical seizures, and hysteroepilepsy. We prefer to use the term "pseudoseizure" or "nonepileptic event." We avoid the term "psychogenic *seizure*," which many patients have difficulty differentiating from epileptic seizures. It is not infrequent for clinicians to hear patients say: "Do I or don't I have seizures?" even after they have been given ample explanations on the nature of their events.

CLINICAL CHARACTERISTICS OF PSYCHOGENIC PSEUDOSEIZURES

Prevalence

The frequency of pseudoseizures among patients referred to epilepsy centers has ranged between 17% and 30% in published series (9–16). These figures probably are skewed, as they are derived from samples of patients referred to comprehensive tertiary epilepsy centers (i.e., patients with more severe disorders) and probably do not represent the actual prevalence of psychogenic pseudoseizures in the general epilepsy population. Differences in prevalence can be identified in selected populations. Golden et al. (16) found that 19% of admissions of adolescents with new-onset seizures had pseudoseizures. In a psychiatric hospital setting, Lelliott et al. (18) found that 17% of admissions to an epilepsy unit had pseudoseizures. The actual prevalence of psychogenic pseudoseizures has yet to be established.

Age

The occurrence of pseudoseizures appears to peak at two different ages: during adolescence from 19 to 22 years, and in early adulthood from 25 to 35 years (13,16,21,23). The occurrence of pseudoseizures before the age of 5 and after the age of 55 is rare. To our knowledge, the youngest patient reported in the literature was 4 years old; the oldest was 77 years old.

Gender

Sex differences have been observed across numerous studies. There is a marked female preponderance, ranging from 66% to 99% of pseudoseizure cases (13,19,21–33). This gender difference also is observed in pediatric populations (73%) (33). The reasons for this obvious gender inequity are poorly understood. Yet, psychogenic pseudoseizures frequently are an expression of a conversion disorder, which is known to be more frequent in women than in men (34).

Neurologic History

Neurologic insults are frequent etiologies of epileptic seizures. It is natural to surmise that an episode is epileptic when associated with a history of neurologic pathology. Yet, many of the patients with psychogenic pseudoseizures have been found to have a positive neurologic history (17,26,35,36). In one study of outpatients with psychogenic pseudoseizures, 23.7% had a neurologic history. The most frequent finding was a history of head trauma with loss of consciousness (17). In a study of adolescent children with psychogenic pseudoseizures, there was a positive neurologic history in 21% of the patients (21). A history of meningitis and arachnoid cysts were the most frequently encountered neurologic maladies in these patients. In one interesting case, a patient developed pseudoseizures after being struck by lightening (21). Therefore, the presence of a neurologic history does not exclude the possibility of pseudoseizures.

Family History

A family history of epilepsy was found in 37.6% of patients with psychogenic pseudoseizures in one study (17). Similar findings were reported by other authors (37), including a study carried out in adolescents (21). One possible explanation for this phenomenon is that these patients had an opportunity to witness the clinical characteristics of epileptic seizures.

Cognitive Factors

Variables in neuropsychological functioning of psychogenic pseudoseizure patients have been examined. Among the different studies, scores ranged from the retarded to the very superior. A full-scale IQ in the low-average or borderline range is a frequent finding. A high incidence of impaired performance on the Halstead-Reitan Neuropsychological Battery has been reported, as more than half the patients scored in the impaired range on more than half of the measures (38). The discriminating ability of neuropsychological testing between psychogenic pseudoseizures and epileptic seizures will be discussed later.

Psychological and Psychiatric Factors

As a group, patients with pseudoseizures have been identified to have a variety of comorbid psychiatric conditions that include, but are not limited to, conversion disorder, somatization disorder, dissociative disorder, personality disorder, anxiety disorder, and mood disorder. Furthermore, there is an increased prevalence of a history of sexual and physical abuse (39–42). These conditions are discussed in great detail in Chapter 25.

Clinical Phenomena

General Observations

The clinical expression of epileptic seizures has a wide spectrum of motor and behavioral phenomena, particularly those involving the complex symptomatology exhibited in temporal and frontal lobe seizures. Thus, reaching a diagnostic impression *solely* on the bases of clinical phenomena may result in erroneous conclusions. For example, in one study that examined 64 patients with suspected pseudoseizures because of atypical phenomena, 12 (18.75%) were found to have epileptic seizures (43). In 23 patients who were thought to have epileptic seizures, video EEG monitoring documented pseudoseizures of psychogenic or physiologic origin in 12 patients. Some studies attempted to categorize pseudoseizures according to the type of epileptic seizures they resemble. In a study of pediatric patients, Holmes et al. (33) suggested that pseudoseizures more frequently resembled generalized tonic-clonic or partial seizures with complex symptoms. Generalized tonic-clonic–like or tonic-like pseudoseizures were observed in 37.5% of patients and partial-like pseudoseizures in 62.3%. Several of the patients had multiple seizure types, but none had absence-like or atonic-like events. A subgroup of eight patients had both epileptic and pseudoseizures; four of these patients had events that resembled epileptic seizures.

Previously held beliefs on the characteristics of pseudoseizures that often preceded the development of EEG monitoring have come under increasing scrutiny (30). More recent studies that relied on video EEG technology demonstrated the presence of epileptic seizures that mimic pseudoseizures (10,43–46) and, vice versa, pseudoseizures that may be indistinguishable from epileptic seizures. Nonconvulsive pseudoseizures are a classic example of the latter. Thus, although clinical phenomena may support suspicion of the presence of psychogenic pseudoseizures, by no means should they be considered absolute. Furthermore, clinical phenomena should never substitute for video EEG monitoring in making a diagnosis. In other words, no matter how suggestive the clinical manifestation of a paroxysmal event may be of pseudoseizures, such diagnosis should never be made without electrographic confirmation.

Unresponsiveness associated with uncoordinated, violent, and very disorganized motor activity are the most frequent clinical behaviors identified in pseudoseizures of adult patients (14,17,35,36,47,48). Generalized trembling associated with unresponsiveness was the second most frequently encountered set of phenomena in one of these studies (17), and unresponsiveness in the absence of any motor phenomena was the third. In other series, motionless stare and unresponsiveness constituted the most frequent clinical pattern (47,48). Verbal unresponsiveness, automatisms, and whole-body flaccidity are phenomena with little discriminating potential between epileptic and nonepileptic events (31).

The clinical characteristics of pseudoseizures appear to be, in general, similar in both children and adult age groups. In one study of 43 children under the age 16 years, 19 had episodes characterized by unresponsiveness associated with generalized violent and uncoordinated movements involving the entire body. Eleven patients had unresponsiveness accompanied by generalized trembling (21).

Typical Clinical Characteristics

Preictal State

With the precise clinical information afforded by video EEG monitoring, other studies examined the events leading up to the pseudoseizure. Benbadis et al. (49) observed that pseudoseizures often arose out of a state that resembled normal sleep by behavioral criteria alone (i.e., motionless patient with eyes closed), whereas the EEG showed evidence of wakefulness (posterior background activity in the alpha frequency, active electromyogram, and rapid eye movement). This new finding was termed "preictal pseudosleep." Patients were divided into two groups based on their seizure type: pseudoseizures and true epileptic seizures. Preictal pseudosleep was seen in 10 of 18 patients with pseudoseizures and in none of 39 patients with epileptic seizures, yielding a sensitivity of 56% and a specificity of 100% for pseudoseizures. Because of its high specificity, preictal pseudosleep may be a useful adjunctive finding to support the diagnosis of pseudoseizures.

The occurrence of a paroxysmal event during true sleep is indicative of an epileptic seizure, a parasomnia, or a movement disorder such as paroxysmal dyskinesia.

Auras

The presence of "auras" has been described in patients with pseudoseizures and certainly is not unique to true epileptic seizures (17,23,35,47). Lancman et al. (17) found "auras" in 23.7% of patients with pseudoseizures. The clinical characteristics of the "aura" were nonspecific, and the duration was variable. Examples of pseudoauras included unusual feelings, light-headedness, sensations of warmth, strange tastes, and headaches (17). Although the "auras" found in patients with pseudoseizures in general are clinically dissimilar than those found in patients with epileptic seizures, these findings are not specific enough to confirm a diagnosis.

Motor Phenomena

In one of the first case-control studies, Gates et al. (31) compared the clinical characteristics of documented convulsive pseudoseizures from 25 patients with the phenomena of generalized tonic-clonic epileptic seizures recorded from a control group of 25 other patients. Upper extremity movements consisting of *in-phase* clonic activity were observed in 96% of the control group compared to 20% for the study group. *Out-of-phase* upper extremity movements, characterized as nonsynchronous movements or movements oriented in multiple directions, were noted in 56% of the study group but in none of the patients in the control group. Similar observations applied to lower extremity movements.

Pelvic Thrusting. Pelvic thrusting has long been associated with pseudoseizures. In the study by Gates et al. (31), high-amplitude forward pelvic thrusting was observed in 44% of the pseudoseizure group compared to no patients in the control group. Retropelvic thrusting (rhythmic movements of the buttocks into the bed while lying on the back) was identified in 12% of the control group with generalized tonic-clonic epileptic seizures but was not present in the study group (31). Forward pelvic thrusting is not specific to pseudoseizures, as it has been recognized in epileptic complex partial seizures of mesial frontal origin (45,46).

Nonmotor Phenomena

Eye Movements. In the same study, Gates et al. (31) classified eye movements as eye fluttering, unilateral winking, and staring. Eighty-eight percent of the pseudoseizure patients exhibited no eye involvement of any kind, whereas 64% of the control group exhibited some form of eye involvement. In another study, eyes were reported to be wide open in more than 90% of patients during the tonic phase of generalized tonic-clonic epileptic seizures. In contrast, a sustained, forceful eye closure with active opposition to opening was present in 41 of 75 cases of psychogenic pseudoseizures with motor symptoms and in 16 of 21 cases with pure unresponsiveness. This relationship was not observed in psychogenic pseudoseizures with only sensory symptoms, as only eight of 72 cases had similar eye closure findings (50).

Staring. Although not frequently encountered, the presence of staring spells should in no way exclude the possibility of a pseudoseizure event. Carmant et al. (51) reported staring spells in two preschool children who were refractory to pharmacotherapy with antiepileptic drugs; these events later were found to be nonepileptic in origin. These episodes were provoked and aborted by suggestion with no concurrent EEG changes, leading to the correct diagnosis. Subsequent testing revealed the presence of a psychological disturbance that was treated with psychotherapy.

Cognitive Phenomena. Cognitive functions during an ictal event can be impaired during epileptic seizures and appear affected during psychogenic pseudoseizures. There appears to be some disparity between the two types of events. In one study, some level of response was detected during 48% of pseudoseizures compared to 18% during complex partial seizures. Items presented during the ictus were recalled after 63% of the pseudoseizure events in contrast to 4% recall after complex partial seizures (52). Complex partial seizures of right mesial temporal origin are a typical example of epileptic seizures during which patients may be, at least, partially responsive. However, patients are invariably amnestic to the events. Thus, cognitive assessment during an ictal event by the clinician provides a limited utility in differentiating between pseudoseizures and complex partial seizures. On the other hand, memory recall appears to correlate highly with pseudoseizures and may be useful in distinguishing these events with more reliability.

Vocalizations. Gates et al. (31) found that only 24% of the control group demonstrated the classic "epileptic cry" at the onset of the seizure; a larger percentage (60%) had an associated cry only after the seizure was well established. This vocalization was limited to the crying sound produced by the involuntary contractions of the muscles of respiration during the tonic or clonic phases of the seizure. For the pseudoseizure group, the sounds observed consisted of a wide assortment of moans, screams, grunts, gagging, snorts, gasps, and retching, as well as understandable verbal statements. As for these sounds, 44% of the pseudoseizure group vocalized at the onset of the event, whereas none had a vocalization after the seizure was well established. In another study, expressions such as crying, yelling, vulgar language, and combativeness were seen only with pseudoseizures (33).

Urinary Incontinence and Bodily Injury. Urinary incontinence and bodily injury are not infrequent components of a true generalized tonic-clonic or partial seizure. Injury to oneself during a pseudoseizure often is considered rare, but studies have shown pseudoseizure patients are capable of inflicting physical injuries, such as tongue bites (14,17,24, 33,35,47,53,54). Biting of the lip or tip of the tongue, as opposed to the side of the tongue, is rare during epileptic seizures and should be suggestive of psychogenic pseudoseizures (50). Some authors have suggested that documented urinary incontinence is virtually nonexistent in pseudoseizures (33), but others have reported its occurrence (17,21,47). It is clear that a reported urinary incontinence by the patient should be viewed with less importance then documented urinary incontinence in the course of video EEG. It has been our impression that reports of urinary incontinence do not occur in early stages of the pseudoseizure history. The repetitive inquiry of this symptom by physicians may account for a "delayed" incorporation of this symptom in the description of pseudoseizures. The increase in complexity of pseudoseizures over time in the same patient has been described extensively (17,21).

Postictal Symptoms. Postictal symptoms in pseudoseizures have been reported by several authors, making this variable unable to differentiate pseudoseizures from epileptic seizures (17,24,35). On some occasions, the duration of the postictal period is shorter in patients with pseudoseizures compared to those with epileptic seizures. More importantly, in pseudoseizures, the postictal period often can be reversed by suggestion (17,24).

Duration. Although pseudoseizures typically are reported as events of long duration

(55,56), this variable is not a reliable discriminator between nonepileptic and epileptic events. In many cases, the duration of either type of event can be highly variable.

Distinguishing Epileptic Seizures that Mimic Pseudoseizures from Pseudoseizures Proper

In a recent study, Parra et al. (43) suggested that as clinicians have become increasingly aware of psychogenic pseudoseizures, an increasing proportion of diagnostic mistakes has resulted from the misdiagnosis of epileptic seizures with atypical features as psychogenic pseudoseizures. Thus, the onus on the clinician is the correct recognition of these two types of paroxysmal events. Fortunately, epileptic seizures that mimic pseudoseizures characteristically are of extratemporal origin, originating and/or involving mesial frontal and/or mesial parietal cortex. These seizures present a number of clinical characteristics that may alert the clinician as to the correct diagnosis: (i) they are very short in duration (less than 30 seconds); (ii) they are stereotypic, including the complex automatisms; (iii) they often occur out of sleep; and (iv) they often display a tonic posturing in abduction of the upper extremities, a sign that was found to be specific to epileptic seizures involving the supplementary sensory-motor area and never seen in pseudoseizures (44). Concurrent electrographic ictal patterns may be elusive, given the location of the source of epileptic activity in relation to the position of recording scalp electrodes. Morris et al. (57) demonstrated the presence of a subtle rhythmic theta pattern in parasagittal leads, buried within muscle and movement artifact. The use of high-frequency filters may be necessary to recognize such a pattern. Thus, the presence of such clinical phenomena in paroxysmal events with atypical features should raise suspicion of epileptic seizures of mesial frontal or parietal origin. Presence of structural lesions on magnetic resonance imaging (MRI) in those regions should be another red flag that should oblige clinicians to review these events with great caution before suggesting a diagnosis of pseudoseizures.

Comorbidity with Epilepsy

It is not uncommon for patients with pseudoseizures to also have a prior or concurrent history of epileptic seizures. The frequency of comorbidity between the two disorders varies widely among different series (17,47, 48,55,58–60). In one of our studies of adults with pseudoseizures, the frequency of epilepsy was 10.7% (17). These results were similar to those of Lesser et al. (60) and Lempert and Schmidt (23). Other authors found significantly higher prevalence rates. In one study that evaluated the frequency of pseudoseizures in children, eight of eleven patients with pseudoseizures also had documented epileptic seizures (33). In a large population-based study Sigurdardottir and Olafsson (61) found that approximately half of the patients with psychogenic pseudoseizures also had epilepsy. Similar high rates of coexisting epilepsy have been found in other studies (18).

In patients with documented pseudoseizures, special care must be taken to ensure the presence or absence of concurrent or prior epileptic seizures. To that end, clinicians must take a careful description of all present and past paroxysmal events. The reported features of the patient's events should be compared with those witnessed during video EEG monitoring, which then should be reviewed with family members who have first-hand knowledge of the patient's seizures. In addition, all reported paroxysmal events should be accounted for during monitoring. If the different events have not been observed, monitoring should be extended. Failure to do so can result in incorrectly limiting the diagnosis to only pseudoseizures while the coexisting true epileptic seizures will go undiagnosed and untreated. Other clues can suggest the existence of a dual diagnosis. These include the presence of interictal phenomena such as spike discharges or focal abnormalities on EEG, and abnormal findings on neuroimaging studies such as MRI, single photon emission computed tomography, and positron emission tomographic studies.

A less frequently encountered and only recently described phenomenon involves the new onset of psychogenic seizures after epilepsy surgery. These patients develop pseudoseizures only after undergoing successful epilepsy surgery. The cause of these episodes is yet to be established. We can speculate on possible explanations for their occurrence, which include the dramatic psychosocial implications of suddenly being rendered seizure-free. For example, patients who once were dependent on government agencies may lose their disability status as a result of becoming seizure-free and be forced to enter the work force. Previous attention from family members because of the patients' intractable seizures may wane in the absence of their once long-standing affliction. This entity may not be as rare as previously thought. In a recently described study, five of 96 patients who had underwent epilepsy surgery experienced postoperative psychogenic pseudoseizures (62). When comparing this group of patients to their surgical cohorts, several trends were observed. Among the patients who went on to develop psychogenic seizures, a higher percentage was found to have had preoperative psychopathologic conditions and operative complications. These patients also were discovered to have lower full-scale IQ scores than their counterparts. The potential development of pseudoseizures in epilepsy surgery patients stresses the need for evaluation with video EEG monitoring in patients with postoperative seizures. This testing would determine the type of events prior to concluding that the patients are epileptic and that surgery has failed.

DIAGNOSTIC EVALUATION

The diagnosis of pseudoseizures can be a daunting task for the clinician. Even the well-trained physician with vast clinical exposure to ictal events often will be uncertain as to the type of a paroxysmal event. More harmful is the well-meaning practitioner who jumps to label an event as a nonepileptic. Those physicians who deal with epileptic patients on a daily basis quickly realize that the spectrum of clinical presentations of epileptic seizures spans the myriad of almost every imaginable process the human brain is capable of producing. Various clinical pearls that have been perpetuated through the years often will lead to misdiagnosis. Characterization of events as pseudoseizures based on clinical observations of thrashing movements of the extremities or retention of consciousness despite bilateral extremity involvement may have some anatomic basis. However, all comprehensive epilepsy centers have witnessed more than one patient having these seizure characteristics that have been proven to represent epileptic phenomena. In particular, seizures arising from and/or involving mesial frontal structures, such as supplementary sensory-motor area, can be extremely difficult to differentiate from pseudoseizures based on clinical criteria (46). For example, epileptic seizures involving this region result in bilateral tonic contraction in abduction of both upper extremities without impairment of consciousness. These movements usually are asymmetric and uncoordinated, leading to the incorrect assumption that these events are psychogenic in nature (see later) (44–46).

In evaluating a patient for possible pseudoseizures, careful analysis of the description of the clinical event can provide some insight, but a final diagnosis should not be made until further confirmatory testing with video EEG monitoring has been performed. Other auxiliary tests include standardized neuropsychological evaluation and measurement of certain hormones, such as prolactin.

Video Electroencephalographic Telemetry

Advances in technology have enabled the physician to accurately assess the electrical activity of the brain during ictal events through the use of video EEG telemetry (63). An epilepsy unit equipped with video EEG monitoring affords the unique opportunity to witness events in a protected medical environment. These units are staffed by physicians, nurses, and technologists who are experts in the field of epileptology. In a typical unit, patients are wired with the standard 10- to 20-electrode array using special adhesives, such as collodion, that allow for prolonged contact of the electrodes to the scalp. Cameras equipped with remote panning hardware and infrared detectors enable the patient to be viewed throughout the day in various environments. When routine monitoring has failed to elicit any events, various methods can be used to hasten their occurrence. Techniques such as withdrawal of antiepileptic medications, hyperventilation, and saline injection with verbal induction often can precipitate a pseudoseizure. Once an event has been captured, a critical review of the EEG and video data often will provide conclusive proof as to the type of paroxysmal event.

Koblar et al. (12) found that, among patients with seizures who underwent video EEG monitoring, 80% had a modification in management as a direct consequence of monitoring. Lancman et al. (64) found that video EEG monitoring is useful for detection of pseudoseizures in populations of patients least suspected of having these events, such as the elderly population.

As important as video EEG monitoring is in the assessment of patients with seizure episodes, it is not without its pitfalls. Although generalized tonic-clonic seizures customarily result in obvious, if not dramatic, EEG abnormalities, partial seizures confined to a restricted region of the cortex can remain electrically silent with standard scalp electrodes. In one study, simple partial seizures revealed EEG abnormalities in only 60% of the recorded events. Repeat recording of the episodes increased the yield of detecting an EEG abnormality to 80% (65). These data suggest that 20% of simple partial seizures may go undetected despite advanced long-term video EEG monitoring. This is because it takes a synchronous activation of a cortical area equivalent to 6 cm^2 before the electrographic activity is detected by scalp recordings. Complex partial seizures may, at times, go undetected by scalp recordings. These usually are seizures originating from mesial frontal, parietal, and at times temporal regions. The lack of detection of ictal patterns is related to the restricted cortical area activated, as well as the angle subtended by the recording electrodes to the epileptic source, the overlying muscle, movement artifacts, or a combination of these factors. The change of high-frequency filters can unmask an underlying electrographic pattern buried within a barrage of movement and muscle artifact. Thus, before diagnosing an event as a pseudoseizure, the physician must always remain cognizant of the fact that certain epileptic seizures may not produce abnormalities on the scalp EEG. To increase the probability of detecting an EEG abnormality, multiple events should be recorded, if possible. An increase in the diagnostic yield of video EEG can be accomplished with the use of special electrodes, such as sphenoidal electrodes and supraorbital electrodes, and the placement of extra electrodes over regions of the brain suspected of being involved in production of the seizure. Sphenoidal electrodes can be used to detect discharges emanating from mesial temporal regions with a small electric field that may preclude its detection by the standard scalp and anterotemporal electrodes.

Neuropsychological Evaluation

A neuropsychological evaluation can provide comprehensive information of a patient's higher cognitive functioning and emotional status. The evaluation is regarded as essential for patients undergoing epilepsy surgery, as reported by the Therapeutic and Technology Assessment Subcommittee of the American Academy of Neurology (66) and can assist in the diagnosis and management of patients with pseudoseizures.

Neuropsychological assessment has been found to be successful in evaluating the functional integrity of brain functioning and providing additional confirmatory data regarding the lateralization and localization of seizure focus (67). Its contribution to distinguishing between patients with pseudoseizures and epileptics has been modest. This may be attributed to (i) the wide heterogeneity of pseudoseizure patients (39); (ii) the presence of identified neuropsychological deficits of attention and memory in patients with conversion disorder and somatization disorder (68,69); and (iii) the presence of identified psychiatric complications in epileptic patients, the targeted comparison group (70).

Despite these difficulties, formal neuropsychological assessment has been found to contribute to the proper diagnosis of these patients. In a recent study, Binder et al. (71) compared the neuropsychological test performance of individuals classified into pseudoseizure, epilepsy, and normal control groups. Significant levels of impairment were found in both seizure groups as compared to the normal controls, but no significant differences were identified between the pseudoseizure and epilepsy groups. Only measures of confrontational naming (Boston Naming Test, $p < 0.02$) and delayed story memory recall (Wechsler Memory Scale-Revised Logical Memory Percent Retention, $p < 0.09$) approached the researchers' predetermined 0.01 level of significance. Upon additional analysis, however, the Minnesota Multiphasic Personality Inventory (MMPI)/MMPI-2 and the Portland Digit Recognition Test (PDRT) were found to be helpful in distinguishing between the pseudoseizure and genuine epilepsy groups. The MMPI-2 (72) and its predecessor, the MMPI, are established measures of personality assessment utilizing a self-report and true/false format, and are the most frequently used tests among neuropsychologists (73). The PDRT (74) is a measure of exaggeration of memory impairment and motivation to perform poorly, and it has been proposed to measure an individual's tendency to embellish or behave in a histrionic manner (42). Binder et al. (71) found that performance on Scales 1 and 2 of the MMPI/MMPI-2 and PDRT was useful in the classification of patients with pseudoseizures and true epilepsy, correctly classifying 48 of 60 (80%) in their clinical sample.

Whereas Binder et al. found significant clinical elevations on Scales 1 and 2 of the MMPI/MMPI-2, others found that pseudoseizure patients could not be characterized by any single MMPI pattern or profile (75). In this sample, the most consistent finding was the unusually high number of patients with several elevated clinical scales. Forty percent of the sample had MMPI profiles with four or more clinical scale elevations, with 91% of those patients having the multiple elevations on both the neurotic and psychotic scales. This further demonstrates the psychological complexity and heterogeneity of this patient population.

Serum Hormone Testing

Various hormones have been studied to aid in the differentiation between true electrical seizures and pseudoseizures. Among these, the most clinically viable has been the measurement of serum prolactin levels. Serum prolactin levels obtained at baseline commonly range between 0 to 15 ng/mL for males and 0 to 20 ng/mL for females. Several studies showed an increase in the peak prolactin level obtained after a true generalized seizure, whereas no significant elevation was noted after a pseudoseizure (76–79). Mehta et al. (76) studied peak serum prolactin levels obtained after different seizure types. Serum prolactin levels were found to be elevated (more than 25 ng/mL) in 68.33% of patients with generalized tonic-clonic seizures and 11.11% in patients with partial seizure events, whereas no patients with pseudoseizures showed a rise in serum prolactin levels. Thus, an elevation of serum prolactin level strongly suggests an event was a true seizure, whereas a normal postictal prolactin level does not exclude the possibility of an epileptic seizure, particularly a partial seizure.

Other studies found interesting associations between prolactin levels and the type of ictal event observed. In one investigation, prolactin levels increased after complex partial seizures that involved motor behaviors and were not increased further by secondary generalization. No increase was demonstrated for nontemporal partial seizures and pseudoseizures (80).

Prolactin levels and their relationship to paroxysmal events such as hypotensive syncope have been studied. Oribe et al. (81) found that nine of eleven patients who sustained tilt table-induced syncope had a greater than four-fold rise in serum prolactin levels after 30 minutes. These data suggest that obtaining prolactin levels after a syncopal event may help in clarifying if the event was truly related to hypotension or was a manifestation of a different process such as a pseudoseizure.

The time of collection of the serum sample after an event is of critical importance. Peak prolactin levels have been found to occur at 30 minutes after the ictal event, with gradual return to baseline during the subsequent hour (76). Additional studies showed slightly different optimal collection times varying between 15 and 20 minutes following a seizure (77).

Other hormones have been investigated for their utility in assessing pseudoseizures. The mean diurnal concentration of adrenocorticotropic hormone was found to be elevated in epileptic patients with temporal lobe seizures, whereas no elevation was noted among patients with pseudoseizures (82). Other hormones, such as cortisol, have not been proven to be useful in differentiating pseudoseizures from generalized tonic-clonic seizures. A rise in cortisol has been found to be nonselectively triggered by both types of events (76).

Induction of Pseudoseizures by Suggestion

In the present era of managed care and limited financial resources that dictate restrictions on the length of hospital stay, the ability to passively observe and wait for a patient to have a spontaneous seizure often is unrealistic. Techniques customarily used in the evaluation of seizure patients to increase the frequency of captured epileptic events during video EEG include the withdrawal of antiepileptic medications and sleep deprivation. Several methods have been established to precipitate the onset of a nonepileptic event and are used frequently in the evaluation of patients with suspected psychogenic pseudo-

seizures. These methods are termed "induction maneuvers" and involve the provocation of psychogenic pseudoseizures through the means of suggestion. Although the induction of an event is suggestive of nonepileptic origin (35), this should not be considered as an absolute rule, as there are reports of epileptic seizures triggered during an induction procedure (43,60,83).

Infusion of intravenous saline solution is the most commonly used method to induce pseudoseizures. Other methods include the application of alcohol pads or ointment creams on the neck or forehead, the use of tuning forks, hyperventilation, and photic stimulation.

Utility of Induction Methods

Several studies proved the utility of induction using intravenous injection of saline in the diagnosis of pseudoseizures (84). In one study of 50 patients suspected of having pseudoseizures, the authors found that 30% of the patients had a spontaneous event during video EEG monitoring and 33% had an event only during saline induction (85). This demonstrates the usefulness of induction in a subset of patients who may not have spontaneous seizure events during monitoring. In another study, 29 of 32 patients with an eventual diagnosis of pseudoseizures were inducible via intravenous saline placebo (59). In the same study, all of the 41 patients with an eventual diagnosis of epilepsy alone were not inducible. Lancman et al. (84) studied the usefulness of this method to diagnose pseudoseizures. They used the technique of an alcohol patch in patients with pseudoseizures compared to patients with epilepsy. The authors found that this method was highly specific, as none of the patients with epilepsy was induced. It also was found to be fairly sensitive, as most of the patients with pseudoseizures were able to be induced. As noted earlier, although these studies suggest that a positive induction is specific to pseudoseizures, such is not always the case, and a electrographic criterion needs to be included in the establishment of all diagnoses of pseudoseizures!

Other studies reported less impressive results. Drake (86) studied 20 patients with suspected pseudoseizures who underwent induction with saline infusion. Eight patients exhibited their characteristic pseudoseizures, but 12 patients failed to respond to saline or had episodes different from their characteristic spells. This suggests that although saline induction may aid in the identification of pseudoseizures and verify their nonepileptic nature, some patients may not be adequately inducible, and others may have events that are different from the events that prompted medical evaluation. This latter subset is of particular concern, as misdiagnosis in patients with coexistent epilepsy may occur. To avoid this error, it is imperative that all induced events be recognized by a family member as being typical for the patient, before a diagnosis of pseudoseizures is considered (see below).

Other studies have questioned the usefulness of induction protocols. Parra et al. (83) investigated the duration of elapsed time for a first diagnostic event to occur spontaneously during video EEG monitoring. The time to first diagnostic event was significantly shorter for psychogenic events than for patients with epileptic seizures. It was found that 77.4% of the patients with psychogenic events had a spontaneous event within the first 24 hours of monitoring. By 48 hours of monitoring, 96.2% of the patients had experienced an episode. Parra et al. (83) suggest that, given the high rates of spontaneous psychogenic events, induction methods as a diagnostic tool should be withheld during the initial 48 hours of video EEG monitoring.

There are no studies comparing the induction potential of the various methods used at the different centers. Based on our experience, there is little difference in their diagnostic yield. The ability to induce a pseudoseizure event appears to rely to a greater degree on the bedside skill of the physician. Attributes that include making the patient comfortable and conveying confidence that an event will happen are often all that separate a provoked pseudoseizure from a failed induction. On the other hand, the use of certain methods may be problematic, as they may be perceived by patients as deceptive practices. This is discussed in greater detail later.

Among the different methods, we prefer the use of hyperventilation to provoke pseudoseizures. The risk of being accused of lying is minimized with this technique, because hyperventilation and photic stimulation are standard activating techniques to facilitate epileptic seizures during routine EEG and video EEG. Patients typically are instructed to hyperventilate for a period of 3 minutes, during which time they are verbally coached. An advantage of this technique is the less invasive nature of the procedure. Potential contraindications to use of this procedure are a history of asthma or heart disease.

An interesting approach to eliciting seizures centered on the use of an intensive psychiatric interview designed to provoke a pseudoseizure during video EEG monitoring (87). Of the 32 patients with unusual or intractable seizures who underwent the procedure, 19 had a pseudoseizure during monitoring. At 3-year follow-up, 22 of 30 patients interviewed recalled the procedure as helpful or benign, and none regarded the experience as negative. The actual utility of this diagnostic technique needs to be determined by further study.

Ethical Issues

Concern often is raised over the ethical issues surrounding the infusion of an innocuous placebo substance that has been misrepresented as a powerful convulsant to the patient. One significant danger involves the risk of damaging the physician–patient relationship, which is an alliance based on trust. This trust, often built over time through countless interactions between physician and patient, can quickly erode even in the hands of an experienced physician. In the opinion of some authors, the actual risk of this occurring is quite small if the patient is presented with the results in a supportive and nonconfrontational manner. On the other hand, patients who may have difficulty accepting a diagnosis of pseudoseizures will try to find reasons to invalidate the diagnosis, including asking the physician what "medication" was used to provoke the pseudoseizure. At that point, the physician will be forced to disclose that intravenous saline was used, which will provide the patient with the "ammunition" to refute the diagnosis and lose trust in future diagnostic evaluations. As noted earlier, this risk is minimized by using photic stimulation and hyperventilation as induction techniques.

Special Considerations

In the evaluation of an induced event, special care must be made to establish that the event is identical to those described in the patient's history. It also is important to know that the event witnessed during monitoring is the only type of event that the patient was having. Therefore, it is imperative that family members verify that the event is typical for the patient by reviewing the videotape. Some of the reasons include the following:

1. A pseudoseizure can be induced in a patient with true epileptic seizures. Failure to identify a seizure event as atypical can result in the potentially catastrophic misdiagnosis of pseudoseizures in a patient with coexistent epilepsy. It is fortunate that these patients are in the minority. Slater et al. (59) found that only one in 29 patients with inducible seizures had a coexistent true epilepsy. Lancman and coworkers (84) did not find any epileptic patients who had induced events.
2. If the episode is not typical of the events that prompted medical attention, the episode may have resulted from high suggestibility. In such cases, the induction is considered negative.
3. In patients with multiple types of events by history, similar discretion is necessary. If the induced episode is characteristic of only one type of event, its relative frequency should be established and a final

diagnosis withheld until the other events are captured. Unfortunately, this may not be possible in one video EEG, and additional studies may be required.

CONCLUDING REMARKS

Psychogenic pseudoseizures now are recognized as a relatively common type of paroxysmal event that needs to be readily distinguished from epileptic seizures. A greater challenge is the ability to properly identify those epileptic seizures that mimic pseudoseizures, as this is becoming a more frequent source of diagnostic error, as clinicians become aware of pseudoseizures. Furthermore, pseudoseizures of organic origin must always be considered as an alternative diagnostic possibility. Although certain phenomena may be specific to epileptic seizures, there really are no signs that can be considered 100% specific for psychogenic pseudoseizures. Thus, even when the diagnosis may be obvious from the patient's clinical description of the event, a thorough evaluation that includes video EEG, MRI, and neuropsychological testing should be performed to confirm the diagnosis, ensure that a concurrent epileptic seizure disorder has not gone unnoticed, and, most importantly, develop a comprehensive treatment plan.

REFERENCES

1. Gumnit RJ, Leppik IE. The epilepsies. In: Rosenberg RN, ed. *Comprehensive neurology.* New York: Raven Press, 1991:311–336.
2. Prensky AL. An approach to the child with paroxysmal phenomenon with emphasis on nonepileptic disorders. In: Dodson WE, Pellock JW, eds. *Pediatric epilepsy: diagnosis and therapy.* New York: Demos Publications, 1992:63–81.
3. Thach BT. Sleep apnea in infancy and childhood. *Med Clin North Am* 1985;69:1289–1315.
4. Pedley TA. Differential diagnosis of episodic symptoms. *Epilepsia* 1983;24[Suppl 1]:S31–S44.
5. Laxdal T, Gomez MR, Reiher J. Cyanotic and pallid syncopal attacks in children (breath-holding spells). *Dev Med Child Neurol* 1969;11:755–763.
6. Meyers WF, Herbst JJ. Effectiveness of positioning therapy for gastroesophageal reflux. *Pediatrics* 1982;69: 768–772.
7. D'Alessandro R, Sacquengna T, Pazzaglia P, et al. Headache after partial complex seizures. In: Ander-

mann F, Lugarese E, eds. *Migraine and epilepsy.* London: Butterworth, 1987:273–328.

8. Brown P, Rothwell JC, Thompson PD, et al. The hyperekplexias and their relationship to the normal startle reflex. *Brain* 1991;114:1903–1928.

9. Liske E, Forster FM. Pseudoseizures: a problem in the diagnosis and management of epileptic patients. *Neurology* 1964;14;41–49.

10. Wilus RJ, Thompson PM, Vossler DG. Bizarre ictal automatisms: frontal lobe epileptic or psychogenic seizures? *J Epilepsy* 1990;3:207–213.

11. Walczak T, Williams DT, Berten W. Utility and reliability of placebo infusion in the evaluation of patients with seizures. *Neurology* 1994;44:394–399.

12. Koblar SA, Black AB, Schapel GJ. Video-audio/EEG monitoring in epilepsy—the Queen Elizabeth Hospital experience. *Clin Exp Neurol* 1992;29:70–73.

13. Krumholz A, Niedermeyer E. Psychogenic seizures: a clinical study with follow-up data. *Neurology* 1983;33: 498–502.

14. Meierkord H, Will B, Fish D, et al. The clinical features and prognosis of pseudoseizures diagnosed using video-EEG telemetry. *Neurology* 1991;41:1643–1646.

15. Lesser RP. Psychogenic seizures. *Neurology* 1996;46: 1499–1507.

16. Golden NH, Bennett HS, Pollack MA, et al. Seizures in adolescence. A review of patients admitted in an adolescent service. *J Adolesc Health Care* 1985;6:25–27.

17. Lancman ME, Brotherton TA, Asconape JJ, et al. Psychogenic seizures in adults: a longitudinal study. *Seizure* 1993;2:281–286.

18. Lelliott PT, Fenwick P. Cerebral pathology in pseudoseizures. *Acta Neurol Scand* 1991;83:129–132.

19. Metrick ME, Ritter FJ, Gates JR, et al. Nonepileptic events in childhood. *Epilepsia* 1991;32:322–328.

20. Wyllie E, Friedman D, Luders H, et al. Outcome of psychogenic seizures in children and adolescents compared to adults. *Neurology* 1991;41:742–744.

21. Lancman ME, Asconape JJ, Graves S, et al. Psychogenic seizures in children: long-term analysis of 43 cases. *J Child Neurol* 1994;9:404–407.

22. Wyllie E, Friedman D, Rothner D, et al. Psychogenic seizures in children and adolescents: outcome after diagnosis by ictal video and electroencephalographic recording. *Pediatrics* 1990;85:480–484.

23. Lempert T, Schmidt D. Natural history and outcome of psychogenic seizures: a clinical study in 50 cases. *J Neurol* 1990;237:35–39.

24. Finlayson RE, Lucas AR. Pseudoepileptic seizures in children and adolescents. *Mayo Clin Proc* 1979;54: 83–87.

25. Duchowny MS, Resnick TJ, Deray MJ, et al. Video EEG diagnosis of repetitive behavior in early childhood and it relationship to seizures. *Pedriatr Neurol* 1988;4: 162–164.

26. Krumholz A, Neidermeyer E, Alkaitis D, et al. Psychogenic seizures: a 5-year follow-up study. *Neurology* 1980;30:392.

27. Lesser RP. Psychogenic seizures. *Epilepsia* 1986;27: 823–829.

28. Gumnit RJ, Gates JR. Psychogenic seizures. *Epilepsia* 1986;27[Suppl 2]:S124–S129.

29. Kristensen O, Alving J. Pseudoseizures—risk factors and prognosis. A case-control study. *Acta Neurol Scand* 1992;85:177–180.

30. Gowers WR. *Epilepsy and other chronic convulsive diseases.* New York: William Wood & Co., 1881.

31. Gates JR, Ramani V, Whalen S, et al. Ictal characteristics of pseudoseizures. *Arch Neurol* 1985;42: 1183–1187.

32. Scott DF. Recognition and diagnostic aspects of nonepileptic seizures. In: Riley TL, Roy A, eds. *Pseudoseizures.* Baltimore: Williams & Wilkins, 1982: 21–34.

33. Holmes GL, Sackellares JC, McKiernan J, et al. Evaluation of childhood pseudoseizures using EEG telemetry and video tape monitoring. *J Pediatr* 1980;97:554–558.

34. Cloninger CR. Somatoform and dissociative disorders. In: Winokur G, Clayton P, eds. *The medical basis of psychiatry,* 2nd ed. Philadelphia: WB Saunders, 1994: 169–192.

35. Cohen RJ, Suter C. Hysterical seizures: suggestion as a provocative EEG test. *Ann Neurol* 1982;11:391–395.

36. Rot A. Cerebral disease and hysteria. *Comp Psychiatry* 1977;18:607–609.

37. Guberman A. Psychogenic pseudoseizures in nonepileptic patients. *Am J Psychiatry* 1982;27: 401–404.

38. Kalogjera-Sackellares D, Sackellares JC. Intellectual and neuropsychological features of patients with psychogenic pseudoseizures. *Psychiatry Res* 1999;86: 73–84.

39. Bowman ES, Markand ON. Psychodynamics and psychiatric diagnoses of pseudoseizure patients. *Am J Psychiatry* 1996; 153:57–63.

40. Bowman ES. Nonepileptic seizures: psychiatric framework, treatment, and outcome. *Neurology* 1999;53: S84–S88.

41. Drake ME Jr, Pakaines A, Phillips BB. Neuropsychological and psychiatric correlates of intractable pseudoseizures. *Seizure* 1992;1:11–13.

42. Binder LM, Salinsky MC, Smith SP. Psychological correlates of psychogenic seizures. *J Clin Exp Neuropsychol* 1994;16:524–539.

43. Parra J, Iriarte J, Kanner AM. Are we overusing the diagnosis of psychogenic non-epileptic events? *Seizure* 1999;8:223–227.

44. Kanner AM, Morris HH, Luders H, et al. Epileptic seizures mimicking pseudoseizures: some clinical differences. *Neurology* 1990;40:1404–1407.

45. Williamson PD, Spencer DD, Spencer SS, et al. Complex partial seizures of frontal lobe origin. *Ann Neurol* 1985;18:497–504.

46. Waterman K, Purves SJ, Kosaka B, et al. An epileptic syndrome caused by mesial frontal lobe seizure foci. *Neurology* 1987;37:577–582.

47. Luther JS, McNamara JO, Carwile S, et al. Pseudoepileptic seizures: methods and video analysis to aid diagnosis. *Ann Neurol* 1982;12:458–462.

48. Gullick TA, Spinks IP, King DW. Pseudoseizures: ictal phenomena. *Neurology* 1982;32:24–30.

49. Benbadis SR, Lancman ME, King LM, et al. Preictal pseudosleep: a new finding in psychogenic seizures. *Neurology* 1996;47:63–67.

50. DeToledo JC, Ramsey RE. Patterns of involvement of facial muscles during epileptic and nonepileptic events: review of 654 events. *Neurology* 1996;47:621–625.

51. Carmant L, Kramer U, Mikati MA, et al. Pseudoseizure manifestations in two preschool age children. *Seizure* 1995;4:147–149.

52. Bell WL, Park YD, Thompson EA, et al. Ictal cognitive assessment of partial seizures and pseudoseizures. *Arch Neurol* 1998;55:1456–1459.

53. Riley TL, Brannon WL. Recognition of pseudoseizures. *J Fam Pract* 1980;10:213–220.

54. Wilkus RJ, Dodrill CB, Thompson PM. Intensive EEG monitoring and psychological studies of patients with pseudoepileptic seizures. *Epilepsia* 1984;25:100–107.

55. Leis AA, Ross MA, Summers AK. Psychogenic seizures: ictal characteristics and diagnostics pitfalls. *Neurology* 1992;42:95–99.

56. Saygi S, Katz A, Marks D, et al. Frontal lobe partial seizures and psychogenic seizures: comparison of clinical and ictal characteristics. *Neurology* 1992;42:1274–1277.

57. Morris HH 3rd, Dinner DS, Luders H, et al. Supplementary motor seizures: clinical and electroencephalographic findings. *Neurology* 1988;38:1075–1082.

58. Shen W, Bowman ES, Markand ON. Presenting the diagnosis of pseudoseizures. *Neurology* 1990;40:756–759.

59. Slater JD, Brown MC, Jacobs W, et al. Induction of pseudoseizures with intravenous saline placebo. *Epilepsia* 1995;36:580–585.

60. Lesser RP, Leuders H, Dinner DS. Evidence for epilepsy is rare in patients with psychogenic seizures. *Neurology* 1983;33:502–504.

61. Sigurdardottir KR, Olafsson E. Incidence of psychogenic seizures in adults: a population-based study in Iceland. *Epilepsia* 1998;39:749–752.

62. Ney GC, Barr WB, Napolitano C, et al. New-onset seizures after surgery for epilepsy. *Arch Neurol* 1998;55:726–730.

63. Lancman ME, Asconape JJ. Clinical usefulness of video-EEG. *Medicina* 1990;50:315–318.

64. Lancman ME, O'Donovan C, Coelho M, et al. Usefulness of video-EEG monitoring in the elderly. *J Neurol Sci* 1996;142:54–58.

65. Barre MA, Burnstine TH, Fisher RS, et al. Electroencephalographic changes during simple partial seizures. *Epilepsia* 1994;35:715–720.

66. American Academy of Neurology Therapeutic and Technology Assessment Subcommittee. Neuropsychological testing of adults: considerations for neurologists. *Neurology* 1996;47:592–599.

67. Rausch R, Le MT, Langfitt JT. Neuropsychological evaluation—adults. In: Engel J Jr, Pedley TA, eds. *Epilepsy: a comprehensive textbook.* Philadelphia: Lippincott-Raven Publishers, 1997:977–987.

68. Almgren PE, Nordgren L, Skantze H. A retrospective study of operationally defined hysterics. *Br J Psychiatry* 1978;132:67–73.

69. Bendefeldt F, Miller LL, Ludwig AM. Cognitive performance in conversion hysteria. *Arch Gen Psychiatry* 1976;33:1250–1254.

70. Perrine K. Psychopathology in epilepsy. *Semin Neurol* 1991;11:175–181.

71. Binder LM, Kindermann SS, Heaton RK, et al. Neuropsychologic impairment in patients with nonepileptic seizures. *Arch Clin Neuropsychol* 1998;13:513–522.

72. Hathaway SR, McKinley JC, Butcher JN, et al. *Minnesota Multiphasic Personality Inventory 2: manual for administration and scoring.* Minneapolis: University of Minnesota Press, 1989.

73. Puente AE. Reimbursement for neuropsychological services. Lecture presented at 19th annual conference of the National Academy of Neuropsychology, San Antonio, Texas, 1999.

74. Binder LM. Malingering following minor head trauma. *Clin Neuropsychol* 1990;4:25–36.

75. Kalogjera-Sackellares D, Sackellares JC. Analysis of MMPI patterns in patients with psychogenic pseudoseizures. *Seizure* 1997;6:419–427.

76. Mehta SR, Dham SK, Lazar AI, et al. Prolactin and cortisol levels in seizure disorders. *J Assoc Physicians India* 1994;42:709–712.

77. Collins WC, Lanigan O, Callaghan N. Plasma prolactin concentrations following epileptic and pseudoseizures. *J Neurol Neurosurg Psychiatry* 1983;46:505–508.

78. Anzola GP. Predictivity of plasma prolactin levels in differentiating epilepsy from pseudoseizures: a prospective study. *Epilepsia* 1993;34:1044–1048.

79. Singh UK, Jana UK. Plasma prolactin in epilepsy and pseudoseizures. *Indian Pediatr* 1994;31:667–669.

80. Laxer KD, Mullooly JP, Howell B. Prolactin changes after seizures classified by EEG monitoring. *Neurology* 1985;35:31–35.

81. Oribe E, Amini R, Nissenbaum E, et al. Serum prolactin concentrations are elevated after syncope. *Neurology* 1996;47:60–62.

82. Gallagher BB, Murvin A, Flanigin HF, et al. Pituitary and adrenal function in epileptic patients. *Epilepsy* 1984;25:683–689.

83. Parra J, Kanner AM, Iriarte J, et al. When should induction protocols be used in the diagnostic evaluation of patients with paroxysmal events? *Epilepsia* 1998;39:863–867.

84. Lancman ME, Asconape JJ, Craven WJ, et al. Predictive value of induction of psychogenic seizures by suggestion. *Ann Neurol* 1994;35:359–361.

85. Bhatia M, Sinha PK, Jain S, et al. Usefulness of short-term video EEG recording with saline induction in pseudoseizures. *Acta Neurol Scand* 1997;95:363–366.

86. Drake ME Jr. Saline activation of pseudoepileptic seizures: clinical EEG and neuropsychiatric observations. *Clin Electroencephalogr* 1985;16:171–176.

87. Cohen LM, Howard GF, Bongar B. Provocation of pseudoseizures by psychiatric interview during EEG and video monitoring. *Int J Psychiatry Med* 1992;22:131–140.

25

Psychopathology and Outcome in Pseudoseizures

Elizabeth S. Bowman

Department of Psychiatry, Indiana University School of Medicine, Indianapolis, Indiana 46202

Pseudoseizures are a psychiatric illness that presents with pseudoneurologic symptoms (i.e., symptoms that resemble organically based seizures but are not due to physiologic dysfunction of the nervous system). They resemble epileptic seizures, so usually they are initially diagnosed by neurologists and subsequently treated by psychiatrists or other mental health professionals. This chapter explores the psychiatric illnesses found in pseudoseizure patients and discusses the prognosis of this troublesome illness.

Of what use is a discussion of the psychiatric illnesses associated with pseudoseizures? Neurologists are unlikely to desire to treat pseudoseizures directly, but they need to know the comorbid psychiatric illnesses when explaining pseudoseizures to patients, screening for psychiatric emergencies in these patients, and making referrals for mental health care.

Understanding the more common pseudoseizure-associated psychiatric illnesses is essential for mental health clinicians who often find themselves faced with the daunting task of sorting out multiple coexisting psychiatric conditions in pseudoseizure patients. For psychiatrists, determination of comorbid diagnoses may play a critical role in treatment outcome, because it is often the emotional pain created by these illnesses that is expressed via pseudoseizures. Reduction of such distress via pharmacologic and psychotherapeutic treatment of depression, panic disorder, or posttraumatic stress disorder (PTSD) can bring an immediate reduction of pseudoseizure frequency. Some "pseudoseizures" appear to be misdiagnosed symptoms of other psychiatric illnesses (e.g., panic attacks or dissociative trances) that require diagnosis and treatment.

HOW COMMON ARE PSYCHIATRIC ILLNESSES IN PSEUDOSEIZURE PATIENTS?

Do persons with pseudoseizures have more psychiatric illnesses than the general population? To clinicians, the answer may appear to be "obviously yes." However, no direct comparison studies have addressed this question. Studies of pseudoseizure patients repeatedly find rates of current psychiatric disorders that greatly exceed those of the general population in the National Comorbidity Survey (NCS) of the United States (1). Table 25.1 shows reported rates of any current psychiatric illness in 16 studies of pseudoseizure patients (2–17). These studies find some kind of psychiatric illness in 43% (2) to 100% (8,11,16, 17) of pseudoseizure subjects.

The methodologic difficulties of comparing the results of pseudoseizure studies are formidable, because the studies used diverse patient populations, differ greatly in the psychiatric illnesses for which they screened, and differ in the methodologic rigor and systematic nature of their screening. For instance,

TABLE 25.1. *Studies reporting prevalence of psychiatric diagnoses, past treatment, and past hospitalization in pseudoseizure patients*

Study reference	Any current diagnosis	Any lifetime diagnosis	Prior psychiatric treatment	Prior psychiatric hospitalization
2	43%	71%		
3	46%			25%
4	47%[a]			
5	60%		50%	30%
6	67%		≥51%	19%
7[b]	67%			
8	[70%][c]			
9	71%		51%[g]	
10	76%			
11	[80%][d]			30%
12	84%			
13	91%			
14	95%			
15	96%			
16	100%			
17	100%			
11	100%[e]		70%	
8	100%[f]			
19			38%	
20				37%
21				32%
29			58%	

[a]Does not include conversion diagnoses.
[b]Systematic SCID diagnoses used.
[c]Does not include mental retardation diagnoses.
[d]Excludes somatoform diagnoses.
[e]Includes somatoform diagnoses.
[f]Includes mental retardation diagnoses.
[g]Prior psychotherapy only.

only three studies listed in Table 25.1 clearly reported data for current psychiatric illness and for a past (lifetime) diagnosis of psychiatric illness (2,6,16). In the remainder of studies, readers are left to presume that only current diagnoses are being reported. Even a choice to include mental retardation as a psychiatric illness greatly changes results. In Pakalnis et al. (8), inclusion of mental retardation raised the psychiatric diagnosis rate from 70% to 100%. However, even a study that excluded mentally retarded persons found a 100% rate of psychiatric illness by doing a comprehensive diagnostic assessment that included a wide array of illnesses (16).

Most pseudoseizures are classified in the *Diagnostic and Statistical Manual of Mental Disorders,* Fourth Edition (DSM-IV) (18) as conversion disorder with seizures, as misdiagnosed panic disorder, or as part of another so-

matoform or dissociative disorder. Thus, it would seem obvious that all persons with pseudoseizures should carry some psychiatric diagnosis, even if it is solely that of conversion disorder. So how can we explain that the median rate of psychiatric diagnoses in 16 studies is 73.5%, rather than 100%? Study aims and methodologies play a huge role. Many studies overlook the fact that the patient has a somatoform (i.e., psychosomatic) disorder and only report findings of illness in other categories such as anxiety, affective, or personality disorders. As shown by the study of Pakalnis et al. (8), when the distinction between nonsomatoform and somatoform disorders is taken into account, the rate of overall psychiatric illness rose from 80% to 100%. This suggests that results from studies in which somatoform illness was not taken into account show a skew in the direction of unrealistically low overall rates of psychiatric illness in pseudoseizure patients. Yet another methodologic bias is failure to study axis II diagnoses (personality and developmental disorders).

The NCS study of the prevalence of psychiatric illnesses in the general U.S. population found that 50% of adults report at least one lifetime mental disorder and that close to 30% report having at least one disorder in the past 12 months (1). NCS studies assessed a wider range of psychiatric illnesses than most of the pseudoseizure studies, so NCS rates of having a current or lifetime mental illness generally would be expected to exceed those found in pseudoseizure studies. Thus, it is striking that the rates of having any mental illness in the NCS study are lower than the lowest rates of psychiatric illness found in the 16 pseudoseizure studies listed in Table 25.1. These data strongly suggest that pseudoseizure patients have far more comorbid psychiatric illness than do people in the general population.

PRIOR PSYCHIATRIC TREATMENT AND HOSPITALIZATIONS

Another way to estimate the level of psychiatric morbidity in pseudoseizure patients is to look at rates of past psychiatric treatment. Only 20% to 40% of people with mental illnesses seek treatment, so rates of treatment seeking seriously underestimate rates of illness (1). Despite this, six studies of pseudoseizure patients listed in Table 25.1 found that an astounding 38% to 70% of patients had previously sought mental health treatment (5,6,9,11,19,20). Four of these studies found treatment rates of 50% or higher. These findings may reflect the unusually severe illness of the tertiary care subject populations in these studies, but they also point to the pseudoseizure patients having multiple and serious psychiatric illnesses. High psychiatric comorbidity in pseudoseizure patients was demonstrated in one study that found a mean of 4.4 current and 6.0 lifetime axis I psychiatric diagnoses (16). Unfortunately, few studies of pseudoseizure patients from primary care settings exist for comparison.

A third way to estimate the frequency and seriousness of psychiatric illnesses in pseudoseizure patients is to assess their rates of past psychiatric hospitalization as an indication of symptoms severe enough to disable or endanger them. Seven studies of past psychiatric hospitalizations (Table 25.1) show rates of 25% to 37% among pseudoseizure patients (3,5,6,11,20–22). No less than one-fourth of them have been psychiatrically ill enough to warrant hospitalization. Whether we examine studies of rates of psychiatric diagnosis, of past treatment, or of hospitalizations, pseudoseizure patients appear to be psychiatrically ill considerably more often than their general population counterparts. It is uncertain but likely that pseudoseizure patients have higher rates of psychiatric illness than general medical or neurologic outpatients.

WHAT TYPES OF PSYCHIATRIC ILLNESSES OCCUR IN PSEUDOSEIZURE PATIENTS?

What kinds of comorbid psychiatric illnesses should clinicians screen for in a newly diagnosed pseudoseizure patient? Studies indicate that more than one type of pathology is likely to be seen. The results of studies of psychiatric diagnoses in pseudoseizure patients need to be interpreted cautiously because of diverse research methodologies and diverse patient populations.

The patient populations studied are diverse in gender proportions, seizure chronicity, proportions with comorbid epilepsy, inpatient versus outpatient status, methods of pseudoseizure diagnosis, age, and specialization of the treatment setting. The majority of studies reflect the relatively symptom-chronic population biases of tertiary care treatment settings. The methods used to diagnose psychiatric illnesses vary greatly in rigor and reliability. The diagnosing clinicians are not always mental health clinicians, so psychiatric diagnostic sophistication varies. Further diagnostic confusion has occurred because different diagnostic systems in North America and Europe result in different diagnostic labels for the same symptoms.

Another methodologic problem is researcher bias. For instance, most studies assess depression and panic attacks because these are common symptoms that are familiar to researchers. Thus, they are assessed and found in more studies than are diagnoses that are less common. It is less common for pseudoseizure patients to be assessed for substance abuse, PTSD, eating disorders, or dissociative disorders because even mental health clinicians overlook these illnesses or are inadequately trained in diagnosing them. This bias in investigation likely skews the literature toward overrepresenting depression, panic disorder, and personality disorders as the most common psychopathologies associated with pseudoseizures because they are the illnesses for which researchers have looked. Few studies have systematically screened for a wide variety of illnesses or used validated and reliable diagnostic instruments, such as the Structured Clinical Interview for DSM-IV (SCID) (23,24). The few studies that took this approach found very high rates of psychiatric illnesses (2,16) and a wider array of diagnoses. Some illnesses may be reported infrequently (e.g., eating, substance, or dissociative disorders) because they are recognized only when patients present with severe and obvious symptoms.

In light of these confounding methodologic problems, studies have yielded a wide range of rates and types of psychiatric illnesses. To answer the question of what specific psychiatric diagnoses are seen with pseudoseizures, we present below summations of literature findings of psychiatric diagnoses in pseudoseizure patients, arranged in clusters of illness types as found in DSM-IV (18). In reviewing these data, keep in mind the distinction between current (met diagnostic criteria within the past month) and lifetime diagnoses (met criteria in the past, with or without current illness). Lifetime rates are always equal to or higher than current illness rates.

MOOD (AFFECTIVE) DISORDERS

Depression is reported in more pseudoseizure studies (19 studies) (Table 25.2) than any other type of psychiatric illness (2,4–7, 9–12,14–17,19–21,25–27). Unfortunately, the definition of "depression" varies too greatly among studies for valid comparisons of their results. Studies that specify DSM-IV major depression or major affective disorder, or use a validated diagnostic instrument, report current rates of depression of 45% to 56% (5,9,16). The range of reported current depression (0% to 100%) illustrates the methodologic problems outlined earlier. The median rate of current depression in these studies is 31%. Thus, clinically significant depression is present in one-third to one-half of persons with newly diagnosed pseudoseizures. Lifetime rates of depression are much higher (36% to 80%), reflecting the recurrent nature of depression.

Other findings in Table 25.2 show that pseudoseizure populations have mood disorders other than major depression. Dysthymia (a chronic low-grade depression) occurs in up to 13% of subjects (2,5,15,16). In many studies, it is likely lumped together with other depressive syndromes, so its true incidence is unclear. Bipolar disorder also accounts for some affective disorder diagnoses, but its occurrence in pseudoseizure patients is uncommon (median 4%) and is near its 1% baseline rate in the general population (1,2,15,16,19, 22,28). This is what would be expected for a mostly genetic illness that likely has a chance association with pseudoseizures.

The 1-year and lifetimes prevalences of major depression in the general population are about 10% and 17%, respectively, and the prevalences for any affective disorder are 11% and 19%, respectively (1). Thus, the high prevalence of depression in the pseudoseizure population is far more than a chance association and suggests that clinicians should always evaluate pseudoseizure patients for depression. Pseudoseizures generally occur in persons who have a life of multiple or severe

TABLE 25.2. Selected [a] affective and anxiety disorders in pseudoseizure subjects

Study reference	Depression/major depression	Dysthymia (current)	Bipolar disorders	Any anxiety disorder	Panic attacks or disorder	PTSD	Any phobia
25	0% Current			22% Current			
12	12% Current			11%			
7	15%[b] Current						
20	16% Current						7% Current
2	21% Current / 36% Lifetime	0%	7% Current and Lifetime		14% Current / 21% Lifetime	14% Current / 36% Lifetime	
10	24%[c] Current			12% Current			
4	25% Current						2% Current
26	33%		4% Current				
19	35%						
27	44%[d]			11%[k] Current			
5	45%[e] Current	5%		10%[j] Current / 80%[l] Current	70% Current		
16	47%[e] Current / 80%[e] Lifetime	13%	2% Current and Lifetime	47%[m] Current / 51%[m] Lifetime	20% Current / 27% Lifetime	49% Current / 58% Lifetime	33% Current / 42% Lifetime
11	50%[f]			19% Current	80% Current		
9	56%[g] Current	7%					
15	60%[e] Current		2% Current		2% Current		
6	65%[d] Lifetime			39%[m] Life	26% Current		16% Current
17	100%[h] Lifetime						
21	58% Lifetime						
14	74%[d,l] Lifetime						
28			4% BP NOS	28%[m] Current / 36%[l] Current	24% Current	8% Current	
22				18% Current / 43%[l] Lifetime			
30			12% Current			10% Current	
31					>90% Lifetime		
33					~33% Current		

[a] For generalized anxiety disorder, obsessive-compulsive disorder, or anxiety disorder not otherwise specified, see discussion in text.

[b] Denotes "major depression or dysthymia."

[c] Denotes "depressive syndrome."

[d] Denotes "depression."

[e] Utilized valid Structure Clinical Interview for DSM-III-R interviews (SCID).

[f] Denotes "current or lifetime mood disorder."

[g] Denotes "major affective disorder."

[h] Denotes "clinical affective syndrome."

[i] Includes bipolar disorder depressions.

[j] Excludes panic subjects.

[k] Defined as "anxiety."

[l] Includes posttraumatic stress disorder (PTSD) and panic.

[m] Excludes PTSD.

stresses (or traumas) or who have a pattern of being unable to express emotions adequately (29). Pseudoseizures are like an emotional "pop-off valve" for relief of pent-up emotional distress. The same losses and stresses that produce pseudoseizures are likely to cause depression. The painful affects associated with depression, in turn, add to the patient's emotional load and may contribute to having more pseudoseizures. When depression is present, it should be treated with antidepressant medications and often with concomitant psychotherapy. Adequate treatment of depression may help decrease pseudoseizures because it decreases the pressure of painful feelings.

ANXIETY DISORDERS

Selected anxiety disorder diagnoses in pseudoseizure subjects are listed in Table 25.2 (2, 5–7,9–12,15,16,22,23,26,28,30,31). Anxiety has been noted often in these patients. This is not surprising, because pseudoseizures are basically a somatic outlet for unmanageably intense feelings such as anxiety, sadness, and anger (32). The range of occurrence of anxiety disorders in pseudoseizure patients is very broad: 0% to 80%. A more useful statistic is the median of the studies' findings: an 18.5% prevalence of current anxiety disorders.

Data on anxiety disorders in pseudoseizure patients are difficult to interpret because studies are inconsistent in which diagnoses were included. Some studies focus solely on panic disorder and generalized anxiety disorder (GAD) (31), whereas others separately included all DSM-IV anxiety diagnoses (16). A particular problem is that PTSD is not included in many diagnostic instruments and was omitted from many studies of other anxiety disorders. Most studies found an anxiety disorder other than PTSD in one-tenth to one-fifth of subjects. When PTSD is included, the rates of any anxiety disorder rise to about 33% to 47%. PTSD is found in 8% to 49% of pseudoseizure subjects (2,16,28,30,33), and an increasing number of investigators are commenting on the association of trauma

with pseudoseizures (2,16,34–36). Some behaviors diagnosed as pseudoseizures are actually dissociative flashbacks of trauma (one of the symptoms of PTSD). Thus, clinicians should screen for PTSD in pseudoseizure patients who have a history of trauma, especially in patients whose seizures resemble abreactions (33,35).

The anxiety disorder most commonly mentioned in pseudoseizure studies is panic disorder, which is found in 14% to 90% of subjects (2,5,6,11,15,16,28,31). The three studies that found high rates of panic disorder focused specifically on this disorder (5,11,31). Studies that assessed panic *disorder* (recurrent panic attacks resulting in dysfunction) rather than isolated panic *attacks* generally find a prevalence of panic disorder in less than one-fourth of subjects. Panic attacks cause symptoms (e.g., trembling, depersonalization, and fear) that often are confused with partial complex seizures, so persons with panic disorder may be mistakenly diagnosed with pseudoseizures (5). Pseudoseizure patients should be questioned about symptoms of panic, keeping in mind the differences in their presentations: severely altered consciousness (i.e., amnesia) is not present during panic attacks, panic usually has a slower onset than pseudoseizures, and diaphoresis is a symptom of panic but not of pseudoseizures.

Some symptoms of generalized anxiety often are observed clinically in pseudoseizure patients, but they often are lumped with symptoms of phobia, panic, and PTSD, and described globally as an "anxiety disorder." Two studies (15,16) each found the DSM-IV (18) diagnosis of GAD, involving pervasive worry with somatic anxiety symptoms, in 9% of pseudoseizure patients as a separate disorder from other anxiety disorders. This is likely the case because DSM criteria dictate that GAD is not diagnosed if anxiety is related to panic, PTSD, obsessive-compulsive disorder, or phobias. Thus, even though many pseudoseizure patients are "worriers," their anxiety may be a symptom of PTSD or panic rather than represent GAD. Clinicians should inquire carefully to assess if anxiety is related to panic or PTSD, because these disorders are treated differently than GAD. Obsessive-compulsive disorder, a largely biologic illness, is found in pseudoseizure patients at a rate of 4% (16), similar to its prevalence in the general population. Anxiety disorder not otherwise specified has been found in 2% (16) to 5% (15) of pseudoseizure subjects.

Pseudoseizure patients suffering from panic or PTSD should receive a selective serotonin uptake inhibitor, such as fluoxetine, paroxetine, sertraline, or citalopram, and they should be referred for psychotherapy. The selective serotonin uptake inhibitor medications are efficacious for depression disorder, panic disorder, GAD, and PTSD. Use of benzodiazepines in GAD, panic disorder, or PTSD patients should be a short-term strategy and should be used in conjunction with seeking psychotherapy. I do not recommend extended use of benzodiazepines without psychotherapy, because this results in medication dependence without resolution of the cause of the anxiety.

SOMATOFORM DISORDERS

Rates of somatoform disorders in pseudoseizure subjects are listed in Table 25.3 (4,5, 7,8,10–12,15,16,19,21,22,25,31,37–39,41). Pseudoseizures are, by definition, a somatic expression of psychological distress that usually falls under the DSM-IV diagnosis of conversion disorder. So how can we explain the findings of Table 25.3 that only one of ten studies found that 100% of pseudoseizure patients carry a somatoform disorder diagnosis, and that the median finding of these studies is that one-third have a somatoform diagnosis?

Research subject recruitment explains a great deal. These patients are diagnosed with pseudoseizures because they have symptoms that result in referral to a neurology clinic. However, they include persons whose symptoms are undiagnosed panic attacks, unrecognized dissociative amnesia, flashbacks of trauma, malingering, factitious symptoms, or difficulties attributed by researchers to per-

sonality disorders. Some subjects have misdiagnosed physical conditions (such as cardiogenic syncope) rather than pseudoseizures (41). None of these subjects would have conversion seizures, and not all would have a somatoform disorder. In addition, somatoform diagnoses can be missed unless researchers systematically ask about other conversion or somatic symptoms.

Conversion seizures account for 33% to 84% of pseudoseizure patients (8,16,25,39). Pseudoseizure patients have strikingly high lifetime rates (42% to 93%) of other types of conversion (10,16,21,31). Conversion seizures and other conversion symptoms exist concurrently in up to one-fifth of subjects. In subjects with concurrent conversion, conversion pseudo-Todd's paralysis, numbness, deafness, and blindness may occur as part of their ictal or periictal presentation. Vein et al. (31) noted a mean of 5.9 conversion symptoms in pseudoseizure subjects. These data suggest that conversion seizure patients are probably a population that recurrently expresses distress via conversion, and who happen to have been studied when they presented with seizure symptoms. Thus, over the patient's lifetime, neurologists might expect to see untreated pseudoseizure patients recurrently with different forms of conversion as life stresses wax and wane. During evaluations, clinicians should ask pseudoseizure patients about other past conversion symptoms and other somatic symptoms.

The seizures of pseudoseizure patients may simply be the presenting symptom of a wider range of somatic symptoms as is found in somatization disorder or undifferentiated somatoform disorder (characterized by fewer somatic symptoms). Two studies found undifferentiated somatoform disorder in 18% (16) and 25% (5) of pseudoseizure subjects. DSM-IV somatization disorder requires eight symptoms in four diagnostic areas, so it is diagnosed less commonly (13%) (16). Intractable headaches are a common form of somatoform pain disorder in these patients. Blumer (22) diagnosed 71% of his subjects with somatoform pain disorder, a proportion that is strik-

TABLE 25.3. Selected somatoform[a] and dissociative[b] disorder diagnoses in pseudoseizure subjects

Study reference	Any current somatoform	Nonseizure conversion	Conversion seizures	Somatoform pain disorder	Any current dissociative disorder	Dissociative disorder NOS	Current dissociative amnesia
10	2%	69% Lifetime					
12	6%	42% Lifetime					
7	17%				11%		
15	22%				22%		
19	23%[c]						22%
37	33%[d,e]	19% Current		14%[d,i]			
38	36%		33% Lifetime		36%	27%[f]	
25	59%			71%			
22	79%						
16	89%	4% Current 82% Lifetime	78% Lifetime	16%[i]	91%	62%[g]	13% Diagnosis 98% Symptom[j]
11	100%						
31		93% Lifetime					53%[f,h]
4		21% Current					
8			55% Lifetime				
39			84% Lifetime				
56				77%	100%		
41				61%[i]			

a For reports of undifferentiated somatoform disorder and somatoform pain disorder, see discussion in text.
b For reports of depersonalization disorder, see discussion in text.
c Defined as Briquet's disorder.
d Pediatric subjects.
e Defined as any nonseizure psychosomatic diagnosis.
f Methods or systematic efforts at diagnosing dissociative disorders are unclear.
g Systematic inquiry using the SCID-D.
h Denotes amnesia during pseudoseizures.
i Defined as chronic headaches. Bowman and Markand (16) found 71% prevalence of headaches but diagnosed somatoform pain disorders in only 16%.
j See text for discussion of differentiating the symptom and the DSM-IV diagnosis of dissociative amnesia.

ingly similar to findings of recurrent headaches in 73% of patients reported by Bowman and Markand (16) and 61% of patients reported by Ettinger et al. (40). These headaches also are seen in persons with nonsomatic presentations of dissociation, and they may be an expression of severe internal conflict or the pressure of suppressed emotional distress. Ettinger et al. (40) also found that somatoform pain was extremely common (77%) in pseudoseizure patients and was found in significantly higher rates in patients whose pseudoseizures persisted on follow-up.

Overall, studies show that about two-thirds of patients diagnosed with pseudoseizures have conversion seizures, about two-thirds have had another type of conversion in the past, and about one-third have a more complex somatoform disorder. Pseudoseizure patients definitely should be screened for somatoform pain, past conversion, and other somatic symptoms.

DISSOCIATIVE DISORDERS

Discussion of dissociation in the pseudoseizure literature presents an odd contradiction. Numerous authors (5,28,30,31,38,39, 42–49) make reference to dissociation as a cause of pseudoseizures, and several authors (36,46–48) have devoted entire papers to arguing that dissociation is the mechanism of action by which conversion seizures occur. In contrast to widespread agreement that dissociation is an important explanatory component for pseudoseizures, very few researchers have formally investigated specific dissociative disorder diagnoses. Most literature references to dissociation in pseudoseizure patients consist of remarks about dissociation as a mechanism of pseudoseizures, or remarks that pseudoseizures can be dissociative trances or depersonalized states that resemble epilepsy.

The connection between dissociation and conversion symptoms stretches back to Pierre Janet (50,51), who coined the term "dissociation" when describing the psychological process involved in conversion and somatization symptoms in patients with hysteria (47). Prior to the DSM-III (52), conversion was classified in DSM-II as a type of dissociative disorder (53). The connection between conversion (formerly called hysteria) and dissociation was less obvious after conversion was classified with the somatoform disorders in DSM-III (52). Nemiah (47) decried the divorce of conversion and dissociation and advocated unsuccessfully for returning conversion to the dissociative disorders section of DSM-IV. He also believed that both conversion and somatization are closely related to dissociative disorders.

Other authors have argued that dissociation explains a subgroup of pseudoseizure patients (35,36,48). Kuyk et al. (36) observed that pseudoseizures could be classified as a somatoform disorder or a dissociative disorder, depending on whether the most prominent symptom was loss of control of motor functions or of changes in memory and consciousness. Harden (48) observed that pseudoseizure patients have features of both dissociation and conversion, but believed that dissociation provides a better diagnostic "fit." Several authors note striking similarities in the characteristics of pseudoseizure or conversion disorder subjects and dissociative disorder subjects, such as high rates of trauma, a similar cluster of comorbid psychiatric abnormalities, amnesia, trauma or sexual abuse histories, high hypnotizability, elevated scores on dissociative disorder instruments, and higher than expected rates of head injuries (16,36,47). Kuyk (36) and Bowman (32,35) separately postulated that pseudoseizure patients are a heterogeneous group, but that dissociation is the appropriate interpretation for a subgroup of them. Harden (48), Torem (46), and Bowman (35) recommended that pseudoseizures patients be assessed for dissociative disorders. This is especially important when trauma or child abuse is reported, or when PTSD or a cluster of concurrent axis I disorders is present (35,48).

The DSM-IV (18) lists five dissociative disorders: amnesia, fugue, depersonalization disorder, dissociative identity disorder (DID), and dissociative disorder not otherwise specified (DDNOS). Authors who mention dissociative disorders in pseudoseizure patients often lump dissociative disorders together and rarely define which ones they diagnosed.

If dissociation is a foundational mechanism of conversion seizures, then why are specific dissociative disorder diagnoses so rarely reported in pseudoseizure studies? Investigator bias and the silent nature of dissociation both are responsible. First, dissociative disorders are underrecognized by mental health professionals because they lack training and experience with these disorders and do not look for dissociative disorders, and because dissociation is inherently difficult to recognize (45,54). Second, common psychiatric diagnostic instruments, such as the commonly used Structured Clinical Interview for DSM-III-R axis I disorders (55), do not include dissociative disorders. Thus, researchers using these instruments do not systematically assess dissociation, even when they note its presence among their subjects (5). Snyder et al. (5) are correct in suggesting that systematic assessment of dissociative disorders in pseudoseizure patients requires use of additional reliable instruments. The most reliable and readily available dissociative disorder diagnostic instrument (Structured Clinical Interview for DSM-IV Dissociative Disorders [SCID-D]) (23,24) has only been used in one study of pseudoseizure patients (16). The absence of dissociative disorder diagnoses in the pseudoseizure literature may be due to a failure to systematically inquire about them.

Third, investigators may overlook dissociative symptoms because they assume that amnesia is simply part of conversion seizures rather than recognizing this amnesia as a dissociative symptom. Fourth, many dissociative symptoms, such as amnesia for childhood or for adulthood events, are symptoms created by a desire to banish material from consciousness. Persons with dissociative disorders wish to avoid awareness of their symptoms and rarely report them spontaneously (16,35). All of these factors make it easy for investigators to miss dissociative symptoms in research and clinical evaluations.

In light of these observations, it is not surprising that significant rates of dissociative disorders in pseudoseizure patients are found only in samples where comprehensive and systematic inquiry occurred. The only study that systematically used a valid diagnostic instrument found that experiences of dissociative amnesia were virtually ubiquitous among pseudoseizure patients (98%) and occurred outside of pseudoseizures in 82% of subjects (16). Even without diagnostic instruments, systematic inquiry found ictal amnesia in 53% of pseudoseizures patients (31).

Rates of any kind of dissociative disorder diagnosis in pseudoseizure patients (Table 25.3) range from 11% to 100% (7,15,16,31, 38,41,56). Gross (56) reported a rate of 100% because he was describing a small series of adolescents with pseudoseizures and dissociation related to incest. Bowman and Markand (16) reported a high rate of dissociative disorders (98%) because they conducted systematic screening with the SCID-D (23,24). The remaining studies appear to demonstrate that blatant dissociative disorders that can be detected without systematic screening occur in 11% to 36% of subjects. These three studies do not help us determine how many patients have less obvious dissociative symptoms.

The *symptom* of dissociative amnesia is common during pseudoseizures and should be differentiated from the DSM-IV *diagnosis* of dissociative amnesia, which requires that amnesia not occur exclusively in the course of somatization disorder or another dissociative disorder. Reports of amnesia in the pseudoseizure literature rarely make this distinction and should be interpreted conservatively as *symptoms,* not disorders. The symptom of dissociative amnesia in pseudoseizure patients is very common, ranging from 53% to 98% (15,16,31). Systematic inquiry about amnesia outside of seizures reveals it to be very common: 82% for adulthood events and 73% for childhood events (16), but the formal diagnosis of dissociative amnesia occurs in a minority of patients, probably because it is usually accompanied by other dissociative symptoms that warrant another dissociative disorder diagnosis.

Depersonalization disorder is rare in the general population (57) and uncommon among pseudoseizure patients. This is not surprising, because depersonalization disorder occurs without the episodic amnesia that occurs during pseudoseizures. Instead, during pseudoseizures, amnesia often combines with transient depersonalization and sometimes with derealization to create DDNOS. Accordingly, DDNOS and dissociative amnesia are the two most common dissociative disorders reported in pseudoseizure patients.

DDNOS includes a variety of atypical dissociative conditions, including "ego state disorder," in which dissociated mental functions act semiautonomously from the patient's usual ego and identity (58). Ego states are similar to the alter personalities of DID patients, but they have less autonomy and identity alteration. Covert ego states (or alter personalities in DID) that contain painful affects related to trauma or interpersonal conflict have been found by investigators from Pierre Janet onward to be the direct cause of pseudoseizures and other conversion symptoms (32,35,46–48,51). Nemiah (47), Torem (46), and Harden (48) cite contemporary and historical cases in which conversion symptoms come and go with dissociative switching among the personality states of DID patients, and I have observed this in pseudoseizure patients and have interviewed alter personalities who stated that they released trauma-related affect via pseudoseizures. Pseudoseizures have been reported to cease permanently after trauma is addressed and dissociated ego states are integrated in psychotherapy (46).

Various authors agree that some pseudoseizures are an expression of dissociated mental content or personality states, or terror or rage from traumatic experiences (16,35,36, 46–48). In 16% to patients, pseudoseizures are related to distinct alter personalities found in DID (16). Nemiah (47) also postulated a connection between DID and conversion, writing, "The data do provide strong evidence that, however different the phenomenologic characteristics of these disorders, both conversion disorder and somatization disorder are closely associated with multiple personality disorder."

What can we conclude from this tangle of studies on dissociative disorders and pseudoseizures? First, true conversion seizures (as opposed to "seizures" that are misdiagnosed panic or other phenomena) are likely a somatic presentation of dissociation (36,45,47). They involve dissociation of consciousness and/or volition from motor control.

Second, the pseudoseizures of one-fourth to more than one-half of patients are a manifestation of a more complex dissociative disorder, such as recurrent trance states, ego state disorder, or DID. With the latter two diagnoses, dissociated traumatic experiences or emotions often being expressed via the seizures. This should not surprise clinicians who are familiar with recurrent findings of elevated rates of child abuse and other traumas in pseudoseizure patients (2,5,16,22,26,32,33, 39,59–62). Third, whereas dissociation is the mechanism of conversion seizures, dissociative disorders are not responsible for all pseudoseizure patients. Persons who are alexithymic or who have intolerable emotional pain from other mental illnesses or life stresses may express their distress dissociatively without having amnesia or a true dissociative disorder.

Fourth, the pseudoseizure literature desperately needs more studies of dissociative disorders that use valid diagnostic instruments. Fifth, research findings confirm that assessment of dissociative disorders in pseudoseizure patients is clearly indicated. This can be accomplished efficiently by screening with a self-report instrument, such as the Dissociative Experiences Scale (63) and following up scores over 20 with diagnostic questions as found in the SCID-D (22–24).

PERSONALITY DISORDERS

Many authors comment on the presence of personality disorders in pseudoseizure patients, but there is no consensus about the frequency or type of personality disorders in this population.

Personality disorders have long been associated with pseudoseizure patients, probably because conversion was once part of the illness "hysteria," which was popularly associated with histrionic personality disorder.

Research studies do not find personality disorders in all pseudoseizure patients. In 15 studies (Table 25.4), the occurrence of any type of personality disorder ranges from 6% to 62%, with a median prevalence of 40% (2, 4,7,8,10,12,15,16,19,20,25–27,64,65). Most studies found personality disorders in 30% to 50%. At least one-third of pseudoseizure patients do not have a personality disorder. When individual personality disorder diagnoses are considered, an exclusive association of conversion seizures with histrionic personality is not supported. The four most common types of personality disorders found in pseudoseizure patients are borderline (2,7,16,25, 65), histrionic (10,16,19,27,65), avoidant (2, 16), and antisocial (7,19,65). Obsessive-compulsive personality and dependent personality disorders are rarely reported in these patients.

Among pseudoseizure patients, the majority do not have a personality disorder, but those who do tend to fall into DSM-IV cluster B disorders (borderline, histrionic, antisocial). A mixture of maladaptive personality traits appears to be more common than single types of personality disorders (16,65). The prominence of borderline personality among pseudoseizure patients is not surprising, as both borderline personality and pseudoseizures are firmly associated with elevated rates of childhood maltreatment (66). It may be that personality disorders, like dissociation, PTSD, recurrent depression, and pseudoseizures, all reflect unstable or abusive early life environments.

MISCELLANEOUS DIAGNOSES

Table 25.5 shows rates of less commonly reported diagnoses in pseudoseizure subjects. Substance abuse or dependence is common in clinical populations, but its diagnosis is easily missed because substance abusers minimize usage and deny abuse. Pseudoseizure studies show that current substance abuse is found in 0% to 28% of subjects and lifetime abuse in 4% to 42% (4,5,7,9,15,16,22). Reported rates of lifetime substance abuse are considerably higher than for current abuse. This may occur

TABLE 25.4. *Selected personality disorders[a] in pseudoseizure subjects (current diagnoses)*

Study reference	Any personality disorder	Histrionic personality disorder	Borderline personality disorder	Avoidant personality disorder	Antisocial personality disorder
4	6%				
10	8%[b]	8%			
26	15%				
7	28%		13%		2%
8	30%				
27	34%	34%			
2	36%		21%	21%	
64	40%				
25	40%		15%		
12	44%[c]				
15	45%				
65	50%	11%	35%		23%
20	>50%[d]				
16	62%[c]	40%[e]	49%[e]	38%[e]	
19	62%	4%			34%[f]

[a] For obsessive-compulsive, dependent, and mixed personality disorders, see discussion in text.
[b] Defined as "hysterical personality."
[c] Primarily chronic pseudoseizure subjects.
[d] Reports that a "majority" of subjects had a personality disorder.
[e] Subjects had these traits rather than full diagnostic criteria.
[f] "Antisocial with borderline traits."

TABLE 25.5. *Miscellaneous psychiatric diagnoses in pseudoseizure patients*

Study reference	Any substance abuse/dependence	Alcohol abuse/dependence	Drug abuse/dependence	Psychotic disorder, any current	Eating disorder, any	Adjustment disorder	Factitious or malingering, current
4	1%[a] Current		1%[a] Current		1%[a] Current		
7	2%[b] Current						
15	4% Lifetime						11% Factitious
5	15%[a] Lifetime	15%[a] Lifetime		2%		13% Current	
22	15%[b] Lifetime			15%	5%[a,f] Current		
9	9%[a] Current			12%[d]			
				9%			
16	11%[c] Current	0% Current	11%[c] Current	0%	9%[e] Current	0% Current	0%
	42%[c] Lifetime	29%[c] Lifetime	24%[c] Lifetime		20%[a] Lifetime	4% Lifetime	
2		28% Current	0% Current			0% Current	
			14% Lifetime				
11		30% Lifetime		10%			
25				0%	7%[g] Current		15% Factitious
39				11%			
28				12%			
19				16%			
12						3% Current	3% Factitious
30							12% Malingering
							20%[h]
38							18% Malingering

[a] Substance dependence.
[b] Substance abuse.
[c] Either abuse or dependence.
[d] Defined as "hallucinatory episodes."
[e] Denotes any eating disorder.
[f] Bulimia.
[g] Anorexia nervosa.
[h] Factitious or malingering.

because current users have more denial than those in recovery, or it may be related to former substance abusers presenting with somatic symptoms when they no longer can utilize substances to mask painful feelings.

The ten studies that assessed psychotic disorders in pseudoseizure patients found low rates (0% to 16% currently) (5,9,11,15,16,19, 22,25,28,39). The median finding for any psychosis is 10.5%. Psychosis may be difficult to assess in pseudoseizure patients because the hallucinations of hysterical psychosis are difficult to differentiate from other psychoses during a brief assessment. In addition, pseudoseizure patients with complex dissociative disorders may be misdiagnosed as psychotic if they report hearing alter ego states or alter personalities as voices inside their heads. Rarely, bizarre symptoms of psychosis may mimic epilepsy and be misdiagnosed. Overall, the literature indicates that psychosis is an uncommon pseudoseizure comorbidity.

Eating disorders appear uncommon (0% to 9%) in pseudoseizure patients (4,5,16,25). This may be due to the patient choosing seizure symptoms rather than eating symptoms as their somatic expression of distress. It also is possible that eating disorders are underdiagnosed in these studies because many clinicians do not routinely inquire about them.

Low rates of adjustment disorders (3% to 13%) in pseudoseizure populations may reflect a sampling artifact (2,12,15,16). Generally, adjustment disorders are diagnosed only if symptoms cease less than 6 months after the end of an acute stressor. In contrast, pseudoseizure research populations usually are tertiary care populations that have chronic symptoms. Thus, it is not surprising that rates of adjustment disorders are low in these study populations. Adjustment disorders may account for the initial onset of pseudoseizures in persons who can identify a clear precipitating stressor, but not all patients can identify a clear precipitant (29).

Malingering and factitious disorders are suspected fairly often but uncommonly diagnosed by clinicians who evaluate conversion disorders. Clinicians may suspect these diagnoses because of their own frustrations with these difficult patients. Certainly some patients malinger seizures when disability payments are involved. However, most pseudoseizure patients are distressed and very inconvenienced by their symptoms. Rates of factitious disorder or malingering may be low because the secondary gain pseudoseizure patients receive in attention from others often is overshadowed by the inconveniences of being embarrassed by the symptoms and their crippling impact on driving and employment. Alternatively, factitious disorder and malingering may be underdiagnosed because clinicians fail to consider them in the differential diagnosis.

OUTCOME/PROGNOSIS FOR PSEUDOSEIZURES

Limitations of Comparing Studies

Table 25.6 lists the results of clinical outcome studies of pseudoseizure subjects, and Table 25.7 lists the characteristics of their study populations (4,6,8–10,12,15,20,21,26, 27,33,37,62,64,67–72). Three outcome groups are commonly mentioned in the literature: subjects who are seizure-free, who are improved (lower seizure frequency), and who show little or no seizure improvement. Studies listed in Table 25.6 are arranged in order of increasing proportions of subjects who were seizure-free. Tables 25.6 and 25.7 illustrate the difficulties of comparing outcome studies. The proportion of subjects in the "seizure-free" outcome group varies from 19% to 87%, and the duration of follow-up is equally broad (3 months to more than 5 years).

Patients with epilepsy and pseudoseizures were included in these studies in proportions from 0% to 100% of subjects. In these patients, epileptic seizures during the follow-up period may skew data toward a poorer outcome. Follow-up studies do not always segregate subjects with concomitant epilepsy from those with solely pseudoseizures when analyzing or reporting outcomes (73). Studies that compared outcome of subjects with and without concomitant epilepsy show mixed re-

TABLE 25.6. *Pseudoseizure occurrence outcome studies[a]*

Study reference	Follow-up duration	Percent seizure-free	"Improved" but seizures continue	Seizures "poor," unchanged, or worse
6	6–9 mo	19%	56%	25%
8	6–12 mo	20%	45%	35%
26	61 mo mean, range 1–12 yr	25%	NR	NR
15	5 mo mean, range 2–6 mo	29%	62%	9%
27	>5 yr	29%	NR	56%
21 (all subjects)	4–24 mo	30% (all subjects)	20% (all subjects)	50% (all subjects)
21 (acute subjects)	5 mo mean, range 0.04–5 yr	60%	40%	0%
21 (chronic subjects)	12 yr mean, range 1–20 yr	0%	0%	100%
20	34 mo mean, range 6–72 mo	33%	42%	25%
10	24 mo mean, range 8–39 mo	34%	NR	56% at 2 yr
19	16 mo mean, range 12–38 mo	35%	655	NR
4	5 yr median, range 1–14 yr	40%	60% improved or no	Change at median 5 yr
67	22 mo mean, range 6–30 mo	41%	34%	25%
68	NR	42%	26%	32%
62	40 mo mean, range to 12 yr	45%	NR	NR
3	5.8 yr median	45%	NR	NR
69	1 yr	34%	NR	NR
	2 yr	43%	NR	NR
	3 yr	48%	NR	NR
	4 yr	51%	NR	NR
	5 yr	58%	NR	NR
70	3 mo mean	50%	19%	31%
	At 1 yr	37%	31%	31%
12	3.5 yr mean, range 0.25–6 yr	50%[b]	28%	NR
71	18 mo mean (SD 10)	52%	43%	5%
64	>2 yr	62%	18%	NR
33	At inpatient discharge	63%		34%
	At 1 yr	31%	14% (1 yr)	(8–12 mo)
37	Immediately after diagnosis	57%	NR	NR
	2.5 yr	78%	NR	NR
72	4 yr	87%	NR	12%

NR, not reported.

[a]Studies are listed in order by increasing proportion of subjects who were seizure-free.

[b]Represents average of outcomes of seizure-free subjects in acute group (15/18, 83%) and chronic group (10/32, 31%).

TABLE 25.7. *Characteristics of pseudoseizure follow-up samples*

Study reference	No. diagnosed/ no. followed-up	Percent with pseudoseizure and epilepsy	Percent receiving psychiatric treatment[b]	Percent adult subjects	Percent female subjects
67	100/61	11%	61%	100%	90%
74	128/121	36%	100%	NR	NR
12	50/50	58%	50%	NR	72%
71	56/56	0%	71%	91%	71%
6	55/43	16%	63%	100%	91%
20	32/19	26%	67%	~93%[a]	74%
21	12/10	0%	NR	100%	83%
64	NR/32	NR	NR	NR	NR
15	45/45	42%	69%	82%	69%
3	28/22	86%	NR	79%	86%
27	41/41	37%	NR	~83%[a]	71%
26	93/63	11%	NR	100%	84%
62	43/22	0%	NR	0%	74%
10	50/41	8%	19%	82%	64%
68	50/19	10%	53%	NR	NR
69	76/74	NR	NR	>95%	74%
70	18/16	50%	100%	~100%[a]	38%
4	110/70	19%	61%	>50%	74%
8	20/16	40%	NR	100%	95%
72	9/8	100%	89%	~89%[a]	89%
9	72/51	33%	80%	NR	84%
37	21/18	0%	79%[c]	0%	71%

NR, not reported.
[a]Estimations are based on percentage of patients older than ages 16–18 years in various studies.
[b]Had ≥1 therapy session.
[c]Had extensive treatment.

sults, but the majority find no difference in outcome between the two groups (6,9,15).

Other limitations of comparing outcome studies include diagnostic uncertainty, and diverse methodologies and subject populations. Recent studies utilize video electroencephalographic diagnosis and are fairly certain of the pseudoseizure diagnosis, but early investigators lacked video electroencephalographic technology (69). Pseudoseizure diagnoses can be erroneous: as many as 8% of pseudoseizure diagnoses are later changed to epilepsy (74). Study populations generally are drawn from the chronic populations of tertiary care centers, so they are biased toward inclusion of patients with long-standing symptoms that are associated with poorer outcomes. The chronicity of subjects varies among studies and varies as much as 20 years within individual studies. The percentage of patients who received psychiatric treatment after diagnosis and the percentage of the sample who were followed (Table 25.7) also vary

greatly among studies and may affect outcome data.

Definitions of a "poor" versus "improved" outcome are not standard, but "improved" usually is defined as a specific percentage drop in seizure frequency. Outcomes defined as a fixed percentage decrease in seizure frequency (e.g., less than 80% baseline frequency) are dependent on the initial frequency of seizures. For example, a decrease from 20 to eight pseudoseizures per month might be rated as improved (a 60% decrease), whereas a drop from six to four seizures (a 33% decrease) per year might confer a better clinical outcome but be rated as unimproved. It is impossible to meaningfully compare results across studies in the "improved" outcome category. The "poor" outcome category consists of patients with minor decreases in seizure frequency, no change, or an increase in frequency compared to the time of diagnosis.

The "seizure-free" category probably is more reliable than the "improved" category, but even its definition in not uniform. Most patients have some seizures after their diagnosis. Not all studies specify how long a subject needed to be seizure-free before the follow-up contact to qualify as seizure-free. Some studies distinguish solely between seizure-free and nonseizure-free subjects (4), and some studies report only those subjects who are seizure-free.

Nearly all studies base outcome on seizure *frequency* because it is easy to measure, but some rely on the subjective patient reports of decreased seizure symptom *severity*. Several studies that included social and psychological well-being as outcome indicators found that occupational, medical, and psychological difficulties were more responsible for poor outcome than were seizure continuation (27,71). Outcomes based solely on seizure frequency do not capture the extent of morbidity associated with this illness.

Outcome studies generally use a cohort of subjects who were diagnosed over a span of time (e.g., over a 3-year span) but contact them only at one follow-up time. Thus, most studies listed in Table 25.6 report outcome at a mean duration since diagnosis rather than studying each patient's outcome at a fixed duration (i.e., at 2 years after diagnosis). These mean durations mask follow-up ranges as long as 20 years (21,69). Reporting follow-up only at mean durations greatly reduces the usefulness of outcome data. The most meaningful data come from studying each patient at several fixed durations after diagnosis (69,70). The only study that conducted multiple serial observations illustrated how seizure-free rates gradually rise over 5 years (69). This field needs studies with serial fixed-time assessments and observation beyond 5 years.

Seizure-Free Outcomes

Despite the limitations of diverse subject populations and averaged outcome durations, a crude estimation of outcomes is available by clumping studies into groups based on short versus long mean durations of follow-up. Seven studies that report seizure-free outcomes for mean durations of less than 1 year found rates vary from 19% to 63% (6,8,15,21, 33,37,70), with the best outcomes associated with immediate posttreatment periods (33, 37). A weighted average at less than 1 year for these seven studies shows that 121 of 264 (46%) subjects followed became seizure-free. How does this compare to longer follow-up periods?

Six studies of adults that reported outcome about 5 years after diagnosis found a range of 0% to 58% seizure-free subjects, with a weighted average of 39% (109 of 280 subjects) seizure-free (3,4,21,27,62,69). When weighted averages of subjects who are seizure-free at 1 year (80 of 246 [32.5%]), 2 years (75 of 155 [48%]), 3 to 4 years (17 of 30 [57%]), and 5 years (109 of 280 [39%]) are examined, the results fall in a range from 39% to 57% seizure-free for all time points, except approximately 1 year after diagnosis. Inclusion of the few teenage subjects in the data does not change the prognosis. In general, it appears that about half of subjects rapidly become seizure-free after diagnosis, then seizures recur in some patients. After 5 years, a chronic group of about 60% of patients continues to have pseudoseizures. Studies that assess a cohort of subjects at a fixed point longer than 5 years are needed.

There are problems with comparing the results of studies with such diverse methodologies and populations. However, pooling their results gives us an estimate of the prognosis of pseudoseizure patients across tertiary care research centers. Tertiary care center patients (studies listed in Tables 25.6 and 25.7) generally are diagnosed long after seizure onset, so their chronicity may confer a poorer outcome. Outcome studies are weighted toward chronic subjects and underestimations of the percentage of patients who become seizure-free. Studies are needed of pseudoseizure patients promptly diagnosed outside tertiary care centers.

"Improved" and "Poor" Outcomes

Fourteen studies report an "improved" category of subjects whose pseudoseizures continued at a significantly decreased frequency (Table 25.6). Three of these studies (9,12,64) did not report on unchanged subjects, and one (4) combined improved and unchanged subjects. The other ten studies report improved outcomes from 3 months to a mean of 22 months' duration. A weighted average of these ten studies shows that 137 of 406 (34%) subjects were improved. The weighted average of 13 studies that report unchanged or poor outcomes reveals that 147 of 488 (30%) subjects have a poor seizure prognosis in the first 3 to 22 months after diagnosis.

Overall, the general trend across subject populations and follow-up durations is that about 45% of pseudoseizure patients become seizure-free, one-third show significant improvement but still experience seizures, and 30% do poorly. These data are helpful in giving general advice to patients, but the data do not tell clinicians the expected outcome for specific patients and what treatments help the most. For that, we must turn to studies of specific factors in prognosis.

Prognostic Factors in Outcome

Nineteen of 22 outcome studies comment on factors associated with seizure outcomes, but their findings are contradictory. Most studies are retrospective analyses that associate outcome with baseline and follow-up characteristics of patients. The most helpful studies are prospective studies that report baseline characteristics that later predict outcome (6,15).

Baseline Medical Factors in Outcome

The results of medical/clinical, patient characteristics, and treatment factors in pseudoseizure outcome are summarized in Table 25.8. Studies of clinical or medical characteristics of the patient at diagnosis have yielded conflicting results, but point toward coexisting epilepsy having little correlation with outcome. Similarly, the presence of other neurologic abnormalities (abnormal result on electroencephalogram or magnetic resonance imaging, or another neurologic condition) does not correlate with outcome, with the exception of one

TABLE 25.8. *Prognostic factors in pseudoseizure outcome*

	Improved outcome	Worse outcome	No outcome correlation
Medical factors			
Coexisting epilepsy	74	4	6, 9, 15
Seizure morphology	74[a]	10[a], 74[a]	9, 62
Shorter duration before diagnosis	9, 10, 12, 21, 62		4, 26, 71
Neurologic abnormality (EEG, MRI, clinical)			15, 26, 62
Higher seizure frequency		62	10, 26
Low intelligence		70	
Baseline patient factors			
Older age at seizure onset		12	6, 10, 52, 71
Any nonconversion psychiatric diagnosis	15[a] (single depression)	9, 10, 12, 21, 15[a] (>1 depression)	4, 6, 26
Personality disorder		8, 15, 64	
Female gender	4		9, 10, 26, 37, 62
History of being abused		64 (sexual abuse)	6,[b] 26
Believes pseudoseizure diagnosis	8, 71		6
Recent or clear-cut precipitating stressor	8, 21		
Treatment factors			
Psychiatric treatment after diagnosis	12, 67		4, 6, 9, 10, 15, 37, 68

EEG, electroencephalography; MRI, magnetic resonance imaging.
[a]See text for discussion of specific symptoms or diagnoses.
[b]Physical or sexual abuse.

study that points to low intelligence worsening the prognosis (70). In contrast, other studies anecdotally cite good outcomes for mentally retarded subjects who were treated with behavioral modification. Two studies of pseudoseizure morphology (10,74) found a worse prognosis for generalized convulsive pseudoseizures that are suspected to be abreactions of childhood sexual abuse (33). Two other studies found no correlation of morphology and outcome. Betts and Boden (74) noted a relatively better prognosis for the swoon (fainting) type of pseudoseizures.

The literature points toward a better prognosis for persons with recent onset of pseudoseizures, but three studies found no correlation between seizure duration and outcome. The lack of correlation is likely related to statistical methods. Studies that found an improved prognosis with shorter seizure duration compared the mean duration of seizure-free and nonseizure-free subjects or compared the proportion of seizure-free subjects in cohorts with seizures longer or shorter than a set duration (e.g., 3 years). Although most authors conclude that patients with seizures of less than 1-year duration do well, there is no consensus on what duration of seizures confers a poor prognosis. The dividing point for better and worse prognoses was 3 years in one study (4) and 5 years in another study (10). The mean duration of seizures associated with a good prognosis was 3.3 years in one study (9), whereas the same duration (3.4 years) was associated with a poorer prognosis in another study (12).

Testing for prognosis based on duration of seizures before diagnosis may be misleading, because associated factors may truly be the determinants of prognosis. For instance, in the study by Guberman (21), the "acute" group with a good prognosis was characterized by several factors: shorter seizure duration, absence of an extensive psychiatric history, and clear-cut stressors preceding seizure onset. In contrast, the group with a poorer prognosis had long-standing seizures, high rates of serious psychiatric difficulties, and an absence of acute precipitating stressors. As the sophisti-

cated prospective study by Kanner et al. (15) illustrates, clusters of patient characteristics and some clinical factors best determine pseudoseizure outcome. Their model of nine psychiatric factors correctly classified 90% of patients into outcome groups.

Baseline Patient Factors in Outcome

After Wyllie et al. (37) reported high rates of seizure cessation in adolescent patients, numerous studies tested the hypothesis that a younger age at pseudoseizure onset conferred a better prognosis. Does preadult seizure onset really have a better prognosis than adult onset? Most studies have not found a correlation between age of onset and prognosis, but they did not explicitly compare adolescent and adult patients. The only studies that studied solely minors differed markedly in outcome (37,62). The study by Lancman et al. of adults (26) and of youths (62) at the same treatment center showed a better prognosis for teens than for adults, but the duration of follow-up of these two studies is not comparable. The study by Lancman et al. (62) found youths have a seizure-free outcome (45%) similar to that of most adults studies, but Lancman et al. used a longer follow-up period than Wyllie et al. (37). It is possible that the findings of a good prognosis reported by Wyllie et al. reflect the shorter-term prognosis of a less chronic group.

The literature points strongly toward a worse prognosis among patients with significant preexisting psychiatric difficulties. Most studies clump all subjects with any previous psychiatric diagnosis. Two excellent studies that reported on the prognosis of patients with specific previous psychiatric problems found that specific preexisting psychiatric diagnoses are associated with different outcomes. Kanner et al. (15) found that a history of only one episode of major depression conferred an improved prognosis, whereas recurrent major depressions worsened the prognosis. Likewise, this study found that dissociative amnesia, chronic abuse (which correlates with dissociative disorders), and personality disorders also worsen the prognosis. Two other studies report that a personality disorder diagnosis is associated with poor outcome (8,64). These three psychiatric diagnoses may correlate with poor pseudoseizure outcome because they (and chronic abuse) are all chronic conditions that can be difficult to treat. Studies of personality disorders in pseudoseizure patients have soundly disproven the assumption that these subjects have high rates of histrionic personality disorders. Studies agree that there is no single personality type associated with pseudoseizures, but any personality disorder worsens the prognosis.

Approximately 75% of pseudoseizure subjects are female (75). Five studies (9,10,26, 37,62) found that female gender does not influence outcome, and one study (4) found improved outcome for women.

Subsequent Psychiatric Treatment

Of nine studies of seizure outcome and post-diagnostic mental health care, seven found no correlation (4,6,9,10,15,37,68). Treatment studies are difficult to compare, because few have quantified the type or amount of mental health care offered. One study looked at the expertise of the treating health professionals and found that patients managed by epilepsy clinic neurologists did as well as those treated by epilepsy clinic psychiatrists, but that community-based mental health professionals had somewhat less positive results (67). They concluded that the expertise of the treater and the treater's certainty about the pseudoseizure diagnosis were helpful in improving outcomes. Unfortunately, little is known about the type of mental health treatment that is most effective for pseudoseizures. Walczak et al. (9) reported that neither psychotherapy nor the number of mental health treatment visits correlated with outcome. A well-designed detailed outcome study found no correlation between outcome and treatment with psychotherapy, psychotropic medications, psychiatric hospitalization, or support groups (6).

Most studies report the results of treatments that are individualized to each patient,

so outcomes reflect an average of all treatments. There are no published controlled treatment trials for pseudoseizures, so it is not possible to know the effectiveness of specific psychiatric interventions. In the literature, there is consensus on four treatment issues. First, psychiatric intervention does not worsen these patients. Second, a minority of recent-onset patients do not require psychiatric treatment. Third, pseudoseizure patients report psychological benefits from psychotherapy for pseudoseizures even if the seizures continue. Fourth, the delivery of clear unambiguous feedback to patients about the psychological nature of their seizures is necessary and should be considered an essential part of treatment. In the study by Aboukasm et al. (67), none of the patients who did not receive diagnostic feedback or psychiatric care had a reduction of seizures, but two-thirds of those who received both feedback and psychiatric treatment did well. The authors emphasize that diagnostic feedback alone is efficacious in terminating the seizures of a minority of patients and that communication of diagnostic uncertainty by treating physicians leads to further diagnostic testing and a poorer outcome.

The variability of outcomes in these studies is likely related to marked variability in the study populations, the individual characteristics and situations of the patients, and the skill and type of treatment rendered by mental health treaters. Most authors agree that there are multiple causes of pseudoseizures, so no single approach to treatment will help all patients. It is possible that the underlying stressor and the patient's psychological resources are powerful prognostic determinants that wash out treatment effects in outcome studies. This field is in great need of comparative trials of specific treatments for pseudoseizures, but large subject populations from multisite studies likely will be required. Across diverse outcome studies, some consensus is emerging: patients have a better outcome if they have recent seizure onset in response to clear-cut stressors, have no personality disorder, and lack complicated or chronic psychiatric problems such as chronic abuse, dissociation, or recurrent depression. Concomitant epilepsy and gender do not appear to affect outcome. The outcome with preadult onset is uncertain.

SUMMARY

In addition to having conversion seizures, pseudoseizure patients have high rates of psychiatric illness (40% to 100%). One-third to two-thirds have previously sought psychiatric treatment, and a minimum of one-fourth have been psychiatrically hospitalized. The most common psychiatric illnesses mentioned in the pseudoseizure literature are those most commonly assessed by researchers (depression, panic disorder, and personality disorder), but these illnesses are not necessarily the most common among pseudoseizure patients. Depression is a very common comorbidity, occurring in one-third to one-half of patients, probably because multiple life stresses contribute to depression and pseudoseizures. Bipolar disorder rarely occurs in these patients.

Anxiety disorders are common in pseudoseizure patients, but only a minority have panic disorder (which can be mistaken for a pseudoseizure). PTSD is the most common anxiety disorder in these patients and occurs as often as depression (in one-third to one-half). PTSD-related flashbacks or abreactions of trauma can be the underlying cause of pseudoseizures. GAD contributes to pseudoseizures in about 10% of patients.

Most pseudoseizures are conversion seizures, but other types of conversion and other somatoform disorders are common in this population. About three-fourths of patients have another type of conversion during their lifetime and may have conversion (paralysis, numbness, etc.) during the pseudoseizure. These patients recurrently use somatic defenses to express distress, but only a minority have true somatization disorder.

Dissociative disorders are quite common but rarely assessed in pseudoseizure patients. Dissociative amnesia is common during the seizures and very common outside of seizures, but patients rarely volunteer these

symptoms. A sizable proportion have complex dissociative symptoms, which include alter ego states that express dissociated affect via pseudoseizures.

Personality disorders occur in slightly less than half of patients and usually fall into DSM-IV cluster B (histrionic, borderline, antisocial). No single personality type predominates. Pseudoseizure patients are rarely psychotic and do not commonly suffer from eating disorders. A small number of persons diagnosed with pseudoseizures are malingering or have a factitious disorder. This is malingering of a physical illness (epilepsy) rather than true "pseudoseizures."

Outcome studies are incredibly diverse and difficult to compare, but generally they find that about 45% of pseudoseizure patients become seizure-free, one-third show significant improvement but still experience seizures, and 30% do poorly. Recent onset of seizures and the absence of extensive trauma and the psychiatric illnesses that accompany it (recurrent depression, somatization disorder, personality disorder, and dissociative disorder) predict a good outcome. Chronic seizures, presence of extensive abuse, and the noted disorders confer a poorer prognosis. The literature is divided about other prognostic factors, but concomitant epilepsy, gender, neurologic abnormalities, and receipt of psychiatric treatment do not predict outcome as well as a combination of psychiatric factors (15).

Controlled treatment trials are nonexistent and cannot guide care, but authors agree that direct unambivalent feedback about the psychological nature of the seizures is absolutely essential to a good outcome. Mental health treatment (pharmacology and/or psychotherapy) from treaters knowledgeable about pseudoseizures appears to confer an improved outcome but may not be superior to feedback alone in persons with recent seizure onset and minimal psychopathology. No consensus exists about the best type of psychotherapy for pseudoseizures, but behavior modification is generally helpful for persons with limited intellect.

Overall, persons with pseudoseizures have a trauma-related cluster of psychiatric diagnoses and should be screened for abuse, recent stressors, depression, PTSD, dissociative disorders, other somatic symptoms, and cluster B personality disorder. Psychiatric treatment then should be individualized to treat these comorbid conditions.

REFERENCES

1. Kessler RC, McGonagle KA, Shanyang Z, et al. Lifetime and 12-month prevalence of DSM-III-R psychiatric disorders in the United States. *Arch Gen Psychiatry* 1994;51:8–19.
2. Arnold LM, Privitera MD. Psychopathology and trauma in epileptic and psychogenic seizure patients. *Psychosomatics* 1996;37:436–443.
3. Kristensen O, Alving J. Pseudoseizures—risk factors and prognosis. *Acta Neurol Scand* 1992;85:177–180.
4. Meierkord H, Will B, Fish D, et al. The clinical features and prognosis and pseudoseizures diagnosed using video-EEG telemetry. *Neurology* 1991;41:1643–1646.
5. Snyder SL, Rosenbaum DH, Rowan AJ, et al. SCID diagnosis of panic disorder in psychogenic seizure patients. *J Neuropsychiatry Clin Neurosci* 1994;6:261–266.
6. Ettinger AB, Dhoon A, Weisbrot DM. Predictive factors for outcome of non-epileptic seizures after diagnosis. *J Neuropsychiatry Clin Neurosci* 1999;11:458–463.
7. Jawad SSM, Jamil N, Clarke EJ, et al. Psychiatric morbidity and psychodynamics of patients with convulsive pseudoseizures. *Seizure* 1995;4:201–206.
8. Pakalnis A, Drake ME, Phillips B. Neuropsychiatric aspects of psychogenic status epilepticus. *Neurology* 1991;41:1104–1106.
9. Walczak TS, Papacostas S, Williams DT, et al. Outcome after diagnosis of psychogenic nonepileptic seizures. *Epilepsia* 1995;36:1131–1137.
10. Lempert T, Schmidt E. Natural history and outcome of psychogenic seizures: a clinical study in 50 patients. *J Neurol* 1990;237:35–38.
11. Rosenbaum DH, Snyder S, Rowan AJ, et al. Outpatient multidisciplinary management of non-epileptic seizures. In: Rowan AJ, Gates JR, eds. *Non-epileptic seizures.* Boston: Butterworth-Heinemann, 1993.
12. Buchanan N, Snars J. Pseudoseizures (non epileptic attack disorder)—clinical management and outcome in 50 patients. *Seizure* 1993;2:141–148.
13. Roy A. Hysterical seizures. *Arch Neurol* 1979;36:447.
14. Blumer D, Montouris G, Hermann B. Psychiatric morbidity in seizure patients on a neurodiagnostic monitoring unit. *J Neuropsychiatry* 1995;7:445–456.
15. Kanner AM, Parra J, Frey M, et al. Psychiatric and neurologic predictors of psychogenic pseudoseizure outcome. *Neurology* 1999;53:933–938.
16. Bowman ES, Markand ON. Psychodynamics and psychiatric diagnoses of pseudoseizure subjects. *Am J Psychiatry* 1996;153:57–63.
17. Roy A, Barris M. Psychiatric concepts in psychogenic non-epileptic seizures. In: Rowan AJ, Gates JR, eds. *Non-epileptic seizures.* Boston: Butterworth-Heinemann, 1993.
18. American Psychiatric Association. *Diagnostic and sta-*
tistical manual of mental disorders, 4th ed. Washington, DC: American Psychiatric Press, 1994.
19. Stewart RS, Lovitt R, Stewart RM. Are hysterical seizures more than hysteria? A research diagnostic criteria, DSM-III, and psychometric analysis. *Am J Psychiatry* 1982;139:926–929.
20. Cohen LM, Howard GF. Provocation of pseudoseizures by psychiatric interview during EEG and video monitoring. *Int J Psychiatry Med* 1992;22:131–149.
21. Guberman A. Psychogenic pseudoseizures in non-epileptic patients. *Can J Psychiatry* 1982;27:401–404.
22. Blumer D. The paroxysmal somatoform disorder: a series of patients with non-epileptic seizures. In: Rowan AJ, Gates JR, eds. *Non-epileptic seizures.* Boston: Butterworth-Heinemann, 1993.
23. Steinberg M, Rounsaviille B, Cicchetti DV. The structured clinical interview for DSM-III-R dissociative disorders: preliminary report on a new diagnostic instrument. *Am J Psychiatry* 1990;147:76–82.
24. Steinberg M. *Structured clinical interview for DSM-III-R dissociative disorders (SCID-D), revised.* Washington, DC: American Psychiatric Press, 1994.
25. Griffith JL. The mind/body problem revisited: pseudoseizure patients. *Fam Syst Med* 1990;8:71–90.
26. Lancman ME, Brotherton TA, Asconapé JJ, et al. Psychogenic seizures in adults: a longitudinal analysis. *Seizure* 1994;2:281–286.
27. Krumholz A, Niedermeyer E. Psychogenic seizures: a clinical study with follow-up data. *Neurology* 1983;33:498–502.
28. Alper K. Nonepileptic seizures. *Neurol Clin North Am* 1994;12:153–173.
29. Bowman ES, Markand ON. A study of the contribution of life events to pseudoseizure occurrence in adults. *Bull Menninger Clin* 1999;63:70–88.
30. Alper K, Devinsky O, Perrine K, et al. Psychiatric classification of nonconversion nonepileptic seizures. *Arch Neurol* 1995;52:199–201.
31. Vein AM, Djukova GM, Vorobieva OV. Is panic attack a mask of psychogenic seizures? A comparative analysis of phenomenology of psychogenic seizures and panic attacks. *Funct Neurol* 1994;9:153–159.
32. Bowman ES. Nonepileptic seizures: psychiatric framework, treatment, and outcome. *Neurology* 1999;53 [Suppl 1]:S84–S88.
33. Betts T, Boden S. Diagnosis, management and prognosis of a group of 128 patients with non-epileptic attack disorder. Part II. Previous childhood sexual abuse in the aetiology of these disorders. *Seizure* 1992;1:27–32.
34. Betts T, Duffy N. Non-epileptic attack disorder (pseudoseizures) and sexual abuse: a review. In: Gram L, Johannessen SI, Osterman PO, et al., eds. *Pseudo-epileptic seizures.* Petersfield, UK: Wrightson Biomedical Publishing, 1993.
35. Bowman ES. Etiology and clinical course of pseudoseizures. Relationship to trauma, depression and dissociation. *Psychosomatics* 1993;34:333–342.
36. Kuyk J, Van Dyck RV, Spinhoven P. The case for a dissociative interpretation of pseudoepileptic seizures. *J Nerv Ment Dis* 1996;184:408–474.
37. Wyllie E, Friedman D, Rothner AD, et al. Psychogenic seizures in children and adolescents: outcome after diagnosis by ictal video and electroencephalographic recording. *Pediatrics* 1990;85:480–484.
38. Ramchandani D, Schindler B. Evaluation of pseudo-

seizures. A psychiatric perspective. *Psychosomatics* 1993;34:70–79.

39. Gross M. Incestuous rape: a cause for hysterical seizures in four adolescent girls. *Am J Orthopsychiatry* 1979;49:704–708.

40. Ettinger AB, Devinsky O, Weisbrot DM, et al. Headaches and other pain symptoms among patients with psychogenic non-epileptic seizures. *Seizure* 1999; 8:424–426.

41. Rothner AD. Not everything that shakes is epilepsy. The differential diagnosis of paroxysmal nonepileptiform disorders. *Cleve Clin J Med* 1989;56[Suppl]:S206–S213.

42. Bjornes H. Aetiological models as a basis for individualized treatment of pseudo-epileptic seizures. In: Gram L, Johannessen SI, Osterman PO, et al., eds. *Pseudoepileptic seizures.* Petersfield, UK: Wrightson Biomedical Publishing, 1993:81–98.

43. Goodwin JM. Childhood sexual abuse and non-epileptic seizures. In: Rowan AJ, Gates JR, eds. *Non-epileptic seizures.* Boston: Butterworth-Heinemann, 1993: 181–191.

44. Kloster R. Pseudo-epileptic v. epileptic seizures: a comparison. In: Gram L, Johannessen SI, Osterman PO, et al., eds. *Pseudoepileptic seizures.* Petersfield, UK: Wrightson Biomedical Publishing, 1993:3–16.

45. Nash, JL. Pseudoseizures: etiologic and psychotherapeutic considerations. *South Med J* 1993;86:1248–1252.

46. Torem MS. Non-epileptic seizures as a dissociative disorder. In: Rowan AJ, Gates JR, eds. *Non-epileptic seizures.* Boston: Butterworth-Heinemann, 1993:173–179.

47. Nemiah JC. Dissociation, conversion, and somatization. *In: American Psychiatric Association review of psychiatry,* Volume 10. Washington, DC: American Psychiatric Press, 1991.

48. Harden CL. Pseudoseizures and dissociative disorders: a common mechanism involving traumatic experiences. *Seizure* 1997;6:151–155.

49. Tomb DA. Psychogenic seizures. *Neurology* 1992;42: 1848.

50. Janet P. *L'automatisme psychologique.* Paris: Félix Alcan, 1889.

51. Janet PF. *The major symptoms of hysteria.* New York: MacMillan, 1907.

52. American Psychiatric Association. *Diagnostic and statistical manual of mental disorders,* 3rd ed. Washington, DC: American Psychiatric Press, 1980.

53. American Psychiatric Association. *Diagnostic and statistical manual of mental disorders,* 2nd ed. Washington, DC: American Psychiatric Press, 1968.

54. Blomhoff S, Malt UF. Psychiatric perspectives on psychogenic seizures and their treatment. In: Gram L, Johannessen SI, Osterman PO, et al., eds. *Pseudoepileptic seizures.* Petersfield, UK: Wrightson Biomedical Publishing, 1993:99–108.

55. Williams JBW, Gibbon M, First MB, et al. The structured clinical interview for DSM-IIIR (SCID), II: multisite test-retest reliability. *Arch Gen Psychiatry* 1992; 49:630–636.

56. Gross M. The clinical diagnosis of psychogenic seizures. In: Gross M, ed. *Pseudoepilepsy: the clinical aspects of false seizures.* Lexington, MA: Lexington Books, 1983:79–96.

57. Simeon D, Gross S, Guralnik O, et al. Feeling unreal: 30 cases of DSM-III depersonalization disorder. *Am J Psychiatry* 1997;154:1107–1113.

58. Watkins JG, Watkins HH. The theory and practice of ego-state therapy. In: Grayson H, ed. *Short term approaches to psychotherapy.* New York: Human Sciences Press, 1979:176–220.

59. Alper K, Devinsky O, Perrine K, et al. Nonepileptic seizures and childhood sexual and physical abuse. *Neurology* 1993;43:1950–1953.

60. Goodwin J. Pseudoseizures and incest. *Am J Psychiatry* 1979;136:1231.

61. LaBarbera JD, Dozier E. Hysterical seizures: the role of sexual exploitation. *Psychosomatics* 1980;21:897–903.

62. Lancman ME, Asconapé JJ, Graves S, et al. Psychogenic seizures in children: long-term analysis of 43 cases. *J Child Neurol* 1994;9:404–407.

63. Bernstein EM, Putnam FW. Development, reliability and validity of a dissociation scale. *J Nerv Ment Dis* 1986;174:727–735.

64. Gumnit RJ, Gates JR. Psychogenic seizures. *Epilepsia* 1986;27[Suppl]:S24–S129.

65. Stewart RS, Lovitt R, Stewart RM. Psychopathology associated with hysterical seizures. In: Gross M, ed. *Pseudoepilepsy: the clinical aspects of false seizures.* Lexington, MA: Lexington Books, 1983:97–108.

66. Zanarini MC, Williams AA, Lewis RE, et al. Reported pathological childhood experiences associated with the development of borderline personality disorder. *Am J Psychiatry* 1997;154:1101–1106.

67. Aboukasm A, Mahr G, Gahry BR, et al. Retrospective analysis of the effects of psychotherapeutic interventions on outcomes of psychogenic nonepileptic seizures. *Epilepsia* 1998;39:470–473.

68. Lesser RP, Lueders H, Dinner DS. Evidence for epilepsy is rare in patients with psychogenic seizures. *Neurology* 1983;33:502——504.

69. Ljungberg L. Hysteria. A clinical, prognostic, and genetic study. *Acta Psychiatr Scand* 1957;32[Suppl 112]: 1–162.

70. McDade G, Brown SW. Non-epileptic seizures: management and predictive factors of outcome. *Seizure* 1992;1:7–10.

71. Ettinger AB, Devinsky O, Weisbrot DM, et al. A comprehensive profile of clinical, psychiatric, and psychosocial characteristics of patients with psychogenic nonepileptic seizures. *Epilepsia* 1999;40:1292–1298.

72. Ramani V, Gumnit RJ. Management of hysterical seizures in epileptic patients. *Arch Neurol* 1982;38: 78–81.

73. Williams DT, Gold AP, Shrout P, et al. The impact of psychiatric intervention on patients with uncontrolled seizures. *J Nerv Ment Dis* 1979;167:626–631.

74. Betts T, Boden S. Diagnosis, management and prognosis of a group of 138 patients with non-epileptic attack disorder. Part I. *Seizure* 1992;1:19–26.

75. Rosenbaum, M. Psychogenic seizures—why women? *Psychosomatics* 2000;41:147–149.

26

Treatment of Psychogenic Pseudoseizures

What to Do After We Have Reached the Diagnosis?

Andres M. Kanner, Susan M. Palac, *Marcelo E. Lancman,
†Christos C. Lambrakis, and ‡Michael I. Steinhardt

*Department of Neurological Sciences, Rush Presbyterian-Saint Luke's Medical Center,
Chicago, Illinois 60612; *Epilepsy Program, Saint Agnes Hospital, White Plains, New York 10605;
and †Northeast Regional Epilepsy Group and ‡Pediatric Neuroscience Institute,
Hackensack University Medical Center, Hackensack, New Jersey 07601*

The advent of video electroencephalographic (VEEG) telemetry has revolutionized the clinicians' ability to properly diagnose psychogenic pseudoseizures (PPS) (1). In contrast to the abundant literature on the phenomenology of PPS, little has been written on their psychopathology and even less has been done to develop treatment strategies for patients with this type of paroxysmal event. The following problems may explain the paucity of available data on the treatment of PPS:

1. The heterogeneity of PPS with respect to their *psychopathogenic* mechanisms.
2. The paucity of published data on the operant psychopathogenic mechanisms of PPS.
3. The lack of established priorities in the treatment process of PPS.
4. The poor communication between neurologists and psychiatrists, a bizarre phenomenon that, sadly, is endemic in many medical institutions in the United States and other countries.

The heterogeneity of PPS psychopathology is clearly reflected in the diverse outcomes that often are independent of the exposure to any therapeutic intervention. For example, in a prospective study of 45 consecutive patients with PPS carried out at the Rush Epilepsy Center, 13 stopped having PPS once presented with the diagnosis; five of these patients did not receive any type of psychotherapeutic intervention (2). A review of the available literature reveals confusing and contradictory results with respect to the results of psychiatric treatment of PPS. Some studies reported better outcome in patients receiving psychotherapy compared to those who did not (3–6). Other studies failed to show any difference in the recurrence of PPS between patients who received psychotherapy and those who did not (7–10). Even with no treatment, 34% to 53% of patients with PPS become event-free over time (3,8,9). A significant number of patients with PPS become event-free shortly after being informed of the diagnosis (5,7,11).

In this chapter, we intend to provide a critical yet practical discussion on what we believe to be the salient issues to consider in the treatment process of patients with PPS. Following a brief review of some of the underlying psychological processes that mediate PPS occurrence, we will attempt to answer the following questions. (i) What should be the first treatment priority, and how can it be reached? (ii) How can the clinician use the data of the patient's psychiatric profile to realistically predict outcome and to plan a proper treatment regimen? (iii) When and how should antiepileptic drugs (AEDs) be discontinued? (iv) When should patients be allowed to drive and be involved in activities that usually are avoided in patients with epileptic seizures? (v) How long should neurologists follow the patient with PPS after a diagnosis has been established?

SOME OF THE PRINCIPAL PSYCHOPATHOLOGICAL PROCESSES UNDERLYING PSYCHOGENIC PSEUDOSEIZURES

Although dependent on specific etiology and individual circumstances, several mechanisms have been proposed to better understand the psychopathologic processes underlying PPS. These include: conversion, somatization, dissociative, factitious, and malingering disorders (12,13). In addition, mood disorders in general, and major depression in particular, as well as anxiety and personality disorders, have been identified as frequently occurring comorbid conditions (12,13). Bowman has reviewed in great detail and critical manner the psychopathology and outcome of PPS (Chapter 25); therefore, we will touch on this topic only in a limited way.

PSYCHOGENIC PSEUDOSEIZURES AS AN EXPRESSION OF CONVERSION DISORDER

These patients experience physical symptoms that affect voluntary motor or sensory functions that are not fully explained by a neurologic or general medical condition, or by the direct effect of a substance (14). Conversion disorder typically consists of a single motor or neurologic symptom (i.e., PPS). A history of other type of somatic symptoms often is encountered in PPS patients, an indication that the patient tends to use somatic complaints as a means of emotional expression. Conversive disorders typically appear during adolescence or early adulthood, but can occur at any age. They are found more commonly in women than in men, with reported ratios ranging from 2:1 to 10:1 (15). Symptoms frequently appear following an acute stressful event; the precipitating stressor sometimes is not readily apparent, however. The *Diagnostic and Statistical Manual of Mental Disorders, Fourth Edition* (DSM-IV) specifies that patients meet criteria of conversion disorder only when the symptoms are not intentionally produced or feigned, as in factitious disorder or malingering (14).

PSYCHOGENIC PSEUDOSEIZURES AS AN EXPRESSION OF SOMATIZATION DISORDER

In contrast to conversion disorder, which primarily involves a limited number of complaints accompanying PPS, somatization disorder is diagnosed when the paroxysmal events are part of a greater constellation of multiple somatic symptoms not fully explained by a known medical condition or use of a substance. As specified in the DSM-IV, the patient's physical complaints must have begun prior to age 30 years, and the constellation must include four pain symptoms, two nonpain gastrointestinal symptoms, one nonpain sexual or reproductive symptom, and one pseudoneurologic symptom (14). Thus, with somatization disorder, the symptoms of PPS are seen in addition to numerous other objective and subjective clinical expressions. Vague reports of ill-defined symptoms are common. Characteristics of this group of patients include a predominance of females, with an onset in adolescence or young adulthood (15). As with conversion disorder, symptomatology may not be intentionally produced or feigned.

PSYCHOGENIC PSEUDOSEIZURES AS AN EXPRESSION OF DISSOCIATIVE DISORDERS

PPS very often are the expression of a dissociative disorder. This group of disorders involves splitting off of normally integrated functions or experiences from conscious awareness. As it pertains to patients with PPS, the dissociative states typically are transient and can present in a manner that can be confused with absence seizures or altered conscious states rather than a primary motor component (16). Patients with PPS can present with symptoms of amnesia, depersonalization, and derealization.

The relatively high frequency of dissociative disorders among patients with PPS is not surprising, as there is a strong historical and conceptual link between dissociative and conversion disorders. One of the early classic cases reported in the psychiatric literature is that of Anna O. This patient of Breuer and Freud (17) clearly displayed both somatoform and dissociative features. The close relationship between these disorders is reflected in the most recent revision of the International Classification of Diseases (ICD-10), in which conversion disorder is not included as a somatoform disorder, but has been reincorporated as a combined dissociative (conversion) disorder (18). It has been posited that the psychological process of dissociation forms the basis of a conversion disorder (19). A history of sexual and physical abuse is another commonality found among both patient groups, as well as in patients with PPS. In one study, trauma was reported by 84% of the subjects, with 67% experiencing sexual abuse, 67% experiencing physical abuse, and 73% having experienced "other" traumas (12). In another study, 43% to 57% of PPS patients described a history of sexual or physical abuse on a self-report questionnaire compared to 13% to 18% in the control group (20).

PSYCHOGENIC PSEUDOSEIZURES AS AN EXPRESSION OF FACTITIOUS DISORDER AND MALINGERING

As noted earlier, when assessing a patient for the presence of a somatoform disorder, the possibility of a patient intentionally producing the symptoms should be considered. With factitious disorder, the motivation for the behavior is solely to become identified as "a patient" or "ill," but the motivation of symptom production may have an external incentive (i.e., monetary gains) (14). In factitious disorder by proxy (Munchausen syndrome by proxy), seizures are the most common presentation (16). In this syndrome, the caretaker, typically the mother, either reports or induces an illness that requires medical attention and/or hospitalization.

A common example of PPS presenting as an expression of malingering can be encountered among prisoners who "fake" seizures so that they will be taken to the community hospital. Other examples include patients who are involved in litigation and feign illness for the financial incentives associated with their case. Proving malingering at times can be extremely difficult, however (Chapter 4).

What Should Be the First Priority in the Treatment Process of Psychogenic Pseudoseizure Patients?

As with any medical and psychiatric disorder, the immediate goal of therapy is to remove any threat to the patient's physical well-being. In the case of PPS, that threat is the continuous potential that physicians may continue to misdiagnose them as epileptic seizures. As is often the case, PPS usually are construed and managed as if they were refractory epilepsy. This, in turn, unnecessarily exposes patients to high-dose AEDs that can result in serious—and unnecessary—*iatrogenic* morbidity. In one study, about 53.8% of PPS patients were receiving AEDs and 66.7% had taken these drugs in the past (21). The percentages are even higher in other series (22,23). The worst-case scenario is that of PPS patients presenting to the emergency room with suspected status epilepticus and who can be aggressively treated with intravenous AED therapy. Pakalnis et al. (24) investigated 20 patients with continuous repetitive PPS simulating status epilepticus. In over 50% of these patients, seizures continued until respiratory arrest and intubation occurred. There are reports of patients with PPS who died after aggressive treatment with anticonvulsants and anesthesia with intubation to control seizures that were not actually epileptic in nature. Thus, the immediate goal of therapy is to ensure that both patient and family have *accepted the fact that the spells are not epileptic.* This will preclude the patient going (or being taken) to an emergency room after having PPS and, thus, minimizes the risk of potentially serious iatrogenic problems. It should be recognized, however, that the acceptance that the paroxysmal events are not epileptic *does not necessarily* require the *initial* acceptance by the patient of a psychogenic cause.

In our opinion, the latter should be the second and *not necessarily* the first goal of the therapeutic process. Acceptance that the paroxysmal events are not epileptic and acceptance of a psychogenic cause are both dependent on the way the diagnosis is presented to the patient.

PRESENTATION OF PSYCHOGENIC PSEUDOSEIZURES DIAGNOSIS

Shen et al. (25) developed a protocol for presentation of the diagnosis of PPS that is now considered classic by many epilepsy centers. This protocol contains six main points, which we list (in italics) below and comment upon.

1. *A review of the recorded events with the patient and family to ensure that the captured event is typical for the patient.* This is of utmost importance as patients (even with epileptic seizures) may be highly suggestible and have events during VEEG that differ from their typical spells. Such a mistake can result in a false-positive diagnosis of PPS in patients with epileptic seizures.
2. *Explanation in "positive terms" of the nature of the spells, i.e., their nonepileptic cause and hence the possibility of discontinuing AEDs.* Note again that Shen et al. are not introducing the psychogenic cause of the events at this time.
3. *An acknowledgement that the nature of the event is yet to be established and that*

its cause may not always be found. This is, in our opinion, of the essence if we expect the patient and family to trust what we have to say. First, because the statement is true! In many cases, we cannot find a psychogenic cause of the PPS or a psychiatric profile that is indicative for a risk of conversive disorders. Second, a patient should never be told that their PPS is psychogenic before having objective evidence to support such suppositions.

4. Following the outline statement 3, Shen et al. make the observation that, *in many cases, such events may be of psychogenic origin, with an added explanation that the causes may be related to "upsetting emotions" that remain unconscious (i.e., and therefore the patient is unaware of) and that an evaluation by a psychiatrist, psychologist, or counselor may be indicated.* We use the same statement at our center, but we again add: "At this point in our evaluation, we cannot tell you whether or not these observations are applicable to you." However, we do not suggest at this point that the patient undergo a psychiatric evaluation; instead, we wait to the end, as very often patients will volunteer on their own a psychogenic causality for their events in the course of the following points (see later). When a patient reaches the conclusion that his or her spells are psychogenic, it has a significantly more powerful impact on outcome than if this is suggested by the clinician.
5. Shen et al. emphasize that *having these types of conflicts in no way implies that the patient may be "crazy."*
6. Next, the authors make the observation that *a history of sexual abuse often is encountered in patients with these events.* We introduce as well this concept at this point of our discussion, but we do not restrict the association to a history of sexual abuse. We also include any history of physical and emotional trauma and offer the example of veterans of the Vietnam War. At this point, we offer the explanation that "exposure to very traumatic ex-

periences *demands* that the mind take extreme measures to protect itself from the overwhelming pain associated with the traumatic experience, by disconnecting itself from the surrounding environment." And we add: "If our mind could not protect itself in that manner, we would not be human but superhuman." Such explanation conveys to patients the sense that they have nothing to be ashamed of and gives patients with a prior history of abuse an opening to acknowledge their own history of abuse without having to feel ashamed or guilty. It has been our experience that, following this statement, most patients with such a history volunteer that information spontaneously, without our having to ask them if they have ever been a victim of abuse or crime of any type.

7. Finally, Shen et al. tell their patients that *the spells may spontaneously resolve on their own and that, although one component is subconscious in nature, "one can exert a conscious voluntary effort to abort these attacks."* Although we also tell our patients that their spells may stop occurring just by knowing that they are not epileptic in nature, we do not suggest to them that they can exert a conscious voluntary effort to abort these attacks. Our reasons are threefold. First, unless the patient is malingering (which is a minority of the cases), we do not believe that the patients have a conscious control over the occurrence of their events, at least at the beginning. Second, patients (and family members) often may interpret such observation as a suggestion that they are voluntarily faking the events, which raises their resistance to accept the diagnosis further. Third, we are convinced that the exertion of control of the events occurs eventually, as a result of the treatment (see below).

It is only after these explanations are given that we ask patients if they think that their episodes may be related to a psychogenic process, if they have not yet volunteered that observation on their own. From this point on, we guide the discussion according to the answer we get from the patient:

A. If patients accept the possibility of a psychogenic process as a cause of their spells, we encourage them to elaborate on their reasons and to cite examples that may illustrate potential conflicts. We suggest that they undergo complete neuropsychological and psychiatric evaluations.

B. If patients acknowledge a history of abuse or having been victims of traumatic experiences, we ask them to recall how they "dealt" with such situations, at the time of their occurrence. It has been our experience, and that of others, that most patients have no recollection of the actual traumatic event(s). We use that "personal" experience to illustrate the phenomenon of dissociation, by again reiterating the fact that "when an individual is facing a traumatic experience, their mind will automatically protect itself by blocking any awareness of their surroundings." We then add, "This is similar to what may happen when you are having a spell" and go on to explain that, after repeated traumatic experiences, one's mind may learn to automatically "shut out" the outside world, *even in the presence of less traumatic situations.* We repeat the statement: "There is only so much trauma one person can endure before fending the traumatic experience off one's mind." Usually, patients with a history of abuse can easily relate to these observations. This then becomes the beginning of the therapeutic process. We emphasize to these patients that their process of dissociation most likely will continue until they learn, with the assistance of a counselor, to identify the precipitants, which, by now, need not necessarily be of a traumatic nature.

C. In the case where patients *adamantly refute* the possibility of any psychogenic cause to their events, we suggest that they undergo neuropsychological and neuropsychiatric evaluations to rule out that possibility. We reiterate the unconscious nature of these processes, which may preclude patients from recognizing an underlying psychological process. At the same time, we acknowledge the possibility that their spells may not have a psychogenic cause and that we may not be able to find a cause by the completion of the evaluation. We always add: "If we don't look for it, we'll never find it. It's better to rule out completely a possible psychogenic cause." Patients are told that we would like to continue following them in the clinic, and we ask them to keep a dairy in which they write down the circumstances surrounding the occurrence of future events, were they to continue. Note that we do not push patients to accept a psychogenic cause of their spells when it becomes obvious that they are not ready. In our opinion, the best course to take with such patients is to continue following them in the clinic, strengthening our relationship and their trust in us, while we continue reminding them that their spells are not epileptic (and that no other organic cause has been identified). In our experience, patients eventually accept our recommendation for psychiatric treatment after a few months. During that time, we continue achieving our primary therapeutic goal: averting that their spells be treated as epileptic seizures by other physicians.

D. Occasionally, patients may be adamant about their certainty of some organic or epileptic process triggering their spells, and that we may have erred in our evaluation. Although in such patients we are likely to suspect a factitious or malingering disorder, we try to keep an "open mind." We review the diagnostic process with patients, show the captured events and recordings of epileptic seizures, and graphically demonstrate on the actual paper to both patients and family the differences between the two. If the diagnosis was based on an ambulatory EEG study (Digitrace), we repeat the evaluation in an inpatient VEEG monitoring unit, with the use of sphenoidal electrodes. We have

had three patients in whom an erroneous diagnosis of PPS was reached with ambulatory EEG studies. Two of the three patients had neuropsychological testing that failed to reveal any propensity for conversive disorder. A correct diagnosis of epilepsy was established during VEEG. In short, we must *always* consider the fact that patients may be correct. After all, they know themselves better, notwithstanding the unconscious nature of a potential psychogenic process.

How Can the Clinician Use the Data of the Patient's Psychiatric Profile to Realistically Predict Outcome and Plan a Proper Treatment Regimen?

Elizabeth Bowman provides an outstanding comprehensive review of the studies that have looked at the parameters associated with PPS outcome in Chapter 25. The reader is referred to her chapter for an indepth review of the topic. Understanding the role of certain psychiatric and neuropsychological variables in the PPS outcome of our patients can be of paramount importance in planning treatment strategies. We will illustrate the way in which psychiatric profiles of PPS patients can help understand and predict their outcome and plan treatment strategies.

In a recently published study on neurologic and psychiatric predictors of PPS outcome, we prospectively evaluated the persistence of PPS at 1 and 6 months after diagnosis (2). We identified three outcome patterns of PPS: (i) cessation of PPS since diagnosis; (ii) transient cessation of PPS for a period of at least 3 months with subsequent recurrence; and (iii) uninterrupted persistence of PPS. Here we describe the psychiatric profiles associated with these outcome patterns and treatment plans.

Patients with Uninterrupted Persistence of Psychogenic Pseudoseizures

Twenty of the 45 patients had an outcome pattern consisting of uninterrupted PPS. These patients were more likely to have a history of abuse (physical, emotional, sexual, mixed), a history of recurrent major depression, personality disorder, and a history of dissociative disorder (not presenting as PPS). Given the frequent history of abuse, it is reasonable to expect that PPS is an expression of a dissociative process. This observation is supported further by the higher frequency of a history of dissociative disorder that preceded and presented as forms other than PPS. Thus, the uninterrupted persistence of PPS in these patients is not surprising, as the mere fact of being told that they do not have epilepsy is meaningless to them. As long as the PPS is the expression of a dissociative state and patients have not found other means of dealing with stress, PPS is expected to persist. Furthermore, having made the connection that their PPS is a dissociative process does not necessarily result in cessation of PPS. Of interest is that, despite their severe psychopathology, 17 of these 20 patients readily accepted the psychogenic nature of their events and were able to recognize their PPS as a form of dissociation soon after their diagnosis was discussed with them *(vide supra)*.

The following would be potential treatment plans for patients with this type of psychiatric profile:

1. First and foremost, we help the patient recognize that PPS is an expression of a dissociative state that may not necessarily occur in the presence of traumatic experiences. In our experience, patients with prior history of abuse can easily recognize the link between their PPS and a dissociative process (see earlier). We have used, however, a cognitive strategy in this endeavor. Patients are asked to keep a dairy and to report the circumstances surrounding the occurrence of a PPS. Very soon, patients recognize their tendency to avoid situations that engender feelings of anger, hopelessness, etc.

2. Once the patients are able to identify potential triggers, they are taught relaxation techniques that can be used when they recognize a situation that makes them feel uncomfortable in any way. Through this process (and not by just telling them that the have control over their PPS), patients may be able to abort PPS. This achievement is reflected in the following statement of one of our patients with a long history of abuse: "Doc, sometimes I have the urge to dissociate. I just can't help it!"

3. Together with this type of cognitive strategy, psychopharmacologic interventions are considered in the presence of comorbid affective, anxiety, or other psychiatric disorders that merit pharmacologic treatment. Often, AEDs are used as prophylactic agents in bipolar disorders. Nevertheless, in such cases we make sure that patients and families understand that the AED is prescribed as a mood-stabilizing agent and not because of a suspicion of epileptic seizures.

4. The next phase of treatment consists of long-term psychotherapy and pharmacotherapy, tailored by the treating psychiatrist to the individual issues at hand.

Patients with Transient Cessation of Psychogenic Pseudoseizures for a Period of at Least Three Months

Twelve of the 45 patients had this outcome pattern. They differed from those with the two other outcomes in two areas. First, they were more likely to deny the presence of any psychiatric or psychological problems. Eight of the 12 patients with this outcome refused a recommendation to start psychiatric treatment. All patients accept that their events were not epileptic, however. Second, patients in this group were more likely to develop new somatic complaints after the diagnosis of PPS was established. In these patients, we suspect that somatoform/conversive disorders are mediating their PPS, in contrast to patients with persistent PPS who were more likely to have a dissociative process underlying their PPS. In these patients, the treatment plan included the following steps:

1. We ensured that patients accepted that they did not suffer from epileptic seizures and proceeded to discontinue their AEDs.

2. We offered the option of getting a second opinion at a different center.
3. Their refusal of our recommendation of psychiatric treatment was a clear indication that they were not ready to accept and face their psychological problems. We chose to follow them in the clinic on a regular basis, for the sole purpose of strengthening the trust between them and us. We expected this stronger relationship to result in the patients' ability to follow our recommendations. Five of the eight patients eventually accepted a referral to a psychiatrist/psychologist. Until this time arrived, we wanted to intervene, in case of PPS recurrence, before the patient was restarted on AEDs by clinicians who would fail to recognize the PPS.

Of note, one of these 12 patients with an old history of epilepsy that had been controlled for 2 years was found to have recurrence of epileptic seizures after a diagnosis of PPS was established.

Cessation of Psychogenic Pseudoseizures Since Diagnosis

Paradoxically, this group of patients is the most puzzling from a psychiatric standpoint. Most had psychiatric disorders of mild severity, but in five of the 13 patients, no current psychopathology was identified during the psychiatric and neuropsychological evaluations. In those cases, we did not suggest any psychiatric treatment, and we followed them in the clinic with visits every 3 months initially and then every 6 months. In the other patients, treatment was tailored to the nature of the identified psychiatric disorder, after we ensured that the patients accepted that their events were not epileptic. One of the 13 patients refused referral for psychiatric treatment; yet, there was no PPS recurrence up to the time of the last follow-up visit.

In summary, among the 45 patients, one refused to accept the diagnosis of PPS and 13 initially refused recommendations of psychiatric treatment. As stated earlier, patients with a transient cessation of PPS were more likely to refuse pursuing psychiatric treatment. Three of the 45 patients continued to be brought to the emergency room upon recurrence of PPS. Two of these patients, however, had a concurrent epileptic seizure disorder.

LITERATURE REVIEW OF PSYCHOGENIC PSEUDOSEIZURE TREATMENT

The aim of treatment must include improvement of the overall quality of life of our patients, as PPS can have a significant impact on patients' lives. Lempert and Schmidt (8) reported that 42% of PPS patients lost their job or were receiving Social Security. In a series of 62 patients who were employed before developing PPS, 34 were not working at the time of the diagnosis (21). In another study, it was found that when PPS patients were free of their events, their quality of life improved significantly. Performance and attendance in school or work, as well as the degree of independence, were noted to be improved (26).

The financial burden placed on patients and health care providers is noteworthy. In a research study in which the financial cost of caring for patients with PPS was analyzed, the cost was immense (27). Many of the patients had several prolonged hospitalizations as well as numerous tests, including EEGs, computed tomography, and magnetic resonance imaging. This expenditure of resources illustrates the importance of aggressive measures in obtaining an accurate diagnosis and initiating treatment as soon as possible.

Several investigators studied the efficacy and prognosis of various treatment strategies in patients with PPS. In one study, 50 patients underwent treatment consisting primarily of confrontation of the diagnosis with additional psychotherapeutic interventions of various degrees of intensity (6). Overall, 46% of the patients taking anticonvulsants either discontinued their medication or had reductions in dosage. When divided into acute or chronic groups, 80% of the patients in the acute group became free of PPS, whereas only 28% of the patients in the chronic group reached a similar control. This supports the contention that early diagnosis and intervention of PPS can have a high rate of success, whereas less favorable outcomes occur in patients with more protracted histories. It is unclear why the patients were maintained on AEDs. This study merits an additional comment. In our opinion, if a patient does not have evidence of epileptic seizures (past or present), AEDs should be discontinued when PPS diagnosis is established. Maintaining patients on AEDs, unless they are used as mood-stabilizing agents, can be very confusing and gives the patient a "double message" (see below).

In another study that analyzed retrospectively the effects of psychiatric interventions on patients with PPS, psychotherapy or feedback provided by comprehensive epilepsy program professionals with experience in epilepsy was found to be superior to other or no interventions (5). Eleven of 16 (68%) patients who received five or more counseling sessions, including review of the videotaped recording of the nonepileptic event by the comprehensive epilepsy program psychotherapist, had cessation or reduction of their episodes. Twelve of 25 (48%) patients who received counseling by a noncomprehensive epilepsy program psychologist or psychiatrist had a cessation or reduction of episodes. Of five patients who received no intervention, none had improvement in their condition. In another study of 33 patients, only seven patients (25%) reported that their events had ceased after a minimum of 23 months from diagnosis. Eight of these patients continued taking AEDs. Of 13 patients who were referred and received psychotherapy, six became free of PPS. Of the patients who were referred for psychotherapy who did not participate in the treatment plan, the results were dismal. All of these patients continued to have PPS (28).

The impact of treatment over time appears to persist. McDade and Brown (29) studied patients with a diagnosis of PPS who agreed to complete a therapeutic program. Eight of 16 patients were PPS-free, and three of 16 had only occasional events at the conclusion of treatment. At 1-year follow-up, no increase in PPS frequency was apparent. Improvement in social functioning and a marked reduction in demands on health service resources also were noted.

Children and adolescents with PPS tend to have a better prognosis than adults. Wyllie et al. (7) found that of 18 children and adolescents, 81% were PPS-free after 3 years. This is in contrast with the group of 20 adults studied, of whom only 40% were PPS-free after the same time period (7). Lancman et al. (26) found that 45% of children and adolescents studied were free of events after a mean follow-up of 40 months. In another study, Lancman et al. (21) reported that only 25% of adult patients with PPS were free of events after a mean follow-up of 60 months. The reason for the more favorable outcome among children and adolescents is unknown, but is likely in part related to greater effectiveness with early intervention (30).

When and How Should Antiepileptic Drugs Be Discontinued?

As stated earlier, the use of AEDs should be restricted to patients with concurrent or past epileptic seizures or patients with affective disorders in whom AEDs are used for its mood-stabilizing properties as a prophylactic drug to prevent recurrence of depressive or manic episodes. AEDs also are useful in patients with PPS who have recurrent flashbacks caused by a history of severe abuse or a posttraumatic stress disorder. Carbamazepine and valproic acid are the AEDs known to block the occurrence of flashbacks in these patients. In the absence of any of these circumstances, we recommend discontinuing AEDs once a diagnosis of PPS has been established. If patients are kept on AEDs for psychiatric reasons, we make sure that they and their family have a clear understanding of the reasons they must continue taking these drugs.

Mode of Discontinuation

One concern of clinicians is the occurrence of withdrawal seizures in *nonepileptic* patients resulting from the rapid discontinuation of AEDs. To the best of our knowledge, these are likely to result from a rapid discontinuation of benzodiazepines and barbiturates, but not of other AEDs.

Other precautions need to be kept in mind: acute discontinuation of AEDs with mood-stabilizing properties can unmask a latent affective and/or panic disorder (31). This observation is relevant in PPS patients, as the incidence of recurrent major depression is known to be high in these patients. When discontinuing AEDs, we use the following guidelines.

When a diagnostic VEEG is performed because of the suspicion of PPS, we keep patients on their baseline doses of AEDs for the initial 48 hours. In a recently published study, we demonstrated that PPS occurs within the initial 48 hours in 86% of patients. In the absence of events, AEDs without mood-stabilizing properties are stopped on day 3, with the exception of benzodiazepines, as withdrawal, psychotic, or anxiety episodes or seizures may result from the abrupt discontinuation of this family of AED. In the case of barbiturates, we try, whenever possible, to begin a slow taper before admission. We try not to stop abruptly AEDs with mood-stabilizing properties in patients with any psychiatric history. Unfortunately, increasing limitations in the duration of VEEG force us to accelerate the discontinuation process of AEDs, in which case we monitor very closely for the resurgence of psychiatric symptoms, at which time we slow down or abort the tapering process.

If AEDs are to be discontinued on an outpatient basis, we recommend tapering the dose in a stepwise manner with the following schedules: carbamazepine by 200 mg per week; valproic acid by 250 to 500 mg per week; phenytoin by 100 mg per week; phenobarbital and primidone by 30 mg and 250 mg every 3 weeks, respectively; gabapentin by 600 mg per week; lamotrigine by 100 mg per week; topiramate by 100 mg per week;

tiagabine by 4 to 8 mg per week; and oxcarbazepine by 300 to 600 mg per week.

When Should Patients Be Allowed to Drive and Be Involved in Activities that Usually Are Avoided in Patients with Epileptic Seizures?

That patients do not suffer from epilepsy does not mean that they are not at risk of hurting themselves or others if they drive or use heavy machinery in the midst of PPS. Such concern applies above all to patients in whom PPS is the expression of a dissociative state. Our approach with these patients is to withhold their driving privileges until they have reached a PPS-free state or can control in a convincing manner the occurrence of their events. Hence, the decision to lift the usual "seizure precautions" has to be individualized. Having said this, we must recognize the total lack of data on this issue, which explains why it remains the source of much debate among clinicians.

How Long Should Neurologists Follow the Patient with Psychogenic Pseudoseizure After a Diagnosis Has Been Established?

This is an issue that, in our opinion, deserves to be addressed, as it remains a controversial issue. It is common practice among many neurologists and epileptologists to discharge patients from their practice as soon as the diagnosis of PPS is established. Yet, more often than not, many patients may not be prepared to be discharged from their neurologist's care, especially when they have a long working relation. In our opinion, discharge of PPS patients from their neurologist's practice should not take place before they have an opportunity to complete the transition of their care to the psychiatrist or psychologist to whom they are referred. We usually tell our patients to decide when they want to stop coming to see us. A "premature" discharge may contribute to the patients' resistance to accept the diagnosis of a psychogenic process. Clinicians must realize that when patients are told "you don't have epileptic seizures; you need to be followed by a psychiatrist or a psychologist" and are immediately discharged from the neurologist's care, they may perceive it as a rejection that they attribute to the fact that "they must be crazy."

There are other important reasons not to rush the discharge of these patients. For one, a certain percentage of patients with PPS may have had epileptic seizures that were controlled with AEDs. Thus, recurrence of these seizures can take place as early as a few weeks to several months following the discontinuation of AEDs. Therefore, we believe that neurologists and epileptologists should follow patients with completely normal VEEG for at least 6 months after discontinuing AEDs. Patients in whom VEEG recordings revealed interictal epileptiform activity should be suspected of having had seizures in the past and should not be discharged from the neurologist's care.

CONCLUDING REMARKS

PPS is a relatively common paroxysmal disorder that we have learned to diagnose with increasing accuracy since the advent of VEEG. Unfortunately, the treatment of patients with PPS is still in its infancy. In this chapter, we attempted to highlight some of the key issues that come into play when considering a treatment plan for these patients. There is no doubt that collaboration between neurologists and psychiatrists will be essential to overcome the myriad of remaining problems. Because PPS requires the intervention of both disciplines, we hope that neurologists and psychiatrists alike will overcome whatever barrier prevents them from communicating with each other and join their efforts to find solutions for this complex clinical problem.

REFERENCES

1. King DW, Gallagher BB, Murvin AJ, et al. Pseudoseizures: diagnostic evaluation. *Neurology* 1982;32: 18–23.
2. Kanner AM, Parra J, Frey M, et al. Psychiatric and neurologic predictors of psychogenic pseudoseizure outcome. *Neurology* 1999;53:933–938.
3. Meierkord H, Will B, Fish D, et al. The clinical features and prognosis of pseudoseizures diagnosed using video-EEG telemetry. *Neurology* 1991;41:1643–1646.
4. Krumholz A, Niedermeyer E. Psychogenic seizures: a clinical study with follow-up data. *Neurology* 1983;33: 498–502.
5. Aboukasm A, Mahr G, Gahry BR, et al. Retrospective analysis of the effects of psychotherapeutic interventions on outcomes of psychogenic nonepileptic seizures. *Epilepsia* 1998;39:470–473.
6. Buchanan N, Snars J. Pseudoseizures (non epileptic attack disorder)—clinical management and outcome in 50 patients. *Seizure* 1993;2:141–146.
7. Wyllie E, Friedman D, Luders H, et al. Outcome of psychogenic seizures in children and adolescents compared with adults. *Neurology* 1991;41:742–744.
8. Lempert T, Schmidt D. Natural history and outcome of psychogenic seizures: a clinical study in 50 patients. *J Neurol* 1990;237:35–38.
9. Storzbach D, Binder LM, Salinsky MC, et al. Improved prediction of nonepileptic seizures with combined MMPI and EEG measures. *Epilepsia* 2000;41:332–337.
10. Walczak TS, Papacostas S, Williams DT, et al. Outcome after diagnosis of psychogenic nonepileptic seizures. *Epilepsia* 1995;36:1131–137.
11. Berkhoff M, Briellmann RS, Radanov BP, et al. Developmental background and outcome in patients with nonepileptic versus epileptic seizures: a controlled study. *Epilepsia* 1998;39:463–469.
12. Bowman ES, Markand ON. Psychodynamics and psychiatric diagnoses of pseudoseizure patients. *Am J Psychiatry* 1996;153:57–63.
13. Bowman ES. Nonepileptic seizures: psychiatric framework, treatment, and outcome. *Neurology* 1999;53: S84–S88.
14. American Psychiatric Association. *Diagnostic and statistical manual of mental disorders,* 4th ed. Washington, DC: American Psychiatric Press, 1994.
15. Cloninger CR. Somatoform and dissociative disorders. In: Winokur G, Clayton P, eds. *The medical basis of psychiatry,* 2nd ed. Philadelphia: WB Saunders, 1994:169–192.
16. Andriola MR, Ettinger AB. Pseudoseizures and other nonepileptic paroxysmal disorders in children and adolescents. *Neurology* 1999;53:S89–S95.
17. Breuer J, Freud S. Studies on hysteria (1893–1895). In: Strachey J, ed. *The Complete Psychological Works of Sigmund Freud,* Volume 2. London: Hogarth, 1955: 1–311. Strachey J, translator.
18. World Health Organization. *Diagnostic and management guidelines for mental disorders in primary care: ICD-10 chapter V primary care version.* Gottingen, Germany: Hogrefe & Huber, 1996.
19. Kuyk, J, Van Dyck R, Spinhoven P. The case for a dissociative interpretation of pseudoepileptic seizures. *J Nerv Ment Dis* 1996;184:468–474.
20. Shen W, Bowman ES, Routledge B, et al. Sexual and physical abuse in the pseudoseizure population. *Ann Neurol* 1991;30:293.
21. Lancman ME, Brotherton TA, Asconape JJ, et al. Psychogenic seizures in adults: a longitudinal study. *Seizure* 1993;2:281–286.

22. Luther JS, McNamara JO, Carwile S, et al. Pseudoepileptic seizures: methods and video analysis to aid diagnosis. *Ann Neurol* 1982;12:458–462.

23. Gullick TA, Spinks IP, King DW. Pseudoseizures: ictal phenomena. *Neurology* 1982;32:24–30.

24. Pakalnis A, Drake ME Jr, Phillips B. Neuropsychiatric aspects of psychogenic status epilepticus. *Neurology* 1991;41:1104–1106.

25. Shen W, Bowman ES, Markand ON. Presenting the diagnosis of pseudoseizure. *Neurology* 1990;40:756-759.

26. Lancman ME, Asconape JJ, Graves S, et al. Psychogenic seizures in children: long-term analysis of 43 cases. *J Child Neurol* 1994;9:404-407.

27. Lancman ME, Gibson P, Asconape JJ, et al. Financial cost of delayed diagnosis of pseudoseizures. Presented at the 21st International Epilepsy Congress, Sydney, Australia, September 1995. *Epilepsia* 1995;36[Suppl 3]:S179.

28. Jongsma MJ, Mommers JM, Renier WO, et al. Follow-up of psychogenic, non-epileptic seizures: a pilot study—experience in a Dutch special centre for epilepsy. *Seizure* 1999;8:146–148.

29. McDade G, Brown SW. Non-epileptic seizures: management and predictive factors of outcome. *Seizure* 1992;1:7–10.

30. Gumnit RJ. Psychogenic seizures. In: Wyllie E, ed. *The treatment of epilepsy: principles and practice.* Philadelphia: Lea & Febiger, 1993:692–696.

31. Ketter TA, Post RM, Theodore WM. Positive and negative psychiatric effects of antiepileptic drugs in patients with seizure disorders. *Neurology* 1999;53[Suppl 2]:S53–S67.

Subject Index

Note: Page numbers in *italics* indicate figures; page numbers followed by t indicate tables.